WOMEN'S HEALTH IN CANADA:
CRITICAL PERSPECTIVES ON THEORY AND POLICY

Edited by Marina Morrow, Olena Hankivsky, and Colleen Varcoe

In recent years greater attention has been paid to the different health care needs and concerns of men and women. Women's health, in particular, has emerged as a distinct concept and discipline in the last two decades. However, there has not been much in the way of a comprehensive text on the subject of women's health in Canada. This volume fills that gap by providing a resource for teachers, students, practitioners, and others concerned with women's health care in this country.

The volume brings together an interdisciplinary group of experts in the fields of economics, anthropology, sociology, nursing, political studies, women's studies, and psychology to provide a far-reaching examination of important issues relating to women's health. Drawing on the rich history of the women's health movement in Canada, and on emergent theory, policy, and practice in the field, it highlights scholarship that explores ways to implement this knowledge in health care and policy. The collection adopts an intersectional approach, taking into account social factors such as gender, race, ethnicity, class, sexuality, and gender identity. Contributors focus primarily on the social, economic, and cultural contexts of women's lives and their physical, spiritual, and mental well-being. Providing much-needed discussion from a critical, feminist, and anti-racist perspective, this wide-ranging volume makes an important contribution to the current research and literature on women's health.

MARINA MORROW is an assistant professor in the Faculty of Health Sciences and is co-director of the Institute for Critical Studies in Gender and Health at Simon Fraser University.

OLENA HANKIVSKY is an associate professor in the Public Policy Program and is co-director of the Institute for Critical Studies in Gender and Health at Simon Fraser University.

COLLEEN VARCOE is an associate professor in the School of Nursing at the University of British Columbia.

Women's Health in Canada

Critical Perspectives on Theory and Policy

EDITED BY
MARINA MORROW, OLENA HANKIVSKY,
AND COLLEEN VARCOE

UNIVERSITY OF TORONTO PRESS
Toronto Buffalo London

© University of Toronto Press Incorporated 2007
Toronto Buffalo London
Printed in Canada

Reprinted in paperback 2008

ISBN 978-0-8020-3939-2 (cloth)
ISBN 978-0-8020-9638-8 (paper)

Printed on acid-free paper

Library and Archives Canada Cataloguing in Publication

Women's health in Canada : critical perspectives on theory and
policy/ edited by Marina Morrow, Olena Hankivsky, and Colleen Varcoe.

Includes bibliographical references.
ISBN 978-0-8020-3939-2 (bound). – ISBN 978-0-8020-9638-8 (pbk.)

1. Women – Health and hygiene – Canada. 2. Women's health services –
Canada. 3. Medical policy – Canada. 4. Women – Health and hygiene –
Sociological aspects. I. Morrow, Marina, 1963– II. Hankivsky, Olena
III. Varcoe, Colleen, 1952–

RA564.85.W666867 2007   613' .042440971   C2007-900047-9

University of Toronto Press acknowledges the financial assistance to
its publishing program of the Canada Council for the Arts and the
Ontario Arts Council.

University of Toronto Press acknowledges the financial support for
its publishing activities of the Government of Canada through the
Book Publishing Industry Development Program (BPIDP).

I would like to dedicate this book to my mother, Isabella, my two sisters, Leah and LuAnne, and my niece Tatiana – three generations of women whose wisdom and support both teach and inspire me.

Marina Morrow

This book is dedicated to all the women in my family and in my life – especially my mother, Roma, my cousins Ruslana and Ircia, and my sister-in-law Alicia – whose strength, integrity, and resilience nurture, sustain, and inspire me.

Olena Hankivsky

I dedicate this book to my mother, Marion Evelyn Varcoe (1927–2005) – my strength and the source of my passion for my work. Every day I miss her love and enthusiasm for life.

Colleen Varcoe

Contents

Acknowledgments

The idea of this book was born over glasses of wine and heady discussion about our respective research into women's health, and specifically about our concern that so much of the innovative and interesting feminist scholarship we had each encountered had not been showcased in a way that reflected the breadth and depth of Canadian scholarship on these issues. We have been extremely lucky to have found and worked with so many wonderful people in putting this collection together. Each contribution uniquely represents exciting and emerging scholarship in women's health. We also wish to thank Liz Blackwood and Rodney Hunt for their assistance and support. The publication of this book would not have been possible without the financial contributions of the University Publications Fund and the Faculty of Health Sciences at Simon Fraser University.

Acknowledgments

The idea of this book was born over glasses of wine and heady discussion about our respective research into women's health, and specifically about our concern that so much of the innovative and interesting feminist scholarship we had each encountered had not been showcased in a way that reflected the breadth and depth of Canadian scholarship on these issues. We have been extremely lucky to have found and worked with so many wonderful people in putting this collection together. Each contribution uniquely represents exciting and emerging scholarship in women's health. We also wish to thank Liz Blackwood and Rodney Hunt for their assistance and support. The publication of this book would not have been possible without the financial contributions of the University Publications Fund and the Faculty of Health Sciences at Simon Fraser University.

Acknowledgments

WOMEN'S HEALTH IN CANADA

Introduction: Beyond Gender Matters

COLLEEN VARCOE, OLENA HANKIVSKY,
AND MARINA MORROW

The very idea of women's health is a 'concept' in the making (Anderson, 2004). As a concept, it engenders increasingly complex questions and debates which have not been adequately addressed or resolved. Concern with the limited ways in which women's bodies have been understood, and focus on the ways social conditions and inequities shape health, have driven the emergence and development of women's health as a field of study. Within the last several decades, approaches to women's health have developed significantly through the efforts of a wide range of theorists, researchers, grassroots activists, politicians, policy makers, and women more generally. These efforts have influenced and transformed understandings, practices, and policies and have challenged and shaped the very paradigms within which research is designed and conducted. And yet, social and health inequities persist for all women, and particularly for women disadvantaged by multiple forms of oppression. Such inequities demand a critical analysis of the adequacy of 'women's health' as a generic category and framework for health research, policy, and practice. These inequities demand analyses of women's health that are not restricted to gender alone, but rather contextualize women in their diverse social and economic circumstances and understand gender as inseparable from other forms of social difference such as race, ethnicity, culture, class, sexual orientation, gender identity, and ability. As Green (2002) asks, 'What has been left out of our analysis because of the current (often unarticulated) definitions of women's health that we use?' (p. 6).

Canada often has been suggested as a model for advances in health care generally and women's health specifically. The central role of health care within the Canadian national identity, and our national self-identity as a country with a strong human rights record, means that Canada often is cited as an innovator in discussions of human health and well-being. Despite this reputation, the health of Canadians and health care reflect structural inequities, and these inequities permeate women's experiences. Canada's history as a colony and colonizing power, its approach to 'multiculturalism' and its history as a destination for immigration by people from around the globe, means that the circumstances that shape women's health in Canada have relevance beyond our national borders. The successes, failures, and contradictions related to women's health in Canada offer lessons for improving health as well as a basis for comparative work in other countries.

The purpose of this book is to expand the meanings and boundaries of women's health through critical analysis and re-conceptualization of theory, policy, and practice within the Canadian context. Considering women's health within a Canadian context offers unique opportunities for putting forward new ideas and furthering a women's health agenda at a research and policy level, both nationally and internationally. In what follows we highlight some of the key characteristics and features of women's health in Canada, and outline the theoretical perspectives taken in this book. We position ourselves within a dynamic and rapidly evolving theoretical landscape, a landscape that we both seek to understand and to shape.

Women's Health in Canada

While Canada has a relatively high standard of living and health, these standards do not extend evenly across the population. Living in a wealthy Western country it is no surprise that Canadian women rank as some of the healthiest and longest-living in the world. Canadians in general, and Canadian women specifically, enjoy particularly good health as reflected by life expectancy rates. According to the World Health Organization (WHO, 2002), Canada had the ninth highest life expectancy in the world for both sexes, only 2.1 years behind Japan, which has the longest life expectancy in the world at 81.4 years. In 2001 life expectancy at birth was estimated at approximately 76 years for men and 81 years for women, giving Canada the seventh highest life expectancy for men and the eleventh highest life expectancy for women in the world, and a life expectancy very similar to other wealthy, industrialized countries. By 2004 life expectancy in Canada had increased to 78 years for men and 83 years for women (WHO, 2006).

Both Canada's social welfare state and largely public health care system have contributed to this enviable record. Yet, beneath this apparently positive picture, there are important gender differences and significant health inequities. Although life expectancy is longer for women than for men, differences between men's and women's health largely are not in the favour of women. Differences in life expectancy between women and men in Canada are mostly attributable to men dying from 'external causes,' especially motor vehicle accidents and suicide (Health Canada, 1999a). Although women live longer, they:

- die prematurely from largely *preventable* conditions such as cervical cancer and lung cancer;
- *die in the prime of life* in greater numbers than men, largely because of breast cancer and other cancers;
- experience *higher levels of disability* than men, especially in later life (see Text Box I.1).

Text Box I.1 Gender Matters in Canada

- Women have a larger death burden due to sex-specific causes of death (e.g., breast cancer) than men (e.g., prostrate and testicular cancer). Age-adjusted mortality rates were 40.55 per 100,000 per annum for women and 29.15 per 100,000 per annum for men in 1997–1999 (Desmeules, Turner, & Cho, 2003).
- In 2000–2001, over 4 million women compared with under 3 million men reported having two or more chronic conditions (Desmeules, Turner, & Cho, 2003).
- In 2000–2001, over 500,000 more women than men reported having disabilities based on an assessment of their functional health (Desmeules, Turner, & Cho, 2003).
- In 2000, incidence rates of cancer were higher among women than men between 20 and 54, and mortality rates for cancer are higher for women than men aged 35–54, although mortality rates were higher among men than women for all other age groups (National Cancer Institute of Canada, 2004).

Further, significant social inequities for both men and women exacerbate gender differences. For example, income alone is an important factor. In 1996, life expectancy for high-income women was 1.6 years longer than for low-income women; life expectancy for high-income men was five years longer than for low-income men. (Wilkins, Berthelot, & Ng, 2002). People living in the poorest urban neighborhoods had an infant mortality rate 1.6 times higher than the rate for people in the richest urban neighborhoods (Wilkins, Berthelot, & Ng 2002). Geography is another important determinant of inequity. Life expectancy varies significantly among Canada's provinces and territories, from a high of 83 years for women in British Columbia to a low of 71 years for women in Nunavut (Canadian Population Health Initiative, 2004). Various influences interact, as illustrated by the dramatic inequities between Aboriginal and non-Aboriginal people that reflect the interacting effects of colonialism, racism, income, and geography. For example, life expectancy for Aboriginal women is 76.2 years compared to 81.0 years for non-Aboriginal women. Aboriginal women experience higher rates of circulatory problems, respiratory problems, diabetes, hypertension, and cancer of the cervix than the rest of the general female population (Health Canada, 1999b, 2000), disparities that exist because of continuing economic, political, and social disparities (Adelson, 2003).

Following several decades of neo-liberal policies in Canada, social inequities and health inequities are deepening. The income gap between the wealthiest and the poorest Canadians is widening, with the proportion of those living in poverty steadily increasing and with people who have recently immigrated, Aboriginal people, and single-parent families at the greatest risk of living in poverty (Kerr & Michalski, 2005; Myles & Picot, 2002; Picot & Myles, 2004; Statistics Canada, 2004, 7 April; Statistics Canada, 2004, 23 December). The numbers of people who are homeless are rising steadily and there are concomitant rises in health issues associated with poverty and homelessness. These trends affect women and men differently, differences that will be explored in detail by Reid in Chapter 7, and built upon throughout this book.

Simultaneous with these social changes, the health care system in Canada is under increasing pressure. Corporatization and privatization have been touted as both the cause and the answer to problematic health care resource allocation strategies, increasing acuity of health care problems, and the declining ability of the health care system to meet the expectations of Canadians.

Women's Health and the Canadian Health Care System

Women's health in Canada has been shaped in part by the particularities of the Canadian health care system. The system is seen as especially capable of ensuring that health care of good quality is accessible to all Canadians. The commitments of the Canada Health Act and the services that are provided mean that most women in Canada have some access to a range of health care services (see Text Box I.2). There are, of course, some exceptions, such as women who do not have legal immigration status. And, as Bilkis Vissandjée and her colleagues point out in Chapter 8, 'access' for women who migrate to Canada is complex and involves multiple barriers. Further, despite the commitment to equity, as the life expectancy data indicates, inequities persist in relation to factors such as geography, poverty, and ethnicity.

Further, not all services are covered by the Canada Health Act. The ability to secure private insurance or to pay for services privately varies with income. For example, recent studies have shown that among self-employed women, who in comparison with men tend to be in lower paying, part-time work and concentrated in service industries, less than half have supplementary health coverage (Delage, 2002; Rooney, Lero, Korabik, & Whitehead, 2003). And among these women, individuals with a previous health condition, those generating low income, those considered to be in 'high-risk' occupations, home-based workers, and seasonal workers found it difficult to obtain private insurance (Rooney et al., 2003). Indeed, 'women, on average, earn less than men, have lower incomes and are more likely to live in poverty. Women are less likely to have supplementary health insurance coverage through their paid employment. As a result, women face greater financial barriers when health care costs are privatized' (National Coordinating Group on Health Care Reform and Women, 2000, p. 3).

Between 85 and 90 per cent of all caregiving activity is provided informally (Cranswick, 1997; Denton 1997) and studies show that it is women who do the bulk of society's informal care work, which includes the care of children, the elderly and those with disabilities or chronic illnesses (Gregor, 1997; Stobert & Cranswick, 2004; Zukewich, 2003). As Armstrong (Chapter 20) argues, recent changes to the Canadian health care system have included significant shifts from institutionalized care to home and community care, thus markedly increasing such work by women. In sum, the Canadian health care system has contributed to Canadian women being among the healthiest in the

---

Text Box I.2 Key Features of the Canadian Health Care Systems

Although often talked about as publicly funded, Canada's health care system can best be understood as a public/private mix with the public aspects of the system accounting for 70% of health care provision (CIHI, 2005). The legal framework for the system is the Canada Health Act with its principles of a universal, public, accessible, portable, and equitable health care system. The act is operationalized with a national health insurance program, composed of 13 interlocking provincial and territorial health insurance plans, all of which share certain common features and basic standards of coverage, with slight differences. The act covers insured health care services, including medically necessary hospital services, physician services, and surgical dental services, and some extended health care services, including some aspects of long-term residential care, home care, and ambulatory care.

Services that are not covered by public funding range from those that are generally considered 'necessary,' such as pharmaceuticals and dental care, to those that are considered optional, such as some forms of cosmetic surgery. Some Canadians, particularly those people who are employed in the public sector or in private corporations that provide benefits, have private insurance (or 'supplementary converage') for those services not publicly covered. Private payment is required for those services not covered by public or private insurance, and over the past few decades, provinces have cut back publicly funded services, introduced more private payment in forms such as user fees, and 'delisted' services.

The Canadian health system also relies heavily on philanthropy, volunteerism, and informal care, much of which is led or enacted by women. Community boards, volunteer organizations, municipalities, or regional health authorities run most hospitals.

---

world. However, there are significant differences between men and women's health and health care access in Canada, and significant inequities among women depending on factors such as where they live, their access to income, and their membership in groups stigmatized by issues such as racism, heterosexism, ableism, ethnocentrism, and so on.

These differences and inequities are the central focus of this book. Such focus demands theoretical perspectives that take difference and inequity into account.

Evolving Theoretical Perspectives on Women's Health

As the preceding discussion of women's health in the Canadian context illustrates, research has produced evidence on conditions unique to women and to sex and gender differences in health. With such evidence, researchers, policy makers, and practitioners increasingly recognize that without explicit attention, gender inequities and differences are often overlooked. In turn, such research has challenged and influenced the very paradigms within which research is designed and conducted (Pinn, 2003; Wizemann & Pardue, 2001) and the ways in which women and health are understood. The very idea of 'women's health' raises questions and debates: Why women separately from men? Who are 'women'? Are women more similar to one another across circumstances than they are to men in similar circumstances? Spurred by such questions, approaches to women's health have developed significantly within the last several decades, gaining increasing currency and complexity through the work of a wide variety of stakeholders, including grassroots activists, health care practitioners, theorists, politicians, policy makers, and women themselves.

Women's health as a specific area of focus and study first gained currency during the second wave of feminism when women increasingly critiqued the ways in which the medical and scientific establishment had ignored women's health concerns in favour of men's, or had narrowly defined women's health in biological and reproductive terms. Many decades of women's health activism and research later, the understanding of and support for the usefulness of considering women's health has grown rapidly in Canada, as it has elsewhere. These ideas have been shaped by and have shaped social structures and policy, research and practice. Feminist, postcolonial, and queer theories have advanced consideration of concepts such as woman, sex, and gender and called for an understanding of health that 'reframes current discourse and is inclusive' (Anderson, 2000). Specifically, these theories have highlighted the importance of intersectional analyses in health that contextualize women in their diverse social and economic circumstances and understand gender as inseparable from other forms of social difference such as race, ethnicity, culture, class, sexual orientation, gender identity, and ability.

In the context of these advancements, different and sometimes conflicting definitions of women's health have been used, reflecting an analytical and material fragmentation of the ways women's health has been investigated and pursued (Green, 2002, p.1). Increasing demands for conceptual clarification have been accompanied by a growing critical analysis of the adequacy of 'women's health' as a generic category and framework for health research and policy. Without doubt, traditional conceptualizations of women's health have been limited, particularly by their focus upon women as reproductive beings and by their failure to take the diversity of women into account. Even though women's health is an important idea, applying generalizations based on *some* women to *all* women can have detrimental consequences. If we take seriously that women's health needs are socially heterogeneous, it becomes crucial to consider what, if anything, women have in common, and in particular, on what basis there can be 'women's health' (Schofield, 2004). Currently, one of the central issues in women's health internationally is trying to understand diversity among women while at the same time maintaining a commitment to women's collective interests (Schofield, 2004; Young, 1994).

The challenge then becomes, how do we frame women's health? According to Schofield (2004), sorting out the following questions is integral: 'Is it still the case that women are united by a generalized relationship of social inequality between men and women? Is health care a major and active arena in which such inequality is generated?' (p. 5). We argue that gender is a significant determinant of all women's lives, so that understanding their health must take gender into account. An example helps to illustrate this. Women with mental illness have often had experiences of male violence and abuse. And yet, because policy and practice frequently do not recognize the importance of gender as a determinant of health, this aspect of women's lives is often overlooked. For instance, mental health services commonly do not prioritize safety from threat of violence or offer women-specific services to deal with violence. As the foregoing suggests, certain generalizations are required to ensure that women's health problems and their determinants are visible. That is, gendered health inequities and health problems 'can only be remedied if they are recognized' (U.S. Department of Health and Human Services, 2004).

At the same time, it is essential to question whether 'women's' health is adequate for reflecting and responding to the diversity of women's health care needs. Feminist theory provides directions for rethinking conventional understandings of 'women' that go beyond an all encompassing monomorphic category defined in binary opposition to 'men.' Butler (1995) argues that the term 'women' can be understood as a site of permanent openness and resignificability' (p. 50). Fraser and Nicholson (1990) argue: 'Instead of thinking that there must be a common meaning to "woman" across contexts or that there merely exists a disparate assortment of such meanings with no connection, we can instead understand the meaning of the male/female distinction across cultures in another way. We can see it as encompassing a complex web of distinctions evidencing threads of overlap within a field of discontinuities' (p. 35). Similarly, Young (1994) proposes a concept of 'gender as seriality' as 'a way of thinking about women as a social collective without requiring that all women have common attributes or a common situation' (p. 723).

We argue that this kind of understanding of women as a reasonable and defendable social category also is needed within the field of women's health. That is, the health field requires an understanding in which there is space for a more flexible and elastic understanding of 'women' and one where the intersections of gender with other forms of social and material inequity (such as race, class, sexuality, ability) are better theorized. There is therefore ample room for expanding the meaning and boundaries of women's health. In turn, this justifies maintaining a focus on women's health, as this collection does, albeit striving for a reformulated approach that can affect and transform research and policy at international and national levels. To understand what is needed to move the women's health agenda forward in the Canadian context, however, requires an overview of how the field has evolved and an understanding of key issues, debates, and approaches.

Sex and Gender

Foundational to the debates regarding how to understand 'women' and the evolving approaches to women's health, are changing understandings of the terms *sex* and *gender*. While social science and humanities researchers have made distinctions between sex and gender, researchers in health continue to confuse and conflate the two terms (Green, 2002). In English (at least in Canada and the United States) gender is closely associated with, but distinguished from, 'sex.' This distinction has been absorbed into bureaucratic structures. For example, Health Canada defines gender as referring to 'the array of socially determined roles, personality traits, attitudes, behaviours, values, relative power and influence that society ascribes to the two sexes on a differential basis' and distinguishes gender from 'sex, which refers to biological characteristics such as anatomy (e.g., body size) and physiology (e.g., hormonal activity or functioning of organs)' (Health Canada, 1999a, p. 35). Status of Women Canada (1998) defines gender a little differently, saying that gender refers to 'the culturally specific set of characteristics that identifies the social behaviour of women and men and the relationship between them. Gender, therefore, refers not simply to women and men, but to the relationship between them, and the way it is socially constructed' (p. 3).

'Gender' is, however, a highly contested term. Gender generally refers to social experiences and differences that arise from the social environment, and has been used to distinguish the influence of 'culture' from the influence of 'nature' in the culture/nature binary (Haraway, 1991). However, both the binary of culture/nature and the idea that gender is a binary (i.e., male/female) have long been challenged (Bordo, 1994; Haraway, 1991). Haraway (1991) points out that, like all words and ideas, 'gender' has a history, and its usage reflects 'interwoven modern histories of colonial, racist and sexual oppression' (p. 131). Throughout this book various authors take up aspects of these debates, drawing attention to the ways that gender is both a useful concept and a constraining one.

Inherent in the concept of women's health is the paradoxical challenge that differences *among* women are often greater than the differences *between* women and the implied binary opposite, men. As we have suggested, the division of sex and gender into binaries – men/women, male/female –increasingly has been challenged (Butler, 1999; Fraser & Nicholson, 1990; Jaggar, 1983; Scott, 1988). In particular, theory emerging from the experiences of inter-sexed and transgendered persons has disrupted essentializing and dichotomizing tendencies and pointed to the diversity among those categorized as female and women (Califia, 1997; Fausto-Sterling, 2000). Women are neither biologically nor socially uniform. Therefore, women's health cannot be understood solely as biologically determined, nor decontextualized from the ways women's social positions are shaped by circumstances and factors beyond gender. While gender is an important category, it must be understood in relation to multiple intersecting categories of analysis, including, but not limited to, race, class, geography, ability, gender identity, and sexuality, each of which presents similar conceptual challenges. In sum, women's health is concerned with sex and gender as important categories of analysis, but critical perspectives recognize that these are not sufficient combined or alone, and that sex and gender are often less salient than other influences such as poverty, geography, racism, and ability in determining women's health. Attention to sex and gender is increasingly a component of approaches to women's health, and understanding sex and gender as intersecting with other categories of analysis is the current critical challenge in these evolving approaches.

Four Approaches to Women's Health

Alongside the conceptual debates, four approaches to thinking about women's health have co-existed and evolved (see Text Box I.3). As elsewhere, these four approaches have been taken up within the Canadian context in various ways, and unevenly among different jurisdictions, disciplines, researchers, and areas of concern. First, the health of women has often been invisible, and not considered as distinct from the health of people in general. Using a 'gender neutral' stance, research, policy, and practice have overlooked the unique needs of women, often with the consequence that men's health has been used as a proxy for women's health (CIHR, 2004; Marks, 2002; Rogers, 2004). Second, when women have been considered, often women's health has been associated simply with reproductive function. Third, recognition of the limi-

---

Text Box I.3 Four Approaches to Thinking about Women's Health

- Gender neutral approach: Sex and gender seen as irrelevant to health
- Biological and reproduction determinism: Women's health narrowly focused on reproductive capacity and biology.
- Sex and gender analysis: Social determinants of health recognized and seen as critical to women's health
- Intersectional analysis: Sex and gender understood as inseparable from other forms of social difference and attention paid to difference

---

tations of associating women's health with reproductive function and the shortcomings of this view within the biomedical paradigm have led to sex and gender analyses that consider how social circumstances and systematic gender inequities profoundly influence women's lives and health. Fourth, and finally, recognition of the complex influences of the intersections of multiple social determinants and more sophisticated and complex understanding of concepts such as sex and gender in relation to women's health have created new bodies of knowledge and shifts in policy and programs. Nationally and internationally, these trends have generated increasing attention to alternative frameworks and theories that now inform research, policy, and practice. At the same time, as previously suggested, these shifts in thinking have raised critical questions regarding the use of women's health as an analytic category.

Gender Neutral Approaches: Seeing Sex and Gender as Irrelevant

When differences between men and women are not taken into account, women are often inappropriately grouped with and treated 'the same as' men, making the health of women invisible, overlooking the unique needs of women, and inappropriately basing women's health care upon the study of men's health (CIHR, 2004; Marks, 2002; Rogers, 2004). This inappropriate grouping is based on the assumption that a disease or condition and the effects of treatment are the same for women and men (Health Canada, 1999a). An excellent example of this is coronary artery disease, which Lynne Young takes up in more detail in Chapter 17. Until recently, recognition of myocardial infarction (heart attack) and angina in women was based on studies involving only men, with the result that symptoms more common to women were often overlooked and disregarded. In relation to cardiac disease, women are still more likely to be misdiagnosed, have greater delay to treatment, have fewer benefits from treatment, and poorer outcomes (e.g., Agvall & Dahlström, 2001; Crawford, Meana, Stewart, & Cheung, 2000; Dong & Ben-Shlomo, 1998; Harrold et al., 2003; Norris et al., 2004; Watson et al., 2001). The effects of overlooking women's unique experiences and relying on knowledge derived from studies involving only men are compounded by the gender-biased attitudes and practices of health care providers and women themselves. For example, Canadian women often think that breast cancer poses the greatest risk to them, without realizing that, in fact, cardiovascular disease poses greater risk (Health Canada, 1999a).

Biological and Reproductive Determinism: Seeing Women as Reproductive Beings

Women's reproductive health, in part because it had either been ignored or poorly understood, was the initial focus of women's health. However, concentrating on women's biology and reproductive processes and overlooking cultural, political, and environmental influences has led to pathologizing and over-medicalization of normal processes. The term *pathologizing* refers to seeing a normal process as pathological, and *medicalization* means bringing that process under the control of medicine. A good example of this is menopause, explored in Chapter 16 by Cindy Patton and Brian Richter. Women's normal processes of aging, which include the cessation of menses, are often depicted as pathological and brought under medical control through treatment with various surgeries and drug and hormone treatments. This narrowness of focus can be seen in a preoccupation with reproduction (especially a preoccupation with maternity) in woman's health, and can be seen in the emphasis on health defined and operationalized within the health care system as an absence of illness (Health Canada, 1999a).

A narrow, biomedical focus can also be seen in the uptake of certain ideologies in frameworks and approaches to practice. For example, as explained by Hankivsky in Chapter 2, despite intending to widen understanding, lifespan frameworks often reflect a continuing reliance on biomedical understandings. Similarly, health care providers may operate predominantly on biomedical understandings of women's health. For example, an analysis of women's health papers indexed by CIHAHL (the Cumulative Index for Health and Allied Health Professionals) found that women's health was viewed in these publications from narrow, stereotypical, and biomedical perspectives (Raftos, Mannix, & Jackson, 1997): 'Women were referred to as fragmented bodies, body parts and diseases, and were depicted as being passive and silent' (p. 1142). Thus, within the health care system the focus on women's health is often on pathophysiology. So, for example, if a woman with osteoporosis breaks her hip, the fracture may be dealt with, but her nutrition, need for safe housing, and assistance with the tasks of daily living may be ignored, perhaps at greater cost to the health care system and the woman.

Sex and Gender Analysis: Seeing Women as Different from Men

Taking sex and gender into account in the study of health and health care highlights the differences between women and men, and permits comparisons of these differences internationally. Use of this approach in Canada not only has resulted in the investigation of patterns of difference in illness, disease, and mortality, but also in study of patterns of difference in experiences of illness, in the effects of risk factors, and in interactions with the health system (Health Canada, 1999a).

The importance of differences in experiences of illness is highlighted by the example of women's experiences of HIV/AIDS. Although women represent an increasing proportion of reported cases of HIV in Canada (Gatali & Archibald, 2003; Health Canada Centre for Infectious Disease Prevention and Control, 2001; Health Canada, 2003), only recently have women's experiences been addressed. Standard prevention strategies such as condom use, knowing your partner's sexual history, and negotiation of safe sex practices are largely irrelevant to many women given the dynamics of women's risk factors for HIV, such as violence (Canadian AIDS Society, 2000; Gielen et al., 2000; Kirkham & Lobb, 1998; Summers, 1997; Zierler & Krieger, 1997) and sexual abuse (Harlow et al., 1998; Johnsen & Harlow, 1996; Mullings, Marquart, & Brewer, 2000; Zierler & Krieger, 1997). Although HIV has been studied in relation to women, such study has been limited, and programs, policies, and prevention strategies tend to be gender neutral. These issues and the importance of attending to these different patterns and experiences in the particular context of HIV/AIDS are taken up in more detail in Chapter 14 by Meredith Raimondo, who points out how prevention and screening strategies are troubled by the historical tendency to focus on women as reproductive beings and the failure to focus on the role of gender and inequities as determinants of both health and informed consent.

Analyses that take sex and gender into account also have shown gender differences in the effects of risk factors and the social, cultural, economic, and personal determinants of health, as the example of HIV/AIDS illustrates. Such analyses highlight how women's biological and social characteristics and experiences interact to create different effects on women in relation to a range of health issues such as violence, teen pregnancy, and smoking (Health Canada, 1999a). Smoking is a most compelling demonstration of gender differences in risk factors. According to Health Canada (1999c), the number of young women who smoke is increasing, and there is an overall slower decline in the rate of smoking among women compared to men, trends that are echoed globally (World Health Organization, 2004). Health Canada reported that 31 per cent of women aged 15 to 19 smoke compared to 27 per cent of men the same age. The World Health Organization (WHO) warns that globally smoking has increased risks of lung cancer to the point that lung cancer now surpasses breast cancer as the leading cause of cancer among women, a trend that has been noted in Canada since 1994 (Health Canada, 1999a). WHO also notes that evidence is mounting that breast cancer risk itself is increased with smoking. Importantly, smoking dynamics are different for women than for men. Graham and Greaves (Graham, 1995; Graham & Der, 1999a, 1999b; Greaves, 1996) have argued that smoking functions as a form of social control for women, as a tool for dealing with stress, motherhood, and poverty. Smoking also affects women differently than it does men. For example, smoking among women is linked to lower fertility, cancer of the cervix, osteoporosis, and menstrual and menopausal problems (Health Canada, 1999c). These differences in risk factors also highlight the importance of attending to the unique features of women's health.

Differences between men and women's experiences of and interactions with the health system also are identified through sex and gender analyses (Health Canada, 1999a). First, because caregivers of children and elderly, ill, or disabled persons are most often women, they are frequently interacting with the health care system on behalf of relatives and friends. Second, when women experience health problems themselves, these problems are often compounded by their caregiving work. For example, authors of the Women's Health Strategy note that 'as patients, women's early discharge from hospital can have different consequences than for men and often takes place in the absence of an understanding on the part of the health system that more women than men live alone or will return to a family situation where they are the primary executor of household duties and are likely to be without a family caregiver' (Health Canada, 1999a, p. 15). Finally, gendered assumptions often shape health care interactions. Health care providers often erroneously 'assume that women will assert themselves as readily as men do when interacting with the health system, and therefore do not encourage active participation in care and treatment decisions'

(Health Canada, 1999a, p. 15). Paradoxically, being a woman is considered a characteristic of 'the difficult patient,' a pervasive notion that can result in women's health concerns being minimized or dismissed (Carveth, 1995; Johnson & Webb, 1995a, 1995b; Werner & Malterud, 2003).

All of these differences – in patterns and experiences of illness, disease, and mortality, in risk factors and in health care experiences – point to the critical importance of women's health and the value of gender analyses. However, as Hankivsky explains in Chapter 5, when gender analyses are used in the absence of an understanding of the differences between sex and gender, and in the absence of attention to the differences among women more widely, the knowledge that is created can be seriously limited in its generalizability. At the same time as a focus on gender remains critical, the differences among women often overshadow the differences between women and men.

Intersectional Analyses: Seeing Differences Among Women

Although gender remains a useful lens through which to view women's health, sole attention to gender carries the risk of treating all women the same; essentializing sex and gender; overlooking the fluid and changing nature of gender; overlooking the ways in which economics, race, ability, geography, ability, sexuality, and other influences shape and intersect with gender; and diverting attention away from differences among women. For example, while one of the areas of greatest difference between women and men is their respective profiles of mental health disorders (Health Canada, 1999a; Kornstein & Clayton, 2002), differences among women profoundly affect women's mental health. While research has repeatedly reported higher levels of depression among women, higher rates of psychiatric hospitalization, and more frequent suicide attempts (Gold, 1998; Health Canada, 1999a; Prior, 1999), rates and types of mental health problems experienced by women are also influenced by factors such as racism and poverty (Boyer, Ku, & Shakir, 1997; Saraceno & Barbui, 1997). For example, the ongoing effects of colonialism and residential schooling in many Aboriginal communities have resulted in rates of depression, alcoholism, suicide, and violence in these communities far above national rates (Dion Stout, 1998; Dion Stout & Kipling, 2002; Health Canada, 1999b; Kirmayer, Brass, & Tait, 2000). As the foregoing illustrates, in both theory and practice we require intersectional models and approaches to understanding women's health.

Intersectionality refers to the idea that gender is experienced by women simultaneously with their experiences of class, race, sexual orientation, size, and other forms of social difference. Intersectionality is the interaction between forms of oppression (for example, racism, classism, sexism, homophobia) in ways that are complex and compound one another (Brewer, 1993; Collins, 1993; Crenshaw, 1994; George, 1998; Meyers, 2004; Re'em, 2001). That is, for example, the experience of being poor (or subjected to racism, or disabled, or aged) is not simply an 'added' form of oppression for a woman; rather, being poor compounds the oppression inherent in being a woman, without gender necessarily being the primary determinant. Being subjected to racism compounds poverty, as does disability; being poor shapes the effects of racial discrimination and rural inequities, and so on. Intersectionality addresses the ways in which various forms of inequity and oppression are inseparable, reinforcing each other and interacting. Thus, for example, an Aboriginal family whose members cannot find employment because of racism is forced to remain in poverty. Or, as Mathieson shows in Chapter 10, vulnerability is amplified when the experience of being bisexual or lesbian is compounded by other forms of discrimination. As she points out, people with varied gender attractions are from diverse ethnic, religious, and class backgrounds, with neither sexual identity nor gender subsuming other identities. Using the idea of intersectionality to consider women's health turns attention to the differences *among* women and the ways in which geography, ability, racism, poverty, sexuality, and other influences intersect with gender to affect health.

Women's Health: Current Issues and Challenges

While these strategies and initiatives and the conceptual shifts in thinking about women's health are important, they have not resulted in consistent progress with respect to the study of women's health, women's health policy, or women's health status. Despite the fact that Canada is seen as a world leader and innovator in health care and policy, and in women's health specifically, women's health in Canada faces multiple challenges that cross research, theory, and policy. While these challenges have characteristics specific to the Canadian context, many reverberate internationally with other countries and health care systems.

First, the process of health care reform continues without adequate attention being paid to the gendered effects of such change (Armstrong et al., 2001; Grant, 2002). Culminating with the completion of the

Romanow Commission on the Future of Health Care in Canada in November 2002, the Canadian health system has been widely debated in the last few years. Commenting on the final report of the commission, the National Coordinating Group on Health Care Reform and Women (NCGHCRW) (2003) concluded that 'the Report is fundamentally flawed. By not offering a gendered analysis, it fails to consider women's places in the health care system and the consequences of health care reforms for women in different locations throughout the system' (p. 7). Health reform is a global trend and intimately linked to globalizing processes, many of which have been shown to have a deleterious effect on women, and, as intersectional analyses show, have different effects on different women according to their situations (Anderson, 2000; Hankivsky & Morrow, 2004).

Second, since the mid-1990s, the Canadian federal government has reduced program spending in all policy areas in ways that are unmatched in any other advanced industrialized nation (Yalnizyan, 2004). Public goods, services, and programs, such as those that address violence, promote economic security, ensure access to legal aid, housing, and appropriate health care, are being eliminated or reduced. These trends have not been reversed even though since 1997 the federal government has reported a budget surplus (Day, McMullen, & CFAIA, 2004). In particular, social welfare reform and declining social conditions have had detrimental health impacts for women, especially women who face intersecting forms of oppression.

Third, the commitments and initiatives in the area of women's health have not been fully supported politically, adequately resourced, or implemented wholly or evenly, and there are few comprehensive evaluations of their impact and effectiveness. For example, the Women's Health Strategy and the Gender-Based Analysis Policy have not undergone any formal evaluation. In general, it is difficult to determine with any certainty the efficacy of existing health policies, programs, and services, or policies directed at women in other sectors that directly affect health (Hankivsky, 2005). Innovations like the Centres of Excellence for Women's Health have not been consistently resourced. Further, women's health policy units provincially have lost funding in recent years, and in some instances have been amalgamated into different government departments.

Fourth, in Canada, as in other jurisdictions, the lay public is beginning to think that women's health has received enough attention and there appears to be growing resistance and even backlash against women's health as a specific field of research (Legato, 2000). According to Grant (2002, p. 1), while the need for gender-based analysis in the area of health and health care continues, there is resistance and outright hostility to this strategy. The ability of the public and health care researchers to understand women's health is further hindered by the focus on biomedicine over the social determinants of health. Such backlash extends beyond women's health research and is being documented in the area of women's sexual and reproductive rights internationally.

Fifth, despite the growing attention to differences among women, feminists continue to interrogate the concept of women's health and critique essentializing tendencies, especially the way that feminist health theorizing often has given gender primacy as a determinant of health over other key determinants. Within feminist health studies questions are being raised about the limitations of analyses that do not strive for more complex understandings of gender in its intersections with other forms of social difference. The transfer of theoretical advances to research, policy, and practice are, however, limited and uneven. As Hankivsky notes in Chapter 5, this has led to call for a more sophisticated understanding of gender and a new conceptual framework altogether that combines intersecting axes of discrimination, but does not privilege gender over other determinants of health.

And, finally, ways of seeing women and women's health are kept in place by certain ideologies or ways of thinking. Importantly, liberal individualism serves as a profound barrier to seeing women's health at the intersection of multiple relations among people and their environments. Individualism is the defining feature of liberalism, and advances the idea that people are rational, self-interested, autonomous actors who can be understood separately from their economic, political, or historical context (Browne, 2001; Burt, 1995). Liberalism is linked to a free market economy in which each individual (regardless of her or his socio-cultural position) is believed to have the same freedom to exchange goods and to access resources. This ideology has been buttressed globally by economic policies, which are driven by cost containment and an ideology of individual responsibility for health. These ways of thinking, which dominate Western thinking, limit analysis of structural inequities and construct health as an individual attribute. Thus, these ideologies run counter to understanding the complexity of women's lives, their interrelationships with others and their environments, and the impact of those interrelationships. Closely allied with liberalism are a range of discourses that limit analysis of inequities based on race. Henry, Tator, Mattis, and Rees (2000) argue that in Canada liberal democratic racism, in which Canadian values for fairness, equality, and social justice coexist with discrimination and institutionalized racism, deflects attention from such inequities.

Now is the time for critical reflection – not only on the concept of women's health and its utility, but also upon the understandings that arise from an intersectional analysis of health, and upon the potential for translating knowledge into meaningful improvement in the lives of women.

An Overview of This Book

This book brings together diverse authors who engage critically with key research and debates concerning women's health within the Canadian context. The integration of key strands from theory, research, policy, and practice is intended to create synergistic new knowledge. Each author provides a synopsis of the current state of knowledge in a given area, situating the issues within the wider international context, and draws upon and extends critical perspectives on social determinants of health and emerging understandings of gender and women's health. In particular, authors use the idea of intersectionality implicitly or explicitly. Within each specific area of concern, the authors turn attention to the impact of multiple interacting forms of disadvantage, oppression, and marginalization on women's health.

This book reflects the transitions among the various approaches to thinking about women's health. Research on various issues within women's health has progressed at different rates, and researchers within diverse disciplines have taken up theories and understandings of women's health differently. Such uneven development is influenced by multiple factors, including policy priorities, ideological pressures, disciplinary traditions and methodological norms, media attention, funding availability, community action, international pressure, and particular health crises. Mindful of this unevenness and the particularities of the Canadian context, we have chosen contributors committed to improving the health of women by grappling with issues of sex and gender, the social determinants of health and intersectionality. We also have chosen health issues that highlight some of the key concerns and tensions in the development of thinking in women's health and that will have relevance nationally and internationally. Every chapter thus reflects the state of knowledge development particular to each selected area of concern.

The chapters are organized into four parts. In the two chapters of Part 1: Locating Ourselves, we further locate women's health in Canada by documenting the history of the women's health movement, and by considering the importance of a lifespan approach to women's health. In Part 2, Theory and Methods, we expand upon current debates regarding sex and gender and highlight theoretical and methodological responses, including the need for broader, interdisciplinary, and collaborative approaches to the challenges and possibilities raised by these debates. Part 3, The Social Determinants of Health, explores in greater detail the key influences shaping women's health and health care, with specific, but not exclusive, attention to women in Canada. Finally, in Part 4, Key Issues in Women's Health, we present data and analyses that extend current and emerging debates of national and international relevance.

To date there has not been such a collection. We believe that this book represents a contribution towards a paradigm shift in the understanding of women's health, towards research, policy, and practice that take into account the complexity of women's lives. In contributing to this shift in thinking, as Morrow's chapter on the women's health movement shows, we stand on the shoulders of many activists, theorists, researchers, service providers, and community members. If such a shift is to be strengthened, then these various constituents must continue to work together. If women's health is truly to be fostered, research methodologies must not only take sex and gender into account; rather, the complex interactions among the biological, environmental, social, political, and economic influences on women's lives must be considered in each study. Similarly, policy and service provision must be developed from such complex understanding. And such understanding requires partnerships beyond academia and service provider communities.

This book will be an essential resource for Canadian readers interested in understanding the state of women's health in Canada and the related challenges and debates. Because international discourse regarding women's health emphasizes the importance of social determinants of health, and because work in Canada has prioritized such a perspective, this collection will also be of value to international readers, including those undertaking comparative research. The successes, limitations, and challenges of women's health in Canada both echo international trends and offer points of comparison. Thus, the purpose of this book is to provide students, teachers, researchers, service providers, activists, and policy makers with critical analyses of the theories, research, and issues most salient to women's health in Canada within the wider international context.

REFERENCES

Adelson, N. (2003). *Reducing Health Disparities and Promoting Equity for Vulnerable Populations: Aboriginal Canada:* Synthesis paper. Ottawa: Canadian Institutes for Health Research.

Anderson, J.M. (2000). Gender, 'race,' poverty, health and discourses of health reform in the context of globalization: A postcolonial feminist perspective in policy research. *Nursing Inquiry, 7*, 220–229.

Anderson, J.M. (2004). Lessons from a postcolonial-feminist perspective: Suffering and a path to healing. *Nursing Inquiry, 11*(4), 238–246.

Agvall, B., & Dahlström, U. (2001). Patients in primary health care diagnosed and treated as heart failure, with special reference to gender differences. *Scandinavian Journal of Primary Health Care, 19*(1), 14–19.

Armstrong, P., Amaratunga, C., Bernier, J., Grant, K., Pederson, A., & Willson K. (Eds.) (2001). *Exposing Privatization: Women and Health Care Reform in Canada.* Health Care in Canada Series. Aurora, ON: Garamond Press.

Bordo, S.R. (1994). Feminism, postmodernism and gender skepticism. In A.C. Hermann & A. Stewart (Eds.), *Theorizing Feminism: Parallel Trends in the Humanities and Social Sciences* (pp. 458–482). Boulder, CO: Westview Press.

Boyer, M., Ku, J., & Shakir, U. (1997). *The Healing Journey: Phase II Report- Women and Mental Health: Documenting the Voices of Ethnoracial Women Within an Anti-Racist Framework.* Toronto: Across Boundaries Mental Health Centre.

Brewer, R.M. (1993). Theorizing race, class and gender: The new scholarship of Black feminist intellectuals and Black women's labour. In S.M. James & A.P.A. Busia (Eds.), *Theorizing Black Feminisms: The Visionary Pragmatism for Black Women* (pp. 13–30). London: Routledge.

Browne, A.J. (2001). The influence of liberal political ideology on nursing practice. *Nursing Inquiry, 8*(2), 118–129.

Burt, S. (1995). The several worlds of policy analysis: Traditional approaches and feminist critiques. In S. Burt & L. Code (Eds.), *Changing Methods: Feminist Transforming Practice* (pp. 357–378). Peterborough, ON: Broadview.

Butler, J. (1999). Performativity's social magic. In R. Shusterman (Ed.). *Bourdieu: A Critical Reader.* Oxford: Blackwell.

Califia, P. (1997). *Sex Changes: The Politics of Transgenderism.* San Francisco: Cleis Press.

Canadian AIDS Society. (2000). *Women and HIV/AIDS*. Ottawa: Canadian AIDS Society.

CIHI Ottawa: (2005) *Exploring the 70/30 Split: How Canada's Health Care System is Financed*. Canadian Institute for Health Information. http://secure .cihi.ca/cihiweb.

CIHR Institute of Gender and Health. (2004). *What's Sex and Gender Got to Do With It? Integrating Sex and Gender into Health Research*. Final report (27 February – 1 March 2003).

Canadian Population Health Initiative. (2004). *A Snapshot of Population Health Trends in Canada*. Ottawa: Canadian Institute for Health Information.

Carveth, J.A. (1995). Perceived patient deviance and avoidance by nurses. *Nursing Research, 44*(3), 173–178.

Collins, P.H. (1993). Toward a new vision: Race, class and gender as categories of analysis and connection. *Race, Sex and Class, 1*(1), 23–45.

Cranswick, K. (1997). Canada's caregivers. *Canadian Social Trends*. Ottawa: Statistics Canada.

Crawford, B.M., Meana, M., Stewart, D., & Cheung, A.M. (2000). Treatment decision making in mature adults: Gender differences. *Health Care for Women International, 21*(2), 91–104.

Crenshaw, K.W. (1994). Mapping the margins: Intersectionality, identity politics, and violence against women of color. In M.A. Fineman & R. Mykitiuk (Eds.), *The Public Nature of Private Violence* (pp. 93–118). New York: Routledge.

Day, S., McMullen, N., & the Canadian Feminist Alliance for International Action (FAFIA – AFAI). (2004, November). *A Decade of Going Backwards: Canada in the Post-Beijing Era*. A report prepared by S. Day and N. McMullen in response to UN Questionnaires on the Implementation of the Beijing Platform for Action (1995) and the Outcome of the Twenty-Third Special Session of the General Assembly (2000). Ottawa: FAFIA – AFAI.

Delage, B. (2002). *Results from the Survey of Self-Employment in Canada*. Ottawa: Human Resources Development Canada, Applied Research Branch.

Denton, M. (1997). The linkages between informal and formal care of the elderly. *Canadian Journal of Aging, 16*(1), 17–37.

Denton, M., Prus, S., & Walters, V. (2004). Gender differences in health: A Canadian study of the psychosocial, structural and behavioural determinants of health. *Social Science & Medicine, 58*(12), 2585–2600.

Desmeules, M., Turner, L., & Cho, R. (2003). Morbidity experiences and disability among Canadian women. In M. Desmeules, D. Stewart, A. Kazanjian, H. Maclean, J. Payne & B. Vissandjée (Eds.). *Women's Health Surveillance Report: A Multidimensional Look at the Health of Canadian Women*. Ottawa. Canadian Institute for Health Information.

Dion Stout, M. (1998). Aboriginal Canada: Women and health: A Canadian
   Perspective. Retrieved 29 April 1998, from http://www.hc-sc.gc.ca/canusa/
   papers/indigen.htm
Dion Stout, M., & Kipling, G.D. (2002). Aboriginal Health, *Sharing the Learning
   – The Health Transition Fund Synthesis Series*. Ottawa: Health Canada.
Dong, W., & Ben-Shlomo, Y. (1998). Gender differences in accessing cardiac
   surgery across England: A cross-sectional analysis of the Health Survey for
   England. *Social Science & Medicine, 47*(11), 1773.
Fausto-Sterling, A. (2000). *Sexing the Body: Gender Politics and the Construction
   of Sexuality*. New York: Basic Books.
Fraser, N., & Nicholson, L.J. (1990). Social criticism without philosophy: An
   encounter between feminism and postmodernism. In L.J. Nicholson (Ed.),
   Feminism/Postmodernism (pp. 19–38). New York: Routledge.
Gatali, M., & Archibald, C. (2003). Women and HIV. In M. Desmeules, D.
   Stewart, A. Kazanjian, H. Maclean, J. Payne, & B. Vissandjée (Eds.),
   *Women's Health Surveillance Report: A Multidimensional Look at the Health of
   Canadian Women*. Ottawa: Canadian Institute for Health Information.
George, U. (1998). Caring and women of colour: Living the intersecting
   oppressions of race, class, and gender. In C.T. Baines, P.M. Evans, & S.M.
   Neysmith (Eds.), *Women's Caring: Feminist Perspectives on Social Welfare* (2d
   ed., pp. 69–83). Toronto: Oxford University Press.
Gielen, A.C., Fogarty, L., O'Campo, P., Anderson, J., Keller, J., & Faden, R.
   (2000). Women living with HIV: Disclosure, violence, and social support.
   Journal of Urban Health, 77(3), 480–491.
Gold, J.H. (1998). Gender differences in psychiatric illness and treatments:
   A critical review. *Journal of Nervous and Mental Disease, 186*(12), 769–774.
Graham, H. (1995). Surviving by smoking. In S. Wilkinson & C. Kitzinger
   (Eds.), *Women and Health: Feminist Perspectives*. London: Taylor & Francis.
Graham, H., & Der, G. (1999a). Influences on women's smoking status: The
   contribution of socioeconomic status in adolescence and adulthood. *Euro-
   pean Journal of Public Health, 9*(2), 137–141.
Graham, H., & Der, G. (1999b). Patterns and predictors of smoking cessation
   among British women. *Health Promotion International, 14*(3), 231–239.
Grant, K. (2002, January). *Gender-Based Analysis: Beyond the Red Queen Syn-
   drome*. Presentation at the Gener-Based Analysis Fair. Ottawa.
Greaves, L. (1996). *Smoke Screen: Women's Smoking and Social Control*. Halifax:
   Fernwood.
Green, M. (2002). *Defining Women's Health: An Interdisciplinary Dialogue*.
   Background draft. Retrieved 15 April 2002, from http://www.fas.harvard
   .edu/womenstudy/events/proposal.htm

Gregor, F. (1997). From women to women: Nurses, informal caregivers and the gender dimension of health care reform in Canada. *Health and Social Care in the Community, 5*(1), 30–36.

Hankivsky, O. (with the Canadian Women's Health Network). (2005). *Women's Health in Canada: Beijing and Beyond.* Retrieved 18 March 2005, from http://dawn.thot.net/cwhn_beijing_response-health.htm.

Hankivsky, O., Morrow. M. (with P. Armstrong). (2004). *Trade Agreements, Home Care and Women's Health.* Ottawa: Status of Women Canada.

Haraway, D.J. (1991). 'Gender' for a Marxist dictionary: The sexual politics of a word. In D.J. Haraway (Ed.), *Simians, Cyborgs and Women.* New York: Routledge.

Harlow, L.L., Rose, J.S., Morokoff, P.J., Quina, K., Mayer, K., Mitchell, K., et al. (1998). Women HIV sexual risk takers: Related behaviors, interpersonal issues, and attitudes. *Women's Health, 4*(4), 407–439.

Harrold, L.R., Esteban, J., Lessard, D., Yarzebski, J., Gurwitz, J.H., Gore, J.M., et al. (2003). Narrowing gender differences in procedure use for acute myocardial infarction. *JGIM: Journal of General Internal Medicine, 18*(6), 423.

Health Canada. (1999a). *Health Canada's Women's Health Strategy.* Ottawa: Health Canada.

Health Canada. (1999b). *The Health of Aboriginal Women*: Fact sheet. Ottawa: Health Canada.

Health Canada. (1999c). *Women and Tobacco.* Ottawa: Women's Health Bureau.

Health Canada. (2000). *Statistical Profile on the Health of First Nations in Canada.* Ottawa: Health Canada.

Health Canada. (2003). *HIV/AIDS in Canada: Surveillance Report to June 30, 2003.* Ottawa: Centre for Infectious Disease Prevention and Control, Surveillance and Risks Assessment Division.

Health Canada Centre for Infectious Disease Prevention and Control. (2001). *HIV/AIDS Epi Updates.* Retrieved 26 October 2001, from http://www.hc-sc.gc.ca/hpb/lcdc/bah/epi/epi_e.html#HIV.

Henry, F., Tator, C., Mattis, W., & Rees, T. (2000). *The Colour of Democracy: Racism in Canadian Society.* Toronto: Harcourt Brace.

Jaggar, A.M. (1983). *Feminist Politics and Human Nature.* Lanham, MD: Roman & Littlefield.

Johnsen, L.W., & Harlow, L.L. (1996). Childhood sexual abuse linked with adult substance use, victimization, and AIDS-risk. *AIDS Educational Preview, 8*(1), 44–57.

Johnson, M., & Webb, C. (1995a). The power of social judgement: Struggle and negotiation in the nursing process. *Nurse Education Today, 15*, 83–89.

Johnson, M., & Webb, C. (1995b). Rediscovering unpopular patients: The concept of social judgement. *Journal of Advanced Nursing, 21,* 466–475.

Kerr, D. & Michalski, J. (2005). *Income poverty in Canada: Recent trends among Canadian families 1981–2002.* Discussion paper 05–02. London, ON: Population Studies Center: University of Western Ontario.

Kirkham, C.M., & Lobb, D.J.T. (1998). The British Columbia Positive Women's Survey: A detailed profile of 110 HIV-infected women. *Canadian Medical Association Journal, 158,* 317–323.

Kirmayer, L.J., Brass, G.M., & Tait, C.L. (2000). The mental health of Aboriginal peoples: transformations of identity and community. Canadian Psychiatric Association. *Canadian Journal of Psychiatry,* 45(7) 607-616.

Kornstein, S.G., & Clayton, A.H. (2002). *Women's Mental Health: A Comprehensive Textbook.* New York, NY: Guilford Press.

Legato, M. J. (2000). *Women's Health: Not For Women Only.* Columbia University seminar. http://www.fathom.com/course/10701010/.

Marks, D.F. (2002). *Perspectives on Evidence-Based Practice.* Public Health Evidence Steering Group. HAD Contract no 02/042, Project 00477. London: Health Development Agency,

Meyers, M. (2004). African American women and violence: Gender, race, and class in the news. *Critical Studies in Media Communication, 21*(2), 95–118.

Mullings, J.L., Marquart, J.W., & Brewer, V.E. (2000). Assessing the relationship between child sexual abuse and marginal living conditions on HIV/AIDS-related risk behavior among women prisoners. *Child Abuse and Neglect, 24*(5), 677–688.

Myles, J., & Picot, G. (2002). Neighbourhood inequality in Canadian cities. *Horizons, 5*(1), 8–10.

National Cancer Institute of Canada. (2004). *Canadian Cancer Statistics 2004.* Toronto: National Cancer Institute of Canada.

National Coordinating Group on Health Care Reform and Women. (2000, rev. 2002). Women and Health Care Reform. Ottawa: Women's Health Bureau, Health Canada.

National Coordinating Group on Health Care Reform and Women. (2003). Reading Romanow: Implications of the final report of the Commission on the Future of Health Care in Canada for Women. NCGONHCR: http://www.cewh-cest.ca.

Norris, C.M., Ghali, W.A., Galbraith, P.D., Graham, M.M., Jensen, L.A., Knudtson, M.L., et al. (2004). Women with coronary artery disease report worse health-related quality of life outcomes compared to men. *Health and Quality of Life Outcomes, 2*(1), 21–25.

Picot, G., & Myles, J. (2004). Income inequality and low income in Canada. *Horizons, 7*(2), 9–18.

Pinn, V.W. (2003). Sex and gender factors in medical studies. *Journal of the American Medical Association, 289*(4), 397–400.

Prior, P.M. (1999). *Gender and Mental Health.* New York: New York University Press.

Raftos, M., Mannix, J., & Jackson, D. (1997). More than motherhood? A feminist exploration of 'women's health' in papers indexed by CINAHL 1993–1995. *Journal of Advanced Nursing, 26*, 1142–1149.

Re'em, M. (2001). The politics of normalcy: Intersectionality and the construction of difference in Christian-Jewish relations. *International Journal of Qualitative Studies in Education (QSE), 14*(3), 381–397.

Rogers, W. (2004). Evidence-based medicine and women: Do the principles and practice of EBM further women's health? *Bioethics, 18*(1), 50–71.

Rooney, J., Lero, D., Korabik, K., & Whitehead, D.L. (2003). *Self-Employment for Women: Policy Options that Promote Equality and Economic Opportunities.* Cat. no. SW21-108/2003E-PDF. Ottawa: Status of Women Canada.

Saraceno, B., & Barbui, C. (1997). Poverty and Mental Illness. *Canadian Journal of Psychiatry, 42*, 285–290.

Schofield, T. (2004). *Boutique Health? Gender and Equity in Health Policy.* Commissioned paper. Series 2004/08. Sydney: Australian Health Policy Institute, University of Sydney.

Scott, Joan W. (1988). *Gender and the Politics of History.* New York: Columbia.

Statistics Canada. (2004, April 7). Low income in census metropolitan areas. *Statistics Canada – The Daily.* Ottawa: Statistics Canada.

Statistics Canada. (2004, 23 December). Study: Rural-urban income gap. *Statistics Canada – The Daily.* Ottawa: Statistics Canada.

Status of Women Canada. (1998). *Gender-Based Analysis: A Guide to Policy-Making.* Ottawa: Status of Women Canada.

Stobert, S., & Cranswick, K. (2004). Looking after seniors: Who does what for whom? *Canadian Social Trends,* (74), 2–6.

Summers, M. (1997). *The Intersection of Domestic Violence and HIV Disease in Women.* Paper presented at the 10th Annual BC AIDS Conference, Vancouver.

U.S. Department of Health and Human Services, Health Resources and Services Administration (2004). *Women's Health USA 2004.* Rockville, MD: U.S. Department of Health and Human Services.

Watson, R.E., Stein, A.D., Dwamena, F.C., Kroll, J., Mitra, R., MacIntosh, B.A., et al. (2001). Do race and gender influence the use of invasive procedures? *JGIM: Journal of General Internal Medicine, 16*(4), 227–235.

Werner, A., & Malterud, K. (2003). It is hard work behaving as a credible patient: Encounters between women with chronic pain and their doctors. *Social Science & Medicine, 57*(8), 1409–1419.

Wilkins, R., Berthelot, J.M., & Ng, E. (2002). Trends in mortality by neighbourhood income in urban Canada from 1971 to 1996. In *Health Reports – Supplement* (Vol. 13, pp. 1–28.). Ottawa: Statistics Canada.

Wizemann, T.M., & Pardue, M.L. (2001). *Exploring the Biological Contributions to Human Health: Does Sex Matter?* Washington, DC: National Academy Press.

World Health Organization (2002). *The World Health Report 2002: Reducing Risks, Promoting Health Life.* Geneva: WHO.

World Health Organization (2004). *Tobacco Free Initiative: Women's health.* Retrieved 1 August 2004 from www.who.int/tobacco/en.

World Health Organization. (2006). *World Health Statistics.* Geneva: WHO.

Yalnizyan, A. (2004). *Canada's Commitment to Equity: A Gender Analysis of the Last 10 Federal Budgets 1995–2004).* Ottawa: Feminist Alliance for International Action (FAFIA–AFAI)

Young, I.M. (1994). Gender as seriality: Thinking about women as a social collective. *Signs, 19*(3), 713–738.

Zierler, S., & Krieger, N. (1997). Reframing women's risk: Social inequalities and HIV infection. *Annual Review of Public Health, 18,* 401–436.

Zukewich, N. (2003). Unpaid informal caregiving. In *Canadian Social Trends* (pp. 14–19). Ottawa: Statistics Canada.

PART ONE

Locating Ourselves

1 'Our Bodies Our Selves' in Context: Reflections on the Women's Health Movement in Canada

MARINA MORROW

While much attention has been paid to documenting the history of the women's movement in Canada, there has been less of a concerted effort to chronicle the women's health movement. The very nature of this movement – a key feature of which is to expand the definition of what is commonly understood as health – means that it overlaps substantially with the key events and issues raised by the larger women's movement. Throughout the following discussion, the women's health movement will be examined both as a distinct body of theorizing and activism and as an area integrally related to and embedded in the larger women's movement. For example, both are concerned with challenging dominant paradigms while at the same time building a body of theory and practice to influence policy and responses to women's concerns.

Prior to the emergence of the women's movement, women's health issues in Canada were either patently ignored or relegated to narrowly defined reproductive health concerns. The dominance of the medical and health sciences by male researchers and practitioners and the rise of biomedicine in the nineteenth century greatly contributed to these occlusions both by placing a greater focus on the needs and concerns of men and by neglecting to pay attention to the social determinants of health and the ways in which social inequities affect health.

This chapter begins with a brief discussion about the ways in which women's bodies have been understood throughout Western intellectual history. This discussion sets the stage for understanding the impetus for the women's health movement. What follows next is a historical discussion of the political and activist strategies used to educate health professionals about women's bodies, to challenge androcentric, ethnocentric and racist research paradigms, to develop women-centred care models, and to enhance women's reproductive rights and access to specialized care. The tensions that arise from women's differing experiences in the health care system are also highlighted, with a special focus on the critical contributions of women with disabilities, immigrant women, Aboriginal women, and women of colour. Concluding the chapter is a discussion of the current challenges to Canadian health policy arising from national and international trends such as globalization, and of the strengths that transnational feminist activism is bringing to the women's health movement.

Women and the Body

Throughout Western history, beliefs about the body – particularly those beliefs about the fundamental differences between women's and men's bodies – have greatly influenced the development of contemporary Western science and medical practice. Thus, some reflection on the ways in which the body has been understood is a necessary starting point for understanding the impetus for the women's health movement.

Within Western intellectual traditions the body has often been ignored, dismissed, or regarded as the 'site of unruly passions and appetites that might disrupt the pursuit of truth and knowledge' (Price & Shildrick, 1999, p. 2). Indeed, the transcendence of the body over the mind is a vaulted goal in the Western tradition. Within the intellectual traditions of Judeo-Christian thought, the body was tolerated as a commonplace route to higher spirituality; however, in the post-Cartesian period the body is rejected as a barrier to pure rational thought. Women's roles as nurturers and caretakers, and their own 'messy' bodies which menstruate, lactate, and give birth, gave way to a gendered association of women with the body and men with the mind and transcendence of the body (Bordo, 1993; Dinnerstein, 1975). (Thus, women historically have been understood as less capable than men, who were thought to be ruled by reason and capable of achieving 'higher' spiritual states of being.) Somatophobia, or fear of the body, was therefore heightened in discussions about women's bodies, that is, female bodies were seen as being out of control and in need of regulation. In contrast, the male body was understood to be ordered and self-contained, and was seen in Western history as the standard or the norm against which women's bodies were to be compared. One historical example of the ways in which the feminine body has been marked with irrationality, is the ancient association of hysteria with the womb (Laquer, 1990; Price & Shildrick, 1999).

The body has not only been associated with the feminine but has also been racialized and classed; that is, the association of the body with irrational physicality has also extended to working-class people and to people of colour. Indeed, historically, the bodies of people of colour and poor people were often seen as morally suspect and as 'embodying deviance' (Gilman, 1985; Urla & Terry, 1995; Young, 1999). Thus, while the ability to effect transcendence (of mind over body) has been gender marked as an attribute of men alone, only certain kinds of men (white, heterosexual, healthy, etc.) were said to have this ability. Schiebinger (1999) argues that scientific racism depended on the 'chain of being' thesis[1] – that is, that a hierarchy of species was natural and absolute – whereas scientific sexism depended on radical biological divergence. In other words, that men and women were opposites and therefore relegated to different social spheres.

Because the body has been understood in different ways in different times, it is difficult to make broad generalizations without reference to particular historical time periods (Laquer, 1990; Price & Shildrick, 1999). For example, although somatophobia, or fear of the body – especially in association with the feminine – is a recurring phenomenon, it has to be conceptualized in terms of different paradigms of the body over time (Laquer, 1990; Price & Shildrick, 1999). That is, Platonic thought was focused on concern about the state of the embodied soul, whereas in medieval times, there was a greater concentration on the physical aspects of the body, such as pain, death, and decay (Price & Shildrick, 1999). During the Enlightenment, discussions turned to the transcendence of the mind over the body, while present-day preoccupations are with the biological body, the genetic makeup of the body, and with prolonging life. Thus, the questions feminists have asked about the body have been set within the concerns and context of particular historical moments (Price & Shildrick, 1999).

The rise of medical science in the nineteenth century, and the subsequent medicalization of women's bodies, provides background for understanding contemporary feminist concerns with women's health. One of the key underlying assumptions of early medical science was that men's and women's bodies differed biologically and that men's bodies were the standard by which women's bodies were to be compared. Another is biological determinism; that is, that people's abilities and roles in society were assumed to be attributable to their biology. Freud's famous dictum that 'anatomy is destiny' has often been used to relegate women to specific gendered roles in society – for example, as wives and mothers. In medical science, these assumptions went unchallenged for long periods of time, and the result was that discussions of women's health focused narrowly on women's obvious physiological differences from men (e.g., menstruation, the ability to give birth, lactation, and menopause).

Prior to the professionalization of medicine, women were primarily responsible for their health and for the health of their families and communities (Ehrenreich & English, 1978; Mitchinson, 1993). The knowledge that women gained through this work was overridden by medical science and the vaulted status it gave to doctors, who were seen as the true experts concerning women's bodies.

Feminists themselves have theorized and understood women's bodies in a variety of ways, and this, in turn, has influenced their understanding of women's health. Broadly speaking, the move in feminism has been from an initial desire to transcend the body – except for issues related to sexuality and reproduction – through to an affirmation of the body and a recognition of body politics, to a contemporary focus on the relationship between embodiment, power, and knowledge (Price & Shildrick, 1999). Each of these periods produced different activist strategies with regard to women's health concerns.

The Impetus for the Women's Health Movement in Canada

The women's health movement in Canada developed both parallel to and as part of the women's movement as a whole. In turn, these movements are linked to larger historical forces and to the social concerns of the present day (Carroll, 1997). The impetus for the women's health movement came both from the ways women's bodies have been understood historically in the western intellectual tradition and as a result of identifying women's subordinate social status. Indeed, one of the key defining features of the women's health movement is that ... 'women's health is about much more than particular reproductive organs and secondary sex characteristics ... It is defined by, and shaped in, social, psychological, and economic environments and relationships ... This means that health is a social issue and a social contract rather than simply a medical and technical problem to be addressed by experts' (Armstrong, 1998, p. 249).

Although the issues differ in each historical time period, several overarching themes are consistent throughout the women's health movement. These include women's health issues, women's roles as caregivers, and women's labour issues in the health professions. As such, the women's health movement has been focused in a variety of spheres of activity, including grassroots community-based organizations, universities, hospitals, labour unions, and government institutions. Likewise, the movement has included a variety of strategies, including direct action and protest, work to influence government health and social policy, and the development of health education.

The women's movement is often understood to have occurred in waves or 'peaks' of activity. Although critics suggest that this approach obscures the continuity of women's activism, it is still useful to highlight the themes and key issues associated with different historical time periods if one bears in mind that women have continually campaigned for change – even during times of conservative backlash against women. This holds true for the women's health movement, which has had times of intense but also enduring activity.

In what follows, a more detailed analysis of the first (late 1800s to 1940s), second (1960s to 1980s), and third (late 1980s to the present) waves of the women's movement is provided with attention to the corresponding social context and the evolving understanding of the body in each period. The key issues of focus are discussed for each time period along with significant trends and ongoing challenges. A summary of key events in the women's health movement can be found in Text Box 1.1 at the end of this chapter.

The First Wave

Early first wave feminists were focused primarily on gaining access to formal political systems vis-à-vis the campaign for the franchise. The political power of predominately white middle- and upper-class women from this time period came from their involvement in the moral reform movement which focused on a host of social issues including housing, public health, child welfare, temperance, and religious instruction (Errington, 1993). The commitment of most women reformers to their own race and class interests meant that they ignored many of the concerns of working-class women and that they also focused some of their work on the regulation (including a preoccupation with hygiene) of immigrants, working-class people, and people of colour[2] (Valverde, 1991). Women's arguments at this time – which carry over into the second wave – were twofold: (1) that their bodies should not prevent them from being able to participate in political decision-making (the refutation that women's bodies made them inferior thinkers); and, connected to this, (2) the idea that women's roles as mothers and wives placed them in a special category vis-à-vis social mores and thus they should bring this knowledge and experience to bear in political decision-making.

With respect to health-related issues, some women were concerned with poverty as evidenced through campaigns for better housing, especially for single women, and by concerns expressed about maternal and infant mortality and other public health issues that affected the lives of poor women.

Women have always played a central role in caring for the health needs of their families and in providing care to elderly and sick people (Oakley, 1993). Even prior to the nineteenth century, women played a public role in health care in their work as healers, midwives and nurses. The rise of the medical establishment in the nineteenth and twentieth centuries undermined these roles, effectively driving women from the field (Biggs, 1983). As outlined in Chapter 19 (this collection) by Benoit, Carroll, and Westfall, the medical monopoly over childbirth was an integral part of European colonization through which Aboriginal women, in particular, were displaced from their traditional roles as midwives and healers. There were also attempts during this time period to expand the scope of practice for nurses. For example, the Victorian Order of Nurses was founded by the National Council of Women in 1897 in order to aid women in rural communities who had limited access to physicians (Mitchinson, 1993). This care was originally meant to include midwifery but doctors vehemently opposed this (Michinson, 1991; Mitchinson, 1993). Women also met with resistance when they attempted to get into the practice of medicine because the established professionals and the male guardians of universities argued that women were not physically or mentally strong enough to study to be doctors[3] (Kealy, 1979; Mitchinson, 1993).

For most of the nineteenth century, the prevailing belief was that women were the weaker sex both mentally and physically (Agnoito, 1977). Women's physical and mental health problems were routinely attributed to their reproductive organs, and the goal of the medical profession was to uphold women's roles as wives and mothers. For example, there was a prevailing focus on maternal mortality, not out of concern for women, but out of concern for their role as the bearers of children (Mitchinson, 1993). Further, once women entered into puberty they were seen as emotionally and mentally weaker than men as a result of the normal processes of menstruation. Later, as women aged, menopause was also seen as a sign of this weakness.

During this time period there was increased professionalization of medicine, which pushed many women out of their traditional caregiving roles, and increased the medicalization of the body. Medicalization meant that natural bodily processes and conditions began to come under the control of the medical establishment, effectively undermining women's own traditional knowledge about things such as childbirth, sexuality, and menopause (Findlay & Miller, 2002). This medicalization extended to women's minds, where the discourse of medical science in the form of psychiatry was used to pathologize women who did not conform to norms of femininity and traditional gender roles (Boehnert, 1993; Chesler, 1972; Penfold & Walker, 1983; Perkins Gilman, 1899).

Women were also concerned about issues related to the physical and sexual exploitation of women (e.g., Miles, 1985; Stanko, 1986). A closer look at some of the first wave of feminist activism suggests an emerging analysis of male dominance that focused on a women's right to bodily integrity and the right to say 'no' to sexual advances (Bland, 1983; Gordon, 1988). In Britain, some of this activism took the form of protesting against government regulation of prostitution and condemning the random medical examinations of women in the sex trade (Dubois & Gordon, 1983). Drawing on the work of the birth control advocate Margaret Sanger in the United States,[4] Canadian women also began to demand information about reproduction and birth control.

On the whole, activists in the first wave of feminism began to make a case for women's equality with men by challenging the notion that women's biology made them intellectually inferior to men. Further, women's concerns with public health, violence, and birth control were all issues that became critical in the second wave of feminism. So although there was no consciously defined women's health movement, women had already begun to pave the way for sustained activism on women's health.

The Second Wave

Writers in the early part of the second wave of feminism focused on critiquing the ways in which women had been characterized as less than fully human by male philosophers/thinkers because of their bodies (a challenge to the idea that 'anatomy is destiny'). The most systematic refutation of the idea that differences between men and women can be attributed to some natural and eternal 'feminine essence' came from the French feminist, Simone de Beauvoir, author of *Le Deuxième Sexe* written in 1949 and subsequently published in English as *The Second Sex* in 1952. De Beauvoir's claim that 'one is not born a woman, one becomes one' (de Beauvoir, 1952) laid the ground for understanding women's particular circumstances through a social rather than biological lens.

Early second wave feminists, including de Beauvoir, held on to the belief that women's bodies were somehow 'troublesome,' and that equality would be achieved when women could go 'beyond' their bodies and take up intellectual pursuits. Thus, these thinkers failed to refute the idea that women's bodies tied them to nature and were somehow more burdensome than men's (Young, 1989). A classic example is the work of Shulamith Firestone in *The Dialectic of Sex* (1970) where she takes up de Beauvoir's call for an escape from the immanence[5] of the reproductive female body. Firestone argued that the 'disabilities' and dependencies of pregnancy made women vulnerable to male domination, and that progress in technology, such as extra-uterine reproduction, would prepare the way for women's liberation (Firestone, 1970).

The second wave of feminism coincided with an intense period of social upheaval in North American and European society, which in turn spawned a host of social movements including the peace movement, the civil rights movement, a strengthening of the labour movement, the movement for Aboriginal self-government, and, in Canada, the Québec movement for sovereignty. Women who were disenchanted with the ways in which many of these movements either ignored or accepted sexism began to meet and form consciousness-raising groups where they could talk about their experiences and come to understand them in a larger social context. The slogan 'the personal is political' accurately captures this emerging awareness. In other words, that which had been previously understood as individual personal problems, were in fact larger social and political issues for women. A natural extension of this thinking was for women to actively reclaim their bodies and to begin to give a central place to the material body in Western thought.

The second wave is often characterized as a period of activism dominated by the concerns of white, middle-class, able-bodied, heterosexual women. While this is true, it is also the case that Aboriginal women, lesbians, women with disabilities, women of colour, and immigrant women were actively working in their communities and were a driving force in the second wave of feminism – especially in terms of critiquing naive notions of shared 'sisterhood' by pointing to the inequities between women (Anzaldua & Moraga, 1981; Bannerji, 1987; Davis, 1981). The autonomous organizing of these groups led to the establishment of a number of women's organizations in Canada that included health as one of their concerns. This included the Toronto-based Centre for Spanish Speaking Peoples in 1973, Women Working with Immigrant women in 1974, Women's Health in Women's Hands in 1988, the National Association of Native Women in 1973, and, the DisAbled Women's Network (DAWN) in 1985. As women from a variety of communities began to voice their specific health-related concerns, the women's health movement was pushed to develop a deeper analysis of the differing needs and concerns of women.

A number of key issues galvanized the women's movement during the second wave, including reproductive health issues, violence against women, sexuality, and issues related to women's roles in the health care sector. As each of these issues are discussed below, it will become apparent that the medicalization of women's bodies and the concern that women should be seen as active agents in their own health care rather than just as passive patients of the medical system, provided momentum for activism during this time period (Sherwin, 1992).

Coinciding with these developments, at a national policy level Canada was beginning to embrace health-promotion frameworks which recognized the role of social justice and equity as prerequisites for health. The establishment of the Ottawa Charter for Health Promotion in 1986 focused on promoting health through the recognition of the effects of the physical and social environment on people's health, as well as promoting the idea of 'healthy public policy.'

In feminist writing, theorists spoke about the body as a site of knowledge ('embodied' knowing) (Bartky, 1993). For example, in contrast to early second wave feminists' attempts to transcend the body through technology, feminists in the later part of the second wave began to take up women's experiences of childbirth and maternal caregiving as transformative experiences that could provide a model that would displace masculinist spheres of government and the economy (Ruddick, 1983). For example, the valuing of women's unpaid caregiving could shift how we think about labour and economics. This line of thinking and the subsequent development of an 'ethic of care' began to dramatically change women's relationships to their bodies, to their traditional roles as caregivers, and to politics (Gilligan, 1982; Hankivsky, 2004).

This shift in thinking was crystallized in women's campaigns for control over their own bodies, and women began to protest institutions of the state, religion, law, and pharmaceutical companies, and the violence women endured at the hands of men (Roach Pierson, 1993). Women's organizations proliferated to include the establishment of rape crisis centres, shelters, women's centres, and centres specific to women's health (e.g., the Vancouver Women's Health Collective; the Regina Immigrant Women's Centre, Naissance Renaissance Outaouais, DES Action, the Fredericton Women's Centre). Women's health centres provided women-only space where women could come to get health information and support. The development of self-help groups supporting women with mental health problems, breast cancer, endometriosis, and exposure to the drug DES[6] helped women to explore a range of alternative approaches to care (Boscoe, 1994). Women's health centres also actively worked to help women make links between their social positioning and their health.

Publications about women's health formed an important part of the women's health movement. In 1968, a student initiative at McGill University produced the *Birth Control Handbook* (McGill Student's Union Collective, 1969) and spawned the Montreal Health Press, which produced numerous health-related works. In the early 70s, the Boston Women's Health Course Collective was started in the United States, and in 1971 it published its now famous health guide, *Our Bodies, Our Selves: A Course by and for Women*, which provided women with information about their bodies and their health (Boston Women's Health Course Collective, 1971). Although Canada's health press preceded the Boston Collective, *Our Bodies, Our Selves*[7] became an enormously popular book in Canada and inspired similar self-help initiatives.

Pressure from feminist organizations resulted in the establishment of the Royal Commission on the Status of Women in 1967. The commission was charged with documenting the situation of Canadian women with the goal of establishing recommendations that would further women's equality. Although health was not an explicit focus of the commission, by the time its report was tabled in the House of Commons in 1970, it contained recommendations related to abortion (e.g., abortion should be available to women on demand before 12 weeks) and on other health related issues (e.g., laws against sexual harassment)

(O'Neill, 2003). One result of the commission was the establishment of the National Action Committee on the Status of Women. Other advisory councils on the status of women were formed in each province at this time, ostensibly to ensure that the recommendations of the Royal Commission were implemented.

Early on, women's groups across the country identified the need for inter-regional ties, and a number of local and provincial groups were developed (e.g., Le Regroupement des Centres de Santé des Femmes du Québec). Attempts were made to establish a national committee on women's health as early as 1982. Around this time, the idea for a play on the theme of women and pharmaceuticals was conceived at a workshop in Quebec hosted by Inter Pares, an Ottawa-based development agency. The resulting play, *Side Effects,* toured the country in 1985 and sparked further interest in a Canada-wide women's health network (Boscoe, 1994). In 1986, at an informal gathering of women attending a health and welfare conference on women and addictions, a draft funding proposal for developing a women's health network was put together (Boscoe, 1994). What followed was a series of consultations and proposals which resulted in support from Health Canada for a three-year project to develop the Canadian Women's Health Network, which was formally established in 1993. The mandate of the network was to support *Healthsharing* magazine and develop a Canada-wide database identifying groups and resources on women's health issues. The funding was also to be used to conduct a Canada-wide consultation of women's groups to develop strategies for building and sustaining the network (Boscoe, 1994).

REPRODUCTIVE CHOICE

Reproductive health became a key issue for the second wave of feminism, in part spurred by the use of thalidomide as a treatment for morning sickness for Canadian women during the 1960s, a treatment that resulted in the birth of babies with severe damage to their limbs.[8] This tragic event helped to galvanize women's activism on issues related to reproduction. Women began to demand the legalization of birth control, campaign for reproductive choice, and expose the dangers of newly developed drugs for use during pregnancy and for contraception.

Prior to 1969, birth control and distributing information about birth control was illegal. One of the key actions related to this was the aforementioned production of the *McGill Birth Control Handbook* by feminist activists at McGill University, who, despite threats of arrest, published and circulated this material widely. Pressure from organizations like Planned Parenthood resulted in the legalization of birth control; however, abortion was still illegal in all except very exceptional cases (Roach Pierson, 1993). Protest against this law was the main impetus behind the 1970 Abortion Caravan Rally that went from Vancouver to Ottawa to call for the decriminalization of abortion.

The Canadian Association for Repeal of the Abortion Law was founded in 1974, later changing its name to the Canadian Abortion Rights Action League/Association Canadienne pour le Droit a l'Avortement (CARAL/ACDA). CARAL/ACDA's purpose was to 'ensure that no woman in Canada is denied access to safe, legal abortion,' and to put forward 'the right to safe, legal abortion as a fundamental human right' (Roach Pierson, 1993, p. 102). This national organization inspired similar provincial organizations throughout Canada such as the Ontario Coalition of Abortion Clinics, which fought to protect women's rights to legal, safe abortions. CARAL/ACDA continues to raise issues related to reproductive choice for women.

Aboriginal women, women of colour, lesbians, and women with disabilities challenged white, able-bodied heterosexual women to develop an analysis of reproductive choice that recognized how poverty, race, and disability curtailed women's choices (Disabled Women's Network, 1988; Egan & Gardener, 1994). For example, Aboriginal women and women with disabilities were more vulnerable to involuntary sterilizations, and lesbians were generally barred from being able to adopt children and often lost custody of their own children in marriage breakdowns (Agger, 1976; Bourne, 1993).

Feminist activists also took up the issue of new reproductive technologies (NRTs), which became more widely available in the 1980s. The concerns primarily focused on the potential dangers of fertility drugs and invasive procedures, but also encompassed concerns that health resources were being directed towards helping infertile women, while ignoring some of the common causes of infertility such as chlamydia (Roach Pierson, 1993). A call to investigate the physical and moral repercussions of NRTs resulted in the establishment in 1987 of the Canadian Coalition for a Royal Commission on the New Reproductive Technologies. The commission was formed in 1989 and unfolded amidst much controversy before it tabled its report in 1993. Critics charged that the commission's work had been biased in favour of medical professionals and pharmaceutical companies, and many feminists who originally called for the commission later protested against it (Roach Pierson, 1993).

MEDICALIZATION AND THE SOCIAL DETERMINANTS OF HEALTH
Feminist scientists and social scientists launched a sustained critique of the androcentric, ethnocentric & racist biases embedded in medical and psychological research, arguing that scholarship that did not take the context of women's lives into account was potentially detrimental to women's health (Harding & O'Barr, 1987). Feminists argued that health had to be understood holistically, and that addressing the social determinants of health, such as poverty, racism, experiences of violence, and other forms of social inequality was critical. For example, women's disproportionate poverty was an issue on the women's health movement agenda (see Chapter 7 by Reid, this collection) and women lobbied for governments and health care professionals to address poverty so that women, especially lone mothers, elderly lone women, Aboriginal women, and women with disabilities could have their basic needs met for maintaining health.

Also tied to this position was a critique of medicalization. One of the foci of this discussion was on birthing practices in North America – particularly with regard to the dominance of medical doctors and medical interventions in birthing. A movement to return to 'natural' childbirth, which included promoting breastfeeding, was begun and women organized birthing classes, campaigned for home births and started breastfeeding support groups (e.g., La Leche League). As part of this activism, women moved to restore midwifery practice (see Chapter 19 by Benoit, Carroll, & Westfall, this collection).

The critique of medicalization extended to both psychology and psychiatry, and, in the 70s and 80s, feminists drawing on the work of antipsychiatry activists began to develop an analysis of the 'psychiatric paradigm' and to raise concerns about the abuses of psychiatry and its claims to objective knowledge (Burstow, 1992; Chesler, 1972; Penfold & Walker, 1983). Feminists pointed to the ways in which women historically had been pathologized by psychiatry, and argued that women's subordinate social positioning and disproportionate poverty led to mental health problems (Penfold & Walker, 1983). Still others exposed Western psychiatry as based on racist assumptions (Boyer, Ku, & Shakir, 1997). This critique led to the establishment of peer-support groups for women and the increased use of women's organizations as sources of support for women with mental health problems, who wanted either to avoid or recover from psychiatric treatment (see Chapter 13 by Morrow, this collection). The reaction to the medicalization of women's bodies resulted in a wide range of self-help models and supports for women who were eager to understand their own bodies and health needs in ways that would empower rather than disempower them in their interactions with the medical system.

SEXUALITY

Since the beginning of the 60s and the so-called 'sexual revolution,' feminists had been actively involved in reclaiming women's sexual pleasure, both through exposing the myths about women's sexuality that had been proliferated by the medical and psychological establishments, and by actively promoting lesbian sexuality. Drawing on the work of feminists who provided a critique of 'compulsory' heterosexuality (Millet, 1970; Rich, 1980), and, bolstered by the release of several important research studies on sexuality such as the Kinsey report on female sexuality in 1953 (Kinsey, Wardell, Pameroy, Martin, & Gebhard, 1953), the report by Masters and Johnson in 1966 (Masters & Johnson, 1966), and the Hite report in 1976 (Hite, 1976), women were able to develop a better understanding of the range of women's sexual pleasure. To this end, workshops by women about sexuality became popular and feminists challenged the psychological and medical professions for pathologizing lesbian sexuality. For example, in 1972 the gay liberation movement succeeded in pressuring the psychiatric and psychological professions into removing homosexuality as a diagnosis from the Diagnostic and Statistical Manual (the DSM).

VIOLENCE AGAINST WOMEN

Connected to the exploration of women's sexuality was the recognition of sexual exploitation. Protests exposing male violence, battery, and the sexual abuse of female children brought violence against women into the spotlight for the first time (Butler, 1980; MacLeod, 1980; Stanko, 1986). In 1980, Linda MacLeod's report, *Wife Battering in Canada: The Vicious Circle*, commissioned by the Canadian Advisory Council on the Status of Women was widely publicized. In MacLeod's estimation, 1 in 10 Canadian women was a victim of male battering (MacLeod, 1980). Despite the gravity of her findings, in 1982 when Margaret Mitchell (MP for Vancouver East from 1979 to 1993) stood in the House of Commons to ask the federal government how it was going to respond to the report, which had been tabled by the Standing Committee on

Health, Welfare and Social Affairs, the male-dominated assembly erupted in laughter (Roach Pierson, 1993). This event galvanized feminist activists across the country to demand more support for initiatives to help women and to prevent violence. Organizations were developed to shelter and advocate for women, and feminists ardently campaigned to change legal and social policy to recognize violence as a serious social problem. The serious health implications of violence began to be documented at this time, and violence against women as a health issue was firmly established by the late 1980s (see Chapter 18 by Hankivsky & Varcoe, this collection).

Activism on violence against women was connected with a growing understanding of the role of the media in proliferating images of women that sexualized or normalized violence. MediaWatch, originally a subcommittee of the National Action Committee on the Status of Women, formed in 1981 to monitor the media for offensive images of women (Roach Pierson, 1993). Further, feminists began to look to media representations of women as a way of understanding many women's dissatisfactions with their bodies and the troubling number of eating disorders that women displayed. Thus, weight and shape issues became an important area of exploration for feminists and a key health issue (Bordo, 1993; Ciliska & Rice, 1989; Nopper & Harley, 1986).

WOMEN'S LABOUR

Women's activism on health extended to labour concerns within the health care professions themselves. Thus, feminists challenged women's concentration in health care jobs with the least status and remuneration, and argued that men effectively dominated the medical professions. The relationship between feminists and nurses has not always been an easy alliance because of tensions between nursing's patriarchal roots and the goals and aims of feminism (Chinn & Wheeler, 1985; Vance, Talbot, McBride, & Mason, 1985). For example, feminists have claimed that the nursing profession has not always adequately recognized its own power relative to other female job ghettos (Nelson, 1997) and that race and class inequities continue to prevail in the profession (Varcoe & McCormick, 2002). Despite this, the nursing profession increasingly is drawing on feminist theories to develop its practice (David, 2000).

Feminists' concerns with health care labour extended to the unpaid labour of women who provide the majority of care to children, elderly people, and sick people. They argued that this unpaid work was essentially unrecognized by governments and society and that this had serious implications for women who expressed the need for help in caring for others (Heller, 1986).

The Third Wave

Many of the issues that were central to women's health activism in the second wave remain concerns for women in the third wave of feminism. However, contemporary feminists have become active players in both the development of women's specialized health programs and in the development of health policy in Canada. Women of colour, immigrant women, and Aboriginal women have been on the cutting edge of critiquing the role of colonialism in its long-lasting effects on Aboriginal health and the health of racialized populations. Thus, feminist postcolonial health studies is now a burgeoning field (see Chapter 5 by Browne, Smye, and Varcoe, this collection). Feminist health studies and activism have also come to encompass globalization and to analyse how the changing nature of migration, the trade in goods and services across borders, the increased privatization in the health care sector, and the governance of international bodies are effecting women's health and domestic health policy (Hankivsky & Morrow, 2004; Koivusalo, 2003; Spieldoch, 2001; White, 2001).

While much of second wave feminism worked within a modernist framework and struggled primarily with the heritage of cultural devaluation of the female body, the third wave has been marked by an increasingly sophisticated postmodern analysis of the familiar binaries (such as man/woman, nature/culture) that have shaped the structure of Western thought. In other words, categories such as 'man' and 'woman' are socially constructed and cannot be understood as polar opposites. Feminist theorists in the third wave see their task as one of reclaiming the marginalized female/feminine body without reinstating it as a closed, unified, and given category (Butler, 1999). Alongside the deconstruction of binary thinking, another widely influential aspect of postmodernist thought is the emphasis given to the relationship between embodiment, knowledge, and power.

Since de Beauvoir, many feminists have argued that gender is a cultural configuration that is often understood as natural. However, no one doubted that there was a biological substrate (i.e., sex) independent of culture. Thus, although feminists challenged the degree to which men and women's physiology differs, most have agreed that there are certain biological sex differences between men and women (such as pregnancy). Judith Butler, however, throws this into question by arguing that sex as well as gender belongs to the realm of discourse – just as earlier feminists tried to deconstruct gender, Butler's aim is to deconstruct sex (Butler, 1999). Essentially, feminists have come to understand that much of biological 'science,' as well as our very experience of the body is filtered through language and metaphor. The result has been feminist health scholarship that is taking apart the language of science to expose the ways in which it constructs illness and disease (see Richter's and Patton's Chapter 16, this collection). Further, feminists have been challenged to expand their understanding of the concepts of sex and gender through the recognition that masculinity and femininity is expressed and experienced differently by different ethnic and cultural groups. Feminist theorists also have been confronted by the work of Queer theorists[9] who argue that sexual orientation and gender identity are fluid rather than static concepts. Some of this work has resulted in increased attention to the lives and health of transgendered people (Cope & Darke, 2002; Mira Goldberg, 2004) (also see Chapter 10 by Cynthia Mathieson, this collection).

Activism in the third wave is characterized by increased involvement of women in bureaucratic and institutional structures. With this has come increased influence over the development of women's health initiatives, policy, and research. However, it has also meant that some of the more radical and progressive aspects of the women's health movement have become co-opted to fit various government and institutional agendas. Although the co-option of women's movement agendas by governments' has been explored extensively, especially with respect to its impact on the anti-violence movement (e.g., Barnsley, 1995; Walker, 1990), little analysis has focused explicitly on the impact on the women's health movement. It is fair to say that the tensions between institutional and feminist demands will remain a central part of activism in the third wave.

Another related feature of the third wave is the degree to which feminist agendas are reactive to government and institutional agendas. That is, many of the organizations and initiatives established in the second wave of feminism have seen their funding cut as part of a general trend in Canada towards less social spending (Bashevkin, 1998; Burt & Mitchell, 1998; Morrow, Hankivsky, & Varcoe, 2004). The ways in which the women's health movement has handled these changes includes finding opportunities where available and launching a sustained critique of government cutbacks and the privatization of health services. For example, in the mid-1990s the Canadian Women's Health Network (CWHN) began to take on a central role in helping women's health groups communicate across the country, share information and resources, promote women's involvement in health research and participatory research models, and act as a 'watchdog' on emerging issues that impact on women's health. The network, launched in the aftermath of federal cutbacks to women's organizations (such as in the 90s the cuts to the Secretary of State Women's Program) and during the establishment of the Beijing Platform for Action, saw its political role as not only sharing information, but also critiquing government cutbacks to health and social services, countering attacks on Medicare, and opposing the privatization of health services (Boscoe, 1994). In light of more recent federal cutbacks (2006) to organizations like Status of Women Canada, CWHN is poised to play an enduring activist role.

Activism and lobbying by women's organizations has resulted in an intensification of activity with respect to developing women's health research and women's health policy. In 1990, the Federal/Provincial/Territorial Working Group on Women's Health released their report, *Working Together for Women's Health: A Framework for the Development of Policies and Programs;* and in 1994, the Medical Research Council Advisory Committee on Women's Health Research Issues conducted a survey of women's research areas in health (Medical Research Council of Canada, 1994). In the same year, the Canadian Advisory Council on the Status of Women held a national symposium, Working in Partnership: Working Towards Inclusive, Gender-Sensitive Health Policies (Canada Advisory Council on the Status of Women, 1995). In 1996, the Canada-USA Women's Health Forum was held and recommendations about key women's health issues (including environmental health, occupational health, violence against women, health issues relevant to Aboriginal women) were put forward. In 1999, Health Canada's Women's Health Strategy recognized the importance of both these recommendations and Canada's international commitments to women's health and equality.

The Canadian government has also officially endorsed national and international documents that outline women's rights to equity and health (e.g., the *Canadian Charter of Rights and Freedoms* (1982); *Setting the Stage for the Next Century: The Federal Plan for Gender Equality* (1995); *Canada Health Council: Building on the Legacy, National Forum on Health* (1997); *The Beijing Platform for Action, Report on The Fourth World Conference on Women* (1995)[10]; and *The Women's Health Strategy* (1999)). The women's health movement has used these endorsements to remind the Canadian government of its commitments to women and their health.

In the 1990s, the Centres of Excellence for Women's Health Program was established by Health Canada (the Women's Health Bureau) in five regions in Canada (BC, Ontario, Manitoba, Quebec,[11] and Nova Scotia). The centres' initiative was spearheaded by the CWHN and became operative in 1996. The mandate of the Centres of Excellence program is to improve the health status of Canadian women by enhancing the health system's understanding of, and responsiveness to, women's health issues. The work conducted at the centres is policy-oriented and involves collaborative partnerships with academics, researchers, health care providers, and community-based women's organizations. The CWHN coordinates the networking components of the centres. A number of national groups have come together under the Centres of Excellence, including the National Coordinating Group on Health Care Reform and Women and the Women and Health Protection Working Group.

In 2000, the federal government established the Canadian Institutes of Health Research (CIHR) as part of its plan to make Canada one of the top five research nations in the world. The CIHR is an arm's-length organization that reports to the Minister of Health. In the time leading up to the establishment of the 13 institutes that make up the CIHR, a group of women's health researchers/activists began campaigning for the establishment of a women's health research institute and for the CIHR to integrate the health concerns of women into each of its institutes (Greaves, Hankivsky, et al., 1999). The result was the CIHR inclusion of an Institute of Gender and Health (IGH) that prioritized a lifespan approach to women's health (see Chapter 2 by Hankivsky, this collection). Although the IGH does not have an explicitly feminist agenda it arguably has increased the capacity of researchers to investigate questions related to gender and health.

Below, three key issues – health reform and health care restructuring, women-centred care, and health as a global issue – are discussed as current examples of the work of third wave feminists.

Health Reform and Health Care Restructuring

At the same time as governments are adopting new initiatives in health, especially with respect to health research, cutbacks in health have occurred and have been accompanied by massive health care service restructuring in the 1990s. Regionalization of most health care systems in Canada (Ontario being the exception) has been accompanied by other changes, including controlling public expenditures on health care,[12] closure of hospitals and the shift to community and home-based care, the privatization of the delivery of health care services, and the adoption of private sector management practices (Armstrong et al., 2002). The implications for women have been enormous, and have entailed more women taking on unpaid caregiving work, the degradation of women's working conditions in the health care sector, and the inability of many women to access the health care they need (Armstrong et al., 2002; Armstrong et al., 2004; Aronson & Neysmith, 1997; Cohen, 2001; Cohen & Cohen, 2004; see also Armstrong, Chapter 20, this collection). Although theoretically in a regionalized system, decisions about how health care dollars are spent can be made closer to communities, these analyses suggest that the negative consequences for women are significant. Thus, women's issues are not consistently on the table in all health regions and the lack of clear provincial standards regarding women's health in many provinces means that whether women's health initiatives are supported at all is largely dependent on individuals who sit on regional health boards, and on political will.

When the Commission on the Future of Health Care in Canada was struck to examine health care in Canada, feminists, along with a myriad of groups, had the opportunity to contribute their concerns to the commission. The resulting report (Romanow, 2002) has since been used by politicians as the blueprint for Canadian health care policy and delivery. Concerns have been raised, however, that the report does not adequately reflect the lives and concerns of women, and feminists continue to try to make their voices heard at federal/provincial and territorial levels of government on health issues (Armstrong et al., 2003). Likewise, the reports emerging from the Standing Senate Committee on Social Affairs, Science and Technology led by Senator Michael Kirby concerning mental health and mental illness in Canada have not adequately addressed the mental health concerns of women. (For a feminist response to the Kirby report see http://www.cwhn.ca/resource/cwhn/mentalhealth.html.)

Women-Centred Care Models

Part of the work of the women's health movement was to provide a critique of health service delivery models. Activists argued that the health care system over-medicalized women's concerns and did not provide a variety of care options that reflect a more holistic approach to health. One response to this was to develop 'women-centred' care models (Doyal, 1998). Women-centred models aim to shift traditional models of care by focusing on women, encouraging the involvement and participation of women in their care, and operating from the principles of empowerment, respect, and safety (Barnett, White, & Horne, 2002). Further, services that are women-centred should address the complexities of women's lives, be inclusive of diversity, and utilize an integrated service delivery model.

What distinguishes women-centred care models from patient-centred care models is the assertion that the provision of health care has to be contextualized with respect to the social, political, and economic situation of women. Additionally, women-centred care recognizes that both sex (biological) and gender (social) differences between men and women will impact on the health care needs of both. Thus, these models recognize that men and women sometimes differ in terms of the kinds of social determinants that impact on their health; in their patterns and experiences of illness, disease, and mortality; in how they interact with the health system; and with respect to which programs and treatments ensure the best health outcomes.

Many examples of women-centred health care models now exist in the Canadian context. Some of these are institutionally based (for example, in women's hospitals or health care institutions), but the majority are community-based clinics and programs. Critics, however, argue that women-centred care models have a tendency to give primacy to concerns about sex and gender and therefore do not always adequately address the differences between women and health care issues related to race, ethnicity, culture, sexual orientation, gender identity, and class.

Health as a Global Issue

International feminist activism began to establish itself in the second wave of feminism, with the UN declaration of the Decade of Women in 1975. In the third wave, this activism has intensified, and as mentioned earlier has benefited from a deeper analysis of the role of colonialism and imperialism on women's lives and women's health. Transnational feminist activism now includes extensive links between women's organizations all over the world and includes a growing critique of the processes of globalization with respect to its effects on, among other things, health and the environment (Naples & Desai, 2002; Shiva & Mies, 1993). The growing awareness between local health issues and global health issues can be illustrated by the feminist activism surrounding HIV/AIDS. Feminists – especially lesbians working alongside gay men – have been very active in the movement to raise awareness about HIV/AIDS in Canada, particularly with respect to the ways in which the particular expression of HIV symptoms in women went largely unnoticed until many women had already died (see Chapter 14 by Raimondo, this collection). Contemporary feminist activists have been at the forefront of raising awareness about the rising rate of HIV/AIDS among heterosexual women in the developing world and have made links between poverty, HIV/AIDS, and racialization, particularly in Aboriginal and Black communities in North America and internationally.

Additionally, new work is examining the impact of free trade agreements on women's health and women's health policy both in Canada (Hankivsky & Morrow, 2004) and in the international context (Spieldoch, 2001). This work critically examines the trend towards privatization in Canadian health care and assesses how opening health care to the market has specific implications for women's health and women's health care labour (Armstrong et al., 2002; Cohen, Ritchie, Swenarchuk, & Vosko, 2002).

Challenges for the Future

Despite the impressive evidence illustrating the relationship between the biological and the social, women's health advocates still find themselves up against a medical system that is biomedical in focus and treats women 'as a set of parts to be fixed by practitioners who alone know what is best for women' (Armstrong 1998, p. 251). Biological sciences are still seen as representing 'objective' truths. The human genome project has brought with it an increased focus on genetics, which in turn marginalizes the study of the social determinants of health. These challenges, along with globalization and its deleterious effects on the health and the environment, health care restructuring, and the fears that Canada may be losing its public health care system to increased privatization, continue to motivate the women's health movement.

Conclusion

Contemporarily, women's health activism and research has been built on the shoulders of the women before us who reclaimed the centrality

---

Text Box 1.1 Selected Events in the Women's Health Movement

1883 Entry of first women into medical schools in Canada
1897 Victorian Order of Nurses established
1967 Royal Commission on the Status of Women
1969 Publication of the *McGill Birth Control Handbook*
1970 Abortion Caravan
1972 Removal of 'homosexuality' as a mental illness from the DSM
1974 Establishment of the Canadian Abortion Rights Action League/Association Canadienne pour Le Droit à l'Avortement (CARAL/ACDC)
1980 Release of Linda MacLeod's report on wife battering in Canada
1981 Establishment of Media Watch
1985 Production of the play Side Effects
1985 Establishment of the Disabled Women's Network
1989 Royal Commission on New Reproductive Technologies
1990 Release of report of the Federal/Territorial/Provincial Working Group on Women's Health, *Working Together for Women's Health: A Framework for the Development of Policies and Programs*
1993 Establishment of the Canadian Women's Health Network
1995 Beijing Platform for Action
1996 Establishment of the Centres of Excellence for Women's Health
1999 Canadian Women's Health Strategy
2000 Establishment of the Institute of Gender and Health as part of the Canadian Institutes of Health Research

---

of the material body in Western thought and campaigned passionately for women's reproductive rights, opposed medicalization of childbirth and menopause, and raised issues related to violence, poverty, and racism as critical determinants of women's health. Today, women's organizations still struggle with some of the same key issues that prompted the women's health movement: the medicalization of women's bodies, the failure of medical science to consistently include sex and gender as part of their analysis, and the implementation of health policies by governments that fail to adequately recognize women's roles as caregivers. However, third wave feminists are continually pushing analysis of women's health by calling into question the 'existence' or security of the so-called 'natural body' and by providing more comprehensive challenges to essentialized differences between men and women (Haraway, 1989; Nicholson, 1990). This increased emphasis on the differences among women and on the importance of theorizing gender, race, class, sexuality, and gender identity in an integrated way when talking about health, has the potential to move the women's health agenda forward in new and unique ways.

NOTES

1 'Scientific' theories of race in the eighteenth century relied on the paradigm of 'the great chain of being' which postulated that a species could be arrayed along a fixed and vertical hierarchy stretching from God down to the 'lowliest' sentient being. This led to the idea that the hierarchies observed in society are natural and unchanging.

2 For example, some well-known first wave Canadian feminists, such as Emily Murphy, supported the eugenics movement.

3 The first medical schools in Canada to allow women entry were the University of Toronto and Queen's University in 1883.

4 Margaret Sanger, who worked actively in the U.S. during the 20s, 30s, and 40s, was responsible for establishing the principle that a woman's right to control her body is a human right. Among Sanger's many accomplishments was the reversal of federal and state 'Comstock laws' that prohibited publication and distribution of information about sex, sexuality, and contraception.

5 De Beauvoir discusses the tension between 'immanence' and 'transcendence' for women. That is, social definitions of womanhood condemn women to 'immanence' or 'being-for-others' in socially prescribed roles; whereas 'transcendence' allows an escape from the physical body to higher intellectual states.

6 DES is 'diethylstilbestrol,' a synthetic estrogen prescribed to women between 1938 and 1971 to prevent miscarriages and avoid other pregnancy problems. Children born to women exposed to DES have suffered from a range of problems including vaginal cancer in women and noncancerous testicular growth in men. See http://www.cdc.gov/DES/consumers/about/history.html.

7 This book has recently been updated by the Boston Women's Health Collective and re-released as *Our Bodies, Ourselves: A New Edition for a New Era* (2005). New York: Touchstone.

8 Although thalidomide was pulled from the Canadian market in 1962, it is still used in developing countries as a treatment for leprosy and is being tested for a variety of medical uses in Canada and the U.S., including in the treatment of AIDS. See http://www.tv.cbc.ca/witness/thalidomide/extracome.htm.

9 Queer theory is a body of theory that emerged in the 1990s and is attractive to feminists because of its focus on sex, sexual orientation, and gender identity.

10 One of the strategic objectives in the Beijing Platform for Action was to 'promote research and disseminate information on women's health research.'

11 The centre in Quebec was closed in 2001.

12 In 1995, the federal government substantially reduced federal transfers for health care, education, and social services. The result was cutbacks to health services; increased private payment, such as user fees; deductibles; and co-payments and the delisting of some health services by removing them from public coverage.

REFERENCES

Agger, E. (1976). Lesbians fight to keep kids. *Body Politic* (*December/January*). Repr. R. Roach Pierson & M. Griffen Cohen. (1993). *Canadian Women's Voices*. Vol. 2: *Bold Visions Twenty-Five Years of Women's Activism in English Canada* (pp. 76–78). Toronto: James Lorimer Press.

Agnoito, R. (Ed.). (1977). *History of Ideas on Women*: Pedigree Books.

Anzaldua, G., & Moraga, C. (Eds.). (1981). *This Bridge Called My Back: Writings by Radical Women of Colour*. New York: Kitchen Table Press.

Armstrong, P. (1998). Women and health: Challenges and changes. In N. Mandell (Ed.), *Feminist Issues: Race, Class and Sexuality* (2nd ed., pp. 249–263). Scarborough, ON: Prentice Hall, Allyn & Bacon.

Armstrong, P., Amaratunga, C., Bernier, J., Grant, K., Pederson, A., & Wilson, K. (2002). *Exposing Privatization: Women and Health Care Reform in Canada*. Aurora, ON: Garamond Press.

Armstrong, P., Boscoe, M., Clow, B., Grant, K., Pederson, A., Wilson, K., Hankivsky, O., Jackson, B., & Morrow, M. (2003). *Reading Romanow: The Implications of the Final Report of the Commission on the Future of Health Care in*

Canada for Women. Ottawa: National Coordinating Group on Health Care Reform and Women.

Armstrong , P., Grant, K., Amaratunga, C., Boscoe, M., Pederson, A., & Wilson, K. (Eds.). (2004). *Caring For/ Caring About Women, Home Care and Unpaid Caregiving.* Aurora, ON: Garamond Press.

Aronson, J., & Neysmith, S. M. (1997). The retreat of the state and long-term provision: Implications for frail elderly people, unpaid family carers and paid home care workers. *Studies in Political Economy, 53*(Summer), 37–66.

Bannerji, H. (1987). Introducing racism: Notes towards an anti-racist feminism. In B. Crow & L. Gotell (Eds.), *Open Boundaries: A Canadian Women's Studies Reader, 2000* (pp. 26–32). Toronto: Prentice Hall, Allyn & Bacon.

Barnett, R., White, S., & Horne, T. (2002). *Voices from the Front Lines: Models of Women-Centred Care in Manitoba and Saskatchewan.* Winnipeg, MB: Prairie Women's Health Centre of Excellence.

Barnsley, J. (1995). Co-operation or co-optation? The partnership trend of the nineties. In L. Timmins (Ed.), *Listening to the Thunder: Advocates Talk about the Battered Women's Movement* (pp. 215–222). Vancouver: Women's Research Centre.

Bartky, S.L. (1993). The feminine body. In A. Jagger &. S. Rothenberg (Eds.), *Feminist Frameworks–Alternative Theoretical Accounts of the Relations between Women and Men* (pp. 454–461). New York: McGraw Hill.

Bashevkin, S. (1998). *Women on the Defensive.* Chicago: University of Chicago Press.

Biggs, C.L. (1983). The case of the missing midwives: A history of midwifery in Ontario from 1795–1900. *Ontario History, 65*(2), 21–35.

Bland, L. (1983). Purity, motherhood, pleasure or threat? Definitions of female sexuality 1900–1970. In L. Bland (Ed.), *Sex and Love: New Thoughts on Old Contradictions* (pp. 8–29). London: Women's Press.

Boehnert, J. (1993). The psychology of women. In S. Burt, L. Code, & L. Dorney (Eds.), *Changing Patterns: Women in Canada* (pp. 452–487). Toronto: McClelland & Stewart.

Bordo, S. (1993). *Unbearable Weight: Feminism, Western Culture and the Body.* Berkeley: University of California Press.

Boscoe, M. (1994). *The Strength of Links: Building the Canadian Women's Health Network.* Report on the Canadian-Wide consultation meeting held in Winnipeg, MB, 21–24 May 1993.

Boston Women's Health Book Collective. (2005). *Our Bodies, Ourselves: A New Edition for a New Era.* New York: Simon & Schuster.

Boston Women's Health Course Collective. (1971). *Our Bodies, Our Selves. A Course by and for Women.* Boston: Women's Health Course Collective.

Bourne, P. (1993). Women, law and the justice system. In R. Roach Pierson M. Griffin Cohen, P. Bourne, & P. Masters (Eds.), *Canadian Women's Issues. Volume One: Strong Voices – 25 Years of Women's Activism in English Canada* (pp. 322–392). Toronto: James Lorimer.

Boyer, M., Ku, J., Shakir, U. (1997). *The Healing Journey: Phase II Report – Women and Mental Health: Documenting the Voices of Ethnoracial Women Within an Anti-Racist Framework*. Toronto: Across Boundaries Mental Health Centre.

Burstow, B. (1992). *Radical Feminist Therapy: Working in the Context of Violence*. Newbury Park, CA: Sage.

Burt, S., & Mitchell, C. (1998). What's in a name?: From sheltering women to protecting communities. In L. Pal (Ed.), *How Ottawa Spends 1998–99 Balancing Act: The Post-Deficit Mandate* (pp. 271–291). Don Mills, ON: Oxford University Press.

Butler, J. (1999). *Gender Trouble: Feminism and the Subversion of Identity*. New York: Routledge.

Butler, S. (1980). Incest: Whose reality, whose theory? *Aegis: Magazine on Ending Violence Against Women*, (*Summer/Autumn*), 49.

Canada Health Council. (1997). Canada Health Council: Building on the Legacy. Vol. 1 National Forum on Health. Ottawa: Health Canada.

Canadian Advisory Council on the Status of Women. (1995). *What Women Prescribe: Report and Recommendations from the National Symposium Women in Partnership: Working Towards Inclusive Gender-Sensitive Health Policies*. Ottawa: Canadian Advisory Council on the Status of Women.

Carroll, W. (Ed.). (1997). *Organizing Dissent: Contemporary Social Movements in Theory and Practice*. Toronto: Garamond Press.

Chesler, P. (1972). *Women and Madness*. New York: Avon Books.

Chinn, P.L., & Wheeler, C.E. (1985). Feminism and nursing: Can nursing afford to remain aloof from the women's movement? *Nursing Outlook, 33*(2), 74–77.

Ciliska, D., & Rice, C. (1989). Body image/body politics. *Healthsharing, 10*(3), 13–17.

Cohen, M. (2001). *Do Comparisons Between Hospital Support Workers and Hospitality Workers Make Sense?* Vancouver: Hospital Employees Union.

Cohen, M., & Cohen, M. (2004). *A Return to Wage Discrimination: Pay equity Losses Through Privatization in Health Care*. Vancouver: Canadian Centre for Policy Alternatives.

Cohen, M., Ritchie, L., Swenarchuk, M., & Vosko, L. (2002). Globalization: Some implications and strategies for women. *Canadian Woman's Studies/ les cahiers de la femme: Women, Globalization and International Trade, 21*(22), 6–14.

Cope, A., & Darke, J. (2002). *Trans Inclusion Manual for Women's Organizing: A Report for the Trans/Women Dialogue Planning Committee and the Trans Alliance Project*. Vancouver: Trans/Women Dialogue Planning Committee and Trans Alliance Project.

David, B.A. (2000). Nursing's gender politics: Reformulating the footnotes. *Advances in Nursing Science, 23*(1), 83–93.

Davis, A. (1981). *Women, Race and Class* (2nd ed., 1983). New York: Random House.

De Beauvoir, S. (1952). *The Second Sex*. New York: Bantam Books.

Dinnerstein, D. (1975). *The Mermaid and the Minotaur: Sexual Arrangements and Human Malaise*. New York: Harper & Row.

Disabled Women's Network. (1988). DAWN: Toronto fact sheet on reproductive rights. In R. Roach Pierson, M. Griffen Cohen, P. Bourne, & P. Masters (Eds.), *Canadian Women's Issues: Volume I Strong Voices: Twenty-Five Years of Women's Activism in English Canada* (pp. 131–132). Toronto: James Lorimer.

Doyal, L. (1998). *Women's Health Services*. Buckingham, UK: Open University Press.

Dubois, E.C., & Gordon, L. (1983). Seeking ecstasy on the battlefield: Danger and pleasure in 19th-century feminist sexual thought. *Feminist Studies, 9*(1), 7–25.

Egan, C., & Gardener, L. (1994). Race, class and reproductive freedom: Women must have real choices. *Canadian Women's Studies, 14*(2), 95–99.

Ehrenreich, B., & English, D. (1978). *For Her Own Good: 150 Years of Expert's Advice to Women*. New York: Anchor Press, Doubleday.

Errington, J. (1993). Pioneers and suffragists. In S. Burt, L. Code, & L. Dorney (Eds.), *Changing Patterns: Women in Canada* (2nd ed., pp. 59–91). Toronto: McClelland & Stewart.

Federal/Provincial/Territorial Working Group on Women's Health. (1990). Working Together for Women's Health: A Framework for the Development of Policies & Programs. Ottawa: Health Canada.

Findlay, D.A., & Miller, D.L. (2002). Through medical eyes: The medicalization of women's bodies and lives. In B.S. Bolaria & H. Dickinson (Eds.), *Health, Illness and Health Care in Canada* (3rd ed., pp. 185–210). Toronto: Nelson.

Firestone, S. (1970). *The Dialectic of Sex: The Case for Feminist Revolution*. New York: Farrar, Straus & Giroux.

Gilligan, C. (1982). *In a Different Voice: Psychological Theory and Women's Development*. Cambridge: Harvard University Press.

Gilman, S.L. (1985). Black bodies, white bodies: Toward an iconography of female sexuality in late nineteenth-century art, medicine, and literature. *Critical Inquiry,* Autumn(12), 204–242.

Gordon, L. (1988). *Heroes of Their Own Lives: The Politics and History of Family Violence: Boston 1880–1960.* New York: Viking.

Greaves, L., Hankivsky, O., et al. (1999). *CIHR 2000: Sex, Gender and Women's Health.* Vancouver: British Columbia Centre of Excellence for Women's Health.

Hankivsky, O. (2004). *Social Policy and the Ethic of Care.* Vancouver: University of British Columbia Press.

Hankivsky, O., & Morrow, M. (2004). *Trade Agreements, Homecare and Women's Health.* Ottawa: Status of Women Canada.

Haraway, D. (1989). *Primate Visions: Gender, Race and Nature in the World of Modern Science.* New York: Routledge.

Harding, S., & O'Barr, J. (Eds.). (1987). *Sex and Scientific Inquiry.* Chicago: University of Chicago Press.

Health Canada. (1999). *Women's Health Strategy.* Ottawa: Health Canada.

Heller, A.F. (1986). *Health and Home: Women as Health Guardians.* Ottawa: Canadian Advisory on the Status of Women.

Hite, S. (1976). *The Hite Report: A National Study of Female Sexuality.* New York: Seven Stories Press.

Kealy, L. (1979). *A Not Unreasonable Claim: Women and Reform in Canada 1880–1920.* Toronto: Women's Educational Press.

Kinsey, A., Wardell, B., Pomeroy, C., Martin, E., & Gebhard, P. (1963). *Sexual Behaviour in the Human Female.* Bloomington: Indiana University Press.

Koivusalo, M. (2003). Assessing the health policy implications of WTO trade and investment agreements. In K. Lee (Ed.), *Health Impacts of Globalization: Towards a Global Governance* (pp. 161–175). Hounsdmills, Basingstoke, Hampshire, UK: Palgrave Macmillan.

Laquer, T. (1990). *Making Sex: Body and Gender from the Greeks to Freud.* Cambridge, MA: Harvard University Press.

MacLeod, L. (1980). *Wife Battering in Canada: The Vicious Circle.* Ottawa: Advisory Council on the Status of Women.

Masters, W.H., & Johnson, V.E. (1966). *Human Sexual Response.* Boston: Little Brown Books.

McGill Student's Union Collective. (1969). *Birth Control Handbook* Montreal: Montreal Health Press.

Medical Research Council of Canada. (1994). *Report of the Advisory Committee on Women's Health Research Issues* Ottawa: MRC.

Michinson, W. (1991). *The Nature of Their Bodies: Women and Their Doctors in Victorian Canada*. Toronto: University of Toronto Press.

Miles, A. (1985). Feminism, equality and liberation. *Canadian Journal of Women and the Law, 1*, 42–61.

Millet, K. (1970). *Sexual Politics*. Garden City, NY: Doubleday.

Mira Goldberg, J. (2004). *First Year Report Transgender Health Program*. Vancouver: Transgender Health Program, Three Bridges Community Health Centre, and Vancouver Coastal Health.

Mitchinson, W. (1993). The medical treatment of women. In S. Burt, L. Code, & L. Dorney (Eds.), *Changing Patterns: Women in Canada* (2nd. ed., pp. 391–421). Toronto: McClelland & Stewart.

Morrow, M., Hankivsky, O., & Varcoe, C. (2004). Women and violence: The effects of dismantling the welfare state. *Journal of Critical Social Policy, 24*(3), 358–384.

Naples, N., & Desai, M. (Eds.). (2002). *Women's Activism and Globalization: Linking Local Struggles and Transnational Politics*. New York: Routledge.

Nelson, S. (1997). Reading nursing history. *Nursing Inquiry, 4*, 229–236.

Nicholson, L. (Ed.). (1990). *Feminism/Postmodernism*. New York: Routledge.

Nopper, S., & Harley, J. (1986). How society's obsession with thinness is consuming women. *Herizons: Women's News and Feminist Views, 4*(7), 24–27.

Oakley, A. (1993). *Essays on Women, Medicine and Health*. Edinburgh: Edinburgh University Press.

O'Neill, B. (2003). *Royal Commission on the Status of Women: Looking Back, Looking Forward*. Unpublished paper.

Penfold, S., & Walker, G. (1983). *Women and the Psychiatric Paradox*. Montreal: Eden Press.

Perkins Gilman, C. (1899). *The Yellow Wallpaper*. Boston: Small & Maynard.

Price, J., & Shildrick, M. (Eds.). (1999). *Feminist Theory and the Body: A Reader*. New York: Routledge.

Rich, A. (1980). Compulsory heterosexuality and lesbian existence. *Signs: Journal of Women in Culture and Society, 5*(4), 631–660.

Roach Pierson, R. (1993). The politics of the body. In M. Griffen Cohen, R. Roach Pierson, P. Bourne, & P. Masters (Eds.), *Canadian Women's Issues, Volume I: Strong Voices, Twenty-Five Years of Women's Activism in English Canada* (pp. 98–185). Toronto: James Lorimer.

Romanow, R. (2002). *Building on Values: The Future of Health Care in Canada*. Ottawa: Commission on the Future of Health Care in Canada.

Ruddick, S. (1983). Maternal thinking. In J. Trebilcot (Ed.), *Mothering: Essays in Feminist Theory* (pp. 213–230). New Jersey: Rowan & Allanheld.

Schiebinger, L. (1999). Theories of gender and race. In J. Price & M. Shildrick (Eds.), *Feminist Theory and the Body: A Reader* (pp. 21–31). New York: Routledge.

Sherwin, S. (1992). *No Longer Patient: Feminist Ethics and Health Care.* Philadelphia: Temple University Press.

Shiva, V., & Mies, M. (1993). *Ecofeminism.* Halifax, NS: Fernwood.

Spieldoch, A. (2001). *GATS and Healthcare: Why Do Women Care?* International Gender and Trade Network – Secretariat. Retrieved 6 June 2002, from http://www.genderandtrade.net/GATS/GATS%20and%20Healthcare.pdf.

Stanko, E. (1986). *Intimate Intrusions: Women's Experiences of Male Violence.* London: Routledge & Kegan Paul.

Status of Women Canada. (1995). *Setting the Stage for the Next Century: The Federal Plan for Gender Equality.* Ottawa: Status of Women Canada.

United Nations (1995) The Beijing Platform for Action, Report on the Fourth World Conference on Women. Geneva, Switzerland: UN.

Urla, J., & Terry, J. (1995). Introduction: Mapping embodied deviance. In J. Urla & J. Terry (Eds.), *Deviant Bodies* (pp. 1–18). Bloomington and Indianapolis: Indiana University Press.

Valverde, M. (1991). *The Age of Light, Soap and Water: Moral Reform in English Canada: 1885–1925.* Toronto: McClelland & Stewart.

Vance, C., Talbot, S., McBride, A., & Mason, D. (1985). An uneasy alliance: Nursing and the women's movement. *Nursing Outlook, 33*(6), 281–285.

Varcoe, C., & McCormick, J. (2002). Racing around the classroom margins. In L. Young & B. Patterson (Eds.), *Learning Nursing: Student-Centered Theories, Models, and Strategies for Nurse Educators* (pp 439–446). Philidelphia: Lippincott, Williams & Wilkins.

Walker, G. (1990). *Family Violence and the Women's Movement: The Conceptual Politics of Struggle.* Toronto: University of Toronto Press.

White, M. (2001). GATS and women. *Foreign Policy in Focus, 6*(2), 1.

Young, I.M. (1989). Throwing like a girl: A phenomenology of feminine body comportment, motility and spatiality. In J. Allen & I.M. Young (Eds.), *The Thinking Muse: Feminism and Modern French Philosophy* (pp. 51–70). Bloomington and Indianapolis: Indiana University Press.

Young, L. (1999). Racializing Femininity. In J. Arthurs & J. Grimshaw (Eds.), *Women's Bodies: Discipline and Transgression* (pp. 67–90). London and New York: Cassell.

2 More Than Age and Biology: Overhauling Lifespan Approaches to Women's Health

OLENA HANKIVSKY

An international push to conceptualize women's health across the lifespan is a fairly recent phenomenon, having started in the 1990s. The introduction of a lifespan perspective can be interpreted as a direct response to a number of factors: persistent conflations of women's health with reproductive and gynecological health (Pinn, 2003; Healy, 1991); the need to better document, comprehend, and respond to the specific challenges and contributing factors that influence girls' and women's lives from birth to death; and the need to ensure that appropriate policies and programs are developed, monitored, and evaluated so that 'all women across life stages have access to reasonable care that emphasizes health promotion and disease prevention' (Correa-de Araujo, 2004, p. 31). The development of this longitudinal approach in Canada is in its nascent stages. And yet, with the Institute of Gender and Health prioritizing research on health across the lifespan and Health Canada recently announcing that it will be 'working towards the development of a renewed plan of action on women's health with targeted objectives to focus research and policy work on life cycle and diversity issues' (Standing Committee on the Status of Women, 2005), this particular framing of women's health is a growing priority in research, policy, and practice.

The 'scientifically interesting' (Kuh & Hardy, 2002, p. 410) lifespan approach does have significant potential to reveal largely unexamined aspects of women's health, provide new insights into the causes of health problems, and identify important themes and patterns that cut across all age groups. For the potential to be realized, however – in Canada and elsewhere – a number of conceptual and methodological shortcomings need to be overcome, especially the current focus on age and life stages which prioritize disease and illness within narrow confines of a biomedical perspective. Efforts have been made to make lifespan frameworks more comprehensive by including, for example, social factors and psychological processes that shape health. And yet, these additional considerations are simply grafted into existing frameworks, falling short of what is needed: a transformation of current modes of analysis.

In this chapter, the existing lifespan paradigm and its resultant shortcomings are examined. Specifically, biomedical hegemony and its related priorities are shown to cause narrow and often incorrect conceptualizations of women's health across the lifespan. The argument put forward is that an alternative, more flexible and fluid framework is needed. This alternative must reflect the reality that women's health is socially produced and biologically embedded (Smith, 2003, p. xxix). It has to synthesize biomedical factors *as well as* broader determinants of health, including the political, economic, social, and cultural constructs of women's lives. As Kuh and Hardy (2002) argue, 'A common framework is ... needed to combine the life course perspective with its emphasis on long-term temporal processes and the eco-social perspective which draws attention to the hierarchy of factors operating at any one time at different levels, from the macroeconomic to the molecular (p. 397). Most importantly, however, as was argued in the Introduction, multiple axes of analyses (e.g., gender, 'race'/ethnicity, class, sexuality, ability), which illuminate the health effects of intersections among a wide variety of social categories and factors, must be explicitly recognized and fully integrated for any lifespan framework to be inclusive and responsive to the diversity of women's health.

Theoretical Background

The life course/span perspective arose in sociology and psychology in the 1960s and has since then been used by economists, demographers, anthropologists, geographers, gerontologists, historians, epidemiologists, and women's health researchers (Johnstone, 2001; Elder & O'Rand, 1995; Kertzer, 1991). It prioritizes a framework that implies a notion of human life that is structured predominantly by age. It looks at the distinctive series of roles and experiences that an individual progresses through as s/he proceeds from birth to death. It focuses on investigating pathways and connections between different life phases rather than seeing any one phase in isolation (Moen, Dempster–Mclain, & Williams

1992, p. 1614). This perspective is advantageous because it seeks to contextualize lives and demonstrate the processes and consequences of change at different stages of a person's life. As Elder and O'Rand (1995) explain: 'Life course theory is temporal and contextual in locating people in history through birth years and in the life course through the social meanings of age-graded events and activities. The perspective also directs inquiry to processes by which life change occurs and to studies following people over time' (p. 454).

In the context of health, the explanatory power of the lifespan perspective lies in its ability to locate individuals by chronological and physiological age, organized by period and by cohort (Kuh & Hardy, 2002). The approach seeks to further the understanding of life changes and specifically to ' better characterize the relative importance of influences acting at different stages of life to the generation of inequalities in health in adulthood' (Smith, 2003, p. xv). In terms of physical health, age is a particularly important facet of life course position since there is a strong relationship between age and health and age and mortality (Kaplan, 1996). Of course, there is also considerable heterogeneity in the health status of individuals of any given age – as a function of differential stress exposure, access to resources, and biological vulnerability (House et al., 1990). Nevertheless, in the process of establishing a common methodological framework, there is a tendency to assume that there are key life stages through which all individuals pass (e.g., infancy, childhood, adolescence, etc.), and from which certain generalizations about health can be made.

A lifespan approach to women's health aims to inform and 'better structure policies that address the specific circumstances and problems women face at various stages of their lives, as well as issues that are universal among women' (Wyn & Solis, 2001, p. 148). First and foremost, it is intended to expand notions of women's health beyond the reproductive years to include pre-adolescence through to and beyond menopause (Weisman, 1997). In so doing, its objective is to elucidate how and why women's health risks and concerns change throughout the course of their lives. Conceptualizing health across the lifespan holds much promise for better understanding the full complexity, including pathways and key intersecting factors, which influence and uniquely shape women's health. Compared to men, women do have different lifespans and patterns of illness. Understanding such differences is important to developing new approaches to prevention, diagnosis, and treatment (Wizemann & Pardue, 2001). And yet, a lifespan approach moves beyond an understanding of how women's health compares to that of men. It is motivated by a more fundamental concern about how women as a distinct group develop and by concern regarding how to improve knowledge about the full range of health risks, unique diseases, illnesses, experiences, and challenges they face throughout their lifespan (Collins, Bussell, & Wenzel, 1997).

Evolution of the Lifespan Approach in Women's Health

The call for a more expansive view of the 'totality' of women's lives was driven by a growing awareness of the aging baby boom generation about health issues in midlife and later years (Weisman, 1997). The lifespan approach was also a response to the general need for information that is specific to women in terms of their age, lifestyle, and current life events (Johnstone, 2001). Internationally, different interpretations of the lifespan approach have been embraced by a growing number of organizations and countries, including the United Nations. For example, according to the Fourth World Conference on Women held at the UN in September 1995:

> Women's right to the enjoyment of the highest standard of health must be secured throughout *the whole life cycle* in equality with men [emphasis added]. Women are affected by many of the same health conditions as men, but women experience them differently. The prevalence among women of poverty and economic dependence, their experience of violence, negative attitudes towards women and girls, racial and other forms of discrimination, the limited power many women have over their sexual and reproductive lives and lack of influence in decision-making are social realities which have an adverse impact on their health. Lack of food and inequitable distribution of food for girls and women in the household, inadequate access to safe water, sanitation facilities and fuel supplies, particularly in rural and poor urban areas, and deficient housing conditions, all overburden women and their families and have a negative effect on their health. Good health is essential to leading a productive and fulfilling life, and the right of all women to control all aspects of their health, in particular their own fertility, is basic to their empowerment.

Other than the United Nations, the World Health Organization (WHO) has recognized and used this approach (Bonita, 1996). The Global Commission on Women's Health, established in 1992 under the auspices of the WHO, has also adopted 'health security for women throughout the lifespan' (World Health Organization [WHO], 1996) as the platform for its future advocacy efforts.

The lifespan approach has been popularized in the United States and accepted, for example, by the Office of Research on Women's Health (ORWH) (National Institutes of Health, 1992) as an overarching theme for research on women's health: 'The health of girls and women is affected by developmental, physiological, and psychological age. Women's lives are marked by continuum from intrauterine life to the elderly years: infancy, childhood and adolescence, menarche, reproductive life, the menopausal transition, postmenopausal years, the elderly and frail years' (ORWH, 2004, p. 1). Women's Health Victoria (WHV) in Australia, an independent statewide women's health promotion, advocacy, and health information service also utilizes such an approach to collect data on women's health (Johnstone, 2001).

In Canada, *Health Canada's Women's Health Strategy* (Health Canada, 1999), embedded within a population health framework[1] that prioritizes three life stages of childhood and adolescence, early to mid-adulthood, and later life. According to Health Canada 'throughout their lives – as children, in middle adulthood and as seniors – women face life conditions and health issues specific to their biology and social circumstances' (Health Canada, 1999, p. 2). More recently, Health Canada's *Women's Health Surveillance Report* concluded that 'our understanding of women's health would benefit from increased knowledge in this area, and more emphasis should be placed on health across life stages' (Health Canada 2003, p. 70). Currently, lifespan approaches are priorities in both research and policy, because it is generally understood that health status and the aging process are responsive to some degree of intervention (NIH, 1992).

Even though the value of a lifespan approach has been accepted, it is not used to its full advantage. Johnstone (2001) has argued that 'in health, particularly in the policy and planning arenas, the importance of life cycle stages may be recognized but are rarely applied in a systematic way' (p. 7). This is especially true in the case of Canada. However, before full-scale systematic incorporations are contemplated, the adequacy of current frameworks needs to be considered and critically evaluated to reveal both the substantive shortcomings and concomitant changes that are required for the lifespan approach to be used in an effective and inclusive fashion to inform research, policy, and practice.

Lifespan Framework: Current Practices and Proposed Reforms

Those who have examined current frameworks have argued that they are not well articulated or described (Johnstone, 2001). In general, there is a need to better conceptualize and organize the categories used in lifespan frameworks. For example, the categories and content of age cohorts differ, as there is no set standard regarding how these should be determined (Wyn & Solis, 2001). Moreover, there is a definite lack of longitudinal data on women's health, which of course is essential for any effective lifespan analysis (Kuh & Hardy, 2002). Data that does exist is not methodically organized into lifespan frameworks. And in many cases, even when there are attempts to collect and synthesize available data, the mode of analysis does not explain fully why and how health is the product of a very broad range of experiences across the life course (Bierman, 2003).

In what follows, a number of specific shortcomings of current lifespan approaches are examined. All are linked to biological hegemony, which gives primacy to the physical body and factors related to age and biology including illness and disease. By focusing on biological explanations, lifespan frameworks assume that the best points of intervention are individual level behavioural changes and medical treatments, overlooking the possibilities for more systematic social interventions to improve the health of the population (Bird & Rieker, 2002, p. 114). Current lifespan framings are problematic also because they underestimate the importance of a range of social determinants, marginalize gender, and in particular gloss over differences among women across all life stages. All these issues, as the discussion below details, need to be acknowledged and addressed to develop an effective approach that is capable of understanding and responding to the diversity of women's longitudinal health issues.

Biomedical Hegemony

To begin, despite the extensive body of literature that demonstrates the relationship between social factors and health, lifespan approaches to women's health remain largely determined by a biomedical model. The explanatory power of this model prevails because, as Eckman (1998) has argued, 'biological sex, extended throughout the whole of a woman's body, has been repositioned as the foundational truth from which health research should start' (p. 149). Accordingly, 'currently, women's health research primarily focuses on life stage (adolescence, midlife, and later years) organ systems (reproductive health), or disease (breast cancer, HIV/AIDS, heart disease) (Bierman, 2003, p. 202). Not surprisingly, the hegemony of biomedicine is also superimposed on lifespan frameworks.

Diabetes illustrates the problems associated with the current lifespan approach, especially when it is the sole or even dominant frame for understanding women's health. The existing biomedically informed approach would suggest that obesity and genetic factors are the most important determinants of morbidity in diabetes, and that making lifestyle changes, including better diet and more exercise from early life on, is the most effective means of combating diabetes. The narrowness of such an explanation glosses over other contributing factors and issues that influence the onset and complications associated with diabetes. For example, diabetes is disproportionately prevalent among Aboriginal communities in Canada, even though it was virtually unknown in these communities 50 years ago (Health Canada, 2000). Thus, the disease cannot simply be attributable to genetic factors. Moreover, simple solutions for diabetes reduction do not take into account the factors that affect this disease within First Nations communities, such as early onset, greater severity at diagnosis, high rates of complications, and lack of accessible services compared to the general Canadian population (Health Canada, 2000). Further, the traditional framing of diabetes does not necessarily illuminate the higher rates among First Nations women. Not only are the rates for diabetes higher for Aboriginal women than the female non-Aboriginal population, but two-thirds of First Nations people diagnosed with diabetes are women (Bobet, 1997) who in turn are at higher risk for cardiovascular disease and blindness (Thompson-Reid, Beckles, & Jones, 2001). Few such women have access to culturally appropriate curative and preventative services. Any framework that continues to be determined by biological hegemony with an attendant focus on individual health and with superficial attention to social determinants, including gender and its intersection with other categories of experience, will not capture such complex dynamics. Current lifespan approaches often do not focus on the right issues, ask the right kinds of research questions, collect appropriate data, or result in a comprehensive or inclusive analysis that could inform interventions across the lifespan that are truly able to improve *all* women's lives as they age. This is evidenced first and foremost by the organizational categories used to capture each cohort's health status, health behaviours, and specific age-related issues.

The Organization and Conceptualization of Life Stages

Health Canada's *Women's Health Surveillance Report* (2000) provides a fairly typical typology and classification that is used to arrange women's health across the lifespan. It illustrates the often-used life stages (e.g., fetal life, childhood, adolescence, early adult life, midlife, and later adult life) and related biomedically focused health issues and research priorities, which tend to organize around reproductive health (including pre-reproduction and menopause), and prioritize concerns relating to morbidity and mortality (2003). Although factors beyond biomedicine are included, they tend to be presented as secondary in importance to the primary focal points of analysis. To illustrate in more detail, starting with early life stages, lifespan approaches consider fetal life and childhood in terms of risk factors later associated with chronic diseases and disorders (Kuh & Hardy, 2002). These include effects of exposure to drugs during prenatal and perinatal stages of development, long-term and short-term effects of drugs on the fetus and child, and the impact of environmental agents on fetal development. Dominant frameworks also focus on childhood factors such a calcium intake, mineral supplementation, malnutrition, and physical activity. According to the Office of Research on Women's Health (1999), 'research on the prenatal, infancy, and childhood years can focus on identifying the short and long-term effects of drugs on unborn infants and young children; and normal physical, behavioural, and psychological development, including the influence of genes and the environment' (p. 25). Related studies in this early life stage also seek to determine sex and gender differences in response to stress and nutrition, critical stress points, and the development of coping behaviours.

During adolescence (onset of puberty to approximately 17 years of age), issues that are noted consistently include menarche, sexual behaviour, pregnancy, HIV/AIDS, sexually transmitted illnesses (STIs), substance use, eating disorders, violence, and family disruption. In early adult life, the focus tends to be on reproduction and issues related to contraception, pregnancy, and STIs. Diseases and conditions for which reproductive-age women are at risk include cardiovascular diseases, autoimmune disorders, female cancers, infertility, endometriosis, uterine fibroids, mental health disorders, substance abuse, stress-related digestive orders, and obesity (ORWH, 1999, p. 25). Lifespan frameworks also mark this stage in life by development concerns such as employment, finding a partner, having and raising children. Again, diseases often are considered decontextualized from the wider issues that shape them.

In midlife – as women move into their forties – lifespan frameworks continue to focus on chronic diseases. Issues relating to infertility, late unintended pregnancy, menopause, family, and employment issues join these foci. This time in a woman's life is marked by the onset of menopause, defined as the time when a woman stops menstruating. Menopause is seen as one of the most critical physiological changes for women, often associated with an increase in depressive symptomology. Cardiovascular disease and osteoporosis are also significant health risks. Much research at this stage attends to the effects of hormones on menopause, psychological aspects of menopause, links between menopause and coronary heart disease, and societal attitudes towards menopause (ORWH, 1999, p. 25). And finally in late adult life (65+), the focus changes to functional health and especially osteoporosis, osteoarthritis, cardiovascular disease, diabetes, cervical and breast cancer, urinary incontinence, and hypertension. Further, issues relating to vision, hearing, and cognitive decline are illuminated. Depression as triggered by factors relating to physical and mental health (Alexander, Larosa, & Bader, 2001) and toxic drug reactions are also identified as prime concerns for elderly women.

The life stages briefly outlined above reflect typical biomedical hegemony with its focus on the interplay between age and sex, and manifest in disease and illness patterns, and, specifically, on excesses in female morbidity and mortality. According to the Institute of Medicine in Washington, DC (2001), 'scientific evidence of the importance of sex differences throughout the life span abounds' (p. 1). Biological sex does matter, as does age. However, favouring age- and sex-specific explanations, even when others may be noted or considered, does not provide a sufficient analytic frame for examining women's health across the lifespan. In fact, it leads to a number of problematic assumptions and interventions starting with an overly individualistic focus on responsibility for health.

Individualizing Responsibility for Health

Biomedicine is fixated on individuals, their risks factors, and behaviours that are expressed through the body (Kuhlmann & Babitsch, 2002, p. 437). As such, a lifespan approach is intended to give women 'a more complete and coherent understanding of the ways in which their health risks change as they move through life' and significantly, 'how personal behaviours in one phase of life can affect health status in subsequent years' (Collins et al., 1997, p. iii). It has been established for example, that 'lifestyle' in midlife predicts morbidity and mortality among older women (Bierman, 2003). Many interventions are focused on encouraging women to modify their behaviour by reducing or ceasing to smoke, stopping substance use, maintaining normal body weight, exercising regularly, and eating a healthy diet (Collins et al., 1997). Without doubt, individual agency and autonomy are important. There is, however, a real danger in presenting all choices that women make in their lives as freely determined 'personal choices.' Using this individualistic approach can lead to blaming women for apparent 'lifestyle' choices and concomitant behaviours over which they may have little or no control. As Green (2002) explains: 'The analytic separation of the individual from her larger social situation is, of course, one of the classic distinguishing features that separates the approaches of biomedicine and public health. These distinctions may be important for developing interventions to treat or avert disease or disability, but it is precisely in this gap between individuals and the wider social context that many researchers locate the inadequacies of biomedicine to address the health needs of many populations' (p. 7).

Health inequalities cannot simply be reduced to 'the unconstrained adoption of insalubrious lifestyle choices' (Smith, 2003, p. xvi). Kuh and Hardy (2002) raise the difficulties for life course research in this regard within the context of maternal and child health. Victim blaming of mothers can occur when possible interventions during pregnancy are focused on individual women (e.g., smoking, drinking, poor maternal nutrition). A similar problem arises in the case of violence, where women are often blamed for 'choosing' to stay with their partners, rather than making the 'decision' to escape their abusive situations. In such instances, what remain unquestioned are the social hierarchies and how they 'mediate an individual's power, personal agency, and available choices relating to their health' (Inhorn & Whittle, 2001a, p. 554).

Recognizing the effects of lifestyle factors may be important but ineffectual if these factors are not properly situated in a broad social context (Jones & Rothney, 2001). To be sure, individually focused models have proven unable to bring about high-risk behaviour change (Smedley & Symes, 2000). Numerous factors may not be modifiable by the individual but instead require attention to the breadth of socioeconomic factors that affect women's health and predispose many women to disease throughout their lives. Emerging evidence suggests that health inequalities begin from economic disadvantage early in life and accumulate throughout the lifespan (Wamala, Lynch, & Kaplan, 2001). Choices are rarely autonomous but instead are shaped by our interdependent and relational existence in society. As Bird and Rieker (2004) explain: 'Women's opportunities and choices are to a certain extent constrained by decisions and actions taken by families, communities, and government policies,' and, moreover, 'these connections between broader social contexts and individual choices are rarely transparent and their health consequences are often underestimated and overlooked.' (p. 23). What any lifespan framework therefore requires is an explicit incorporation of the determinants of health that inform the context of all women's lives and health. Krieger, Rowley, Herman, Avery, & Phillips (1993) have made a similar argument using a metaphor of a spider's web: '[F]or research to set the basis for effective disease prevention policies, it must address the structural determinants of health, not simply factors labeled as 'lifestyle choices.' Continuing merely to catalog individual risk factors from an amorphous 'web of causation' no longer can suffice. If our goal is to alter the web rather than merely break its strands, it is time to look for the spider' (p. 109).

Undervaluing Determinants of Health

The association between socioeconomic determinants and health is recognized and yet this knowledge is not fully or consistently integrated into lifespan frameworks (Mishra, Ball, Dobson, & Byles, 2004; Prus, 2003; Lock, 1998). The universalized natural female body, which dominates the biomedical framing of women's health, remains the 'gold standard of hegemonic social discourse' (Haraway, 1989, p. 355). Moreover, interdisciplinary methods and knowledge about health determinants emerging from the social sciences and humanities are seen as inferior to dominant approaches and marginalized. For example, in the *Agenda for Research on Women's Health for the 21st Century*, the chairs of the taskforce wrote that 'social and behavioural science needs to communicate the principles of its discipline to the longer-established and more "mainstrean" medical disciplines. It is not a familiar resource or partner for conventional research' (ORWH, 1999, p. 14). Consequently, concerns beyond biological workings in research, policy, and lifespan frameworks are often 'added on if and as needed' (Eckman, 1998, p. 158).

While it is important not to lose sight that some diseases are largely genetic in origin, most originate from a range of factors that are genetic, environmental, bacterial, viral, and behavioural. After all, 'human beings do not age as specimens in laboratories' (Riley & Bond, 1983, p. 245). Health extends beyond the physical body and fundamental causes of health differences during the lifespan are rooted in economic, political, historical, and social arrangements. Such connections were first noted sometime in the mid-nineteenth century with the rise of the public health movement (Kaufert, 1996). In Canada, Health Canada (1999) has recognized that income and social status, employment, education, social environments, physical environments, healthy child development, personal health practices, and coping skills, health services, social support networks, biology and genetic endowment, and culture as well as gender are key determinants of health. The health determinants perspective 'is intended to lead to better understandings of health disparities by pointing to a range of social, behaviours and predisposing genetic and biological pathways to positively or negatively influence health' (Benoit, 2005, p. 3).

Understanding the influence of various determinants is absolutely essential if the lifespan framework is to contribute to a meaningful change in how women's health is understood. To start with, more attention needs to be paid to key economic and social challenges. For example, of great importance is the enduring nature of poverty in Canada and the links between poverty and ill health. Poverty is known to contribute to poor health through inadequate environments, poor housing, lack of food security, and by creating barriers to accessing affordable, quality health care. To illustrate, First Nations, Inuit, and Métis women suffer from different forms of poverty: poverty of subsistence, poverty of sexual and reproductive health, poverty of identitty, poverty of safety and security, poverty of mental health, poverty of civic participation, and poverty of power and knowledge (Aboriginal Women's Health and Healing Research Group, 2005). Because major determinants of health such as poverty lie outside the health care sector, an approach that can draw on multiple perspectives to contextualize health with respect to a range of sectors, experiences, and events is required (Bierman, 2003).

Further, lifespan health researchers need to consider the consequences of trends like social welfare state retrenchment and economic globalization on social safety nets and publicly delivered services including education, social services, and health. In Canada, the effects of cost containment and reduced public expenditures on the health care system and related social support have been documented (Morrow,

Hankivsky & Vacoe, 2004; Strobino, Grason & Minkovitz, 2002; Armstrong et al., 2001). Demographic trends are also altering human life courses. In the United Kingdom it has been observed that 'shifts in employment, family formation and government policy have combined to reconfigure the lifecourse pathways along which individual socio-economic position is determined' (Graham, 2002, p. 2011). Political events are equally life-altering. For instance, the dramatic changes in Eastern Europe after the fall of the Soviet Union have had both short- and long-term effects on women's health, as did the end of apartheid in South Africa (Jones & Kumssa, 2000). Moreover, social exclusion, that is discrimination, stigmatization, and hostility, is experienced by various groups of women. Although it is not explicitly or consistently reflected in how women through the lifespan are analyzed, social exclusion undermines all aspects of citizenship and results in a range of health problems (Marmot & Wilkinson, 2003).

Even when attempts have been made to move beyond a focus on specific illnesses to broader factors that affect health and on health promoting activities (e.g., Alexander et al., 2001; Allen & Phillips, 1997), lifespan frameworks have not paid adequate attention to the social determinant of gender. Like both age and sex, gender is a fundamental dimension throughout the lifespan. According to Wyn and Solis (2001) 'there are both social and medical markers that change as women age, such as child and family responsibilities, work commitments, economic security, and health status' (p. 148). Similarly, the Office of Research on Women's Health (2004) has recognized that 'the health of girls and women is affected by developmental, physiological, and psychological age' (p. 1). And, Health Canada (2003) has noted that biological, psy-chological, and social factors interact to influence women's health. Any explication of determinants of women's health needs to encompass the role of gender and in particular, how women's living conditions, dis-crimination, and complexities of their lives on their health and well-being.

Marginalization and Misconceptualization of Gender

Biomedical explanations that dominate existing lifespan approaches are limited in what they can tell us about what makes women sick because they marginalize the extent to which gender inequality and discrimination harm girls' and women's health directly and indirectly throughout the life cycle (Doyal, 1995). In some instances, the 'interactions between sex linked and gender-based factors' (Greaves, Hankivsky et al., 1999) are noted. For the most part, however, biological sex remains central while gender-blindness prevails. Referring to the NIH's agenda for future research in the United States, which is embedded in a lifespan approach, Green (2002) argues that the concept of women's health put forward in the plan leaves little conceptual room for gender analysis despite the fact that social scientists have determined that the different roles and responsibilities prescribed for women and men based on cultural conventions and expectations have important health implications (Grant, 2002, p. 12).

In Canada, for example, 'women continue to experience inequalities in their lives, manifested in abuse and violence, the double day, and the gendered imbalance in status in compensation in the workplace (Williams & Garvin, 2004, p. 30). Moreover, 'gender inequalities within one life stage may influence and be predicated on gender inequalities in another' (Arber & Cooper, 1999, pp. 124–125). Gender inequalities contribute to the manifestation, severity, frequencies, and social and cultural responses to disease (Greaves & Hankvsky et al., 1999, p. 2). In particular, women and men may be differentially exposed to a variety of health risks, differentially vulnerable to aspects in their physical and social environments, and have different access to resources and support systems (Vissandjee, Desmeules, Cao, & Abdool, 2004, p. 3). Given such evidence, it is not justifiable to privilege a biomedical perspective in the framework of women's health across the lifespan, especially when such a perspective tends to marginalize the importance of gender.

Even when gender as a central organizing feature of life and society is taken into account, its meaning and significance are often misunderstood. Current accounts of gender tend to result in essentialist and deterministic ideas about women's health. For example, surveys and studies that have used a lifespan approach often observe constant gender effects on health across various age groups (Macintyre, Hunt, & Sweeting, 1996). They report numerous similarities in women's health. For instance, parallel health status gaps by income, high levels of depressive symptoms, and patterning of chronic conditions have been argued as universal concerns that cut across age groups (Wyn & Solis, 2001). Health Canada's *Women's Health Strategy* (Health Canada, 1999) states that in most age groups, women suffer more than men from chronic conditions, particularly migraines, allergies, arthritis, and rheumatism. And others have suggested that adverse physical and psychosocial environments in early life have a direct affect on diseases, disorders, and damaging health behaviour in later life stages for most if not all women (Kuh & Hardy, 2002, p. 397). Identifying similar patterns in women's health may be of some value, but on balance, this approach does not attend to differences among women in any sufficient way. The notion of gender as the most important category of women's experiences 'flattens out important differences' (Marshall, 2000, p. 47). It results in viewpoints and conclusions that 'downplay diversity among women' and ultimately fall victim to 'treating all women as biologically equivalent' (Weisman, 1997, p. 183). Thus women's health across the lifespan cannot be properly explained by appealing solely to gender in a way that results in 'categorical hegemony' (Friedman, 1995). Gender must remain an important category; however, its relationship to other categories of analysis must be acknowledged and further interrogated.

The Invisibility of Difference

Perhaps the most important shortcoming of lifespan frameworks is their failure to adequately recognize the diversity in women's lives (Johnstone, 2001, p. 4). Writing in the Canadian context, Anderson (1993) reminds us that, 'as we speak about women's health across the lifespan ... we need to be clear about who these women are, and we need to keep reminding ourselves of the diversity within this nation' (p. 1). Arguably, current issues of concern are limited and limiting because they predominantly focus on age, sex, and sometimes gender, albeit inadequately conceptualized. Allowing these factors to dominate masks the operation and interdependence of other categories of experience. As Greaves, Hankivsky, et al. (1999) have noted, 'Our gendered experiences of health, illness, and health care are a complex blend of our maleness or femaleness mixed in with our cultural identity and social and generational locations' (p. 2). What is needed is a conceptual shift in which age, sex, and gender are analysed as 'inextricably imbricated' with 'race'/ethnicity, class, nationality, religion, ability, sexuality, and power (Eckman, 1998, p. 135).

For any lifespan framework to be inclusive, it is essential that the diversity and variation within age cohorts be made front and centre. Indeed, while biological explanations need to be enjoined by social explanations of gendered health disparities, it cannot be assumed that all women will experience similar patterns of health over the lifetime. There is a need to interpret age and developmental considerations in a way that is meaningful for the diverse situations of women. This necessitates investigating how women of different backgrounds with different life opportunities and experiences may have unique risks, health conditions, and health outcomes. Just as women's health researchers have shed light on the differences in health status between women and men, it is equally important to acknowledge that there are both similarities *and* crucial differences in experiences of health among women based on numerous social divisions (Jones & Rothney, 2001, p. 6). As Bierman (2003) explains, 'Huge inequalities in health and health status among women by socioeconomic status, race/ethnicity, and geography persist' (p. 201).

For example, some groups of women – those belonging to the middle and upper classes – typically enjoy health advantages over those who are poor, unemployed, precariously employed, or suffering from various forms of discrimination such as racism and homophobia (Kaufert, 1996). In the United States, health disparities among African American, Hispanic, and Asian American Women in comparison to white women have been established (United States Department of Health and Human Services, 2000; ORWH, 1999). For instance, African American women in general live five years less than white women (Arias, 2002). Not surprisingly, it has been argued that in the United States, 'issues of inequality in health care are often related more to race/ethnicity and socioeconomic status than to gender' (Collins et al., 1997, p. 21). That said, significant gaps remain as to what is known about women who are marginalized. For example, little is known about lesbian health in midlife and old age (Appleby & Anastas, 1998).

In Canada, the approach to understanding differences among women differs but is nonetheless in nascent stages of development. For instance, the life expectancy of Aboriginal women is less than 77 (as compared to over 81 for the general Canadian female population). As mentioned earlier, Aboriginal women have higher instances of diabetes. They die more often as a result of violence and have higher rates of smoking, disability, and suicide (Donner, 2000; Janzen, 1998). Although 'the reasons for this difference is "unquestionably complex," it is known that their socio-economic marginalization, along with the poor health status, poverty, violence, substance abuse, and lack of adequate child care help to skew the end results' (Stout, Kipling, & Stout, 2001, p. 12). And yet, these multiple burdens have not been adequately examined. Organizing frameworks, including lifespan frameworks, have not been 'respectful of Aboriginal women's multiple burdens,' their 'linguistic and cultural diversity,' (pp. 2–4) or the cumulative effects of colonialism over the course of their lives. This gap, together with the current trend towards population diversification in Canada, including predictions that one in five Canadians will belong to a visible minority group by 2017 (Statistics Canada, 2005), necessitates a substantial reframing and broadening of women's lifespans in health-focused frameworks.

Intersectionality as an Explanatory Resource

As described in the Introduction, this collection, an important resource for health researchers interested in developing lifespan frameworks that integrate knowledge of multiple dimensions of oppression and which make diversity their cornerstone is the growing body of litera- ture by feminists and other critical thinkers around the idea of 'inter- sectionality' (e.g., Anthias, 2002; Collins, 2000; Bannerji, 1995; Brewer, 1993; Crenshaw, 1991; hooks, 1984). Emerging from Black, Third-World feminism, queer and postcolonial theory, intersectionality – as pre- sented in the Introduction, this collection, utilizes interactive analyses of several categories of experience and their operation in specific cul- tural and social contexts to understand and tackle women's subordina- tion in all its forms (Oxman-Martinez & Hanley, 2005). In other words, this analysis moves beyond single or dual categories of analysis (e.g. gender or gender/'race') to ask questions about 'deprivation, privilege, discrimination, and aspirations, to permit characterizing people more fully, and as more than the sum or product of their parts' (Zierler & Krieger, 1995, p. 253). Weber and Parra-Medina (2003, p. 184) provide an excellent synthesis of the broad questions that drive an intersectional analysis. These are:

1 What is the meaning of race, ethnicity, class, sexuality, and other systems of inequality across the ideological, political, and economic domains of society in institutional structures and individual lives?
2 How are these co-constructed systems of inequality simultaneously produced, reinforced, resisted, and transformed – over time, in different locations, and in different institutional domains (e.g., health, education, economy, religion, polity, family)?
3 How can our understanding of the intersecting dynamics of these systems guide us in the pursuit of social justice?

This approach has inspired the development of new conceptual frame- works and methodologies to understand the implications of diversity and the construction of power and privilege, including intersecting domains of inclusion, exclusion and inequality (Shookner & Chin-Yee, 2003).

Examinations of how intersections of gender, 'race'/ethnicity, class, and other axes of difference, including but not limited to age, sexuality, disability, immigration, and religion, effect women's health are in their nascent stages of development. Moreover, there is little empirical work that examines intersectional differences between multiple social categories, and models that move beyond the notion of a 'generic' woman that are able to measure and simultaneously investigate multiple intersectionalities are only beginning to be developed (Carter, Sellers, & Squires, 2002, p. 112). Nevertheless, the important, albeit largely theoretical work to date (e.g., Krieger et al., 1993; Ruzek, Oleson, & Clarke, 1997; Zambrana, 2001) has 'problematized and sought to revision women's health in a more complex and inclusive way by taking seriously the intersectional processes that co-construct inequality and women's health' (Weber & Parra-Medina, 2003, p. 185).

The current challenge is how to translate conceptual approaches to intersectionality to inform the practical requirements of lifespan frameworks. New methodologies that are able to capture and address the problems of intersectional discrimination are necessary. To begin with, as Allen and Phillips (1997) have suggested, 'Given the heterogeneity among women, future research [in terms of lifespan issues] endeavors must use samples of women representative of the various cultural, ethnic and socioeconomic backgrounds' (p. 34). One possible practice to draw upon is the lifecycle framework used by Women's Health Victoria, in Australia. The framework includes subsections within each life-cycle stage that 'allow for the organization of diverse data on a range of health issues and for a range of different population groups' (Johnstone, 2001, p. 6). These include socio-economic correlates and indicators, women in rural and remote regions, indigenous women, women from culturally and linguistically diverse backgrounds, pregnancy and childbirth, sexual and reproductive health, sexuality, mental and emotional health, physical health, disability and chronic illness, violence against women, behaviours adversely affecting health, and caring responsibilities.

Intersectional lifespan frameworks also require determining which factors should be included in the analysis and how multiple factors can be examined to capture the interactive complexity of different experiences (Carter, Sellers, & Squires, 2002, pp. 112, 118). In so doing, researchers must resist using white women as a reference group against which all other women are measured (Weber & Parra-Medina, 2003, p. 196). In addition, using such an approach also forces us to deal with certain tensions, including the fact that most individuals occupy both dominant and subordinate positions at the same time (p. 204). And, as much as we want to avoid essentialist assumptions about gender, the same extends to other categories as well. Not only are between-group differences important, within-group differences, including 'dominant and subordinate groupings and categories' (Anthias, 2002), must also be attended to so that various categories of analysis are not overly simplified and homogenized.

Finally, any framework committed to understanding and addressing issues of diversity would also recognize 'the validity of women's life experiences and women's own beliefs about and experiences of health' (Phillips, 2002, p. S22). Lived experiences should inform the generation of knowledge used in lifespan approaches. Women who are at the intersection of multiple systems of inequality are, after all, in a unique position from which to understand systems of oppression, and the meaning and interpretations of different social categories (Collins, 2000). Their insights can be derived from a variety of methodologies, including mixed-method and qualitative research that incorporates humanistic and social science techniques and collects data using approaches such as open-ended interviews, participant observation, and life histories (Kertzer, 1991; Weber & Parra-Medina, 2003). To be consistent with an intersectional paradigm, research must do more than further knowledge; it must also lead to social changes in women's health.

Conclusion

In conclusion, a lifespan approach offers a conceptual framework for organizing the study of health and for developing policy interventions that are intended to be responsive to women's health needs at each life stage. Being able to understand how women's lives are 'formed in and by a rapidly changing world' (Elder & O'Rand, 1995, p. 469), to identify themes in each life stage, as well as to recognize issues that may affect all ages, is important. To be effective, however, any lifespan framework must synthesize the insights about women's lives to create some sense of 'whole knowledge' about the complexities of women's health. Whole knowledge, however, cannot be realized within current frameworks that are dominated by biomedical perspectives or by approaches that have attempted to simply modify or build upon these perspectives.

Understanding women's health across the lifespan requires more than an age and biological focus, which reflects 'mechanistic views of the body, health and illness' (Inhorn & Whittle, 2001b, p. 150). An interdisciplinary approach, which enables dialogue between biomedical and social scientists, is necessary (Bird & Rieker, 2004). While researchers from both biomedical and social determinant paradigms have noted the importance of a life course perspective, there is much work left for there to be a convergence of these often competing streams of research. What is especially absent is the prioritization and critical understanding of health determinants, gender, and issues of diversity. In particular, drawing on the growing body of literature on intersectionality can provide a way to break new ground regarding the complexities and differences in women's lives and their experiences of health.

While an intersectional analysis holds promise, its application to health is only starting to be explored, and its application to lifespan framing remains largely uninvestigated. More sustained and sophisticated work therefore will be needed to understand the interactions between age, sex, health determinants, gender, and other social axes of discrimination and disadvantage within a lifespan framework However, unless the multiplicity of interactions are successfully incorporated and a broader perspective is taken on how to understand the diversity of women's health, we will not succeed in knowing how to develop effective interventions, when they should be introduced, and for whom they may be most useful.

NOTE

1 This approach concerns itself with the entire population or large subgroups and rests on a body of research demonstrating that a combination of personal, social, and economic factors, in addition to health services, plays an important role in achieving and maintaining health.

REFERENCES

Aboriginal Women's Health and Healing Research Group. (2005, Fall). Canada needs a Health and Healing Strategy for First Nations, Inuit, and Métis women. *Canadian Women's Health Network Magazine, 8*(1/2), 15.

Alexander, L.L., Larosa, J.H., & Bader, H. (2001). *New Dimensions in Women's Health*, 2nd ed. Sudburg, MA: Jones & Bartlett.

Allen, K.M., & Phillips, J.M. (1997). *Women's Health Across the Lifespan: A Comprehensive Perspective.* Philadelphia: Lippincott.

Anderson, J.M. (1993). Reflections on women's health in a pluralistic society. Paper presented at Women's Health Across the Lifespan Conference, 16–8 October 1992. University of British Columbia Centre for Research in Women's Studies and Gender Relations, Vancouver.

Anthias, F. (2002). Beyond feminism and multiculturalism: Locating difference and the politics of location. *Women's Health International Forum, 25*(3), 275–286.

Appleby, G.A., & Anastas, J.W. (1998). *Not Just a Passing Phase: Social Work with Gay, Lesbian, and Bisexual People.* New York: Columbia University Press.

Arber, S., & Cooper, H. (1999). Gender and inequalities in health across the lifecourse. In E. Annandale & K. Hunt (Eds.), *Gender Inequalities in Health* (pp. 123–149). Buckingham, UK: Open University Press.

Arias, E. (2002). United States life tables 2002. *National Vital Statistics Reports, 51* (3), 1–39.

Armstrong, P., Amaratunga, C., Bernier, J., Grant, K., Pederson, A., & Willson K. (Eds.). (2001). *Exposing Privatization: Women and Health Care Reform in Canada.* Health Care in Canada Series. Aurora, ON: Garamond Press.

Bannerji, H. (1995). *Thinking Through: Essays on Feminism, Marxism, and Anti-Racism.* Toronto: Women's Press.

Benoit, C. & Shumka, L. (2007). *Gendering the Population Health Perspective: Fundamental Determinants of Women's Health.* Final Report prepared for the Women's Health Research Network, a Population Health Network Funded by the Michael Smith Foundation for Health Research.

Bierman, A. (2003). Climbing out of our boxes: Advancing women's health for the 21st century. *Women's Health Issues, 13* (6), 201–203.

Bird, C.E., & Rieker, P.P. (2002). Integrating social and biological research to improve men's and women's health. *Women's Health Issues, 12*(3), 113–115.

Bird, C.E., & Rieker, P.P. (2004). Rethinking gender differences in health: What is needed to integrate social and biological perspectives? Paper presented at Health Inequalities Across the Life Course Conference, State College Pennsylvania, 6–7 June.

Bobet, E. (1997). *Diabetes among First Nations People: Information from the 1991 Aboriginal Peoples Survey Carried Out by Statistics Canada.* Ottawa: Medical Services Branch, Health Canada.

Bonita, R. (1996). *Women, Aging and Health: Achieving Health Across the Lifespan*. Geneva: World Health Organization.

Brewer, R. (1993) Theorizing race, class and gender: The new scholarship of Black feminist intellectuals and Black women's labour. In S.M. James & A. Buisa (Eds.), *Theorizing Black Feminisms: The Visionary Pragmatism of Black Women* (pp. 13–30). London and New York: Routledge.

Carter, P., Sellers, S.L., and Squires, C. (2002). Reflections on race/ethnicity, class, and gender inclusive research. *African American Perspectives, 8*(1): 111–124.

Collins, K.S., Bussell, M.E., & Wenzel, S. (1997). *The Health of Women in the United States: Gender Differences and Gender-Specific Conditions*. Commonwealth Commission on Women's Health. New York: Columbia University Press.

Collins P.H. (2000). *Black Feminist Thought: Knowledge, Consciousness and the Politics of Empowerment*. 2nd ed. New York: Routledge.

Correa-de-Araujo, R. (2004). A wake-up call to advance women's health. *Women's Health Issues, 14*(2), 31–34.

Crenshaw Williams, K. (1991). Mapping the margins: Intersectionality, identity politics, and violence against women of color. *Stanford Law Review, 43*(6): 1241–1299.

Donner, L. (2000). *Women, Poverty and Health in Manitoba: An Overview and Ideas for Action*. Prepared for Women's Health Clinic, Winnipeg, MB.

Doyal, L. (1995). *What Makes Women Sick: Gender and the Political Economy of Health*. London: Macmillan.

Eckman, A.K. (1998). Beyond 'the Yentl Syndrome': Making women visible in post-1990s women's health discourse. In P.A. Triecker, L. Cartwright, & P. Penley (Eds.), *The Visible Woman: Imaging Technologies, Gender and Science* (pp. 131–158). New York: New York University Press.

Elder, G.H., & O'Rand, A. (1995). Adult lives in a changing society. In K.S. Cook, G.A. Fine, & J.S. House (Eds.), *Sociological Perspectives on Social Psychology* (pp. 452–475). Needham Heights, MA: Allyn & Bacon.

Friedman, S.S. (1995). Beyond white and other: Relationality and narratives of race in feminist discourse. *Signs, 21*(1), 1–49.

Graham, H. (2002). Building and interdisciplinary science of health inequalities: The example of lifecourse research. *Social Science & Medicine, 55*(11), 2005–2016.

Grant, K. (2002). GBA: Beyond the Red Queen Syndrome. Presentation at the GBA Fair. Ottawa: Congress Centre. 31 January 2002.

Greaves, L., Hankivsky, O., Amaratunga, C., Ballem, P., Chow, D., De

Koninck, M., Grant, K., Lippman, A., Maclean, H., Maher, J., Messing, K., & Vissandjee, B. (1999). *CIHR 2000: Sex, Gender and Women's Health*. Vancouver: British Columbia Centre of Excellence for Women's Health.

Green, M. (2002). *Defining Women's Health: An Interdisciplinary Dialogue*. Background draft. Retrieved 15 April 2002, from http://www.fas.harvard.edu/womenstudy/events/proposal.htm.

Haraway, D. (1989). *Primate Visions: Gender, Race, and Nature in the World of Modern Science*. New York: Routledge.

Health Canada. (1999). *Health Canada's Women's Health Strategy*. Ottawa: Minister of Public Works and Government Services Canada

Health Canada. (2000). *Diabetes Among Aboriginal (First Nations, Inuit and Métis) People in Canada: The Evidence*. 10 March 2000.

Health Canada. (2003). *Women's Health Surveillance Report: A Multi-dimensional Look at the Health of Canadian Women*. Ottawa: Canadian Population Health Initiative, Canadian Institute for Health Information.

Healy, B. (1991).The Yentl Syndrome. *New England Journal of Medicine, 325*, 274–276.

hooks, b. (1984). *Feminist Theory: From Margin to Centre*. Boston: South End Press.

House, J., Kessler, R., Herzog, R., Mero, R., Kinney, A., & Breslow, M. (1990). Age, socio-economic status and health. *Millbank Quarterly, 68*, 383–411.

Inhorn, M., & Whittle, L.K. (2001a). Feminism meets the 'new' epidemiologies: Toward an appraisal of antifeminist biases in epidemiological research on women's health. *Social Science & Medicine, 53*, 553–567.

Inhorn, M., & Whittle, L. (2001b). Rethinking difference: A feminist reframing of gender/race/class for the improvement of women's health research. *Social Construction of Health and Disease, 3*(1), 147–165.

Institute of Medicine. (2001). *Exploring the Biomedical Contributions to Human Health: Does Sex Matter?* Washington, DC: National Academy Press.

Janzen, B.L. (1998). *Women, Gender and Health: A Review of the Recent Literature*. Saskatoon, SK: Prairie Women's Health Centre of Excellence.

Johnstone, K. (2001). A life cycle approach to Women's health data collection: Development and application. Paper presented at the 4th Australian Women's Health Conference, 19–21 February.

Jones, E., & Rothney, A. (2001). *Women's Health and Social Inequality*. Ottawa: Canadian Centre for Policy Alternatives.

Jones, J.F., & Kumssa, A. (2000). *The Cost of Reform: The Social Aspect of Transitional Economies*. New York: Nova Science.

Kaplan, H.B. (1996). *Psychosocial Stress: Perspectives on Structure, Theory, Life-Course, and Methods*. San Diego, CA: Academic Press.

Kaufert, P. (1996). Gender as a determinant of health: A Canadian perspective. Paper commissioned for the Canada-USA Women's Health Forum, 8–10 August. Ottawa.

Kertzer, D. (1991). Household and gender in a life-course perspective. In E. Masini & S. Stratigos (Eds.), *Women, Households and Change*. Tokyo: United Nations University Press. Retrieved 18 August 2004, from http://www .unu.edu/unupress/unupbooks/uu10we/uu10we00.htm#Contents.

Krieger, N., Rowley, D., Herman, A.A., Avery B., & Phillips, M.T. (1993). Racism, sexism, and social class: Implications for studies of health, disease and well-being. In D. Rowler & H. Tosteson (Eds.), Racial differences in preterm delivery: Developing a New research paradigm. *American Journal of Preventative Medicine, 6* (Suppl. 9), 82–122.

Kuh, D., & Hardy, R. (2002). *A Life Course Approach to Women's Health*. Oxford: Oxford University Press.

Kuhlmann, E., & Babitsch, B. (2002). Bodies, health, gender – Bridging feminist theories and women's health. *Women's Studies International Forum, 25*(4), 433–442.

Lock, M. (1998). Anomalous women and political strategies for aging societies. In S. Sherwin (Ed.), *The Politics of Women's Health: Exploring Agency and Autonomy* (pp.178–204). Philadelphia: Temple University Press.

Macintrye, S., Hunt, K., & Sweeting, H. (1996). Gender differences in health: Are things really as simple as they seem? *Social Science & Medicine, 48,* 49–60.

Marmot. M., & Wilkinson, R. (Eds.). (2003). Social determinants of health: The solid facts. 2nd ed. WHO 2003. Retrieved 28 August 2004, from www.who .dk/document/e59555.pdf.

Marshall, B. L. (2000). *Configuring Gender: Explorations in Theory and Politics.* Peterborough, ON: Broadview Press.

McDonough, P., & Walters, V. (2001). Gender and health: Reassessing patterns and explanations. *Social Science & Medicine, 52*(4), 547–559.

Mishra, G., Ball, D.K., Dobson, A.J., & Byles, J.E. (2004). Do socioeconomic gradients in women's health widen over time and with age? *Social Science & Medicine, 58*(9), 1585–1595.

Moen, P., Dempster-Mclain, D., & Williams, R.M. (1992). Successful aging: A life-course perspective on women's multiple roles and health. *American Journal of Sociology, 97*(6), 1612–1638.

Morrow, M., Hankivsky, O., & Varcoe, C. (2004). Women and violence: The effects of dismantling the welfare state. *Critical Social Policy, 24*(3), 358–384.

National Institutes of Health. (1992). Women's health over the lifecourse: Social and behavioural Aspects. *NIH Guide, 21*(34).

Office of Research on Women's Health. (1999). *Agenda for Research on Women's Health for the 21st Century: New Frontiers in Women's Health.* Vol. 7. Bethesda, MD: ORWH.

Office of Research on Women's Health. (2004). *FY 2004 NIH Research Priorities for Women's Health.* Bethesda, MD: ORWH. Retrieved 20 July 2004, from http://www4.od.nih.gov/orwh/2004ResearchPriorities.pdf.

Oxman-Martinez, J., & Hanley, J. (2005). Health and social services for Canada's multicultural population: Challenges for equity. Canada 2017: Policy Forum. Retrieved 5 April 2005, from http://www.pch.gc.ca/multi/canada2017/4_e.cfm.

Phillips, S. (2002). Evaluating women's health and gender. *American Journal of Obstetrics and Gynecology, 187,* S22–4.

Pinn, V.W. (2003). Sex and gender factors in medical studies. *Journal of the American Medical Association, 289*(4), 397–400.

Prus, S.G. (2003). A life course perspective on the relationship between socio-economic status and health: Testing the divergence hypothesis. SEDAP Research Paper No. 91. Hamilton, ON: McMaster University.

Riley, M., & Bond, K. (1983). Beyond ageism: Postponing the onset of disability. In M. Riley, B.B. Hess, & K. Bond (Eds.), *Aging in Society: Selected Review of Recent Research* (pp. 243–252). Hillsdale, NJ: Erlbaum.

Ruzek, S., & Olesen, V., & Clarke, A. (Eds.) (1997). *Women's Health: Complexities and Differences.* Columbus: Ohio State University Press.

Shookner, M., & Chin-Yee, F. (2003, June). An inclusion lens: Looking at social and economic exclusion and inclusion. Paper presented at the Canadian Social Welfare Policy Conference, Ottawa. Retrieved 23 November 2004, from http://ccsd.ca/cswp/2003/papers/abstracts/shookner-chin-yee.htm.

Smedley, B.D., & Symes, S.L. (2000). *Promoting Health: Intervention Strategies from Social and Behavioural Research.* Institute of Medicine Report. Washington, DC: National Academy Press.

Smith, G.D. (2003). *Health Inequalities: Lifecourse Approaches.* Bristol, UK: Polity Press.

Standing Committee on Status of Women. (2005, April). *Gender-Based Analysis: Building Blocks for Success.* Report of the Standing Committee on Status of Women, Anita Neville, MP chair. Retrieved 15 June 2005, from http://www.parl.gc.ca.

Statistics Canada. (2001). *How Healthy Are Canadians?* 2001 annual report. Ottawa: Minister of Industry.

Statistics Canada. (2005). Study: Canada's visible minority population in 2017.

The Daily. Retrieved 22 March 2005, from http://www.statcan.ca/Daily/ English/050322/d050322b.htm.

Stout, M.D., Kipling, G.D., & Stout, R. (2001, May). Aboriginal Women's Health Research Synthesis Paper: Final Report. Prepared for the Centres of Excellence for Women's Health Research Synthesis Group.

Strobino, D., Grason, H., & Minkovitz, C. (2002). Charting a course for the future of women's health in the United States: Concepts, findings and recommendations. *Social Science & Medicine, 54,* 839–848.

Thompson-Reid, P., Beckles, G., & Jones, W. (2001). *Diabetes and Women's Health Across the Life Stages: A Public Health Perspective.* Atlanta, GA: Department of Health and Human Services, Centers for Disease Control and Prevention, National Center for Chronic Disease Prevention and Health Promotion, Division of Diabetes Translation.

United Nations Fourth World Conference on Women. (1995). *Platform for Action.* Section C. New York: United Nations.

United States Department of Health and Human Services. (2000). *Healthy People 2010.* Washington, DC: U.S. Department of Health and Human Services.

Vissandjee, B., Desmeules, M., Cao, Z., & Abdool, S. (2004). 'Integrating socioeconomic determinants of Canadian women's health. *BMC Women's Health, 4* (Suppl. 1), S34.

Wamala, S.P., Lynch, J., & Kaplan, G.A. (2001). Women's exposure to early and later life socioeconomic disadvantage and coronary heart disease risk: The Stockholm female coronary risk study. *International Journal of Epidemiology, 30,* 275–284.

Weber, L., & Parra-Medina, D. (2003). Intersectionality and women's health: Charting a path to eliminating health disparities. In M. Texler Segal, V. Demos, & J. Kronenfeld (Eds.), *Gender Perspectives on Health and Medicine: Key Themes.* Oxford: Elsevier.

Weisman, C.S. (1997). Changing definitions of women's health: Implications for health care and policy. *Maternal and Child Health Journal, 1*(3), 179–189.

Williams, A., & Garvin, T. (2004). Taking stock: Geographic perspectives on women and health in Canada. *The Canadian Geographer, 48*(1), 29–34.

Wizemann, T.M., & Pardue, M.L. (2001). *Exploring the Biological Contributions to Human Health: Does Sex Matter?* Washington, DC: National Academy Press.

World Health Organization. (1996). Global commission on women's health to promote 'Health Security Throughout the Lifespan.' Press release 32. WHO/32. 22 April. Retrieved 18 June 2004, from http://www.who.int/ archives/inf-pr-1996/pr96-32.html.

Wyn, R., & Solis, B. (2001). Women's health issues across the lifespan. *Women's Health Issues, 11* (3), 148–159.

Zambrana, R.E. (2001). Improving access and quality for ethnic minority women: Panel discussion. *Women's Health Issues, 11*(40), 354–359.

Zierler, S., & N. Krieger, N. (1995). Accounting for the health of women. *Current Issues in Public Health, 1*: 251–256.

PART TWO

Theory and Methods

3 Feminist Methodology and Health Research: Bridging Trends and Debates

MARINA MORROW AND OLENA HANKIVSKY

In this chapter, we bridge recent trends and debates within feminist methodology and link these to women's health research. Attention is paid to the challenges of operationalizing critical feminist perspectives and methodologies, especially as these relate to understanding the lives of women marginalized through relations of gender, race, class, and other forms of social difference. Within this context we discuss self-reflexivity in relation to power differentials between researchers and those whom they research. Specifically, the challenges of bringing inter-sectional analyses to research are explored. In so doing, the interplay between theory and research is brought to the fore and the potential for interdisciplinary research, and the use of a variety of methods to improve our understanding of women's health is interrogated.

It is generally understood that there is a need for more research to strengthen, develop, and increase the understanding of diseases and health conditions that affect women. Further, research that analyses health care systems' responses to women, the social determinants of women's health, and women's experiences and relationships to their own health and the health of their communities are also seen as critical. It is recognized by many health researchers that approaches that combine both biomedical and social science perspectives are required in investigations of women's health. In particular, there is growing concern about expanding the understanding of health disparities between women and men and among different groups of women. Less attention, however, has been paid to the various dimensions of research – from knowledge creation, defining research agendas, choosing methodological approaches, facilitating the involvement of research participants, social action, and linking research with policy. Epistemological and methodological issues regarding 'how to understand the intersectionality of race, class, gender, and other structural features of societies; about inappropriate essentializing of women and men; about phenomena that are both socially constructed and fully 'real'; and about the apparent impossibility of accurate interpretation, translation, and representation among radically different cultures' (Harding & Norberg, 2005, p. 2011) are relevant and increasingly pressing across all fields, including health research.

Creating Knowledge

In view of the historical fact that women were systematically excluded from scientific inquiry as 'knowers' and that the paradigms guiding scientific endeavors were androcentric and ethnocentric, the feminist challenge to Western sciences initially took on two interconnected projects: that of recovering women as agents/producers of knowledge and that of challenging the sexism and racism inherent in scientific studies.[1] This has been particularly critical in the male-dominated research fields of medical science and psychiatry but is also relevant across the health sciences disciplines. Feminist inquiries thus have raised fundamental challenges to the paradigms of science and in so doing have made critical contributions to our understanding of ontology and epistemology. According to Harding and Norberg (2005), 'In challenging conventional epistemologies and their methodologies, both of which justified problematic understandings of research methods, feminists have contributed to the epistemological crisis of the modern West, or North' (p. 2010).

The critique of the Western epistemological project as androcentic (e.g., reason as masculine) led to claims about the epistemological significance of the knower (e.g., Harding, 1987a; Bordo, 1987; Code, 2000; Stanley & Wise, 1993). From this, feminists put forth the importance of positionality and self-reflexivity in the act of knowledge production (Hallam & Marshall, 1993). That is, rather than aspiring to produce universalizing truths that apply to all women, they argue that personal biographical factors and social context play an important role in the production of knowledge. Self-reflexivity, meaning self-examination of one's biases and assumptions, is thus seen as foundational to multivocal feminist knowledge production. Further, some feminists have made claims about the 'epistemic' privilege of knowledge that comes from groups marginalized in society (Collins, 1991; hooks, 1984).

Epistemology, as a theory of knowledge, is the foundation for methodology and methods. Following in the Kuhnian[2] tradition, feminists make the point that science is a social process. Foundational to this are challenges to the notion of scientific objectivity and attempts to illustrate the ways in which science is socially and historically located and therefore influenced by social relations of power, politics, and the social and cultural mores of the day. Feminists especially have challenged the artificial split between objective and subjective knowledge that is central to scientific paradigms. Much of the early feminist critique argued that 'objectivity' is an inherently masculine construct. In such a paradigm, facts speak for themselves and the social, moral, and political implications and consequences upon which these facts rest are suppressed. The goal was thus to expose the 'lie' of objectivity and to call attention to the ways in which social bias made itself into research at every stage of the research endeavor (e.g., Harding, 1987b). Contemporary feminist debates focus on the ways in which objectivity and subjectivity are inextricably linked and on finding ways to 'resuscitate' or 'save' objectivity in order to strengthen knowledge claims and make them relevant to broad constituencies (Scheman, 2001). Harding (1991) refers to this scientific goal as 'strong objectivity.' Haraway (1988) uses the concept 'situated knowledges,' and discusses the importance of researchers striving to 'see well' (objectively), while acknowledging that everyone does not see things in precisely the same way.

Feminist Methodology

According to Fonow and Cook (2005), ' feminist methodology involves the description, explanation, and justification of techniques used in feminist research and is an abstract classification that refers to a variety of methodological stances, conceptual approaches, and research strategies' (p. 2213).

Despite a convergence with respect to critiquing traditional paradigms in research, feminists have argued that there is no distinctively feminist approach to methodology (Harding, 1987c) and thus no ontological or epistemological position that is distinctly feminist. That is, 'feminist researchers do not consider feminism to be a method. Rather they consider it to be a perspective on an existing method in a given field of inquiry or a perspective that can be used to develop an innovative method' (Reinharz, 1992, p. 241). Indeed, there are methodological disputes within feminism that stem from the differences within feminist theory and activism. These differences have been categorized in a number of different ways. For example, Harding (1987c) used the following taxonomy for describing differences in feminist research:

Feminist Empiricism:

- Feminists who adhere to some of the tenants of empiricism. For example, knowledge as *found* not *made*, 'knowers' as separate and interchangeable, and bias as an aberration that can be eradicated. Some, like Helen Longino (1990) suggest a 'contextual empiricism' which recognizes the influence of social values in science and results in a 'softening' of the empirical stance.

Feminist Standpoint Theories:

- Feminists who argue that empiricism cannot offer a radical enough analysis of the historical-material circumstances that produce both subjectivities and knowledge. Standpoint theorists honour the material, domestic, and emotional labour of women and see these as practices that are constitutive of knowledge and subjectivity. While empiricists see the knower as a separate individual (or communities of individuals), standpoint theorists see subjectivities as socially produced within power-saturated structures of dominance.

Feminist Postmodernism:

- Feminist postmodernists contest the 'enlightenment ideal project' and the apparently apolitical aims of modernity. Postmodernists refuse any one theoretical stance and assert that the multiplicity of knowledge-making practices do not result in a universal meta-narrative. Interactions with reality are mediated by conceptual frameworks or discourses, which are historically and socially situated.

To Harding's taxonomy we would add *Feminist Postcolonial Theory* (see Chapter 4, by Brown, Smye, and Varcoe, this collection), which sees colonialism and imperialism as critical and necessary axes of analysis when theorizing about women's lives and experiences. Additionally, the categories in this taxonomy should not be seen as mutually exclusive; that is, any one feminist research project may encompass more than one type of research approach.

Thus, even within feminism, there is no agreement regarding 'the meaning and consequences of experience, justice, power, relationships, differences and morality' (Ramazanoğlu & Holland, 2002, p. 3). Further, the reliance on the undifferentiated category of 'woman' has been challenged by postmodernism and poststructuralist thought and also through the contributions of postcolonial feminist researchers. Diverse perspectives also result in the variety of ways that feminist researchers develop questions and collect and analyse data (Naples, 2003). Feminist methodologists continue to engage in debates about the nature of science, truth, epistemology, and details of fieldwork and research practices (Cook & Fonow, 1990; Fonow & Cook, 2005; Harding & Norberg, 2005).

At the same time there are converging areas of concern. Olesen (2003) asserts: 'Without in any way positing a global, homogeneous, unified feminism, qualitative feminist research in its many variants, whether or not self-consciously defined as feminist, centers and makes problematic women's diverse situations as well as the institutions that frame those situations' (p. 333). Rienharz (1992, p. 240) also identifies a number of defining features of feminist research, including:

- It strives to represent human diversity;
- It aims to create change;
- It involves ongoing criticism of non-feminist scholarship; and,
- It frequently attempts to develop special relations with the people studied (in interactive research).

The interconnected nature of ontology (theories of being), epistemology (broadly, the study of knowledge), methodology (the theory and analysis behind research), and methods (the techniques for gathering data) are key for feminist researchers. Thus, one of their central challenges is to bear these interconnections in mind when they are defining research agendas that are able to elucidate the social context of women's lives and attend to differences among groups of women. In so doing, there are many available approaches and methods, all of which have the potential to help feminists design women's health research. The key to optimizing the potential of approaches and methods is to understand their strengths and limitations and to determine how they can contribute to the development of an adequate knowledge base for meeting women's health needs. Of course, this can be understood as the key challenge of feminist methodology more generally. As Ramazanoğlu and Holland (2002) explain, 'Any researcher who sets out to understand gender relations and grasp their impact on people's lives has to consider: how (or whether) social reality can be understood; why conceptions of sexuality and gender have some meanings rather than others; how people make sense of their experiences; and how power inhabits knowledge production' (p. 2).

Women's Health Research

Contemporarily, feminist researchers have translated their philosophical concerns into concrete applications for the study of women's health. In Canada, the need to improve health research gained significant momentum with the release of the Medical Research Council of Canada's report on women's health research issues in 1994. Among its many recommendations, the report emphasized the need to expand on traditional biomedical research approaches, support research that will attend to health differences between men and women, and eliminate barriers to women's participation in health research (Medical Research Council of Canada, 1994). Six years later, with the establishment of the Institute for Gender and Health (IGH) within the Canadian Institutes of Health Research (CIHR), these recommendations were at least partially addressed. The mandate of the IGH is 'to support research to address how sex (biological factors) and gender (socio-cultural experiences) interact with other factors that influence health and create conditions and problems that are unique, more prevalent, more serious or different with respect to risk factors or effective interventions for women and girls, men and boys.' The IGH also has provided leadership in advancing the careers of women scientists (CIHR, 2005).

The feminist research enterprise, both in Canada and elsewhere, has become increasingly complex (Olesen, 2003). In view of this, feminists have experimented with a range of methodological approaches and methods, including those that involve mixed methods and/or interdisciplinary collaborations. Concomitantly, the health field itself is continually changing and there is a greater recognition that new knowledge creation requires new conceptual frameworks and new ways of doing research (CIHR, 2004). This requires bringing together a range of issues: epistemological; ethical; and, in the language of the CIHR (2004), 'the political economy of health and cross-pillar research production'[3] (p. 19). At a national level it has also been explicitly recognized that gender, sex, and health – in all their complexity – need to be brought to the forefront of research in Canada (Spitzer, 2004, p.4). A key strategy in this regard has been gender-based analysis, which is explored by

Hankivsky in Chapter 5, this collection. An ongoing challenge is to ensure that researchers interested in sex, gender, and health adopt explicitly feminist understandings of women's health, including development of a conceptual framework that furthers the understanding of health inequalities beyond gender to capture differences among women (Ruzek, Olesen, & Clarke, 1997).

Diversity and Difference: Reconceptualizing Women's Health Research

As earlier chapters in this collection have illustrated, the need for incorporating diversity and the inequalities between women that are caused by racism, colonialism, ethnocentrism, heterosexism, and able-bodiedism has been acknowledged by feminist health researchers. However, as Catterall-Ironstone et al. (1998) acknowledge, 'recognizing the diversity of women poses special problems for women's health' (p. 16) because it challenges the singular political strategy used for generating change. Not surprisingly, the adoption of a strategy which sees gender as the primary analytic category through which to view health has meant that exclusionary practices in health research continue. It is therefore imperative to recognize that new conceptual frameworks that are being developed for researching women's health must also address and be responsive to the diversity of the lived experiences of Canadian women. As Anderson (2000) argues, 'If we are to conduct health research that is applicable to all people, then we must reframe the discourse, and strive for an inclusive scholarship' (p. 226).

Some of the first challenges to feminist research came from Black and South Asian feminists who were writing against 'imperialist' feminism (e.g., Amos & Parmar, 1984; Collins, 2004; Hill-Collins, 1991; Mohanty, 2003; Mohanty, Russo, & Torres, 1991), and, in particular, the problem of speaking for 'Third World women' (Mohanty, 1988; Spivak, 1988). From this has emerged feminist anti-racist and postcolonial research frameworks which aim to employ intersectional analyses and to 'decolonize methodologies' (Battiste & Youngblood Henderson, 2000; Sandoval, 2000; Tuhiwai Smith, 1999).

Tuhiwai Smith (1999) documents the emerging spaces for indigenous research (in the academy and in the community) and the development of a methodological approach that she calls 'Kaupapa Maori research' or 'Maori-centred research.' Her work explores the ways in which research is embedded in institutional and disciplinary structures, and how this has impacted the development of indigenous knowledge. Tuhiwai Smith has cautioned against the 'colonization of methodologies.' Using the example of the Maori people of New Zealand, she observes that traditional research strips away *mana* (our standing in our own eyes) and undermines *rangatiratanga* (an ability and right to determine destiny) (p. 173). She also observes that research often produces knowledge that does not translate into improvement in the lives of those who are the subjects and participants of research.

Similarly concerned with the plight of subordinated communities, Chela Sandoval (2000) has proposed a series of methods ranging from textual analysis, social movement, and identity creation that 'are capable of speaking to, against, and through power' (Davis, 2000, p. xii) in the context of globalization. Sandoval's methodology of emancipation includes five skills: semiotics, deconstruction, meta-ideologizing, democractics, and differential consciousness' (p. 2). These 'methods of the oppressed' are intended to provide a road map for responding to cultural conditions, and, in particular, colonialism in the postmodern world.

In the Canadian context, Dion Stout, Kipling, & Stout (2001) argue that existing health research methodologies are often inappropriate for Aboriginal women. They suggest that researching Aboriginal women's health requires working with Aboriginal women's health researchers, developing culturally appropriate methodologies, and developing a knowledge base of key Aboriginal concepts and principles that are essential to health research within these communities. It also requires a closer examination of the lived experiences of Aboriginal women (Bent, 2004 p. 64). Recently, the Saskatoon Aboriginal Women's Health Research Committee (2002) with support from Prairie Women's Health Centre of Excellence developed ethical guidelines for Aboriginal women's health research. The guidelines explicitly recognize the historically detrimental relationship between Aboriginal peoples and researchers in the research process and are intended to help with the creation of relevant and accurate research.

The challenges of recognizing diversity and working to not conceptually reproduce 'otherness' permeate both feminist theorizing and feminist research, as 'feminists are no more immune than other social researchers to arrogance, ignorance, complacency, academic insecurity, power hunger or limited capacities for self-knowledge, empathy or patient listening' (Ramazanoglu & Holland, 2002, p.109). That is why those who are affected by research must be active participants in shaping the research. This requires a form of responsiveness on the part of researchers which 'requires attending to people's articulations of who they are, what their experiences have been, what their needs are, how these needs have arisen, and how they can best be met' (Hankivsky, 2004, p. 35). As Homi Bhabha (1994) reminds us, we learn the most important lessons from those that have suffered subjugation, domination, and displacement.

Inclusive health research also requires that the voices from differing perspectives and socio-economic locations shape the 'doing' of the research, including the process of interpreting data. The aim is to use a process where research is done 'by, for and on women' (Catterall-Ironstone et al., 1998; Stivers, 1993; Harding, 1991, p. 985). As Hajdukowski-Ahmed, Denton, O'Connor, and Zetytinoglu (1999) remind us: 'Errononous knowledge with regard to women's health, knowledge that passed for science, was sustained by the silencing and ignoring of women's voices' (p. 33).

Equally important is that researchers must reflect on the power imbalances that exist between themselves and those they 'study,' especially in terms of how researchers may create a disconnect, or distance those who are researched from their experiences. It is not enough to acknowledge differences and diversity without understanding how researchers themselves are often implicated in creating relationships of injustice and harm and of creating what Spivak (1988) refers to as the 'epistemic violence' of the discourse of the 'other.' According to Tuhiwai Smith (1999, p. 176):

> When undertaking research, either across culture or within a minority culture, it is critical that researchers recognize the power dynamic which is embedded in the relationship with their subjects. Researchers are in receipt of privileged information. They may interpret it within an overt theoretical framework, but also in terms of a cover ideological framework. They have the power to distort, to make invisible, to overlook, to exaggerate and to draw conclusions, based not on factual data, but on assumptions, hidden value judgments, and often downright misunderstandings. They have a potential to extend knowledge or to perpetuate ignorance.

That said, models in health research that move beyond the 'generic' woman, that are able to consider multiple intersectionalities, and which explicitly reflect on the role of 'feminist researchers as active agents in constructing knowledge' (Fonow & Cook, 2005, p. 2219) are only start-ing to be developed (Carter, Sellers, & Squires, 2002). McCall (2005), for example, argues that 'despite the emergence of intersectionality as a major paradigm of research in women's studies and elsewhere, there has been little discussion of *how* to study intersectionality, that is, of its methodology' (p. 1771).

Without doubt, 'translating the theoretical call for studying the inter-locking systems of oppression and the intersectionality of race, class, and gender into methodological practices is not easy' (Cuádraz & Uttal, 1999, p. 158). Ultimately, intersectionality means the study of a range of complex social relations and multiple categories of analysis that are not limited to the categories above but include sexuality, ability, religion, geography, and so on (McCall, 2005). In the Canadian context, it has been recognized that there is a need for 'targeted research with and on diverse groups' (Bernard, 2002; Hankivsky, 2005; Luce, 2003), and that more funding is required to undertake such work. The goal therefore should be twofold: to develop diversity-specific research and to better integrate diversity within women's health research (Bernard, 2002). Further, and perhaps most importantly, more methodological develop-ment is needed to assist in studying intersectionality. Because women's health is so multidimensional, it is now generally understood that it requires research approaches that cross and combine disciplines, as well as innovative mixes of methodologies and methods.

Research Approaches

Feminist health researchers have been at the forefront of implementing research designs that draw on a variety of disciplines and in working with researchers from a range of traditions. Increasingly, multi-disciplinary, interdisciplinary, and transdisciplinary approaches are being favoured in general health research. Given that these terms are often used interchangeably it is important to distinguish between them.

Rosenfield's (1992) classification of research collaboration among dis-ciplines into three types is useful in this regard:

- Multidisciplinary research: in which researchers work in parallel or sequentially from a discipline-specific base to address the same problem. The risk being, of course, that one simply may redefine the problem and not make the truly innovative or paradigm-shifting approach required for its resolution.

- Interdisciplinary research: in which researchers from two or more disciplines work jointly on a particular problem and collaborate in the design of research strategies and in the analysis of outcomes. Interdisciplinary research is 'a cooperative effort by a team of investigators, each expert in the use of different methods and concepts, who have joined in an organized program to attack a challenging problem.' (Pellmar & Eisenberg, 2000, p. x)

- Transdisciplinary research: in which researchers work jointly from a shared conceptual framework that draws together discipline-specific theories, concepts, and approaches to address a particular problem. Pellmar & Eisenberg (2000, p. x) describe this as 'the development of a common conceptual framework that bridges the relevant disciplines and that can serve as a basis for generating new research questions directly related to the defined problem.' Moving beyond any parallel process, transdisciplinary research produces conceptual frameworks that transcend any one disciplinary perspective.

In general, all approaches that cross disciplines bring together, within a conceptual framework, individual disciplines to bear on research questions (Marks, 2002). A selection of appropriate research methods from a variety of disciplines is valuable in pursuing studies that involve consideration of heterogeneous populations in which sex, gender, race, class, and ethnicity influence health dimensions (Mazure, Espeland, Douglas, Champion, & Killien, 2000). And yet, what is less understood is the time required to understand and develop familiarity with other disciplines. It has been demonstrated that it takes between one and two years for groups of researchers to be able to plan interdisciplinary projects successfully (Marks, 2002).

Time and commitment aside, traditional institutional structures and funding agencies have not always been supportive of interdisciplinary research collaborations. This, however, appears to be slowly changing in the Canadian context. One of the most important developments in the Canadian health research context has been the establishment of the CIHR, the Aboriginal Health Institute, the Gender and Health Institute, and cross-institute funding initiatives. The CIHR purports to be committed to both a problem-based and multidisciplinary approach to health challenges facing Canadians. It seeks to fund research that crosses biomedical, clinical, health systems and services, and population and public health perspectives. According to the Friends of the CIHR – the FCHIR – the intent is to go beyond multidisciplinarity to inter-disciplinary, 'meaning the support and fostering of research in which investigators from various disciplines interact with each other to tackle important research questions that cannot be addressed effectively otherwise' (CIHR, 2001). Although these developments within the CIHR are welcome, it is not yet clear whether they are making a substantive impact on the way in which methodologies and health research is designed in Canada. Indeed, many health researchers con-tinue to undertake disciplinary research, which may provide impor-tant insights but does not always benefit from outside perspectives and approaches.

The challenges of operationalizing interdisciplinary, multidisciplinary, and transdisciplinary research are substantive and are tied not only to the time it takes researchers to familiarize themselves with other dis-ciplines, but also involves more comprehensive discussions about research paradigms. In the section below, we explore some of the foun-dational issues related to working across qualitative and quantitative methodologies and methods and their implications for women's health research. Although this is not the only discussion relevant to examining research approaches, it is of key concern for health researchers whose related disciplines come from both qualitative and quantitative tradi-tions.

Research Methodologies and Methods

The Qualitative/Quantitative Debate

Feminists have argued that different methods are rooted in different epistemological positions (Rose, 2001). One of the central feminist de-bates about methodology has been about the relative usefulness of both qualitative and quantitative paradigms for research. The debates range from early feminist critiques, which argued that methods are gendered and that quantitative methods, which are paradigmatically positivist, reflect 'masculine' positions and points of view (Oakley, 1998; Smith, 1974; Stanley & Wise, 1993) and are therefore inappropriate for feminist research; to discussions about the usefulness of quantitative and mixed method approaches (i.e., approaches that utilize both qualitative and quantitative methods)[4] for feminists (Jayaratne, 1983; Westmarland, 2001). While the debate continues, researchers in women's health acknowledge the need for both quantitative and qualitative methods to address the complexities of women's health (Catterall-Ironstone et al. 1998; Chesney & Ozer, 1995; McCall, 2005; Ruzek, Olesen, & Clarke, 1997).

Quantitative Research

Quantitative research uses methods adopted from approaches used in the physical sciences that draw upon logical positivism and are designed to ensure objectivity, generalizability, and reliability. The purpose of quantitative research is therefore to produce factual, unbiased, and generalizable representations of human experiences (Steckler, McLeroy, Goodman, Bird, & McCormick, 1992). Quantitative approaches to research include the random and purportedly unbiased selection of research participants and the use of standardized questionnaires and statistical methods to analyse relationships between specific variables. Researchers in this process are considered impartial and objective.

   Those who favour quantitative approaches argue that these methods produce quantifiable, reliable data that is usually generalizable to some larger population. The data produced is often effective in terms of influencing policy at all levels of government (Fonow & Cook, 2005; Oakley, 1993), especially in the areas of violence against women and child sexual abuse (Greaves, Hankivsky, & Kingston-Riechers, 1995; Hankivsky & Draker, 2003). Indeed, large-scale surveys can alter public opinion in a way that smaller-scale qualitative studies cannot (Kwan, 2001). Moreover, innovative quantitative feminist research is also transforming traditional methods by emphasizing quantification that is sensitive to a diversity of women's experiences (Hankivsky et al., 2004; Westmarland, 2001). Even though quantitative research may be well placed to capture the experiences of multiply oppressed groups, there is still a need to ensure appropriate sampling in studies concerning the general population (Weber & Parra-Medina, 2003).

   However, feminists have challenged the conception of quantitative research, especially its reliance on concepts such as objectivity. Feminists have highlighted, for example, 'the idea that quantitative data, like qualitative date, is interpreted and often manipulated by the researcher and therefore incorporates subjective acts within a supposedly pure objective analysis' (Westmarland, 2001, p. 3). The greatest weakness of the quantitative approach is that it decontextualizes human behavior in a way that removes the event from its real world setting and ignores the effects of variables that have not been included in the model. Quantitative research 'seeks the *facts* or *causes* of social phenomena with little regard for the subjective state of individuals' (Bogdan & Taylor, 1975, p. 2). Thus, the challenge to those who use quantitative research is to ensure that the research design includes an attention to contextual factors. That is, quantitative measures must be infused with qualitative understandings of the historicity and specificity of the phenomenon researched.

Qualitative Research

Qualitative research methods began to gain significant currency in the 1970s, amidst debates and criticisms of social science research which then still favored research strategies that were based on the quantitative paradigm (e.g., quasi-experimental, correlational, and survey research) (Schwandt, 2003). Qualitative inquiry 'is a "home" for a wide variety of scholars who are often seriously at odds with one another but who share a general rejection of the blend of scientism, foundationalist epistemology, instrumental reasoning, and the philosophical anthropology of disengagement that has marked "mainstream" social science' (p. 293). Historically, feminist researchers were critical of qualitative approaches that did not understand gender and other social dimensions as critical categories of analysis, and were critical of qualitative researchers who were not attentive to the social, economic, and political dimensions of power and how these are structured through relations of gender, race, class, ability, and sexual and gender identity. However, feminist researchers themselves have taken up qualitative inquiry in a range of different ways. Not all of these approaches have been successful with respect to ensuring research rigor and validity, or, indeed, with avoiding the problems related to overgeneralizing results to populations.

Three philosophies are foundational to qualitative research – interpretivism, hermeneutics, and social constructionism – and each of these philosophies determines the aims and methods of qualitative research (Schwandt, 2003). In interpretivism and hermeneutics the concern is with *verstehen*,[5] or '*understanding* human behaviour from the actor's own frame of reference' (Bogdan & Taylor, 1975, p. 2). Feminists have found the use of hermeneutics/interpretivism to be both useful and limiting – useful because it foreground women's 'lived experience,' and limiting because it does not always account for contextual and historical factors.

The concept of social constructionism holds that we are all actively engaged in creating knowledge and that 'we invent concepts, models, and schemes to make sense of experience, and we continually test and modify these constructions in the light of new experiences' (Schwandt, 2003, p. 306). Social constructionists reject the notion that knowledge is apolitical and disinterested, which is one of the reasons it is a particularly compelling philosophical framework for feminist researchers.

In general, qualitative research aims to generate rich and detailed descriptions of events and human experiences. Qualitative methods include participant observations; in-depth, unstructured interviews; and focus groups that use grounded, discovery-oriented, exploratory, descriptive, and inductive approaches. These methods are designed to help researchers understand the meanings people assign to social phenomena while striving to leave participants' perspectives intact. In the health context, qualitative research provides information regarding how people experience health and illness and the context in which people have these experiences.

It has been noted that qualitative studies, especially those that use in-depth interviews and participatory action approaches, have the potential to provide insights regarding the meanings and interpretations of different social categories of experience (e.g., 'race'/ethnicity, gender, class, sexuality) among individuals and between groups (Carter et al., 2002). And yet, the challenge remains how to 'analyze multiple dimensions of individual biography and social structures simultaneously' (Cuádraz & Uttal, 1999; Dyck, Lynam, & Anderson, 1995); that is, how to move from the macro level linking systems of oppression to the micro level of individual and group experiences (Collins, 1995).

The following chart (on page 108) appears in Damaris Rose's (2001, pp. 12–13) paper for Status of Women Canada. It is a useful comparison of qualitative and quantitative methods.

Although historically in traditional research quantitative methods were viewed as more favourable than qualitative ones, this view has changed significantly in the last number of decades (Rose, 2001). The

Quantitative Methodology	Qualitative Methodology
Searches for general laws, empirical regularities	Searches for meanings in specific social/cultural contexts; possibility of theoretical generalization
Adoption of natural science (objectivity as ideal)	Rejection of natural science (subjectivity is valued)
Try to simulate experimental situation	Natural settings
Explanation = prediction of events, behaviour, attitudes ('statistical causality')	Explanation = understanding, interpreting reasons for observable behaviour, sense given to actions ('historical causality')
Large-scale studies (extensive research); random sampling	Studies of small groups; case studies (intensive research); purposive sampling
Deduction	Induction or grounded theory
Survey instruments with predetermined response categories based on theoretical framework	Open-ended research instruments (semi-structured intensive interview, life history, focus group, observation ...) from which theoretical categories may emerge
Numbers (measurement)	Words ('thick description')

result is that many researchers now understand qualitative methods to be critical to our understanding of health. In fact, many scholars have argued that a strictly dichotomous view of quantitative versus qualitative research is inadequate, and have indicated that quantitative methods can be used in ways that are consistent with the goals and values of feminist research (Rose, 2001; Westmarland, 2001). Indeed McCall (2005) asks, 'What happens when particular methods, appropriate to the subject at hand and unlikely to change dramatically, become conflated with particular philosophies of science and potentially prevent freer flows of knowledge across disciplines and among members of the new field as a consequence?' And she argues that this 'limits knowledge in all relevant disciplines but is especially a problem for new fields like Women's Studies, which aspires to be interdisciplinary' (p. 1792).

For example, in her examination of research in the public health field Baum (1995), argues that a polarized debate between traditional epidemiological methods (i.e., those concerned with the etiology of disease) versus qualitative methods concerned with a wider range of health phenomena undermines the need for research that recognizes the complex social, economic, political, biological, and environmental causes of public health problems. She suggests, 'We should recognize the value of an enlarged tool kit so that it can expand rather than limit our understanding of the dynamic of creating and maintaining health for communities and individuals' (p. 467).

Mixed Methods

Fonow and Cook (2005) argue that 'while the gulf between qualitative and quantitative methods is still wide, it is often feminists who have sought to bridge it through their collaborative impulse, their critical stance, their search for more inclusive and nuanced ways to measure complex social phenomena, their location on the continuum of political activism, and their desire to create research that can be used to promote social change' (p. 2226). Accordingly, as feminists rethink the quantitative-qualitative divide, there is a new appreciation of mixed methods research. In fact, according to Weber and Parra-Medina (2003), 'Most feminist researchers now contend that the use of multiple methods makes for the best research' (p. 198).

Although increasingly researchers are looking to the possible benefits of mixed methods approaches for understanding multifaceted health-related phenomena, not all researchers agree that mixed methods are *the* answer to better health research. There is a contrast between researchers like Baum (2003), quoted above, and others (e.g., Carey, 1993), who understand qualitative and quantitative research as simply providing different sets of tools, and those who argue that the underlying assumptions of qualitative and quantitative research are so profoundly different that they are potentially incompatible methodologies (Sale, Lohfeld, & Brazil, 2002). In the first instance, those in support of mixed methods argue that because researchers from either paradigm share the same goals of understanding and improving people's lives, and a dedication to scientific rigour, that mixing methods can help us create better knowledge (Casebeer & Verhoef, 1997; Reichardt & Rallis, 1994). Others suggest that combining research is especially useful for understanding complex health phenomena (Baum, 1995; Clarke & Yaros, 1988; Steckler et al, 1992).

However, Sale et al. (2002) document the ways in which qualitative research is increasingly being held to the same criteria of validity as quantitative research, what they call the, 'growing trend of quantifying qualitative research' (p.50). Further, there is a fear that in the discussion of mixed methods that the philosophical distinctions between qualitative and quantitative research have been so muted that researchers are often led to believe that the differences are merely technical (Sale et al., 2002). Olson (2004), for example, argues that a focus on methods should not drive research, but rather, that a focus on the underlying ontological and epistemological assumptions is critical for guiding research.

In our view, this debate is particularly important for feminist researchers who are challenging the positivist paradigm and who are striving to redefine what counts as good research and good evidence. Thus, with these cautions in mind, we think that mixed methods can best be used for complementary purposes; that is, using the strengths of one method to enhance another (Sale et al., 2002), and that, in at least some instances, good science is characterized by methodological pluralism (Seechrest & Sidani, 1995). The key challenge is how to best combine differing methods to produce more effective knowledge. In this regard, feminists have made particular interventions into the use of mixed methods by importing their concerns with the relations of gender, race, and class, and contextual issues (see Figure 3.1).

The importance of being aware of the range of methodological approaches and tools that are available to analysts and the particular challenges for feminist health researchers are made clear by looking at the following case study on eating disorders.

Eating Disorders

It is generally accepted that eating disorders constitute a wide range of behaviours related to disturbances in eating and that they also include preoccupation with weight and shape (Gucciardi, Celasun, & Ahmad 2003; Health Canada, 2002, 2003; Monro & Huon, 2005; Steiger & Séguin, 1999). Eating disorders are generally classified as anorexia nervosa (inability to maintain a minimally normal body weight), bulimia nervosa

Figure 3.1: Qualitative methods are used to help develop quantative measures and instruments

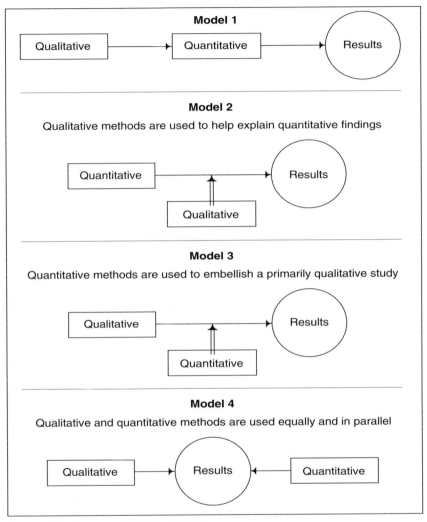

Source: Steckler et al. (1992, pp. 1–8).

(a combination of binge eating and the use of methods to prevent weight gain such as induced vomiting), and binge eating disorder (binge eating that does not include methods to prevent weight gain). Feminist researchers have also widely documented the pressures on women to maintain an 'ideal' body shape and the implications of this for women more generally, which may or may not include serious eating disorders but do include weight preoccupation, body image dissatisfaction, and low self-esteem (Gucciardi et al., 2003; Larkin, Rice, and Russell, 1999; Rice, 2005).

It is now well documented that women have both a higher rate of diagnosed eating disorders than men (Health Canada, 2003) and more concerns generally about weight, shape, and appearance. Prevalence studies in Canada suggest that about 3 per cent of women will be affected by an eating disorder during their lifetime (Health Canada, 2002). Although eating disorders remain primarily a concern for adult women and adolescent women, increasingly eating disorders and body dissatisfaction is being documented in boys and men, although the factors contributing to this may be different than the factors for women (Cohane & Pope, 2001; Mangweth et al., 2003; Presnell, Bearman, & Stice, 2004). For example, there is a correlation between experiences of child sexual abuse and other experiences of violence and either eating disorders or the use of weight control techniques amongst women (Larkin et al., 1999; Rodríguez, Perez, & Garcia, 2005; Romans, Gendall, Martin, & Mullen, 2001; Wonderlich et al., 2001). A burgeoning litera- ture now exists on the prevalence of eating disorders outside of the North American context and the differential features and impact on different cultures and ethnicities in North America (e.g., Humphry & Ricciardelli, 2004; Rodríguez et al., 2005; Rubin, Fitts, & Becker, 2003; Shroff & Thompson, 2004; Wangsgaard Thompson, 1992).

Eating disorders and weight preoccupation have a wide range of psychological, social, and physical effects on women and men. These include heart conditions, electrolyte imbalance, kidney failure, depres- sion, alcohol and other forms of substance dependence, anxiety, and low self-esteem (Health Canada, 2002). The causes of eating disorders are complex and are thought to arise from a combination of biological, psychological, and social factors (Health Canada, 2002). Eating disor- ders are difficult to treat, and, despite a range of research in this area, existing data provides a very limited profile of eating disorders in Canada, especially with respect to the incidence and prevalence of disorders by age, sex, gender and other key variables like ethnicity and socio-economic status (Health Canada, 2002). Further, one of the challenges in this area has been to bring research (largely feminist) that explores the social context of eating disorders together with research that is concerned with the physiological effects of disturbed eating (largely biomedical). These gaps in knowledge and the range of dimensions that eating disorders effect makes mixed methods studies especially attractive. In the examples below, some of the suggested studies have already been undertaken; however, we provide them with a view towards explicating how mixed method models might be useful in research generally.

Quantitative – How Many? What Kind? Strength of Association – The Numbers. Quantitative measures attempt to capture the measurable attributes of human experiences. Data are systematically collected in numeric form and available methods include, for example: clinical and laboratory tests, survey questionnaires, and measurements. Using quantitative methods the following studies could be undertaken:

- Measurement of the prevalence of eating disorders in different groups of women and men
- An epidemiological study to achieve quantitative measures about what pre-existing health factors might be most associated with eating disorders

Qualitative – What? Why? Meaning of Something – The Text. On the other hand, a qualitative research approach which yields detailed description of situations, interactions, personal histories, and direct quotations from people about their experiences (e.g., interviews, focus groups, observational studies, and open-ended questions) may provide us with a certain depth and detail about individual women's and men's experiences. Qualitative methods are also more suitable for understanding the context of women's and men's lives, including, for example, how the social pressures to be thin and/or muscular and socio-economic status might affect women's and men's experiences of their weight and shape, access to resources, and ability to adhere to treatment.

- In-depth interviews with women and men who have been diagnosed with eating disorders to better understand the social context of their lives and their experiences of their bodies.
- A discursive analysis of the medical literature on eating disorders to better understand how the concept of 'eating disorders' has historically and is currently being constructed.

- A survey of the knowledge, attitudes, and beliefs in society about body weight, shape, and size with attention given to how these attitudes and beliefs might operate differently when applied to women and men and across classes and cultures.

Mixed Methods – Combining Qualitative and Quantitative Methods. Because there are strengths and weaknesses in both quantitative and qualitative approaches to researching eating disorders, combining them together in one research project can produce more comprehensive and in some cases more accurate knowledge. Results from one method can shape subsequent methods or steps in the research process. They may also stimulate new research questions or challenge results obtained through one method. There are a number of ways that both methods could be integrated in one study:

- *Qualitative* methods can be used to develop *quantitative* measures and instruments. This could include conducting focus groups, for example, with the group of women or men being studied before developing a structured questionnaire, which could then be used with a much larger sample in order to better understand incidence and prevalence for this group.
- In a *quantitative* study, *qualitative* methods can be used to help interpret and explain the quantitative findings. For example, tabulations from a preliminary survey may reveal interesting patterns of association; detailed qualitative analysis can provide a much richer understanding of why these patterns exist or how they operate. In the example of eating disorders, a survey related to the physiological impact of anorexia might reveal a relationship between specific effects and the age of onset of the eating disorder. In follow-up interviews with the survey participants, the nature and specifics of this relationship might be better revealed.
- *Qualitative* and *quantitative* methods can be used in ways that complement each other and help answer a mix of the questions *'How much?, How?, and Why?'*

In general, a mixed methods approach can increase the quality of final results and provide a more comprehensive understanding of the analysed phenomena. In our case example, the integration of the procedures mentioned above will expand the breadth of the study and likely enlighten the more general debate on women, men, weight, shape, and eating disorders.

Research as Praxis

The contemporary feminist exploration of the use of mixed methods in health research is part of the historical feminist preoccupation with developing research that translates into concrete changes. According to Reinharz (1992) there are five types of feminist change-oriented research: action research, participatory or collaborative research, prevalence and needs assessment, evaluation research, and demystification, the latter of which seeks to address gaps in knowledge. In bringing these to bear on women's health research, researchers need to be self-reflexive, accountable, and understand the complexities of social categories and intersecting forms of oppression and discrimination. These principles are key to realizing any potential for research to make meaningful change. According to Lather (1991, p. 226), a feminist approach requires that 'we consciously use our research to help participants understand and change their situations'. For Anderson (2000), this entails forming networks globally between women in the North and South, and including women from both academia and the grassroots community level, 'so that research will have relevance for policy and action at the local and global levels' (p. 226).

The research policy link has also been conceptualized in this way. Lomas (1997) argues that both researchers and policy makers must interface at various junctures in order for research to be successfully utilized. This view is critical in a policy climate where 'evidence-based' decision-making is highly valued and policy makers look increasingly to researchers to guide their decisions (see Hankivsky and Friesen, Chapter 6, this collection).

If we believe that research findings should be accessible and meaningful to as wide an audience as possible, it is important to recognize that researchers and decision-makers respond to different motivators when it comes to research. Researchers are mainly driven by what they believe to be the scientific importance of a particular line of investigation, whereas decision-makers typically have short timelines and pressing policy issues that must be addressed. Further, policy makers do their work within the wider political context of government decision-making, which brings competing demands. The 'evidence' used by decision-makers includes not only the knowledge acquired through research but also the concerns of the public and a sense of the public acceptability of various potential courses of action. This entails 'studying up'; that is, according to Harding and Norberg (2005), 'studying the powerful, their institutions, policies and practices instead of focusing only on those whom the powerful govern' (p. 2011). It also requires engaging women 'not only as recipients of policy, but as sources of knowledge, influence and power' (Feldberg, 2001).

Conclusion

As Fonow and Cook (2005) remind us, 'Feminists have moved well beyond the analysis of bias and exclusion and toward more contextual forms of theorizing about the intersection of gender with other categories of social difference and with place and time, this inevitably, has led to more sophisticated discussions about methods' (p. 2230). However, this sophistication has not always been adopted in health research, although there are encouraging signs that these issues are being taken up by individual researchers and integrated into research policy discussions at the national level.

NOTES

1 For example, Sherr (2000), in her review of the health literature, found that 95 per cent of research participants are male.
2 Thomas Kuhn, writing in the aftermath of the Second World War, treated the modern sciences as historical, sociological, cultural, and political phenomena, and in doing so launched a revolution in science studies.
3 The CIHR conceives of research as belonging to four pillars: biomedical, clinical, health systems and services, and population and public health.
4 Mixed methods generally refer to the use of two different methods in one research study, whereas multiple methods might be used in any one field of research.
5 *Verstehen* is the German term meaning 'to understand,' and was used by the sociologist Max Weber to refer to the ways in which social scientists try to understand both the context and intention of human behaviour. In philosophical debates about whether or not a distinction exists between the natural and human sciences on the basis of different aims, the term *verstehen* is often used in contrast to *erklären* (explanation) (Schwandt, 2003).

REFERENCES

Amos, V., & Parmar, P. (1984). Challenging imperial feminism. *Feminist Review, 17*(July), 1–19.

Anderson, J. (2000). Gender, 'race,' poverty, and health and discourses of health reform in the context of globalization: A post-colonial feminist perspective in policy research. *Nursing Inquiry, 7*(4), 220–229.

Battiste, M., & Youngblood Henderson, S.K. (2000). *Protecting Indigenous Knowledge and Heritage: A Global Challenge.* Saskatoon, SK: Purich Press.

Baum, F. (1995). Researching public health: Behind the qualitative-quantitative methodological debate. *Social Science & Medicine, 40*(4), 459–468.

Bent, K. (2004). *Anishinaace Ik-We Mino-Aie-Win. Aboriginal Women's Health Issues: A Holistic Perspective on Wellness.* University of Athabasca (Alberta). MAIS 701–702 Final Projects.

Bernard, W.T. (2002). Beyond inclusion: Women's voices. Atlantic Canadian women's contribution to health policy. In C. Amaratunga (Ed.), *Race, Ethnicity and Women's Health.* Halifax: Atlantic Centre of Excellence for Women's Health.

Bhabha, H. (1994). *The Location of Culture.* London: Routledge.

Bogdan, R., & Taylor, S. (Eds.). (1975). *Introduction to Qualitative Research Methods: A Phenomenological Approach to the Social Sciences.* New York: Wiley.

Bordo, S. (1987). The Cartesian masculinization of thought. In S. Harding & J. O'Barr (Eds.), *Sex and Scientific Inquiry* (pp. 247–264). Chicago and London: University of Chicago Press.

Canadian Institutes of Health Research. (2004). *What's Sex and Gender Got to Do with It? Integrating Sex and Gender into Health Research: Final Report.* Workshop (27 February – 1 March 2003). Ottawa: CIHR.

Canadian Institutes of Health Research. (2005). Retrieved from www. cihr-irsc.gc.ca/e/8677.html.

Carey, J.W. (1993). Linking qualitative and quantitative methods: Integrating cultural factors into public health. *Qualitative Health Research, 3*, 298–318.

Carter, P., Sellers, S.L., & Squires, C. (2002). Reflections on race/ethnicity, class, and gender inclusive research. *African American Perspectives, 8*(1), 111–124.

Casebeer, A.L., & Verhoef, M.J. (1997). Combining qualitative and quantitative research methods: Considering the possibilities for enhancing the study of chronic diseases. *Chronic Diseases in Canada, 18*, 130–135.

Catterall-Ironstone, P., McDonough, P., Robertson, A., Payne, B., Rahder, B., Shaver, F., et al. (1998). *Feminist Research Methodology and Women's Health: A Review of Literature.* www.yorku.ca/nnewh/english/pubs/workpap2.pdf.

Chesney, M.A., & Ozer, E.M. (1995). Women and health: In search of a paradigm. *Women's Health Issues, 1*(1), 3–26.

Clarke, P.N., & Yaros, P.S. (1988). Research blenders: Commentary and response. *Nursing Science Quarterly, 1*, 147–149.

Code, L. (2000). Epistemology. In A. Jagger & I.M. Young (Eds.), *A Companion to Feminist Philosophy* (pp. 173–184). Malden, MA: Blackwell.

Cohane, G.H., & Pope, H.G.J. (2001). Body image in boys: A review of the literature. *International Journal of Eating Disorders, 29*(4), 373–379.

Collins, P.H. (1991). *Black Feminist Thought: Knowledge, Consciousness and the Politics of Empowerment*. New York: Routledge.

Collins, P.H. (1995). Symposium: On West and Fenstermaker's 'Doing Difference.' *Gender & Society, 9*(4), 491–494.

Collins, P.H. (2004). *Black Sexual Politics: African Americans, Gender, and the New Racism*. New York: Routledge.

Cook, J., & Fonow, M.M. (1990). Knowlege and women's interests: Issues of epistemology and methodology in feminist sociological research. In J.M. Nielson (Ed.), *Feminist Research Methods: Exemplary Readings in Social Sciences*. Boulder, CO: Westview Press.

Cuádraz, G.H., & Uttal, L. (1999). Intersectionality and in-depth interviews: Methodological strategies for analyzing race, class and gender. *Race, Gender, and Class, 6*(3), 156–186.

Davis, A. (2000). Foreword to C. Sandoval, *Methodology of the Oppressed* (pp. xi–xiii). Minneapolis: University of Minnesota Press.

Dion Stout, M.D., Kipling, G.D., & Stout, R. (2001). *Aboriginal Women's Health Research Synthesis Project. Final Report*. Prepared for the Centre of Excellence for Women's Health Research Synthesis Group, Vancouver.

Dyck, I., Lynam, J.M., & Anderson, J.M. (1995). Women talking: Creating knowledge through difference in cross-cultural research. *Women's Studies International Forum, 18*(5–6), 611–626.

Feldberg, G. (2001). The power of citizen engagement to influence research and policy. *Centres of Excellence for Women's Health Research Bulletin: Voices from the Community, 2*(1).

Fonow, M.M., & Cook, J.A. (2005). Feminist methodology: New applications in the academy and public policy. *Signs: Journal of Women in Culture and Society, 30*(41), 2211–2230.

Friends of the CIHR, Newsletter 2001. Accessed 4 November 2006, from http://www.fcihr.ca/.

Greaves, L., Hankivsky, O., & Kingston-Riechers, J. (1995). *Selected Estimates of the Costs of Violence Against Women*. London, ON: Centre for Research on Violence Against Women and Children.

Gucciardi, E., Celasun, N., & Ahmad, F. (2003). *Eating Disorders*. Ottawa: Canadian Institute for Health Information.

Hajdukowski-Ahmed, M., Denton M., O'Connor, M., & Zeytinoglu, I.U. (1999). Women's voices in health promotion: Theoretical and methodological implications. In *Women's Voices in Health Promotion*. Toronto: Canadian Scholars' Press.

Hallam, J., & Marshall, A. (1993). Layers of difference: The significance of a self-reflexive research practice for a feminist epistemological project. In Mary Kennedy (Ed.), *Making Connections: Women's Studies, Women's Movements, Women's Lives* (pp. 64–78). London and Washington, DC: Taylor & Francis.

Hankivsky, O. (2004). *Social Policy and the Ethic of Care*. Vancouver: UBC Press.

Hankivsky, O. (2005). Gender mainstreaming vs. diversity mainstreaming: A preliminary examination of the role and transformative potential of feminist theory. *Canadian Journal of Political Science*, *38*(4), 977–1001.

Hankivsky, O., & Draker, D. (2003). The economic costs of child sexual abuse in Canada: A preliminary analysis. *Journal of Health and Social Policy*, *17*(2), 1–33.

Hankivsky, O., Friesen J., Varcoe, C., McPhail, F., Greaves, L., & Spencer, C. (2004). Expanding economic costing in health care: Values, gender and diversity. *Canadian Public Policy, 30*(3), 257–282.

Haraway, D. (1988). Situated knowledges: The science question in feminism and the privilege of partial perspective. *Feminist Studies, 14*, 575–599.

Harding, S. (1987a). Introduction: Is there a feminist method? In S. Harding (Ed.), *Feminism and Methodology: Social Science Issues*. Bloomington & Indianapolis: Indiana University Press.

Harding, S. (Ed.). (1987b). *Feminism and Methodology: Social Science Issues*. Bloomington and Indianapolis: Indiana University Press.

Harding, S. (1987c). Conclusion: Epistemological questions. In S. Harding (Ed.), *Feminism and Methodology: Social Science Issues* (pp. 181–191). Bloomington: Indiana University Press.

Harding, S. (1991). 'Strong objectivity' and socially situated knowledge. In S. Harding (Ed.), *Whose Science? Whose Knowledge? Thinking from Women's Lives*. Ithaca, NY: Cornell University Press.

Harding, S., & Norberg, K. (2005). New feminist approaches to social science methodologies: An introduction. *Signs: Journal of Women in Culture and Society, 30*(41), 2009–2015.

Health Canada. (2002). *A Report on Mental Illnesses in Canada*. Ottawa: Health Canada.

Health Canada. (2003). *Canadian Community Health Survey*. Ottawa: Statistics Canada.

Hill-Collins, P. (1991). *Black Feminist Thought: Knowledge, Consciousness & the Politics of Empowerment*. New York: Routledge.

hooks, b. (1984). *Feminist Theory from Margin to Centre*. Boston: South End Press.

Humphry, T.A., & Ricciardelli, L.A. (2004). The development of eating pathology in Chinese-Australian women: Acculturation versus culture clash. *International Journal of Eating Disorders, 35*(4), 579–588.

Jayaratne, T. (1983). The value of quantitative methodology for feminist research. In G. Bowles & R.D. Klein (Eds.), *Theories of Women's Studies* (pp. 283–311). London: Routledge & Kegan.

Kwan, M.P. (2001). Quantitative methods and feminist geographic research. In P. Moss (Ed.), *Feminist Geography in Practice: Research and Methods* (pp. 160–171). Oxford: Blackwell.

Larkin, J., Rice, C., & Russell, V. (1999). Sexual harassment, education and the prevention of disordered eating. In N. Piran, M. Levine, & C. Steiner-Adair (Eds.), *Preventing Eating Disorders: A Handbook of Intervention and Special Challenges* (pp. 194–207). Philadelphia: Brunner/Mazel.

Lather, P. (1991). *Getting Smart: Feminist Research and Pedagogy With/in the Postmodern*. New York: Routledge.

Lomas, J. (1997). Improving research dissemination and uptake in the health sector: Beyond the sound of one hand clapping. Working Paper/Policy Commentary C97–1. McMaster University Centre for Health and Economics and Analysis.

Longino, H. (1990). *Science as Social Knowledge*. Princeton: Princeton University Press.

Luce, J. (2003). Queer women's health research: Methodological questions. *Centres of Excellence for Women's Health Research Bulletin: Voices from the Community, 4*(1).

Mangweth, B., Hausmann, A., Walch, T., Hotter, A., Bieb, W., Rupp, C.I., Biebl, W., Hudson , J.I., & Pope. H.G., (2003). Body fat perception in eating-disordered men. *International Journal of Eating Disorders 35*(1), 102–108.

Marks, D.F. (2002). *Perspectives on Evidence-Based Practice*. HAD Contract no 02/042, Project 00477. London: Health Development Agency, Public Health Evidence Steering Group.

Mazure, C.M., Espeland M., Douglas P., Champion V., & Killien, M. (2000). Multidisciplinary women's health research: The national centers of excellence in women's health. *Journal of Women's Health and Gender-Based Medicine, 9*(7), 717–724.

McCall, L. (2005). The complexity of intersectionality. *Signs: A Journal of Women in Culture and Society, 30*(3).

Medical Research Council of Canada. (1994). *Report of the Advisory Committee on Women's Health Research Issues*. Ottawa: MRC Council of Canada.

Mohanty, C. (1988). Under Western eyes: Feminist scholarship and colonial discourses. *Feminist Review, 30,* 60–88.

Mohanty, C. (2003). *Feminism Without Borders: Decolonizing Theory, Practicing Solidarity.* Durham and London: Duke University Press.

Mohanty, C., Russo, A., & Torres, L. (1991). *Third World Women and the Politics of Feminism.* Bloomington: Indiana University Press.

Monro, F., & Huon, G. (2005). Media-portrayed idealized images, body shame, and appearance anxiety. *International Journal of Eating Disorders* 38(1), 85–90.

Naples, N. (2003). *Feminism and Method: Ethnography, Discourse Analysis, and Activist Research.* New York: Routledge.

Oakley, A. (1993). Some problems of the scientific research method and feminist research practice. In A. Oakley (Ed.), *Essays on Women, Medicine and Health* (pp. 243–264). Edinburgh: Edinburgh University Press.

Oakley, A. (1998). Science, gender and women's liberation: An argument against postmodernism. *Women's Studies International Forum, 21*(2), 133–146.

Olesen, V. (2003). Feminisms and qualitative research at and into the millennium. In N.D.Y. Lincoln (Ed.), *The Landscape of Qualitative Research: Theories and Issues* (pp. 332–397). Thousand Oaks, CA: Sage.

Olson, H. (2004). Quantitative 'versus' qualitative research: The wrong questions.

Pellmar, T.C., & Eisenberg, L. (Eds.). (2000). *Bridging Disciplines in the Brain, Behavioral, and Clinical Sciences.* Washington, DC: National Academy Press.

Presnell, K., Bearman, S.K., & Stice, E. (2004). Risk factors for body dissatisfaction in adolescent boys and girls: A prospective study. *International Journal of Eating Disorders, 36*(4), 389–401.

Ramazanoğlu, C., & Holland, J. (2002). *Feminist Methodology: Challenges and Choices.* London: Sage.

Reichardt, C.S., & Rallis, S.F. (1994). Qualitative and quantitative inquiries are not incompatible: A call for a new partnership. *New Directions for Program Evaluation, 61,* 85–91.

Reinharz, S. (1992). *Feminist Methods in Social Research.* New York: Oxford University Press.

Rice, C. (2005). Between the body and culture: Beauty, ability and growing up female. In B. Crow & L. Gottel (Eds.), *Open Boundaries: A Canadian Women's Studies Reader* (pp. 320–332). Toronto: Pearson.

Rodríguez, M., Pérez, V., & García, Y. (2005). Impact of traumatic experiences and violent acts upon response to treatment of a sample of Colombian women with eating disorders. *International Journal of Eating Disorders, 37*(4), 299–306.

Romans, S., Gendall, K., Martin, J., & Mullen, P.E. (2001). Child sexual abuse and later disordered eating: A New Zealand epidemiological study. *International Journal of Eating Disorders, 29,* 380–392.

Rose, D. (2001). Quantitative versus qualitative methods? The state of the debate. In D. Rose (Ed.), *Revisiting Feminist Research Methodologies: A Working Paper* (pp. 1–13). Ottawa: Status of Women Canada.

Rosenfield, P.L. (1992). The potential of transdisciplinary research for sustaining and extending linkages between the health and social sciences. *Social Science & Medicine, 35,* 1343–1357.

Rubin, L., Fitts, M., & Becker, A. (2003). 'Whatever feels good in my soul': Body ethics and aesthetics among African American and Latina women. *Culture, Medicine and Psychiatry, 27,* 49–75.

Ruzek, S., Olesen, V.L., & Clarke, A.E. (Eds.). (1997). *Women's Health: Complexities and Differences.* Columbus: Ohio State University Press.

Sale, J., Lohfeld, L., & Brazil, K. (2002). Revisiting the quantitative-qualitative debate: Implications for mixed-methods research. *Quality and Quantity, 36,* 43–53.

Sandoval, C. (2000). *Methodology of the Oppressed.* Minneapolis: University of Minnesota Press.

Saskatoon Aboriginal Women's Health Research Committee and Prairie Women's Health Centre of Excellence. (2002*). Ethical Guidelines for Aboriginal Women's Health Research.* Saskatoon, SK: Prairie Women's Health Centre of Excellence.

Scheman, N. (2001). Epistemology resuscitated: Objectivity as trustworthiness. In N.T.S. Morgen (Ed.), *Engendering Rationalities* (pp. 23–52). New York: State University of New York Press.

Schwandt, T. (2003). Three epistemological stances for qualitative inquiry: Interpretivism, hermeneutics, and social constructionism. In N. Denzin & Y. Lincoln (Eds.), *The Landscape of Qualitative Research: Theories and Issues.* Thousand Oaks, CA: Sage.

Seechrest, L., & Sidani, S. (1995). Quantitative and qualitative methods: Is there an alternative? *Evaluation and Program Planning, 18,* 77–87.

Sherr, L. (2000). Women and clinical trials. In L. Sherr & J. St Lawrence (Eds.), *Women, Health & the Mind* (pp. 47–58). Chichester, UK: John Wiley.

Shroff, H., & Thompson, K. (2004). Body image and eating disturbance in India: Media and interpersonal influences. *International Journal of Eating Disorders, 35*(2), 198–203.

Smith, D. (1974). Women's perspective as a radical critique of sociology. *Sociological Inquiry, 44,* 7–13.

Spitzer, D.L. (2004). *What's Sex and Gender Got to Do With It? Integrating Sex and Gender into Health Research.* Final report. Ottawa: Canadian Institute of Gender and Health.

Spivak, G.C. (1988). Subaltern studies: Deconstructing historiography. In G.C. Spivak (Ed.), *In Other Worlds: Essays in Cultural Politics.* London: Routledge.

Stanley, L., & Wise, S. (1993). *Breaking Out Again: Feminist Ontology and Epistemology.* New York: Routledge.

Steckler, A., McLeroy, K.R., Goodman, R.M., Bird, S.T., & McCormick, L. (1992). Toward integrating qualitative and quantitative methods: An introduction. *Health Education Quarterly, 19,* 1–8.

Steiger, H., & Séguin, J. (1999). Eating disorders: Anorexia nervosa and bulimia nervosa. In T. Million, P.H. Blaney, and R. David (Eds.), *Oxford Textbook of Psychopathology* (pp. 365–388). New York: Oxford University Press.

Stivers, C. (1993). Reflections on the role of personal narrative in social science. *Signs: Journal of Women in Culture and Society, 18*(2), 408–421.

Tuhiwai Smith, L. (1999). *Decolonizing Methodologies: Research and Indigenous Peoples.* New York: Zed Books.

Wangsgaard Thompson, B. (1992). 'A way outa no way': Eating problems among African-American, Latina, and white women. *Gender & Society, 6*(4), 546–561.

Weber, L., & Parra-Medina, D. (2003). Intersectionality and women's health: Charting a path to eliminating health disparities. *Advances in Gender Research, 7,* 181–230.

Westmarland, N. (2001). The quantitative/qualitative debate and feminist research: A subjective view of objectivity. *Forum: Qualitative Social Research, 2*(1), 1–12.

Wonderlich, S., Crosby, R., Mitchell, J., Thompson, K., Redlin, J., & Demuth, G. (2001). Eating disturbance and sexual trauma in childhood and adulthood. *International Journal of Eating Disorders, 30,* 401–412.

4 Postcolonial-Feminist Theoretical Perspectives and Women's Health

ANNETTE J. BROWNE, VICTORIA L. SMYE,
AND COLLEEN VARCOE

Recently, the move towards critical inquiry in health has been influenced by a call for postcolonial theoretical perspectives to better understand how gender, class, racialization,[1] and historical positioning intersect to shape the health of individuals, communities, and populations (Anderson, 2000, 2004; Reimer Kirkham & Anderson, 2002). As argued in the Introduction, feminist studies of health are also calling for more complex analyses of gender and its intersection with other forms of social difference. Concepts from postcolonial and feminist theories, when drawn upon in synergistic and complementary ways, have the potential to expand the explanatory powers of each respective theoretical tradition. Building on these traditions, in this chapter we examine the relevance of postcolonial-feminist theories as frameworks for understanding women's health and the factors shaping inequities in health and access to health care. We begin by reviewing the theoretical foundations of postcolonial-feminist theories and consider how these perspectives extend the boundaries of mainstream feminist theorizing to inform critical analyses of women's health. Next, we illustrate how postcolonial-feminist perspectives can be used to analyse women's health concerns using examples related to Canadian Aboriginal[2] women's health as a case in point. We conclude by emphasizing the importance of engaging critically with postcolonial-feminist theories as frameworks for social action aimed at mitigating inequities and promoting social justice in the area of women's health.

Postcolonial-Feminist Theoretical Perspectives: Relevancy to Women's Health

Theoretical Foundations

In its broadest sense, postcolonial theory can be defined as an interdisciplinary family of theories that share a common political and social concern about the legacy of colonialism, and how this continues to shape peoples' lives and life opportunities (Young, 2001). Developed by humanities and social science scholars such as Edward Said (1978), Stuart Hall (1995, 1996), Homi Bhabha (1994, 1995), Leela Gandhi (1998), Paul Gilroy (2000), and Gaytri Spivak (1994), among many others, interpretations and applications of postcolonial theorizing are wide-ranging, and both overlap and are in tension and contradiction with various approaches, including anti-racist theory, feminist theory, and postcolonial indigenous theory. Grounded in diverse disciplinary perspectives (e.g., political science, cultural studies, literary criticism, sociology), postcolonial theories converge on several key points: the need to examine the genesis of racialized, classed, and gendered inequities, both past and present; the need for critical analyses of peoples' experiences of colonialism, and their continuing manifestations; the deliberate decentreing of dominant culture so that the perspectives of those who have been marginalized become starting points for knowledge development; and the need to expand our understanding of how conceptualizations of race, racialization, culture, and Others[3] are constructed within particular historical and current neocolonial[4] contexts (Anderson, 2004; Gandhi, 1998; McConaghy, 2000; Reimer Kirkham & Anderson, 2002). A particularly relevant feature of postcolonial analysis in the realm of women's health is the foregrounding of colonizing and neocolonial practices which continue to construct race and culture as taken-for-granted categories to locate non-European women as the essentialized, often inferior, and subordinate Other (Anderson et al., 2003).

The notion of *post* in postcolonial does not imply that 'colonialism [is] finished business' (Smith, 1999, p. 98), but rather, that new, evolving configurations of power relations are emerging (Hall, 1996). As McConaghy (1998) explains, the postcolonial is perhaps best conceptualized as 'a place of multiple identities, interconnected histories, and shifting and diverse material conditions. It is also a place where new racisms and oppressions are being formed' (p. 1). Postcolonial dis-

---

Text Box 4.1 Application of Postcolonial-Feminist Theories in the Canadian Context

- Recently, postcolonial-feminist theories have been introduced in Canadian health care discourses to refocus on contemporary constructions of race and racialization, and how these intersect with gender, class and socio-historical positioning to shape the lives and well-being of women.
- In the Canadian context, these perspectives have informed recent research addressing the health concerns of diverse populations including Anglo-Canadians, immigrant populations, women of Colour, Aboriginal women, and health care providers.

---

courses thus provide a context for understanding the complexities of health and social inequities by foregrounding issues of race, racialization, culturalism, and Othering, which intersect in different ways among different groups of women to shape life opportunities, health status, and access to health care (Anderson, 2004; Browne, Smye, & Varcoe, 2005) (see Text Box 4.1).

A distinguishing feature of postcolonial theory – which sets it apart from other families of critical theory, for example, critical social theory, liberal feminist theory, or post-structuralism – is its focus on disrupting the enduring history of 'race-thinking' and structural inequities that have been brought about by histories of colonization and ongoing neo-colonial practices (Anderson, 2004; Browne et al., 2005). While we have argued that these analytical perspectives have direct relevance to women's (or men's) health concerns, like some other theories that attend to race or racism, postcolonial theories do not necessarily include a gendered analysis; and some have argued that gender, as an important analytical dimension, has been sorely lacking in some postcolonial scholarship (Gandhi, 1998). To address this gap, some scholars have incorporated perspectives from feminist theories to develop a postcolonial-feminist framework that extends the analytical boundaries of both feminist and postcolonial theories (see, for example, Anderson, 2000, 2002, 2004; McConaghy, 2000; Narayan, 2000; Narayan & Harding, 2000). In addition to refocusing attention on gender, the aspects of feminist theory that are perhaps most relevant to postcolonial analyses relate to the notion of intersectionality (Collins, 2000; Introduction, this collection), and the deliberate decentring of dominant cultural perspectives so that the voices of those who have been marginalized become starting points for inquiry (Anderson, 2000, 2002, 2004), and catalysts and key actors in activism and social change.

As argued in earlier chapters, intersectionality refers to the ability of social phenomena such as race, class, and gender to mutually construct one another; as a consequence, women experience differing constellations of inequities based on their social positioning within hierarchies of power relations (Collins, 2000). For example, when gender interacts with other factors, such as lower levels of education, racialization, or single parenthood, women end up at the bottom of most socioeconomic gradients, with Aboriginal women representing one of the most disadvantaged groups in Canada (Dion Stout & Kipling, 1998). From a postcolonial-feminist perspective, we are directed to consider the intersecting impact of these historically and socially mediated conditions on women's health and human suffering.

Postcolonial-feminist theory also emphasizes the need for critical analyses that are inclusive of multiple voices from diverse socio-historical locations (Narayan & Harding, 2000). The assumption is that voices from the margins – 'those who have suffered the sentence of history' (Bhabha, 1994) – 'produce insights that are intended to interrupt dominant discourses about race, class, gender relations and feminism' (Anderson, 2002, p. 18). With few exceptions, these perspectives have been largely excluded in health policy and research. Instead, issues that marginalize women have tended to be reinterpreted or couched in terms of cultural differences, lifestyle practice, or behavioral choices (Browne & Smye, 2002).

Expanding the Boundaries of Feminist Theorizing

One of the critiques of some forms of feminist theory has been the tendency for analyses to privilege the gendered constraints of women's lives over issues such as racialization or class (Lee & Cardinal, 1998). For example, liberal feminist theory has been criticized for focusing on the problems of relatively privileged – most often white, Western, middle-class, and heterosexual – women (Narayan, 2000). Scholars such as Brewer (1993), Collins (1986, 1993), Mohanty (1992), Ng (1993), and George (1998) have contested the centrality of gender oppression, essentialist conceptions of gender, and the subordination of the experiences of race and class. Following these critiques, as discussed in earlier chapters, feminists have theorized oppression as arising from multiple sites, most expressly including race, class, and gender. Postcolonial-feminist perspectives can be conceptualized as building on these critiques and extending the analytical breadth of feminist theorizing by illuminating how racialized, classed, and gendered positioning, originating in the past and continuing in the present, intersects in different ways to shape (and constrain) women's lives, opportunities, and choices (Anderson, 2000, 2004).

To illustrate these points, we draw on arguments advanced by several Canadian Aboriginal scholars. Monture Angus (1995), for example, takes issue with the fact that the 'women's movement has never taken as its central and long-term goals, the eradication of the legal oppression that is specific to Aboriginal women' (p. 175). For Turpel (1993), the historical oppression levelled against Aboriginal women is 'one of the most important points for feminists to grasp in order to appreciate how state-imposed gender discrimination uniquely affected First Nations women' (p. 180). Stevenson (Johnson, Stevenson, & Greschner, 1993) expresses similar frustrations as she describes the origins of her disillusionment with the feminist movement, which in her view failed to address Aboriginal women's oppression through colonialism. For these reasons (among others) some Aboriginal women scholars have made efforts to construct a gendered identity distinct from non-Aboriginal women and mainstream feminist movements.

For others, postcolonial and feminist theoretical perspectives continue to be useful in emphasizing the inextricable links between racism, sexism, and patriarchy as legacies of colonial oppression. LaRocque (1996), a Métis scholar, draws on postcolonial perspectives to illuminate how colonialism continues to subjugate some Aboriginal women in ways that are distinct from the disadvantages and oppression experienced by other women in Canada. As LaRocque explains, 'Colonization has taken its toll on all Native peoples, but perhaps it has taken its greatest toll on women ... Racism and sexism found in the colonial process have served to dramatically undermine the place and value of women in Aboriginal cultures, leaving us vulnerable both within and outside of our communities ... The tentacles of colonization are not only extant today, but may also be multiplying and encircling Native peoples in ever-tighter grips of landlessness and marginalization, hence, of anger, anomie, and violence, in which women are the more obvious victims' (p. 11–12). As LaRocque's analysis illustrates, drawing on postcolonial *and* feminist perspectives provides the kind of analytical depth required to understand the complexities of factors – for example, political disenfranchisement, racism, historical positioning, and gender – that shape the broad determinants of health.

While postcolonial theories offer a powerful set of analytical tools, it is important to engage critically with theories, and scrutinize what some might consider an imposition of academic, and in some cases, Eurocentric perspectives, onto issues of importance to diverse groups of women (Browne et al., 2005). In the case of women's health, one of the most pertinent to consider is the potential for postcolonial discourses to inadvertently reproduce essentialized portrayals of women. For example, as in other well-intended critical approaches, there can be a propensity in postcolonial theorizing to assume (wrongly) that all women who belong to a particular ethnocultural group share the same experience of oppression (Narayan, 2000). This form of essentialism tends to overlook the diversity within groups, and women's unique experiences and their varying degrees of agency. The well-intentioned imperative to attend to cultural 'differences' can, therefore, result in the perpetuation of assumptions about differences that constitute 'cultural essentialism' (p. 82). The resulting portraits of 'Western women,' 'Third World women,' 'Muslim women,' and the like, as well as the portraits of the 'cultures' that are attributed to these various groups of women, often remain fundamentally essentialist (p. 82). Narayan describes how feminist representations of Third World women have sometimes been modeled on those who are most marginalized and underprivileged (see Text Box 4.2). In the Canadian context, studies have illustrated the extent to which health professionals associate Aboriginal 'culture' with the cultures of poverty, substance abuse, and dependency, giving rise to judgments about Aboriginal women's individual responsibility and choice in shaping their socioeconomic or health status (Browne, 2005; Browne, in press; Browne & Fiske, 2001; Tait, 2000). To counter this tendency to essentialize women's cultural characteristics or experiences, it is imperative to apply postcolonial-feminist perspectives in ways that permit generalizations about shared experiences of racialization, economic marginalization, and other forms of oppression, while, at the same time, focusing attention on differences and particularities of context (Narayan, 2000).

Text Box 4.2 International Perspectives: The Problem with Cultural Essentialism

- As globalization continues, it will be imperative to avoid essentialist portrayals of 'Western women,' 'Third World women,' 'Muslim women,' and similar categorizations, which erase and/or gloss over women's unique experiences, histories, circumstances, and health issues.

As with all theoretical perspectives, it is important to recognize their analytical scope and limitations. We do not want to imply that postcolonial-feminist theories are more valuable than other critical theoretical approaches. Rather, differing theoretical approaches focus one's attention differently on issues of concern to women's health, with postcolonial-feminist theories shedding light on racialization, historical subjugation, culture, and class as social conditions that intersect with gender to shape life opportunities and health in the present. Given these considerations, we turn now to illustrate how postcolonial-feminist perspectives can be used to analyse women's health concerns, using examples pertinent to Aboriginal women's health, each as a case in point. While we draw on examples from Aboriginal women's health, the issues we highlight are relevant to other groups of women as examples of socially organized inequities, inequities that are interwoven into the socio-historical-material fabric of society in varying ways to shape health in its broadest sense.

Examining Women's Health from a Postcolonial-Feminist Perspective

From a postcolonial-feminist vantage point, the entire enterprise of women's health is viewed through a political lens. This interpretive lens recognizes that each life is shaped by history and one's socio-historical positioning within society (Reimer, Kirkham, & Anderson, 2002). In the case of Aboriginal women's health in Canada, a postcolonial-feminist lens would direct us to consider the systematic discrimination levelled against women through colonial laws and policies consolidated in the 1876 Indian Act.[5] Although amendments to the Indian Act have removed many of the overtly racist and sexist policies, it continues to exist as the overarching governing policy for 'Status' or 'Registered' First Nations people in Canada. Under the Indian Act, Aboriginal women continue to be assigned fewer fundamental rights than men (Fiske, 1993, 1995, 2006; Stevenson, 1999). This forms the context in which the social determinants of health exert their effects. From a postcolonial-feminist perspective, these socio-historical conditions are analysed as *determinants* of Aboriginal women's health. For example, one of the most controversial issues has been the enactment of patriarchal state ideology, which, until the 1985 amendments[6] to the Indian Act, stripped women and their children of their Status upon marrying non-Indian or non-Status Indian men (Stevenson, 1999). The effect was to dispossess women, their children, and grandchildren of whatever inherent protections and rights the Indian Act offered (Fiske, 1993, 1995). Even when married to Status Indian men, women were excluded from holding parcels of land under the state-defined system. The denial of property rights directly affected women's capacity to support themselves and their families, exacerbating present-day economic marginalization and the development of welfare colonialism. The links between lower socio-economic status, poverty, and poorer health status are now well established (Canadian Institute for Health Information, 2004). For example, the socio-economic status of many Aboriginal peoples is significantly lower than that of non-Aboriginal Canadians – which provides a context for understanding why the age-standardized mortality rate for all causes among First Nations women is substantially higher compared to other Canadian women (Dion Stout, Kipling, & Stout, 2001).

Postcolonial-feminist theories bring to the forefront issues of 'race,' and how this socially constructed category intersects with gender, culture, and class to structure human relationships. For example, colonizing images of Aboriginal women as irresponsible and negligent contributed to the 'inferiorization of Aboriginal motherhood,' fuelling the widespread removal of Aboriginal children into non-Aboriginal foster homes in the 1960s and 70s (Fiske, 1993, p. 20). More recently, public awareness campaigns portraying fetal alcohol syndrome as an Aboriginal health problem have been critiqued for perpetuating public and professional perceptions of Aboriginal women as abusive and uncaring (Tait, 2000). The marginalizing consequences of negative stereotyping can have far-reaching effects: 'Despite public recognition of past injustices committed against Aboriginal peoples in this country, marginalization and prejudice remain very much present in the daily

lives of many community members. While the effects of this marginalization make themselves manifest in any number of ways, few are
more telling than statistics that place Canada's Aboriginal population
far below their non-Aboriginal counterparts in the United Nations
Human Development Index' (Dion Stout et al., 2001, p. 12). As these
examples illustrate, the explanatory power of analyses informed by
postcolonial-feminist perspectives lies in illuminating enduring histories of discrimination as social conditions that intersect with other
forms of oppression to shape health and social status.

Interpreting Health Status Indicators from a
Postcolonial-Feminist Perspective.

Epidemiological profiles and statistical indicators of health and illness
are invaluable in alerting communities, the health sector, and policy
makers to emerging trends in health status. At the same time, there are
risks inherent in presenting information about groups of people, particularly when it reinforces stereotypes and misconceptions. As O'Neil,
Reading, and Leader (1998) explain, the risk lies in contributing to 'an
understanding of Aboriginal society that reinforces unequal power relationships; in other words, an image of sick, disorganized communities
can be used to justify paternalism and dependence' (p. 230). This is a
paradox that we must confront in presenting health (or other) statistics
that are grouped according to ethnicity.

   From a postcolonial-feminist theoretical stance, it becomes critical to
avoid decontextualized discussions of health statistics. Instead statistics
must be framed in terms of their intersecting social, historical, and
economic determinants. For example, recognizing that the high rates of
diabetes[7] and obesity affecting many Aboriginal women are linked to
overall changes in socio-economic status within entire communities,
and associated diet and exercise patterns, avoids misinterpreting these
conditions as purely 'lifestyle' issues arising from people's unwise
choices. Similarly, substance use problems experienced by some Aboriginal peoples have been linked to intergenerational traumas associated with residential school experiences among other multi-factorial
issues (Royal Commission on Aboriginal Peoples [RCAP], 1996a). While
the underlying causes of these conditions are unquestionably complex,
Dion Stout et al. (2001) argue that more emphasis needs to be placed
on making explicit the linkages between these and other health condi-

tions and 'the realities of gender-based inequity and socio-economic marginalization' (p. 17).

HIV among Aboriginal women represents a case in point. The current crisis caused by extremely high rates of HIV is one of the most devastating manifestations of the cumulative effects of poverty, dispossession, and despair (Spittal & Schechter, 2001). For example:

- HIV infection among Aboriginal populations has increased 91 per cent from 1996 to 1999 (AIDS among Aboriginals, 2001).
- Nationally, from 1998 to 2000, women represented nearly half (45.6 per cent) of all positive HIV test reports among Aboriginal persons (Health Canada, 2002).
- In comparison, women comprised 19.8 per cent of all positive reports for non-Aboriginal persons (Health Canada, 2002).

On the one hand, it is imperative to use statistics to leverage funds and services for prevention, treatment, and social support, and to lobby for actions to address the underlying issues associated with HIV. On the other hand, publicizing these statistics, and the risk factors associated with HIV, can perpetuate images of Aboriginal women as irresponsible, out of control, and identified with drug and alcohol problems. Unless explicit connections are made between the high rates of HIV and the wider determinants of health, it is easy to overlook the complex, intersecting conditions that influence women's everyday lives (Varcoe, Dick, & Walther, 2004). For example, welfare colonialism continues to result in high rates of unemployment and dependency on meager social assistance payments. As documented by the Aboriginal Nurses Association of Canada (1996), exclusion from the wage economy, impoverished living conditions, the links between substance abuse and poverty, and the economic dependence of some women on the sex trade, continue to underlie the current epidemic of HIV among Aboriginal women.

Using postcolonial-feminist perspectives to examine the high rates of cervical cancer mortality among First Nations women in British Columbia represents another case in point. Epidemiologic evidence revealed that mortality between the years 1991 and 2000 was twice as high for Status First Nations women than for other women (British Columbia, 2002). Because cervical cancer is highly preventable and easily detected through Pap screening, questions arise about women's access to health care. 'Risk profiles' are needed to alert health care providers and policy makers to women who should be targeted for screening programs. At the same time, discourses about reproductive risk factors – for example, number of partners, age of onset of sexual activity, and infection with human papilloma virus (factors associated with higher rates of cervical cancer) – can inadvertently reinforce negative stereotypes of Aboriginal women (Browne & Smye, 2002). We are not suggesting that health statistics not be used to lobby for particular programs and services; rather, from a postcolonial-feminist stance, we are directed to discuss health statistics or risk factors in ways that foreground the contexts and conditions that place women at risk. Equally imperative are efforts in writing and research to shift attention away from Aboriginal women as the source of the 'problem' and towards the power differentials in health care that can create patterns of inclusion and exclusion for various groups of women (Browne, in press; Browne & Fiske, 2001).

In summary, postcolonial-feminist perspectives prompt us to engage critically with health information by continually seeking to understand the wider historical, social, economic, and political circumstances that shape women's health. For example, why are some women more susceptible to diabetes, substance use problems, or obesity than other women? What is it about some women's life histories and social circumstances that place them at risk? What are the barriers within the health care system that impede access for some women more than others? By sharpening our critical gaze, we can ensure that health disparities affecting women are not glossed over as lifestyle, behavioural, or cultural issues. From a postcolonial-feminist stance, we can proceed to engage in rigorous scrutiny of the complexities of women's health, and engage in the long-term political activity of social transformation aimed at improving the social determinants of health.

Conclusion: Theory for Social Change

In this chapter, we have highlighted the analytical dimensions that are brought to the forefront from a postcolonial-feminist theoretical perspective. These perspectives extend the boundaries of mainstream feminist theorizing by focusing on the intersection of socio-historical positioning, culture, race, and racialization as intersecting factors shaping the health and social status of women. A distinctive feature of postcolonial-feminist scholarship is its commitment to transformative social change (Anderson, 2002; Reimer Kirkham & Anderson, 2002). In the context of health and health care, knowledge for transformative social action is 'undergirded by critical consciousness on the part of healthcare providers, and that unmasks unequal relations of power and issues of domination and subordination, based on assumptions about "race," "gender," and class relations' (Anderson, 1998, p. 205). Brought into the women's health arena, these goals translate into a commitment to reduce inequities at all levels – interpersonally, between groups, and within society – by (a) supporting the transformation of women's perspectives into action, (b) challenging assumptions about particular groups of women and their 'differences,' (c) resisting various forms of gender and cultural essentialism, and (d) analysing how historical positioning intersects with gender, class, and racialization to influence women's health and well-being.

How can a postcolonial-feminist perspective actually translate into affecting transformative change? One way is to remain vigilant about the ways in which inequities are perpetuated in health care contexts by developing critical awareness of how health care providers, educators, policy makers and other decision-makers respond to notions of 'difference,' and how this can inadvertently portray particular women as deficient (Varcoe & McCormick, 2007). For example, a recent study by Smye (2004) describes a situation involving a young, healthy Aboriginal woman who in the immediate post-partum period was asked by her health care providers to delay breastfeeding until the results of a hepatitis C and HIV test – obtained without her knowledge or consent – were known.[8] This case helps to illustrate how some women can be transformed into 'at risk' patients despite the lack of any risk factors. Postcolonial-feminist perspectives shed light on how this woman is rendered at risk by virtue of her visibility as an Aboriginal woman, illuminating how assumptions about racialized, cultural, and class identities can affect health care practices.

Although this chapter has focused on the relevance of postcolonial-feminist theory to analyses of women's health, it should not be inferred that this perspective ought to be exclusively applied to women's concerns. On the contrary, postcolonial-feminist theory is constructed as an inclusive framework with the potential for wide analytical applications (Anderson, 2004). For example, postcolonial perspectives can be used to frame analyses of physiological health concerns (such as cervical cancer, or wound healing) by drawing attention to class, racialization, historical positioning, and gender as factors that intersect to predispose particular groups of people to certain health conditions (Browne & Smye, 2002; Reimer Kirkham & Anderson, 2002). Applying a postcolonial-feminist lens to biomedical issues would provide direction for (a) critiquing the types of treatments that have gained hegemony in health care settings, (b) considering whose interests are served by the dominance of certain treatment modalities, and (c) analysing which groups have greater access to such treatments than others.

We do not want to imply that postcolonial-feminist theory is *the* definitive theory for women's health. As Anderson (2004) suggests, the greatest analytical 'mileage' may be produced by stitching together insights garnered from differing theoretical perspectives. As we engage with theories as frameworks for informing heath research, policy, and practice, we must consider how constructive they are for unraveling the complexities of inequities and the social determinants of health, and engaging in the political activity of social transformation. The value of drawing on postcolonial-feminist perspectives lies in the direction they provide for critiquing the status quo and generating knowledge that will contribute to social justice in the realm of women's health. By bringing together postcolonial and feminist perspectives, we will be better able to understand and respond to the multiple, intersecting influences on women's health.

NOTES

Funding for several studies discussed in this chapter was provided by the Canadian Institutes of Health Research (CIHR) and Health Canada. Annette Browne and Vicki Smye are supported by New Investigator Awards from CIHR, and Annette is supported by a Scholar Award from the Michael Smith Foundation for Health Research.

1 Fanon (1967) first coined the concept of *racializing* conditions, contrasting them significantly with humanizing ones, to suggest the ways in which racial conceptions and structural conditions order lives and delimit human possibilities (Goldberg & Essed, 2002). The term *racialization* was later adopted by Miles (1989), who defined it as 'a process of delineation of group boundaries and of allocation of persons within those boundaries by primary reference to (supposedly) inherent and/or biological (usually phenotypic) characteristics' (p. 74). Fundamentally, racialization refers to a process of 'categorization, a representational process of defining an Other' (p.75).

2 Consistent with the terminology used by the Royal Commission on Ab-

original Peoples ([RCAP] 1996a, 1996b), the term 'Aboriginal peoples' refers generally to the indigenous inhabitants of Canada including First Nations, Métis, and Inuit peoples, without regard to their separate origins and identities. The commission stresses that the term Aboriginal peoples 'refers to organic political and cultural entities that stem historically from the original peoples of North America, rather than collections of individuals united by so-called 'racial' characteristics' (RCAP, 1996b, p. xii). Specifically, the term *First Nation* replaces the term *Indian* and *Inuit* replaces the term *Eskimo*. The terms Indian or Eskimo, however, continue to be used in federal legislation and policy (e.g., the Indian Act), and in government reports, health reports, and statistical data. In such reports, the terms 'Status' or 'Registered Indian' refer to people who have been registered by the Department of Indian and Northern Affairs Canada as members of a First Nation under the terms of the Indian Act.

3 The notion of Other or Othering refers to the projection of assumed cultural characteristics, 'differences,' or identities onto members of particular groups. These projections are not based on actual identities; rather, they are founded on stereotyped, essentialized, and often racialized identities.

4 'Neocolonial' is the term widely used to refer to current forms of control of prior colonies or populations such as indigenous peoples who continue to live under conditions of internal-colonialism. Neocolonialism is more difficult to detect and resist than historical forms of overt colonialism in large part because it is insidiously maintained by everyday, taken-for-granted structures and processes (Ashcroft, Griffiths, and Tiffin, 1998).

5 The Indian Act, premised on the paternalistic guise of assisting Indians as wards of the state, was intended to civilize and assimilate Indians, and to govern Indians 'until there is not a single Indian in Canada that has not been absorbed into the body politic, and there is no Indian question and no Indian Department' (cited in Manitoba Public Inquiry, 1991, p. 73). The drive to achieve assimilation was pursued on many different levels. For example, classifications of Aboriginal peoples were legislated for the purposes of governing aspects of everyday life: Aboriginal lands were appropriated, Aboriginal peoples were marginalized on reserve lands, cultural spiritual practices were outlawed, and indoctrination into the dominant culture was attempted by force through church or state-run residential schools (Armitage, 1995). A more recent though lesser-known fact is that Status First Nations women, like men, were not permitted, by law, to vote in federal elections until 1960 despite the fact that Aboriginal people were among the most intensively governed members of Canadian society (Furniss, 1999).

6 These amendments, known commonly as Bill C-31, allowed women who had previously lost their status to regain status. However, Bill C-31 did not eradicate gender discrimination (Monture Angus, 1995; Turpel, 1993). Rather, state-defined criteria for who can and cannot be granted status, 'have brought greater state surveillance of women's daily lives and sexual relations' (Fiske, 1993, p. 23).

7 As reported by the Canadian Institute for Health Information (2004), rates of diabetes in the late 1990s were 5.6 times higher for status First Nations women on the reserve compared to other Canadian women (p. 83).

8 Testing pregnant women for hepatitis C and HIV is not mandatory in the province in question (obstetrician, personal communication, November 2003).

REFERENCES

Aboriginal Nurses Association of Canada. (1996). *HIV/AIDS and Its Impact on Aboriginal Women in Canada*. Ottawa: Author.

AIDS among Aboriginals: On the brink of an epidemic? (2001, December). *The First Perspective, 10*(12), p. 7.

Anderson, J.M. (1998). Speaking of illness: Issues of first generation Canadian women – Implications for patient education and counseling. *Patient Education and Counseling, 33*, 197–207.

Anderson, J.M. (2000). Gender, 'race,' poverty, health and discourses of health reform in the context of globalization: A postcolonial feminist perspective in policy research. *Nursing Inquiry, 7*, 220–229.

Anderson, J.M. (2002). Toward a postcolonial feminist methodology in nursing: Exploring the convergence of postcolonial and black feminist scholarship. *Nurse Researcher: The International Journal of Research Methodology in Nursing and Health Care, 9*(3), 7–27.

Anderson, J.M. (2004). Lessons from a postcolonial-feminist perspective: Suffering and a path to healing. *Nursing Inquiry, 11*(4), 238–246.

Anderson, J.M., Perry, J., Blue, C., Browne, A.J., Henderson, A., Lynam, J., Reimer Kirkham, S., Semeniuk, P., & Smye, V. (2003). 'Re-writing' cultural safety within the postcolonial/postnationalist feminist project: Toward new epistemologies of healing. *Advances in Nursing Science, 26*(3), 196–214.

Anderson, J.M., & Reimer Kirkham, S. (1999). Discourses on health: A critical perspective. In H. Coward & P. Ratanakul (Eds.), *A Cross-Cultural Dialogue on Health Care Ethics* (pp. 47–67). Waterloo, ON: Wilfred Laurier University Press.

Armitage, A. (1995). *Comparing the Policy of Aboriginal Assimilation: Australia, Canada, and New Zealand*. Vancouver: UBC Press.

Ashcroft, B., Griffiths, G., & Tiffin, H. (1998). *Key Concepts in Post-colonial Studies*. New York: Routledge.

Ashcroft, B., Griffiths, G., & Tiffin, H. (2000). *Post-colonial Studies: The Key Concepts*. New York: Routledge.

Bhabha, H. (1994). *The Location of Culture*. London: Routledge.

Bhabha, H. (1995). Cultural diversity and cultural differences. In B. Ashcroft, G. Griffiths, & H. Tiffin (Eds.), *The Post-Colonial Studies Reader* (pp. 206–209). New York and London: Routledge.

Brewer, R.M. (1993). Theorizing race, class and gender: The new scholarship of Black feminist intellectuals and Black women's labour. In S.M. James & A.P.A. Busia (Eds.), *Theorizing Black Feminisms: The Visionary Pragmatism for Black Women* (pp. 13–30). London: Routledge.

British Columbia. Provincial Health Officer. (2002). *Report on the Health of British Columbians: Provincial Health Officer's Annual Report 2001. The Health and Well-Being of Aboriginal People in British Columbia*. Victoria, BC: Ministry of Health Planning.

Browne, A.J. (2005). Discourses influencing nurses' perceptions of First Nations patients. *Canadian Journal of Nursing Research 37*(4), 63–87.

Browne, A.J. (in press). Clinical encounters between nurses and First Nations women in a Western Canadian hospital. *Social Science & Medicine*.

Browne, A.J., & Fiske, J. (2001). First Nations women's encounters with mainstream health care services. *Western Journal of Nursing Research, 23*(2), 126–147.

Browne, A.J., & Smye, V. (2002). A postcolonial analysis of health care discourses addressing Aboriginal women. *Nurse Researcher: The International Journal of Research Methodology in Nursing and Health Care, 9*(3), 28–41.

Browne, A.J., Smye, V., & Varcoe, C. (2005). The relevance of postcolonial theoretical perspectives to research in Aboriginal health. *Canadian Journal of Nursing Research. 37* (4), 17–37.

Canadian Institute for Health Information. (2004). *Improving the Health of Canadians*. Ottawa: Canadian Institute for Health Information.

Collins, P.H. (1986). Learning from the outsider within. *Social Problems, 33*(5), 14–32.

Collins, P.H. (1993). Toward a new vision: Race, class and gender as categories of analysis and connection. *Race, Sex & Class, 1*(1), 23–45.

Collins, P.H. (2000). *Black Feminist Thought: Knowledge Consciousness, and the Politics of Empowerment*. 2nd ed. New York: Routledge.

Dion Stout, M., & Kipling, G.D. (1998). *Aboriginal Women in Canada: Strategic Research Directions for Policy Development*. Ottawa: Status of Women Canada.

Dion Stout, M., Kipling, G.D., & Stout, R. (2001). *Aboriginal Women's Health Research: Synthesis Project Final Report*. Ottawa: Centres of Excellence for Women's Health.

Fanon, F. (1967). *The Wretched of the Earth*. C. Farrington (Trans.) New York: Grove.

Fiske, J. (1993). Child of the state, mother of the Nation: Aboriginal women and the ideology of motherhood. *Culture, 13*(1), 17–35.

Fiske, J. (1995). Political status of Native Indian women: Contradictory implications of Canadian state policy. *American Indian Culture and Research Journal, 19*(2), 1–30.

Fiske, J. (2006). Boundary crossings: Power and marginalisation in the formation of Canadian Aboriginal women's identities. *Gender & Development, 14*(2), 247–258.

Furniss, E. (1999). *The Burden of History: Colonialism and the Frontier Myth in a Rural Canadian Community*. Vancouver: UBC Press.

Gandhi, L. (1998). *Postcolonial Theory: A Critical Introduction*. New York: Columbia University Press.

George, U. (1998). Caring and women of colour. Living the intersecting oppressions of race, class and gender. In C.T. Baines, P.M. Evans, & S.M. Neysmith (Eds.), *Women's Caring Feminist Perspectives on Social Welfare* (2nd ed., pp. 69–83). Toronto: Oxford University Press.

Gilroy, P. (2000). *Against Race: Imagining Political Culture Beyond the Color Line* Cambridge, MA: Belknap.

Goldberg, D.T., & Essed, P. (2002). Introduction: From racial demarcations to multiple identifications. In P. Essed & D.T. Goldberg (Eds.), *Race Critical Theories* (pp. 1–11). Malden, MA: Blackwell.

Hall, S. (1995). New ethnicities. In B. Ashcroft, G. Griffiths, & H. Tiffin (Eds.), *The Post Colonial Studies Reader* (pp. 223–227). London and New York: Routledge.

Hall, S. (1996). When was 'the post-colonial'? Thinking at the limit. In I. Chambers & L. Curtis (Eds.). *The PostColonial Question: Common Skies, Divided Horizons* (pp. 242–260). London: Routledge.

Hall, S. (1997). *Representation: Cultural Representations and Signifying Practices*. London: Sage.

Health Canada (2002). *HIV/AIDS Epi Update*. Centre of Infectious Disease Prevention and Control. Retrieved 25 October 2002, from http://www.hc-sc.gc.ca/pphb-dgspsp/publicat/epiu-aepi/hiv-vih/aborig_e.html.

Henry, F., Tator, C., Mattis, W., & Rees, T. (2000). *The Colour of Democracy: Racism in Canadian Society*. Toronto: Harcourt Brace.

Johnson, R., Stevenson, W., & Greschner, D. (1993). Peekiskwetan. *Canadian Journal of Women and the Law, 6*, 153–173.

LaRocque, E.D. (1996). The colonization of a Native woman scholar. In C. Miller & P. Chuchryk (Eds.), *Women of the First Nations: Power, Wisdom, and Strength* (pp. 11–17). Winnipeg: University of Manitoba Press.

Lee, J., & Cardinal, L. (1998). Hegemonic nationalism and the politics of feminism and multiculturalism in Canada. In V. Strong-Boag, S. Grace, A. Eisenberg, & J. Anderson (Eds.), *Painting the Maple: Essays on Race, Gender, and the Construction of Canada* (pp. 215–241). Vancouver: UBC Press.

Manitoba. Public Inquiry into the Administration of Justice and Aboriginal people. (1991). *Report of the Aboriginal Justice Inquiry of Manitoba*. Winnipeg: Government of Manitoba.

McConaghy, C. (1998). *Indigenous Teacher Education and Postcoloniality*. Paper presented at the 1998 Australian Association for Research in Education (AARE) Conference, Adelaide, Australia.

McConaghy, C. (2000). *Rethinking Indigenous Education: Culturalism, Colonialism and the Politics of Knowing*. Brisbane, Australia: Post Pressed.

Miles, R. (1989). *Racism*. London: Routledge.

Mohanty, C.T. (1992). Feminist encounters: Locating the politics of experience. In M. Barrett & A. Phillips (Eds.), *Destabilizing Theory: Contemporary Feminist Debates* (pp. 74–92). Stanford, CA: Stanford University Press.

Monture Angus, P. (1995). *Thunder in My Soul: A Mohawk Woman Speaks*. Halifax: Fernwood.

Narayan, U. (2000). Essence of culture and sense of history: A feminist critique of cultural essentialism. In U. Narayan & S. Harding (Eds.), *Decentering the Center: Philosophy for a Multicultural, Postcolonial, and Feminist World* (pp. 80–100). Bloomington: Indiana University Press.

Narayan, U., & Harding, S. (2000). *Decentering the Center: Philosophy for a Multicultural, Postcolonial, and Feminist World*. Bloomington: Indiana University Press.

Ng, R. (1993). Sexism, racism, Canadian nationalism. In H. Bannerji (Ed.), *Returning the Gaze: Essays on Racism, Feminism and Politics* (pp. 182–196). Toronto: Sister Vision Press.

O'Neil, J.D., Reading, J.R., & Leader, A. (1998). Changing the relations of surveillance: The development of a discourse of resistance in Aboriginal epidemiology. *Human Organization, 57*(2), 230–237.

Reimer Kirkham, S., & Anderson, J. (2002). Postcolonial nursing scholarship: From epistemology to method. *Advances in Nursing Science, 25*(1), 1–17.

Reinert, E.S. (2005). *Development and Social Goals: Balancing Aid and Development to Prevent 'Welfare Colonialism.'* New York: United Nations Development Conference on Millennium Development Goals.

Royal Commission on Aboriginal Peoples. (1996a). *Report of the Royal Commission on Aboriginal Peoples. Volume 3: Gathering Strength*. Ottawa: Author.

Royal Commission on Aboriginal Peoples. (1996b). *Report of the Royal Commission on Aboriginal Peoples. Volume 4: Perspectives and Realities.* Ottawa: Author.

Said, E.W. (1978). *Orientalism.* London: Penguin.

Smith, L.T. (1999). *Decolonizing Methodologies: Research and Indigenous Peoples.* Dunedin, NZ: Otago University Press.

Smye, V. (2004). *The Nature of the Tensions and Disjunctures between Aboriginal Understandings of and Responses to Mental Health and Illness and the Current Mental Health System.* Unpublished doctoral dissertation. University of British Columbia, Vancouver.

Spittal, P.M., & Schechter, M.T. (2001). Injection drug use and despair through the lens of gender. *Canadian Medical Association Journal, 164*(6), 802–803.

Spivak, G.C. (1994). Can the subaltern speak? In P. Williams and L. Chrisman (Eds.), *Colonial Discourse and Postcolonial Theory: A Reader* (pp. 66–111). New York: Columbia University Press. (Reprinted from C. Nelson and L. Grossberg, Eds. 1988. *Marxism and the Interpretation of Culture,* pp. 271–313. London: Macmillan).

Statistics Canada. (2003). 2001 Census. *Aboriginal Peoples of Canada: A Demographic Profile.* Ottawa: Author.

Stevenson, W. (1999). Colonialism and First Nations women in Canada. In E. Dua & A. Robertson (Eds.), *Scratching the Surface: Canadian Anti-Racist Feminist Thought* (pp.49–82). Toronto: Women's Press.

Tait, C. (2000). Aboriginal identity and the construction of fetal alcohol syndrome. In L.J. Kirmayer, M.E. Macdonald, & G.M. Brass (Eds.), *Culture and Mental Health Research Unit Report No. 10: The Mental Health of Indigenous Peoples* (pp. 95–111). Montreal: McGill University.

Turpel, M.E. (1993). Patriarchy and paternalism: The legacy of the Canadian state for First Nations women. *Canadian Journal of Women and the Law, 6,* 172–192.

Varcoe, C., Dick, S., & Walther, M. (2004). *Crossing Our Differences Toward Hope and Healing: Preventing HIV/AIDS in the Context of Inequity and Violence Against Women.* Final report and planning document. Williams Lake, BC: Canadian Mental Health Association.

Varcoe, C., & McCormick, J. (2007). Racing around the classroom margins: Race, racism and teaching nursing. In L. Young & B. Paterson (Eds.), *Learning Nursing: Student-Centered Theories, Models, and Strategies for Nurse Educators* (pp. 439–446). Philidelphia: Lippincott, Williams & Wilkins.

Young, R.J.C. (2001). *Postcolonialism: An Historical Introduction.* Oxford: Blackwell.

5 Gender-Based Analysis and Health Policy: The Need to Rethink Outdated Strategies

OLENA HANKIVSKY

Most research has not been especially attentive to sex, gender, and, in particular, sex/gender interactions even though they intersect to affect health status (e.g., diseases, conditions, and illnesses), the healthcare system (in terms of access and quality), and health policy (e.g., development, implementation, and evaluation). The historic neglect of sex and gender and the resultant lack of evidence have been documented by women's groups and health activists who have analysed health research, policy, and programs to determine the extent to which they meet women's needs (Williams, 1999). These evaluations can be seen as part of an international movement, which started 30 years ago to raise awareness and to encourage governments to develop mechanisms and state machinery to advance women's equality in all areas of policy.

A government strategy that has developed to respond to this shortcoming is that of gender mainstreaming (GM), or what is more commonly known in Canada as gender-based analysis (GBA). GM was formally accepted in 1995 as an international strategy to 'assesses the differential impact of proposed and/or existing policies, programs and legislation on women and men' (Status of Women Canada, 1998, p. 4). It has been particularly significant in the area of health. The World Health Organization (WHO, 2002), for example, has stated that 'gender mainstreaming ... must become standard practice in all policies and programmes.' According to Health Canada (2000), GBA 'will help us secure the best possible health for the women and men and girls and boys of Canada' and moreover, that it 'makes for good science and sound evidence by ensuring that biological and social differences between women and men are brought into the foreground (p. 6).' Others claim that 'mainstreaming can also work positive changes for groups marginalized on the basis of race, ability, sexual orientation or poverty' (Teghtsoonian, 1999, p. 11).

In this chapter, the evolution of GM in the Canadian health context is examined. The role of Health Canada in developing GBA frameworks for identifying, analysing, and addressing gender gaps and inequalities in health research and planning is investigated and assessed. Debates and concerns about current strategies are also discussed. What emerges from this overview is that although considerable strides have been made over the last decade, on balance, policy directions and priorities have not been significantly altered. GBA has been confronted with serious political and implementation challenges. Less understood, however, but equally important, are the inherent conceptual limitations of GBA. As evidenced in existing frameworks, ambiguities surrounding the categories of sex and gender persist; differences *among* women with regard to health status, experiences of the health care system, health behaviours, and other determinants of health are not properly identified or responded to. And, the subject of men and men's health has not been addressed adequately. GBA is therefore at a crossroads. Arguably what is required is a paradigm shift that replaces outdated mainstreaming strategies with approaches such as diversity mainstreaming that are better able to address a broad spectrum of health inequalities and their consequences.

Background

In Canada, the preferred term is *gender-based analysis* (GBA) rather than gender mainstreaming (GM).[1] Since the 1970s, when the idea of GBA was first put forward by the Canadian International Development Agency, the government of Canada has provided what can be considered an 'enabling environment' for GBA. For example, in 1976 a strategy of integration was introduced that required a gendered assessment of all federal initiatives. In 1981, Canada ratified the United Nations Convention on the Elimination of All Forms of Discrimination Against Women, committing to the protection of women's human rights, including those relating to health. One year later, in 1982, the Charter of Rights and Freedoms constitutionally entrenched guarantees of equality through Sections 15 and 28.

In 1995, Canada adopted the United Nations' *Platform for Action*, developed in Beijing at the United Nations World Conference on Women.

It was at the Beijing conference that GM was established as the strategy for promoting gender equality internationally. While definitions vary, GM can be understood as 'a strategy for making women's as well as men's concerns and experiences an integral dimension of the design, implementation, monitoring and evaluation of policies and programmes so that women and men benefit equally and inequality is not perpetu-ated' (Economic and Social Council, 1997). Ultimately, the strategy seeks to address the causes and consequences of inequality and to transform gender relations in society. In so doing, GM represents an important shift from earlier strategies which focused solely on address-ing women's needs and reducing the burdens placed upon them by their multiple roles in society and their disproportionate rates of pov-erty (Department for International Development, 1998).

In the same year as the Beijing conference, the government of Canada adopted a national policy to advance women's equality. The Federal Plan for Gender Equality (1995–2000) stated that all subsequent fed-eral legislation and policies were to include, where appropriate, an analysis of the potential for differential impacts on men and women (1995, p. 18).[2] While the plan was intended to cover all areas of policy, specific attention to women's health was made in Chapter 3: 'Improving the Health and Well-being of Women.' In this chapter the government committed itself to a women's health strategy, which was introduced four years later, in 1999, by Health Canada.

The international commitment made in Beijing to gender main-stream-ing was reinforced in 1997 by the United Nations Economic and Social Council (ECOSOC). Five years after Beijing, at the 2000 Beijing +5 conference, the Ad Hoc Committee of the twenty-third special session of the United Nations General Assembly (United Nations, 2000) made specific recommendations for member countries in terms of integrating GM into the area of women's health:

72. (d) Collect and disseminate updated and reliable data on mortality and morbidity of women and conduct further research regarding how social and economic factors affect the health of girls and women of all ages, as well as research about the provision of health-care services to girls and women and the patterns of use of such services and the value of disease prevention and health promotion programmes for women;

80. Develop and use frameworks, guidelines and other practical tools and indicators to accelerate gender mainstreaming, including gender-based

research, analytical tools and methodologies, training, case studies, statistics and information;

92. (c) In partnership, as appropriate, with relevant institutions, promote, improve, systemize and fund the collection of data disaggregated by sex, age and other appropriate factors, on health and access to health services, including comprehensive information on the impact of HIV/AIDS on women, throughout the life-cycle;

(d) Eliminate gender biases in bio-medical, clinical and social research, including by conducting voluntary clinical trials involving women, with due regard for their human rights, and in strict conformity with internationally accepted legal, ethical, medical, safety, and scientific standards, and gather, analyze and make available to appropriate institutions and to end-users gender-specific information about dosage, side-effects and effectiveness of drugs, including contraceptives and methods that protect against sexually transmitted infections.

More recently at Beijing +10, in 2005, the international community reconfirmed its commitments to gender equality. The WHO has also developed a specific gender policy: Integrating Gender Perspectives. The WHO sees its policy as 'contributing to increasing the coverage, effectiveness, efficiency, and ultimately the impact of health interventions for both women and men, while at the same time contributing to achievement of the broader UN goal of social justice' (WHO, 2002, p. 1). Moreover, key international organizations and government from both Northern and Southern countries have come to endorse GM (Vlassoff & Moreno, 2002), and expressly in the area of health.

GM, Health, and the Canadian Context

It is generally understood that Canada uses a dual strategy of mainstreaming gender through 'integrating a gender perspective in all legislation, policies, and programs; and actions specifically targeted to women and children' (United Nations, 2000, p. 2). Many government departments have now established official protocols and guidelines for GBA; GM has therefore been fairly well institutionalized in Canada. Along with Status of Women Canada, Health Canada is a leader in GBA at the conceptual and policy application level. The Women's Health Strategy of 1999 has been an invaluable contribution in this regard as it set out a comprehensive plan for applying GBA in all of Health Canada's research and policy work. As the plan states: 'In keeping with the commitment in the Federal Plan for Gender Equality, Health Canada will, as a matter of standard practice, apply gender-based analysis to programs and policies in the areas of health system modernization, population health, risk management, direct services and research' (Health Canada, 1999, p. 21). The strategy (Health Canada, 1999, Objective 1) necessitates that

- GBA be applied to policies and programs in the areas of health system modernization, population health, risk management, direct services and research.
- Tools, methods and training material be developed to assist in implementing these gender impact assessments across the department and that senior managers be oriented to the requirements of GBA.
- Women's health issues be taken into consideration in the annual planning exercises of the department, including the development of Business Lines.
- A gender perspective informs Health Canada's approach to ethical issues and that consideration be given to those of particular concern to women.
- The inclusion of gender considerations and differential impacts be one of the criteria when assessing research and demonstration proposals for which Health Canada funding is being sought.
- A plan be developed to mobilize interdepartmental collaboration in identifying objectives and initiatives that will address socioeconomic issues related to health.
- Gender analysis of Health Canada's legal work, including legal advice, litigation, legal policy and legislation, be carried out by the Legal Services Unit, supported by the unit's gender equality specialist designated by Justice Canada.

Besides its Women's Health Strategy, in 2000 Health Canada developed a Gender-Based Analysis Policy. The policy confirms the department's commitment to the implementation of a gender-based analysis and outlines ways in which it is being integrated into the policies and programs of Health Canada. The Bureau of Women's Health and Gender Analysis – with its small GBA unit, located in the Health Policy Branch, oversees the implementation and evaluation of GBA, and ensures that women's health concerns are integrated and responded to appropriately by Health Canada. For example, the unit is mandated 'to build GBA expertise through focused capacity building, including training on the theories and practical application of GBA. It has committed resources to developing women's health indicators and guidelines for the development of gender-sensitive health indicators, pilot projects in relevant policy areas, documentation on concepts of gender and health, coaching-style training that guides staff in applying GBA to real-world case studies, and a quarterly bulleting on GBA' (Standing Committee on the Status of Women, 2005, p 20).

According to Health Canada (2000, p. 6), incorporating GBA into all aspects of health policy and research is critical for the following reasons:

- GBA fulfils the Government of Canada's domestic and international commitments to equality between women and men.
- Gender equality is essential to health as defined by the World Health Organization (WHO): *Health is a state of complete physical, mental and social well-being and not merely the absence of disease or infirmity.*
- GBA helps to actualize Health Canada's mandate to ensure equal access to, and benefits from, the health system for all Canadians.
- GBA is essential to understanding and applying health determinants theory because it explores the relationship between gender and the other determinants of health and how this relationship mediates health and the use of health services.
- Good science makes for good policy. Together they lead to better health for all Canadians.
- Good policy safeguards human rights and Canada's commitments to ensuring that Canadians are served by the best possible health policies, programs and services. Good policy is particularly critical in a period of health system renewal.

More recently, in its *Exploring Concepts of Gender and Health*, Health Canada (2003a) reiterated its pledge to gender equality in health by stating that 'in the context of health, the integrated use of GBA throughout the research, policy and program development processes can improve our understanding of sex and gender as determinants of health, of their interaction with other determinants, and the effectiveness of how we design and implement sex and gender-sensitive policies and programs' (p. 1).

What Does GBA in Health Entail?

GBA seeks to understand how and why inequalities occur in health. Within GBA discourses, there is a certain amount of misunderstanding about what gender equality means. In Canada, it is commonly accepted that formal equality, which focuses on sameness of treatment and benefit, has now been replaced by substantive equality, which focuses on the accommodation of differences and overcoming related experiences of oppression, subordination, and material disparities. Substantive equality, or as it sometimes is referred to as gender equity, recognizes that different approaches vis-à-vis men and women may be needed to ensure equitable outcomes. This is especially true in health where women's and men's needs and experiences often differ and substantive knowledge gaps remain about women's health, in particular regarding differences among groups of women. Research is especially lacking for Aboriginal women, women with disabilities, immigrant women, women of colour, older women, and lesbian women who require special attention and dedicated resources.

To illustrate why health research and health care provision should be based on different needs of women and men, Health Canada's (2003b) internationally recognized *Exploring Concepts of Gender and Health*. This analysis, co-authored by a team of health researchers including Hankivsky and Morrow, provides compelling examples of how being male or female affects health, and proposes a number of questions that need to be carefully considered and responded to in order to understand these differentials. These examples are meant to demonstrate clearly why a gender-based analysis is essential to fully understanding health in diverse populations, and for health planning. This section of the report (Health Canada, 2003a) is reproduced below:

Did You Know?

The same drug can cause different reactions and different side effects in women and men – even common drugs like antihistamines and antibiotics. (Makkar, Fromm, Steinman, Meisner, & Lehmann, 1993)

Are all drugs to be used by both men and women tested for their potentially different effects on both sexes before seeking market approval?

Females are more likely than males to recover language ability after suffering a left-hemisphere stroke. (Shaywitz et al., 1995)

How can additional brain research help us improve the outcomes for men, based upon what we already know about how the female brain processes language?

During unprotected intercourse with an infected partner, women are 2 times more likey than men to contract a sexually transmitted infection and 10 times more likely to contract HIV. (Society for Women's Health Research, 2001)

What can be done to reduce women's risk of contracting sexually transmitted infections?

The death rate from suicide is at least four times higher for men than it is for women. However, women are hospitalized for attempted suicide at about one and one-half times the rate of men (Langlois & Morrison, 2002).

Are there differences between men and women in how they respond to stress and reach out for help? What preventive measures can we take that are sensitive to these differences?

Women who smoke are 20 to 70 per cent more likely to develop lung cancer than men who smoke the same number of cigarettes (Manton, 2000; Shriver et al., 2000).

What is it about female physiology that accounts for this difference?

For Aboriginal women, the rate of diabetes is five times higher than it is for all other women in Canada; For Aboriginal men, the rate is three times higher. (Federal, Provincial and Territorial Advisory Committee on Population Health, 1999)

How can programs aimed at decreasing the incidence of diabetes take this knowledge into account?

In 2000, 70 per cent of all person aged 85 or over were female (Health Canada, 2001). While women live longer than men, they are more likely to suffer from long-term activity limitations and chronic conditions such as osteoporosis, arthritis, and migraine headaches. (Federal, Provincial and Territorial Advisory Committee on Population Health, 1999)

How can policies and programs accommodate the health needs of the growing number of senior women in this country?

To begin the process of trying to answer the kinds of questions that are posed above, GBA requires taking into account the effects of past, current, and emerging social patterns and trends on sex and gender (Health Canada, 2003b, p. 11). It involves asking important background questions relating to health, such as those posed by Watson (2003, p. 24):

- To what extent does gender determine health?
- How does it shape one's contact with the health care system?
- How are those participating in the system socialized with respect to health?
- How do health care providers understand gender and how does this exert itself in the care provided?

In the applied context of research, program and policy development, implementation, and evaluation, more specific questions must be fully integrated and made front and centre, including: What goal does the government want to achieve? For whom? How does the health issue or problem at hand affect men and women differently? What are the expected effects for men and women, girls and boys, as well as different groups of women and men? How will the outcomes be evaluated to ensure gender inclusivity? In approaching such questions, GBA also requires analysts and researchers to be aware and reflect upon the kind of values and biases that they bring to their own work (Status of Women Canada, 1998). Attending to these queries 'brings to view the omission and implications' (Health Canada, 2003b, p.1) of health research and policy. GBA thus seeks 'to better illustrate how gender affects health throughout the lifecycle and to identify opportunities to maintain and improve the health of women and men, girls and boys in Canada' (Health Canada, 2003b, p.1). It is an evidence-based approach that is designed to result in programs and policies which are not biased on the basis of either sex or gender.

Evaluating Success: Implementation and Progress

What would successful mainstreaming look like? According to Dr Olive Shisana, former Executive Director, Family and Health Services, WHO, gender will have been successfully mainstreamed 'when policy planners and researchers have internalized the gender perspective and no longer have to be conscious of their behaviour; when their behaviour pattern has changed and become natural; when they can identify the conditions that affect men and women differently, those that affect men more than women and those that affect women more than men; when they can identify risk factors for men and women for each of their conditions and develop different interventions for men and women accordingly' (United Nations et al., 1999). In general, attempts made by Commonwealth countries including Canada to achieve gender equality in health have been limited and therefore only partially successful (Commonwealth Secretariat, 2002 Hankivsky, 2005). The major achievements are that there is a growing recognition that women's health entails more than just reproductive health, that there are concrete differences between sex and gender even though both interact to affect health, that women's health requires sustained research and attention, and that this requires comprehensive sex disaggregated data and gender indicators. Importantly, multidisciplinary research that integrates biomedicine and the social sciences and which draws upon both qualitative and quantitative measures and tools is seen as essential to understanding the complexities and dimensions of women's health.

In Canada, such progress on issues of women's health can be observed in federal and provincial/territorial initiatives and in the work of Health Canada and the Institute of Gender and Health (IGH) within the Canadian Institutes of Health Research (CIHR). Health Canada's GBA efforts are promoted through the production and dissemination of better knowledge of women's health through the Women's Contribution Program, which supports four Centres of Excellence for Women's Health; research networks focusing on health protection, health reform and Aboriginal health; and the Canadian Women's Health Network (Hankivsky, 2005). In addition, the IGH supports research to address how sex (biological factors) and gender (socio-cultural experiences) interact with other factors that influence health to create conditions and problems that are unique, more prevalent, more serious or different with respect to risk factors or effective interventions for women and for men (Canadian Institutes of Health Research, 2003). It is also important to note that the preamble of the Canadian Institutes of Health Research Act (Bill C-13) stated that health research should 'address the respective health issues of children, women and men and of diverse populations of Canada.' While there has been significant progress in developing both practical and theoretical bases for incorporating gender into health (Vlassoff & Moreno, 2002), a number of obstacles remain, beginning with political challenges.

Political Challenges

Key factors for successful GBA implementation include political commitment; sensitization to gender issues among the public; training for decision-makers, implementers, and other officials; adequate funding; efficient and comprehensive information; and data collection systems (Commonwealth Secretariat, 2002, p. 46). Both Status of Women Canada and Health Canada have worked hard to address such implementation challenges. However, these government departments are operating within non-feminist institutional contexts, which both recognize *as well as* marginalize the importance of GBA (Williams, 1999). GBA has therefore not been consistently incorporated into policy development, implementation, or evaluation (Hankivsky, 2005). In fact, even the government of Canada acknowledges that 'we still face challenges to mainstreaming and institutionalizing the application of gender equality objectives, analyses and processes in the work of governments'(Canada, 2004, p.4).

Health Canada explains the limited effectiveness of GBA by stating that 'progress ... has been uneven, supported by the enthusiasm of some individuals and slowed by the resistance of others' (Standing Committee on the Status of Women, 2005, p. 21). GBA is often resisted and rarely systematically applied in either health research or health policy. This is particularly true in the case of health reform in Canada. As in many Western democracies, transformation of the health care system has been underway at unprecedented levels over the last decade, and yet the gendered implications of these changes have not been considered at all stages of policy development, implementation, and evaluation (Grant, 2002; Armstrong et al., 2001). Of course this is extremely problematic because 'doing gender,' as Bolliger-Salzmann and Margaret Duetz (2003) explain, 'does not refer to one single step in a public health project, but ideally makes part of the every day work routine as a matter of course' (p. 209).

A further challenge relates to difficulties in measuring the overall efficacy of GM. Certainly, GM in health research needs to be carefully monitored and evaluated by established gender-based criteria. Such criteria must be clear and built into any policy planning from the beginning (Schofield, 2004). However, 'it is difficult to assess the impact of gender mainstreaming initiatives or to determine the extent to which the objective of equality of outcomes for both women and men is being achieved' (Commonwealth Secretariat, 2002, p. 48). The political resistance to developing appropriate criteria further compounds this. Consequently, as Pollack and Hafner-Burton (2000) argue, 'the lack of clear measures of mainstreaming has thus far placed limits on our ability to assess progress in gender mainstreaming' (p. 15). This is particularly true in the Canadian context, where no formal evaluations of GBA in the health sector have been undertaken (Hankivsky, 2005).

Another contributing impediment to effective GBA is the multi-jurisdictional nature of Canada. Even though GBA has been established as a key federal policy tool, many provincial policies affecting health have been and continue to be developed without a GBA analysis (Hankivsky, 2005; Williams, 1999). Teghstoonian has argued that a gender analysis is required in federal-provincial negotiations because this is precisely the arena in which a wide range of policies, in health and related areas, are decided (1999). Because health intersects with wider social policies, GBA must be applied across the board in order for broad societal change to be realized. At the same time, this does not negate the need for a sustained application of GBA in health among all levels of government, or the possibility for important transformations to be made within the health care system to challenge gender inequalities (Vlassoff & Moreno, 2002). The absence of a systematic application of GBA in health can lead to mistakes in health research and policy, and can be costly in terms of economic and human costs, including lost opportunities, ill health, suffering, and overall societal loss (Hankivsky et al., 2004; Carriere, 1995).

Conceptual Issues

In addition to existing political challenges, much more attention needs to be paid to a number of key conceptual difficulties underpinning the GBA practices discussed below. Not only are these threatening the overall future potential of this strategy, they also make clear the need for an alternative strategy that can overcome the limitations currently associated with GBA in Canada.

Sex and Gender

Often, sex and gender are conflated even though they are distinct variables. Increasingly, for example, gender is being used inappropriately as a substitute for sex, particularly in the biomedical literature, a tendency which has created confusion (Fischman, Wick, & Koening,

1999). As explained in the Introduction, this collection, sex refers to biological differences between women and men and gender refers to socially and culturally determined differences between women and men, the latter of which are embedded in relationships of power. To be sure, the variable of sex is important in analysing 'diseases and disabilities from which women suffer because of their sex; diseases and disabilities for which both men and women suffer, but which are more prevalent in women or that affect women more severely or that have more adverse effects on women during pregnancy or from which women are less able to protect themselves' (Commonwealth Secretariat, 2002, p. 26). However, as Grant (2002) has argued elsewhere, 'It is simplistic to treat the biological variable sex as if it can capture the full array of social, political and economic forces that both structure and produce (ill) health for women and men, or explain the effects of policy changes on individual recipients and providers of care'(p. 23).

Attention to gender is critical because gender can 'determine different exposures to certain risks, different treatment-seeking patterns, or differential impacts of social and economic determinants of health (Greaves et al., 1999). As argued in earlier chapters, the importance of gender as a determinant of health has been well established and recognized, for example, in the Canadian context by Health Canada. That said, there is still a limited comprehension of what is meant by gender and how it applies to health, and even less understanding of how to measure gender differences in health status (Vlassoff, 2004).

Recently the Canadian Institute of Health Research (CIHR, 2006) introduced a gender and sex-based analysis (GSBA) guide intended to 'contribute to knowledge about the ways in which sex and gender- and the interactions between them- influence the health of men and women' While this is an important development, an incomplete understanding of the relationship between sex and gender still remains even though 'most critical for determining health in Canadian women and men are the interactions between sex-linked and gender-based factors that combine to effect health' (Greaves et al., 1999, p. 1). The challenge of understanding this relationship is not confined to the dominant approaches to GBA in Canada. For all fields of health discourse, there exists an inherent difficulty in understanding where 'sex' stops and where 'gender' begins (Green, 2002). 'Sex' is in a constant state of negotiation (Fausto-Sterling, 2000) and gender is also a contested category. Secondly, determining whether a disease is caused by sex or gender is problematic, and the interplay between biomedical and social science explanations are in their nascent stages of development (Hoffman, 2000). While it is important to be able to ascertain how sex and gender interrelate, less apparent in the literature as argued in earlier chapters is the importance of understanding the differences between sex and gender because 'their range of explanatory validity is not coterminous' (Green, 2002). Green is correct in pointing out that what may distinguish women on the basis of biology does not necessarily characterize all women as gendered beings. And, as the following section demonstrates, the tendency to essentialize women on the basis of gender is also an inherently problematic feature of GBA, one that has significant consequences for social justice in the realm of health research and policy.

Diversity/Difference

Health Canada's *Gender-based Analysis Policy* (Health Canada, 2000) states that the GBA framework should intersect with a diversity analysis which considers factors such as race, ethnicity, level of ability, and sexual orientation. Diversity analysis is a process of examining ideas, policies, programs, and research to assess their potentially different impact on specific *groups* of women and men, girls and boys. It acknowledges that neither men nor women comprise homogeneous groups, but rather that class or socio-economic status, age, sexual orientation, gender identity, race, ethnicity, geographic location, education, and physical and mental ability – among other things – may distinctly affect a specific group's health needs, interests, and concerns. Health Canada's policy, like many others that currently inform GBA, endeavors to reflect an understanding of how gender intersects with other axes of discrimination and disadvantage. And yet, within these frameworks, the hegemony of gender is maintained. As Teghtsoonian (1999) has noted, 'Despite drawing attention to the specific circumstances of multiply-marginalized women, the focus in these documents tends to remain on "gender-in general"' (p. 5). As a result, when differences are taken into account, they are treated as constituting add-on dimensions to the variable of gender, even by women's health researchers. Not only does this marginalize their significance, it often leads to the essentialization and creation of the 'Other,' which perpetuates the privilege that is experienced by affluent, educated, white women (Watson, 2003). The assumptions and biases that get replicated in current GBA lead to incomplete and potentially dangerous analyses. And, as Watson reminds women's health researchers: 'We cannot work towards equity with respect to gender and not be prepared to look at our own intellec-tual, colonialist, and economic advantage and the effect it has on others' (p. 24).

Any worthwhile and effective mainstreaming strategy must assess differences in women's health vis-à-vis other women (Green, 2002). The need to better integrate the various factors that influence health among women has been discussed for some time by researchers. However, 'experience shows that it is difficult to weave gender and other dimen-sions of diversity such as race, sexual orientation and ability into policy analysis, program development and institutional structures' (Teght-soonian 1999, p. 4). The observation made by Krieger, Rowley, Herman, Avery, & Phillips (1993) that an approach for investigating the relation-ship between racism, sexism, classism, and health 'had yet to be synthe-sized into a well-defined paradigm' (p. 99) holds as true for today as when this argument was first made. Such integration is essential to any adequate understanding of the health needs of diverse groups of women.

Take, for example, turberculosis (TB). Recognized globally as a major public health problem (WHO, 2000), research has neglected the gendered aspects of this disease even though TB is a leading killer of women of reproductive age worldwide (WHO, 1999). A traditional GBA analysis may provide better information on how biology and gender affect the risk of infection, progression to disease, diagnosis, social consequences, access to care and cure, and fatality from TB, provided that the catego-ries of sex and gender are not confused. Research of this nature should reveal, for instance, the social stigma for women associated with TB (Long, Johansson, Diwan, & Winkivist, 2001). It would probably also demonstrate that the progression from infection to disease and death are significantly higher for women (Demissie & Lindtjorn, 2003). A GBA analysis may also lead us to consider how different women experience TB, but it would not necessarily lead us to understand fully the layers of complexities associated with TB, for example, within First Nations popu-lations in Canada. This is because gender, more than any other variable is considered *key* to understanding health disparities with a GBA frame-work.

To illustrate: TB rates among Aboriginal populations remain 8 to 10 times higher than overall Canadian rates, and 20 to 30 times higher than Canadian-born, non-Aboriginal rates (Health Canada, 2002). So why is TB so predominant among First Nations and, in particular, for First Nations women between the ages of 25 and 34 (Health Canada, 2003b)? First Nations people experience huge political, economic, and social disparities, and poverty, which all have been linked to TB. Once infected with the TB bacteria, persons in this population are at increased risk of developing TB because of high rates of substance abuse, diabetes, and HIV/AIDS. In addition, overcrowded housing, a common feature on reserves, increases the likelihood that infectious cases will spread TB to others (Health Canada, 2002). Finally, delay in detection and inadequate services also contribute to the overall tuberculosis problem in Aboriginal peoples.

Certainly GBA facilitates a better understanding of how some of these experiences may be gendered within the First Nations community. Neither the National Tuberculosis Elimination Strategy (Health Canada, 1992) nor more recent efforts by Health Canada explicitly call for a gender analysis of TB. However, a typical GBA approach would not necessarily provide us with the contextual understanding of all the social, economic, and cultural variables, many of which are more important than gender in determining differences between non-Aboriginal and Aboriginal women and men. Specifically, oppressive systems of race relations and how these structure the lives of First Nations people, and especially how these shape experiences of both health and disease, are marginalized within current GBA frameworks in Canada.

In the United States, Fee and Krieger (1994) have furthered the understanding of how people's experiences of and responses to discrimination influences their health. As Whittle and Inhorn (2001) explain, they 'demonstrate the importance of looking at social inequalities from multiple locations, in order to make obvious not only how they constitute harmful risks, but also how they confer privileges and benefits that may be protective against disease and ill-health' (p. 158). This type of perspective entails challenging the hegemony of gender as *the* variable, and instead explicitly taking into account the range of variables and contexts which inform explanations of health inequities. As Green argues: 'analysis of multiple axes of difference is not 'optional'; rather, it is central to any comprehensive attempt to understand and alleviate suffering' (Green, 2002). Without doubt, effective TB control cannot be achieved so along as the disease is considered in isolation from the full range of social processes that create the condition (and affect biology), facilitate its spread, and create barriers to care (Demissie & Lindtjorn, 2003, p. 241). But as Teghstoonian (1999) notes, 'Further work needs to be done to weave systematically into gender analysis a focus on race, sexual orientation and ability, and to weave gender into lens-based work on other marginalized groups' (p. 4).

What is needed is an altogether new conceptual framework that combines intersecting axes of discrimination but does not privilege gender over other determinants of health. McDonough and Walters (2001) similarly note that 'we cannot count on a homogeneity of experience for either sex, nor must we generalize about gender or look at gender in isolation' (p. 20). This does require charting new territory because little progress has been made with mainstreaming techniques away from the field of gender (Shaw, 2005). One of the key problems is that 'the discursive effects of [GM] on constructions of gender and equality are not being interrogated. In particular, the potential of recent feminist theory for providing conceptual and analytical knowledge of the complex circumstances involving gender differences, inter-sectionalities, and multiple identities remains largely uninvestigated' (Hankivsky, 2005, p. 2).

As I have proposed elsewhere (Hankivsky, 2005), a viable alternative, one that would pay sufficient attention to differences and power relationships would be 'diversity mainstreaming'.[1] Diversity mainstreaming represents a new direction in the Canadian health policy context. The specific proposal I put forward builds on Iris Marion Young's (1994) notion of 'gender as seriality,' and Kimberlé Williams Crenshaw's (1991, 2000) work on intersectionalities. It also draws on a number of alternative models of mainstreaming developed in the United Kingdom (Donaghy, 2004; Beveridge and Nott, 2002; Rees, 1998). Diversity mainstreaming retains the category of gender, albeit in a qualified manner. Most importantly, it puts front and centre various forms of oppression (e.g., 'race'/ethnicity, class, ability, sexuality, religion) and explores how they interconnect and mutually reinforce one another (Hankivsky, 2005). Referring to this proposal, Shaw (2005) argues that far from diluting GM, the mainstreaming of diversity realizes the transformative potential of the mainstreaming option and prevents its failing and disappointing (p. 24).

Mainstreaming Men

Another related key conceptual challenge in GM is the conflation of gender with women. Feminists, and femocrats alike, are not always willing to explicitly acknowledge that GBA as it is currently understood and applied, is not inclusive of both women and men. In fact, as Chant and Gutmann (2000) argue, 'There is scant evidence of 'male-inclusive' gender initiatives on the ground' (p. 2). Similarly, Doyal (2001) has noted that 'until recently, very little attention has been paid to the impact of gender on men's health' (p. 2). Although some may argue that any attention to men 'represents an unjustifiable detraction from the struggle to make women's concerns as central as men's' (Chant & Gutmann, 2000, p. 4), gender-sensitive standards are needed (Brown, 2001). This is completely consistent with the entire rationale behind GM: the recognition that mainstreaming gender concerns is more effective than focusing only on women, and expecting that it is women who need to change in order to integrate (Saulnier et al., 1999). Indeed as Schofield, Connell, Walker, Wood, & Bultand (2000) argue, 'We need to develop an integrated approach in which men's health and women's health are seen in relation to each other' (p. 254).

This does not mean, however, that women-sensitive or -centred approaches cannot be part of GBA. As the WHO (1998) has rightly observed, 'A mainstreaming strategy does not preclude initiatives specifically directed toward women or toward men.' In most countries, as is the case of Canada, targeted policies may continue to be necessary as women in general continue to experience a disproportionate share of material, social, and civil disadvantage (Chant & Gutmann, 2000). This comparative disadvantage, however, does not negate the fact that mainstreaming gender in health needs to be expanded to include men. For many policy makers, part of what makes GM more palatable than its historic predecessors is the fact that it focuses on evaluating adverse impacts of research, on 'women *and men*' (emphasis added) (Beveridge, Knott, & Stephen, 2000, p. 391). Most importantly, gender is also a health issue for men.

Evidence from many countries and societies demonstrate that gender roles can adversely affect men's health as well as women's health (Commonwealth Secretariat, 2002). For example, the values associated with masculinity, including competitiveness, material success, and engaging in risk-taking behaviour, have health repercussions (Cohen, 2004). The disproportionate levels of accidents, substance abuse, suicide, and violence for males have been noted, although little is known about the relationship between health problems and masculinities (Chant & Gutmann, 2000). Particular health differences among Aboriginal men, men from non-English-speaking backgrounds, gay men, and men of low socio-economic status have been noted (Schofield et al., 2000). Men's reluctance to seek medical help is also linked to gender roles, especially the expectation that they should be strong and capable of suffering without complaint (Vlassoff & Moreno, 2002). And, the mistake is often made to assume that existing health services, because they fall short in meeting women's requirements, are accessible to all men and effective in terms of meeting their unique health needs (Brown, 2001).

The future success of GBA depends on its ability to serve more than just the interests of women. As Annandale (1998) correctly notes, 'In a search for the causes of illness in gendered positions we neglect the similarities in health (and disease) between men and women and the differences within men as a group and within women as a group' (p. 155). If we want GM to be a transformative strategy, we need to rethink how it can be a pluralistic approach that values the diversity of both men and women (Booth & Bennett, 2002). This involves addressing men and masculinities in gender policy and planning, and in particular developing an analytic framework for GM that explicitly recognizes that women and men have different but overlapping gender roles and access and control over resources and health needs (Levy, Taher, & Vouhé, 2000). In sum, if GM is used to its potential, a deeper understanding of sex/gender and other simultaneously interlocking social categories will be gained if men are part of the analysis. As Sweetman (1997) puts it, 'Men and masculinities need to be studied if power relations between the sexes are to be changed for the better' (p. 2).

Conclusion

As evidenced by the discussion in this chapter, GM and specifically GBA in the Canadian context, have made important inroads in terms of women's health. The international and national commitments that have been made by various levels of government demonstrate the extent to which, at the levels of legislation, research, and policy, gender is understood as a significant variable for understanding women's health. At the same time, commitments to gender equality and recognition of the significance of GBA are in themselves inadequate. What is required at this juncture in health policy evolution is critical reflection upon the goals of GBA within the health context, taking, for example, the first objective of Health Canada's *Women's Health Strategy* (Health Canada, 1999), namely to ensure that 'policies and programmes are responsive to sex, gender, and women's health needs.'

Clearly, numerous political obstacles remain which need to be addressed. Even more importantly, issues regarding the conceptual adequacy (which have very real practical implications) of existing approaches and framework need to be challenged. What is required is a paradigm shift. Essential to such a process is resolving conceptual ambiguities regarding sex and gender and their interactions. At the same time, an understanding that sex and gender are not the only and may not be the most important variables for understanding women's health needs to be recognized. Efforts to mainstream equity and bring about important changes in health will require a much more comprehensive understanding of the context of women's lives, especially of those women who have been, and continue to be, marginalized and oppressed within Canadian society and especially in the health care system. What is required is an approach that is able to accommodate more than just sex and gender, but also the numerous variables that interact and produce synergies that impact on health. I have referred to this alternative as a 'diversity mainstreaming' framework rather than a GM framework. Not only will this lead to better responsiveness to all women's health issues, this type of comprehensive approach will also further the understanding of men's health. The kind of shift proposed in this chapter can also be understood as a change in philosophy that requires not only the recognition that 'gender' is not synonymous with 'women or sex,' but also a new lens that allows for the full examination of men and women within the context of their culturally defined roles, constraints, and potentialities (Vlassoff & Moreno, 2002).

NOTES

1 The terms *GBA* and *GM* will be used interchangeably in the chapter.
2 Since then, the government has introduced a subsequent five-year plan: Agenda for Gender Equality (2000–2005).
3 For a fuller elaboration of this approach, see O. Hankivsky (2005).

REFERENCES

Annandale, E. (1998). *The Sociology of Health and Medicine: A Critical Introduction*. Malen, MA: Polity Press.
Armstrong, P., Amaratunga, C., Bernier, J., Grant, K., Pederson, A., & Willson, K. (Eds.). (2001). *Exposing Privatization: Women and Health Care Reform in Canada*. Health Care in Canada Series. Aurora, ON: Garamond Press.

Beveridge, F., & Nott, S. (2002). Mainstreaming: A case for optimism and cynicism, *Feminist Legal Studies, 10,* 299–311.

Beveridge, F., Nott, S., & Stephen, K. (Eds.). (2000). *Making Women Count: Integrating Gender into Law and Policy Making.* Aldershot, UK: Ashgate.

Bolliger-Salzmann, H., & Duetz, M. (2003). Teaching gender mainstreaming in public health. *Soz-Präventivmed, 48,* 209–210.

Booth, C., & Bennett, C. (2002). Gender mainstreaming in the European Union: Towards a new conception and practice of equal opportunities? *European Journal of Women's Studies, 9* (4), 430–446.

Brown, S. (2001). *Mainstreaming Gender in Health: From Theory to Practice.* Melbourne, Australia: Women's Health Victoria.

Canada, Government of (2004). *Canada's Response to UN.* Retrieved 5 March 2005, from http://www.un.org/womenwatch/daw/Review/responses .htm Ottawa, June 2004.

Canadian Institutes of Health Research. (2003). *Institute of Gender and Health.* Retrieved 29 August 2004, from http://www.cihr-irsc.gc.ca/e/11767.html.

Canadian Institutes of Health Research. (2006). *Gender and Sex-based Analysis in Health Research: A Guide for CIHR Peer Review Committees.* http:// www.cihr-irsc.gc.ca/e/32019.html.

Carriere, E. (1995). *Seeing Is Believing: Education Through a Gender Lens.* Vancouver: University of British Columbia.

Chant, S., & Gutmann, M. (2000). *Mainstreaming Men into Gender and Development: Debates, Reflections, and Experiences.* Oxford: Oxfam Publishing.

Cohen, M. (2004, May). The Impact of Gender on Health. Presentation to Northern Ontario Medical School. Retrieved 29 August 2004, from http:// www.normed.ca/events_publications/symposia/.

Commonwealth Secretariat. (2002). *Gender Mainstreaming in the Health Sector: Experiences in Commonwealth Countries.* New gender mainstreaming series on development issues. London: Commonwealth Secretariat.

Crenshaw, K.W. (1991). Mapping the margins: Intersectionality, identity politics, and violence against women of color. *Stanford Law Review, 43*(6), 1241–99.

Crenshaw, K.W. (2000). Background paper for the expert meeting on the gender-related aspects of race discrimination. Zagreb, Croatia. Retrieved 9 March 2004, from http://www.wicej.addr.com/wcar_docs/crenshaw.html.

Department for International Development (DfID). (1998). *Breaking the Barriers: Women and the Elimination of World Poverty.* London: Author.

Demissie, M., & Lindtjorn, B. (2003). Gender perspective in health: Does it matter in turberculosis control? *Ethiopian Journal of Health, 17* (3), 239–243.

Donaghy, T.B. (2004). Applications of mainstreaming in Australia and North Ireland. *International Political Science Review, 25*(4), 393–410.

Doyal, L. (2001). Sex, gender, and science in health research. Forum 5. The 10/90 gap in health research: assessing the progress. Plenary session on Gender and health research: from evidence to practice. (9–12 October 2001), Geneva.

Economic and Social Council (ECOSOC). E/1997/66. Section IA. Adopted by ECOSOC 18 July 1997. Retrieved 29 August 2004, from http://www.un .org/womenwatch/osagi/intergovernmentalmandates.htm.

Fausto-Sterling, A. (2000). *Sexing the Body: Gender Politics and the Construction of Sexuality.* New York: Basic Books.

Federal, Provincial and Territorial Advisory Committee on Population Health. (1999). *Toward a Healthy Future: Second Report on the Health of Canadians.* Ottawa: Minister of Public Works and Government Services Canada. Retrieved 6 May 2003, from http://www.hc-sc.gc.ca/hppb/phdd/report/toward/.

Fee, E., & Krieger, N. (Eds.). (1994). *Women's Health, Power, and Politics: Essays on Sex/Gender, Medicine and Public Health.* Amityville, NY: Baywood.

Fischman, R.J., Wick, J.G., & Koenig, B.A. (1999). The use of 'sex' and 'gender' to define and characterize meaningful differences between men and women. In *National Institutes of Health. Agenda for Research on Women's Health in the 21st Century.* Vol. 1. Washington, DC: Office of Research on Women's Health.

Grant, K. (2002, January). *Gender-Based Analysis: Beyond the Red Queen Syndrome.* Presentation at the Gender Based Analysis Fair. Ottawa.

Greaves, L., Hankivsky, O., Amaratunga, C., Ballem, P., Chow, D., De Koninck, M., et al. (1999). *CIHR 2000: Sex, Gender and Women's Health.* Vancouver: British Columbia Centre of Excellence for Women's Health.

Green, M. (2002). *Defining Women's Health: An Interdisciplinary Dialogue.* Background Draft. Retrieved 15 April 2002, from http://www.fas.harvard .edu/womenstudy/events/proposal.htm.

Hankivsky, O. (2005). Gender mainstreaming vs. diversity mainstreaming: A preliminary examination of the role and transformative potential of feminist theory. *Canadian Journal of Political Science, 38*(4), 00–00.

Hankivsky, O., with the Canadian Women's Health Network. (2005). *Women's Health in Canada: Beijing and Beyond.* Retrieved 18 March 2005, from http:// dawn.thot.net/cwhn_beijing_response-health.htm.

Hankivsky, O., Friesen J., Varcoe, C., McPhail, F., Greaves, L., & Spencer, C. (2004). Expanding economic costing in health care: Values, gender and diversity. *Canadian Public Policy, 30*(3), 257–282.

Health Canada, Medical Services Branch (1992). *National Tuberculosis Elimina-tion Strategy*. Ottawa: Working Group on tuberculosis, 10 June 1992.

Health Canada. (1999). *Health Canada's Women's Health Strategy*. Ottawa: Minister of Public Works and Government Services Canada. Retrieved 29 August 2004, from http://www.hc-sc.gc.ca/english/women/womenstrat.htm.

Health Canada. (2000). *Health Canada's Gender-Based Analysis Policy*. Ottawa: Minister of Public Works and Government Services Canada. Retrieved 29 August 2004, from http://www.hc-sc.gc.ca/english/women/gba_policy.htm.

Health Canada. (2001) *Canada's Seniors, Statistical Snapshot: More Women than Men*. Retrieved 29 August 2004, from http://www.hc-sc.gc.ca/seniors-aines/pubs/factoids/2001/toc_e.htm.

Health Canada. (2002). *TB in First Nations Communities*. Retrieved 8 August 2004, from http://www.hc-sc.gc.ca/fnihb/phcph/tuberculosis/tb_fni_communities.htm.

Health Canada. (2003a). *Tuberculosis in Canada 2001*. Ottawa: Minister of Public Works and Government Services.

Health Canada (with Pederson, A., Hankivsky, O., Morrow, M., & Greaves, L.). (2003b). *Exploring Concepts of Gender and Health*. Retrieved 29 August 2004, from http://www.hc-sc.gc.ca/english/women/exploringconcepts.htm.

Health Canada, Medical Services Branch. (1992). *National Tuberculosis Elimina-tion Strategy*. Ottawa: Working Group on Tuberculosis, 10 June 1992.

Hoffman, E. (2000, November). Women's health and complexity science. *Academic Medicine, 75*(11), 1102–6.

Krieger, N., Rowley, D., Herman, A.A., Avery B., & Phillips, M.T. (1993). Racism, sexism, and social class: Implications for studies of health, disease and well-being. In D. Rowler & H. Tosteson (Eds), Racial differences in preterm delivery: Developing a new research paradigm. *American Journal of Preventative Medicine, 6* (Suppl. 9), 82–122.

Langlois, S., & Morrison, P. (2002). Suicide deaths and suicide attempts. *Health Reports* (Statistics Canada, cat. no. 82-003, pp.9–22). Retrieved 6 May 2003, from http://www.statcan.ca/english/indepth/82-003/feature/hrar2002013002s0a01/pdf.

Levy, C., Taher, N., & Vouhé, C. (2000, April). Addressing men and masculini-ties in GAD. *IDS Bulletin, 31*(2).

Long, N.H., Johansson, E., Diwan, L., & Winkvist, A. (2001). Fear of social isolation as consequences of tuberculosis in Vietnam: A gender analysis. *Health Policy, 58*(1), 69–81.

Makkar, R.R., Fromm, B.S., Steinman, R.T., Meisnner, M.D., & Lehmann, M.H. (1993). Female gender as a risk factor for torsades de pointes associated with cardiovascular drugs. *Journal of the American Medical Association, 270,* 2590–2597.

Manton, K.G. (2000). Gender differences in cross-sectional and cohort age dependence of cause-specific mortality: The United States, 1962–1995. *Journal of Gender-Specific Medicine, 3,* 47–54.

McDonough, P., and Walters, V. (2001). Gender and health: Reassessing patterns and explanations. *Social Science & Medicine, 52,* 547–559.

Pollack, M.A., & Hafner-Burton, E. (2000). Mainstreaming gender in the European Union. *Journal of European Public Policy, 7*(3), 432–456.

Rees, T. (1998). *Mainstreaming Equality in the European Union: Education, Training, and Labour Market Policies.* London: Routledge.

Saulnier, C., Bentley, S., Gregor, F., MacNeil, G., Rathwell, T., & Skinner, E. (1999). *Gender Mainstreaming: Developing a Conceptual Framework for En-Gendering Health Public Policy.* Halifax: Maritime Centre of Excellence for Women's Health.

Schofield, T. (2004). *Boutique Health? Gender and Equity in Health Policy.* Commissioned Paper Series 2004/08. Sydney: Australian Health Policy Institute, University of Sydney.

Schofield, T., Connell, W., Walker, L., Wood, J., Butland, D. (2000). Understanding men's health and illness: A gender-relations approach to policy, research, and practice. *Journal of American College Health, 48*(6), 247–256.

Shaw, J. (2005). 'Mainstreaming equality and diversity in European Union law and policy.' *Current Legal Problems, 38,* 1–46.

Shaywitz, B.A., Shaywitz, S.E., Pugh, K.R., Constable, R.T, Skudlarski, P., Fulbright, R.K., Bronen, R.A., Fletcher, J.M., Shankweiler, D.P., Katz, L., & Gores, J.C. (1995). Sex differences in the functional organization of the brain for language. *Nature, 373,* 607–609.

Shriver, S.P., Bourdeau, H.A., Gubish, C.T., Tirpak, D.L., Davis, A.L., Luketich, J.D., & Siegfried, J.M. (2000). Sex-specific expression of gastrin-releasing peptide receptor: Relationship to smoking history and risk of lung cancer. *Journal of the National Cancer Institute, 92,* 24–33.

Society for Women's Health Research. (2001). *Women and Men: 10 Differences That Make a Difference.* Retrieved 6 May 2003, from http://www.womens-health.org/policy/Priorities/10Differences.htm.

Standing Committee on the Status of Women. (2005, April). *Gender-Based Analysis: Building Blocks for Success.* Report of the Standing Committee on Status of Women. Retrieved 15 May 2005 www.parl.gc.ca.

Status Canada of Women. (1998). *Gender-Based Analysis: A Guide for Policy-*

Making. Retrieved 29 August 2004, from http://www.swc-cfc.gc.ca/pubs/gbaguide/gbaguide_e.html.

Sweetman, C. (1997). Editorial. In C. Sweetman (Ed.), *Men and Masculinity*. Oxford: Oxfam.

Teghtsoonian, K. (1999). Centring women's diverse interests in health policy and practice: A comparative discussion of gender analysis. Prepared for Made to Measure: Designing Research, Policy and Action Approaches to Eliminate Gender Inequity. National Symposium. Halifax, 3–6 October 1999.

United Nations. (2000). Commission on the Status of Women 44th session and preparatory committee for the special session of the General Assembly. *Women 2000: Gender Equality, Development and Peace for the Twenty-first Century*. 28 February – 17 March 2000. New York. Retrieved 29 August 2004, from http://www.swc-cfc.gc.ca/resources/b5-objectives_e.html.

United Nations, WHO, & UNFPA. (1999). *Women and Health: Mainstreaming the Gender Perspective into the Health Sector*. Report of Expert Group Meeting, 28 September–2 October 1998. Tunis (Tunisia).

Vlassoff, C. (2004). *Mainstreaming a Gender-Sensitive Agenda in Health Research: Perspective of International Organizations*. Prepared for the Canadian International Development Agency. Retrieved 29 August 2004, from http://www.globalforumhealth.org/Non_compliant_pages/forum3/Forum3doc951.htm.

Vlassoff, C., & Moreno, G. (2002). Placing gender at the centre of health programming: Challenges and limitations. *Social Science & Medicine, 54*, 1713–1723.

Watson, S. (2003, March). *Gender in Medical Education. A Collaborative Curriculum Project*. Phase 1. Final report. Undergraduate Education Committee. Gender Issues Committee Council of Ontario Faculties of Medicine. Retrieved 29 August 2004, from http://ohs.cou.on.ca/_bin/publications.cfm.

Whittle, L., & Inhorn, M. (2001). Rethinking difference: A feminist reframing of gender/race/class for the improvement of women's health research. *Social Construction of Health and Disease, 3* (1), 147–165.

Williams, W. (1999). Will the Canadian government's commitment to use a gender-based analysis result in public policies reflecting the diversity of women's lives? Prepared for Made to Measure: Designing Research, Policy and Action Approaches to Eliminate Gender Inequity. National Symposium. 3–6 October 1999, Halifax.

World Health Organization (WHO). (1998). *Gender and Health*. Technical paper. Retrieved 29 August 2004, from http://www.who.int/reproductive-health/publications/WHD_98_16_gender_and_health_technical_paper/WHD_98_ 16_table_of_contents_en.html.

World Health Organization (WHO). (1999). Gender and tuberculosis control: Towards a strategy for research and action. Draft strategy paper prepared for Communicable Disease Prevention, Control, and Eradication. Geneva: World Health Organization.

World Health Organization (WHO). (2000). *Global Tuberculosis Report*. Geneva: World Health Organization.

World Health Organization (WHO). (2002). *Director-General's Executive Statement on WHO Gender Policy: Integrating Gender Perspectives in the Work of WHO Integrating Gender Perspectives in the Work of WHO*. Geneva. Retrieved 29 August 2004, from http://www.who.int/entity/gender/mainstreaming/ENGwhole.pdf.

Young, I.M. (1994). 'Gender as seriality: Thinking about women as a social collective.' *Signs 19*(3): 713–738.

6 Engendering Evidence: Transforming Economic Evaluations

OLENA HANKIVSKY AND JANE FRIESEN

Two important issues are currently at the forefront of Canadian health policy: fiscal considerations and gender inequalities in health, particularly those affecting women. In the first instance, the commitment to publicly funded health care in Canada is being scaled back in response to a variety of pressures from within the health care system and to an evolving fiscal culture in which cost containment and reduced public health expenditures are prevalent. As a result, evidence-based medicine (EBM) and evidence-based policy making (EBP), which claim to reduce waste, are seen as essential to the health sector. In the second instance, there is increasing recognition that all policy decisions need to be 'gender aware' and 'diversity inclusive,' and that improving women's health requires a solid evidence base (Correa-de-Araujo, 2004, p. 31). Although it is assumed that EBM and EBP lead to better health care decisions, it is important to question if they lead to better health care for women, and, in particular, whether there are inherent flaws in their methods and application that are leading to the production of incomplete knowledge and potentially misleading information. It is essential to assess whether evidence is robust and gender inclusive, and especially whether it effectively mediates our understandings of intersecting factors that influence differentials in women's health.

In this chapter, we briefly review evidence-based medicine and evidence-based policy decision-making. In so doing we observe that considerable progress has been made to date in revealing the biases in medical research, especially in terms of gender biases. Less progress has been made in the area of health policy research – in Canada or elsewhere – particularly with regard to the economic evaluations that inform evidence-based policy. In particular, cost-effectiveness analysis

(CEA) and cost of illness studies (COI), which have become central to realizing the goals of policy efficiency, have not been subject to the same level of critical analysis. The argument that we make in this chapter is that if evidence-based policy is to be sufficient, effective, and specifically beneficial to women's health, work needs to be done to better understand the gender and diversity biases inherent in the methods of economic evaluations.

Developing methodological approaches that incorporate equity dimensions into economic evaluations has been recognized as a matter of priority (Sassi, Archard, & Le Grand, 2001). To meet this objective, we approach CEA and COI using a feminist ethical perspective that emphasizes social justice and focuses on gender and diversity. Heeding Ruzeck's (1999) observation that feminists will not make meaningful strides unless they are able to recognize the urgency of cost containment and integrate this consideration into their agenda for health reform (p. 304), our goal is not to reject economic evaluations, but instead to explore how they can be strengthened. This approach brings to light much that is limiting, biased, or missing from current approaches, including the uptake of narrow biomedical conceptualizations of health that exclude private-sphere health responsibilities, work, and costs, and CEA and COI methodologies that pay little attention to distributional consequences of health decisions. The proposition of methodological alternatives that are robust, and, in particular, inclusive of women's lives and perspectives in all their diversity, are intended to illustrate the largely uninvestigated potential for evidence-based decision-making and quantitative data, and to bridge the often conflicting goals of equity and efficiency in health policy.

Evidence-Based Medicine

Evidence 'is a particular kind of information, being the knowledge derived from research' (Gray, 1997, p. 1). It is the 'product at the end of a long line of assumptions and choices at the levels of epistemology, theory, methodology and methods' (Crotty, 1998, quoted in Marks, 2002, p. 8). Evidence-based medicine (EBM), originally developed in Canada at McMaster University, has received considerable attention in the past decade (Egger, Davey Smith, & Altman, 2001). Having evolved from clinical epidemiology, evidence-based medicine is 'the conscientious, explicit and judicious use of current best evidence in making decisions about the care of individual patients' (Sackett, Rosenberg, &

Grey, 1996). EBM is premised on the idea 'that scientific medical knowledge exists in some way uncontaminated by social life, and that it can be applied unproblematically to the human being' (Willis & White, 2003, p. 35). Lin explains that EBM entails 'deconstructing, stripping away of contexts, controlling for bias, and searching for universal truth' (Lin & Gibson, 2003, p. 7). Its perceived benefits are improved treatment, greater openness in clinical decision-making, and better informed patients regarding the potential benefits and harms of different treatments (Rogers, 2004).

Considerations relating to quality of evidence, relevance of evidence, and strength of evidence are key in EBM (NHMRC, 2000). Within the EBM movement, the focus on quality of evidence, for example, has been operationalized in the Cochrane and Campbell collaborations,[1] which are systematic reviews of 'high quality' evidence for social and health policy (Dobrow, Vivek, & Upshur, 2004). These reviews are based on the epistemologies of positivist realism[2] (Marks, 2002). The 'best' evidence is usually defined as that which is 'objective,' quantifiable and replicable. RCTs (randomized controlled clinical trials)[3] are considered the gold standard of design validity and reliability; that is, they employ what is widely thought to be the most effective method for determining the effectiveness of treatments and drugs, ensuring 'scientifically agreed protection from error' (McQueen & Anderson, 2001).

Increasingly, the research 'evidence' of EBM is being questioned and contested. For example, the evidence derived from RCTs is seen as necessary but not sufficient for making effective clinical decisions (Willis & White, 2003; Victora, Habicht, & Bryce, 2004). Evidence hierarchies that priorize RCTs are viewed as 'overly prescriptive, restrictive and narrow' (Marks, 2002, p. 4). They are criticized for constraining the full range of potential evidentiary data, including observational studies, qualitative research, and individual clinical expertise on decision-making (Ter Meulen & Dickenson, 2002; Djulbegovic, Morris, & Lyman, 2000). In addition, the objective and value-free claims of EBM are being challenged and the role of moral values in methods and evidence production is being revealed (Biller-Andorno, Reidar, & Meulen, 2002). Feminists have observed that emotion and intuition have little legitimate place in EBM (Armstrong, 2001). And yet, intuitive insights are commonplace in general practice, clinical decision-making, and health care policy making, challenging the notion that decision-making is entirely a logical and deductive process (Champagne, Lemieux-Charles, & McQuire, 2004; Greenhalgh, 2002). As Greenhalgh argues, there exists a false dichotomy between evidence-based medicine and clinical intuition. There is both a science and art to EBM which requires, when available, research evidence as well as 'subjective interpretations of patients' stories from which plausible hypotheses about causation, prognosis, and therapy are generated before being tested against research-derived evidence (Greenhalagh, 2002). And, lastly, the need to involve citizens, as both interest groups and individuals, in terms of setting priorities for research and choosing outcomes measures has been recognized as a means for improving EBM (Tallacchini, 2002; Dickenson & Vineis, 2002).

Rogers (2004) argues that 'in an ideal world, EBM would further the health of all people, including women' (p. 54). What has counted as evidence derived from EBM, and specifically from RCTs, has not always been inclusive or appropriate for women's health. Although EBM has been effective in countering medical 'traditions' in maternal care, the differential effects and biases for different population groups, including women and Aboriginal populations (Rogers, 2004; Armstrong, 2001, NAHO, 2001) have been identified. For example, major studies of cardiovascular disease, including the 1982 Multiple Risk Factor Intervention Trial, the 1986 Coronary Drug Project, and the 1988 Physician's Health Study did not include any female participants, even though the evidence produced in these has informed the treatment and prevention of heart disease. The problem of this gender-exclusive research is two-fold: it perpetuates the myth that cardiovascular disease is a man's disease; and, by applying the findings to the female population, it leads to faulty understanding and responsiveness to women's CVD. The uncritical acceptance of similar empirical evidence on gender and health prevailed for many years in other areas of health research, including HIV/AIDS (Hunt & Annandale, 1999). The generality of the research bias towards male subjects is demonstrated clearly by the fact that 85 per cent of research participants in the United States and 95 per cent of research participants in Canada are male (Sherr, 2000).

Feminists have also observed the incomplete methods and practices of scientific inquiry when it comes to understanding women's health (Marks, 2002). Current approaches to producing evidence reinforce the traditional biases of the biomedical model. As Rogers (2004) observes, EBM 'is superimposed upon current medical practice [informed by a biomedical framework], repeating and reinforcing existing biases against women, both in research and in treatment. The methods of EBM potentially disenfranchise women, both in defining 'the best evidence' and in

developing guidelines. The model of health underpinning EBM ne-
glects gendered differences in the causes of ill health' (p. 54). Moreover,
Rogers also notes the ongoing discriminatory effects of research agendas (e.g., biological essentialism and gender blindness), especially the
deficiencies and lack of appropriate research on diseases that are of
major significance to women. Of course, this has significant implications, as research is the raw material that is the evidence upon which
EBM is based.

Evidence-Based Policy

At the same time that critiques of EBM are intensified in the literature,
its reach is expanding beyond medical care to all areas of public policy.
Building on the premise that decisions need 'a sound evidence base of
the best possible information' (Kelly, Speller, & Meyrick, 2004, p. 3),
evidenced-based decision-making is permeating health policy internationally. Although not always distinguished in the literature, evidence-
based policy (EBP) is 'qualitatively different' from EBM (Black, 2001). It
is different because it concerns decisions at the population-policy level
rather than at the individual-clinical level. As Dobrow Vivek, and
Upshur, (2004) explain: 'decisions are subject to greater public scrutiny
and outcomes directly affect larger numbers of people, heightening the
requirement for explicit justification' (p. 208).

Evidence-based policy making responds to critiques by economists
and health care advocates that health policy reform, including decisions
on health priorities, have been undertaken without the requisite evidence base. Health policies are often seen as being 'wrongly targeted'
and therefore showing 'limited effectiveness' (Niessen et al., 2000, p.
859). Because evidence–based health policy is 'the process of finding,
appraising and interpreting research according to an explicit set of
decision results and statistical and epidemiological techniques' (Lin &
Gibson, 2003, p. xx), it is thought to provide the needed information to
ensure both scientifically sound and fiscally prudent decisions. EBP
encourages investment into treatments, programs, and policies that will
work (Rogers, 2004). In the current policy environment, few people
would argue with the idea that 'that health care should be evidence-
based' and that health policy 'should make full and proper use of
research findings and research methods in policy development, implementation, and evaluation' (Walshe, 2001, p. 1187).

The case for evidence-based policy has clearly been made in Canada.

In 1997, the National Forum on Health concluded that the key goal of the health sector in the twenty-first century would be the 'establishment of a culture of evidence-based decision making, where decision-makers, the public, patients, providers, administrators and policy makers, would use high-quality evidence to make informed choices about health, health care, and the system' (Noseworthy & Watanabe, 1999, p. 228). The Canadian Population Health Initiative (2001) has recognized that evidence can be used as conceptual knowledge (for more research), as instrumental knowledge (for policy and program development), and as persuasive knowledge (for advocacy purposes). Health Canada's *Women's Health Strategy* (Health Canada, 1999) is committed to being 'evidence-based.' More recently, the Romanow Commission on the Future of Health Care in Canada concluded that 'If we are to build a better health care system, we need ... better information ... so that all governments and providers can be held accountable to Canadians' (Romanow Commission, 2002, p. xix).

Within the Canadian context, there has been an increasing demand for transparency and accountability in public policy and programs (Noseworthy & Watanabe, 1999). It is assumed that if policies are not based on sound evidence, they will not be effective or efficient. Because of the growing concern with cost containment in health care, both nationally and internationally, there has been a growing affinity between economic thinking and evidence-based decision-making (Willis & White, 2003). After all, EBP seeks the 'rationalization of rationing and allocating decisions' (Ter Muelen & Dickenson, 2002, p. 234). Increasing cost pressures in health systems are likely to increase the need for evidence-based policy because 'decisions will have to be made explicitly and publicly' (Gray, 1997, p.1). Not surprisingly, a 'cult of efficiency' (Stein, 2001) has come to dominate Canadian health policy.

Evidence-Based Health Policy, Economic Evaluations, and Ethics

In the broadest sense, health policy can be defined as 'those actions of government and other actors in society that are aimed at improving the health of populations' (Niessen et al., 2000, p. 860). Health care policy is also 'concerned with a range of distributional decisions' (Sindall, 2003, p. 83) that allocate 'tangible benefits and services across various interests in society' (Palmer & Short, 2000, p. 46). Rising health care costs, an aging population, growing pressures on the health care system (including those associated with economic globalization), technological advances and treatments, and limited health resources are all contributing to the increased interest in economic information (Niessen et al., 2000). More and more, complex social actions in health care are being translated into a basic set of economic propositions in order that appropriate data can be collected and used to inform allocative decisions about relative costs and benefits of different kinds of expenditures and appropriate budgets for health care (Davis, 1993, p. 120). Economic evidence, derived from full and partial economic evaluations, are increasingly seen as useful and necessary. Of these, cost-effectiveness analysis (CEA) and cost of illness (COI) studies dominate current practice (Kaplan & Groessl, 2002).[4]

CEA reflects a utilitarian approach to decisions, that is, CEA seeks to maximize some total 'good' through the most efficient use of limited resources (Berg, Ter Meulen, & Van Den Burg, 2001). CEA studies are considered full economic evaluations because they measure both the costs of a specific treatment, or other narrowly targeted health intervention, and the expected benefits arising from it. Analysts undertaking CEA purport to identify, measure, and compare all relevant costs to the consequences, often understood as benefits, of addressing a given health problem. Benefits are often measured in terms of QALYs (Quality Adjusted Life Years) and DALYs (Disability Adjusted Life Years).[5] A cost-effectiveness ratio is then computed as the benefit per dollar. This CEA ratio can be compared to other potential treatments for the same or other conditions to determine, in a very narrow and specific sense, where and how scarce health resources can be most efficiently employed. CEA studies provide a close-up perspective on the costs and consequences of specific treatments or health interventions that are necessary for the micro-management of the health care budget within a public system. Being able to compare costs and effectiveness of a number of interventions can guide decision-makers in terms of making scarce resource decisions. They are used widely in a number of areas to compare the effectiveness of alternative forms of treatment for specific medical conditions. For example, CEA studies are now widely required to support the licensing of new pharmaceutical products and to win approval for reimbursement in both public and private health insurance plans.

In contrast to CEA, COI studies are partial economic evaluations, and provide a broad macro perspective on only the current, rather than potential, costs associated with different categories or causes of ill health. COI studies attempt to provide an aggregate measure of all the costs arising from a particular disease or condition, including 'direct' expenditures on prevention, diagnosis, and treatment, and 'indirect' losses of productivity through morbidity and premature mortality. These studies can play a critical role in priority-setting because they provide a comprehensive summary of the wide costs involved in any health issue. The information contained in these studies can provide political justification for conducting other types of studies, and, in particular, for informing cost-effectiveness evaluations (Finkelstein & Corso, 2003; Rice, 2000). Many studies on a variety of health issues have demonstrated the application of this approach and estimated economic costs, including the Global Burden of Disease and Disability Project undertaken by the World Bank and World Health Organization in partnership with the Harvard School of Public Health (Murray & Lopez, 1996). Cost of illness studies are also prevalent in the United States and are used by the National Institutes of Health (Rice, 2000; Varmus, 2000).

In Canada, one of Health Canada's key initiatives has been the Economic Burden of Illness in Canada (EBIC) published in 1991, 1997, and most recently in 2002 (Health Canada, 2002). The primary goal of this program of research 'is to supply objective and comparable information on the magnitude of the economic burden or cost of illness and injury in Canada, based on standard reporting units and methods.' Health Canada maintains that the data produced in this study are 'based on comprehensive, standardized, and valid data' (Health Canada, 2002a, p. 58), and that the cost estimates provide 'the necessary evidence for priority setting, program planning, policy development, and effective allocation of health resources' (p. 59). The results are used extensively, with over 300 hits a day on the Health Canada web site and numerous requests from policy decision-makers, policy advocates, and community decision-makers annually (Desjardins, 2004).

Despite their growing popularity, economic evaluations still require improvement with respect to a number of conceptual, methodological, and practical problems to increase their reliability (Lin & Gibson, 2003; Hoffman, Stoykova, Granville, Misso, & Drummond, 2002). For example, as Niessen et al. (2000) point out, 'At the practical level, there is still large variation in the actual measurement and valuation of costs' (p. 864). According to Hankivsky et al. (2004), what is included in terms of costs and how costs are measured and analysed in terms of their distributional implications reflects an inherently discriminatory methodology that has profound implications for equity – in terms of gender and other intersecting categories of experience. In addition, like other areas of research, 'few studies have the necessary data, sample size, and measures to simultaneously investigate multiple intersectionalities' (e.g., 'race, gender, class, age)' (Carter, Sellers, & Squires, 2002, p. 116). So while CE and COI studies have produced costing data, the question is whether we have the appropriate knowledge base – 'the numbers we need' (Willis & White, 2003) – from which to inform health policies and practices.

One could argue that we do not have the numbers we need largely due to the assumptions that underpin economic evaluations. Value judgments that are implicit in the production and interpretation of evidence are often neglected (Birch, 1997). As Berg et al. (2001) argue, studies such as CEA 'inevitably contain a plethora of assumptions and translations which often *underlie* the 'explications' they bring' (p. 80), and, moreover, 'the rhetoric of the 'objectivity' and 'scientific' character of such tools ... tend to hide the implicit ... ethical aspects ... that are present' (p. 80). In general, normative considerations have typically not been considered within evidence-based health policy debates (Sindall, 2003; Carr-Hill, 1994; Vagero, 1994). And yet, as a growing body of feminist economic literature demonstrates, economic evaluations reflect androcentric values of neoclassical economics, which are often incapable of explaining real world phenomena (Cox, 1993; Barker, 1995; Robeyns, 2000; Barker & Kuiper, 2003).

Recently, important work is emerging at the interface of economics, ethics, moral philosophy, and feminist theory (Hankivsky et al., 2004; Hankivsky, 2004; Shiell, 1997; Mooney, 1999; Sen, 2000). In particular, the value choices and ethical assumptions underlying the production of evidence and more specifically economic evaluations are being interrogated (e.g., Coast, 2004), leading to serious questions about existing methodologies and their practical applications. For example, as Sindall (2003) argues, 'It is well recognized that good policy making should be informed by evidence; but good policies also require explicit and systematic analysis of the values underpinning decisions, and of the ethical consequences of those decisions' (p. 80). The inherent biases in economic evaluations, which undermine policy understandings and valuation of women's lives, are coming to the fore and alternatives to the status quo are being explored. As Marks (2002) points out elsewhere, 'A reliable account of women's lives often requires alternative approaches to inquiry that challenge traditional research routines' (p. 13). This requires, however, not seeing women as one static category but understanding different forms of social inequities in which gender intersects with other identities such as 'race'/ethnicity, age, sexuality, and ability – an intersectional approach that we refer to as a gender and diversity lens.

Applying a Gender and Diversity Lens to Economic Costing Studies

An explicit incorporation of a feminist ethical perspective, which specifically prioritizes social justice and equity, can make more transparent and open to public debate the way in which evidence is developed, counted, and evaluated. In terms of costing studies, applying a gender and diversity lens can assist in interrogating what is measured, how it is measured and analysed, and how the process either reduces or contributes to health inequities, including those associated with gender and its intersectionalities. As Marks (2002) reminds us, 'The knowledge base in science, medicine and health care is not an accident but the outcome of a systematic set of selective biases that operate as "gates" or "filters"' (p. 30). Applying a gender and diversity lens also demonstrates that if health care is to become truly evidence-based, changes are needed in terms of what is counted as evidence. Moreover, the methods for gathering and synthesizing evidence will need to be broadened substantially (p. 44).

In the following section, we focus on a number of specific flaws and limitations that from the perspective of gender equity and diversity appropriateness, undermine the foundation of sound and accountable evidence for health policy:

- First, as has been argued elsewhere in the context of COI studies (Hankivsky et al., 2004), a narrow range of relevant costs has been studied and those that have been measured have used faulty and discriminatory approaches. What is counted and how it is counted does not yet reflect the 'multiplicity of women's identities, interests, and experiences' (Inhorn & Whittle, 2001, p. 160). As Harding (quoted in Thomas, 1991) contends, 'If we start research from women's lives, we will ask different questions, gather different data and end up with a less partial and less distorted picture of the world' (p. 6).
- Second, the narrow emphasis of costing research on treatment rather than prevention of illness and disease is highlighted. Rogers (2004) has similarly argued that 'framing health problems in terms of the

search for evidence of effective interventions tends to maintain discussions of health within the narrow biomedical model, diverting attention and resources away from alternative views' (p. 69).

- Third, as suggested in Hankivsky et al. (2004), the breadth and scope of the current generation of economic costing studies severely limit their usefulness to policy makers who are interested in understanding not only the efficiency of health care resource allocation decisions, but also the extent to which they are equitable. Arguably, any measurement of disease burdens raises issues for equity (Hanson, 1999, p. 1).

In what follows, we elaborate on these three categories of shortcomings and explore how the limitations identified can be overcome by expanding the range of costs included, improving methods of measurement, widening the typically narrow biomedical focus on treatment to include the broader determinants of health and illness, and identifying the distributional consequences of both the costs and benefits of health care policy decisions. What emerges is an expanded set of tools that can generate better-quality evidence that, in turn, provides clearer insights into the efficiency and equity of health policy decisions.

I. Errors and Omissions in Costing Studies

As argued in Hankivsky et al. (2004), in the context of COI studies much of the costing work in the health area reflects the priorities of those primarily concerned with the size of the public health care budget. As discussed in Armstrong's Chapter 20 on home care (this collection), this of course prioritizes the government or state perspective, often obscuring societal perspectives that include individuals, their families, and friends; informal core services; charities; and so on. This tendency is compounded by the inherently biased perspective incorporated into standard costing methodologies, which often seem to render private domestic and caring labour, typically undertaken by women, invisible to researchers. Together these biases lead costing researchers to omit particular types of costs, and to misinterpret or mismeasure others.

Out-of-pocket expenses incurred by people who are ill and by their caregivers exemplify the types of private costs that are often simply omitted from both CE and COI studies. In spite of their obvious place in any complete accounting of health care costs, data on private expenditures for such items as medications, transportation, and caregiving services provided through the market are frequently not collected by researchers. Similarly, the cost of non-market caregiving provided by family, neighbors, and friends, over 80 per cent of which is provided by women, is only sometimes included in COI studies and is regularly overlooked in CE studies. For example, in an apparent effort to draw attention to current expenditures related to obesity in Canada, Birmingham, Muller, Palepu, Spinelli, & Anis (1999) provide estimates of the expenditures on treatment and care associated with this condition; however, they omit both non-market caregiving costs and private out-of-pocket expenses.

When non-market caregiving costs are included in COI studies, they are frequently misinterpreted and therefore misclassified. COI studies typically divide tangible costs into *direct costs* that arise from expenditures to diagnose, treat, and provide care for patients; and *indirect costs* that are associated with partial or unsuccessful treatment of a particular illness or diseases (morbidity and mortality costs). The costs of caregiving clearly represent direct costs, regardless of whether they are incurred by the state or by private individuals, through the market, or in the non-market sphere. However, while market-provided caregiving costs are counted as direct costs, in practice, non-market caregiving costs are typically misclassified as indirect costs when they are counted.

Distinguishing between direct and indirect costs can have important consequences for the development of equitable and effective health care policy. In general, health conditions that are prioritized by society will tend to have higher direct costs, because resources directed towards treating this condition are substantial, and lower indirect costs, because successful treatment reduces the associated loss of life-years. Conversely, those conditions which are not prioritized and successfully treated will have lower direct costs and higher indirect costs; that is, the burden of costs are borne by others, not the state. For example, the direct costs of HIV/AIDS will be lower in marginalized populations such as sex-trade workers, whose fear of stigmatization and consequent loss of employment may mean they seek out and receive relatively little caregiving from family and friends (University of Sussex, 2005). Compared to others, the indirect costs associated with HIV/AIDS for members of this group will be higher if the lack of caregiving they receive shortens their life expectancy. If non-market caregiving costs are misclassified as indirect costs, the lower caregiving costs will be lumped together with the higher mortality costs, so that they offset one another in total. As a result, the extent to which sex-trade workers receive less care and treatment and suffer greater morbidity and mortality than more privileged groups will be obscured.

When non-market caregiving costs, such as family caregiving, are included in COI studies, they are typically measured using the so-called 'replacement method.' This method values non-market caregiving using the price that would have to be paid to purchase an equivalent quantity of caregiving services through the market. However, the true cost to the caregivers is not what they would pay to purchase care in the market, but the value of the time that they themselves had to give up in order to provide the care (Mankiw, 2003). For example, a teacher who takes a year off from paid work to care for a terminally ill family member gives up her income for the year, which may be considerably more than the market rate for comparable caregiving services. Again, given the gendered nature of non-market caregiving, using the replacement method introduces gender bias into costing studies: it will systematically mismeasure costs to a greater degree when a greater share of costs is attributable to non-market caregiving and therefore borne disproportionately by women.

The emphasis in costing studies on costs incurred by the state along with the traditional emphasis within economics on market-based activities, if unchallenged, produces an evidence base that is inaccurate and in particular is biased in the direction of underestimating costs borne by women and expenditures on care for members of marginalized populations. Viewing costing studies through a gender and diversity lens leads us to the consistent application of sound economic methodology to the conceptualization of both market and non-market costs, and to more accurate and complete classification and measurement of these costs. By improving the quality of the evidence produced by costing studies, these modifications can provide the basis for better and more equitable policy decisions.

II. Illness versus Health

CEA studies typically focus narrowly on one or more medical intervention options designed to treat specific illnesses or conditions. Comprehensive health policy strategies must be concerned not only with treatment of illness and disease, but also with its prevention. Here it is important to recall the WHO (1948) definition of health: 'Health is a state of complete physical, mental and social well-being and not merely the absence of disease or infirmity.' The underlying dynamics that lead to the production of health are not necessarily integral to the biomedical model (Ruzeck, 1999). What is required is 'reframing what we mean by the very concept of health and beginning to think about health as located in families and communities, not simply in individual bodies' (Weber & Parra-Medina, 2003, p. 222). In this regard, women have a significant role. Traditionally, and currently – despite shifting and changing gender roles – they are the family members primarily responsible for family health and food preparation and caring for children and ill or elderly family members. Through their multiple roles as parents, spouses, partners, and caregivers, many women impact directly on the life of their family, including their children and other relatives. For example, in a recent U.S. national survey of women's health, mothers were found to take primary responsibility for a range of their children's health care activities and decisions (Wyn, Ojeda, Ranji & Salganicoff, 2003). Moreover, women often share amongst each other information and knowledge that promotes physical, mental, social and spiritual well-being for themselves and their families (Hajdukowski-Ahmed, Denton, O'Connor & Zeytinoglu, 1999, p. 31). Thus, as Hanson (1999) correctly observes, 'So many of women's activities ... are about producing health rather than treating disease' (p. 10).

When the spotlight of evidence is shone on medical responses to ill health through an emphasis on CE studies, the role played by non-market caring and reproductive labour in generating health may be obscured. Health and illness are, after all, 'the result of decisions made in the public and private sphere' (Davis, 1993, p. 133). Taking a broader perspective on the production of health leads us to questions that require a more comprehensive evidence base than is currently provided by CEA studies, and a broader policy response than can be provided by the biomedical community alone. The well-documented rise in obesity rates provides a clear example of the need to understand the role of caring and domestic labour in the production of health, and highlights the potential usefulness of economic evaluations that are broader than CEA studies. Recent data show that almost 15 per cent of Canadians are obese, and over half are overweight or obese (Tremblay, Katzmarzyk, & Willms, 2002). These figures reflect significant increases in obesity rates in Canada that match strong trends towards increasing rates of obesity throughout the world (Raine, 2004). The underlying causes of obesity continue to be an active area of research, but are thought to reflect a combination of environmental, economic, and social forces, including increased working time at the expense of time available to attend to nutrition and food preparation, less active lifestyles, and so on. The growing prevalence of obesity has led to increased incidence of diseases such as type 2 diabetes, hypertension, hyperlipidemia, cardiovascular disease, and cancer (Birmingham et al., 1999).

Developing effective policies to reduce rates of obesity may be critical to containing health care costs in developed economies, and doing so is likely to involve engaging individuals and families to modify the way that they conduct a variety of types of non-market production, including shopping, meal preparation, parenting, and recreational activities. For example, lifestyle modification (i.e. decreases in calorie and fat intake and increased physical activity) leading to even small losses in body weight has been shown to prevent or delay the development of Type 2 diabetes (Knowler et al., 2002). And of course, as highlighted in Chapter 2, this collection, in the discussion of appropriate lifespan approaches to women's health, there must be adequate social supports for individuals to be able to make such changes.

The evidence base necessary to inform policy in this or other areas of health promotion/disease prevention can be produced with a slight expansion of the conceptual framework of CEA studies. Consider first how the standard CEA framework would approach evaluating obesity-prevention policies such as public education campaigns, working time policies designed to give people more time for domestic labour, food-labelling policies, and so on. The cost of the intervention would be measured in a straightforward way, as usual. Compared to standard CEA studies of medical interventions such as coronary bypass surgery that measure benefits in terms of some measure of the value of additional life-years gained, a CEA study of an obesity-prevention study would require a simple intermediate step linking the policy to reduced obesity rates, and reduced obesity rates to reduced incidence and severity of conditions such as diabetes, with the resulting gain of life-years.

However, this simple extension would underestimate the economic benefits of the policy. Unlike a medical intervention, a policy that reduces the incidence of illness or disease achieves not only the resulting savings or improvement in the quality of life-years, but also the costs that would be incurred for diagnosis, treatment, and care of those who are ill. In the case of CVD, for example, a CEA study might compare the costs of bypass surgery to the expected gain in life years. A CEA study of an obesity-prevention policy would compare the costs of the policy to the potential gain in life-years, *plus* the savings arising from the resulting lower incidence of CVD and consequent reduction in the need for treatments such as bypass surgery. The expenses associated with the surgical procedure therefore would be counted on the *benefit* side of a CEA evaluation of a policy aimed at reducing rates of obesity. In other words, reducing the incidence of illness or disease avoids both the direct and indirect costs associated with an episode of illness or disease. Correctly estimating the potential cost savings arising from policies that reduce the incidence of ill health requires data that more closely resemble those produced by COI studies.

III. Accounting for Equity

Ensuring that all aspects of health care and illness are included in economic costing studies and that costs are measured using unbiased instruments is a first critical step towards developing evidence bases and policy tools that will allow us to assess efficiency, and is a first step towards accounting for equity when engaging in policy analysis. If economic evaluations are to respond to the diversity of women and to multiple forms of oppression, the next step must involve mapping the boundary between public and private costs and benefits, and determining the location of this boundary for different groups in society. After being measured, therefore, costs and benefits must be assigned to the public or private sector, by gender and by diversity group. This is an important step because as Sassi et al. (2001) have correctly noted, 'Distributional effects seem to have been completely neglected in existing evaluations, thus ignoring the equity dimension of resource allocation problems' (p. 1).

COI and CE studies that delineate the public/private boundary within costs of illness could lead to areas of illness or particular treatments being given increased priority if it were revealed that current health care practices and funding rules generate inequitable burdens for particular groups. For example, policy decisions about public funding for medications and medical supplies used to manage diabetes will have disproportionate effects on Aboriginal people, because, while estimates for 1991 show the prevalence of diabetes to be only 1.9 per cent in the general population, it is estimated at 5.3 per cent among First Nations people living off-reserve and 8.5 per cent of First Nations people living on-reserve (MacMillan, MacMillan, Offord, & Dingle, 1996). As well as experiencing particularly high rates of diabetes, Aboriginal people are more likely to experience 'early onset, greater severity at diagnosis, high rates of complications, lack of accessible services, increasing trends, and increasing prevalence of risk factors for a population already at risk' (Health Canada, 2002b). Aboriginal women are more than twice as likely as Aboriginal men and five times as likely as non-Aboriginal women to be diagnosed with diabetes (Health Canada, 2002b).

The issue of public funding for medications and medical supplies required to treat diabetes has disproportionate consequences for Aboriginal people, not only because of these higher prevalence rates but also because Aboriginal people experience higher poverty rates than the general population and therefore are more vulnerable to funding decisions, in terms of both social and health policy, that place the burden of these expenses on private individuals. For example, while programs aimed at educating patients to better manage their diabetes through diet and lifestyle modification may appear to be reasonably cost-effective when assessed in the general population, low-income individuals may not have the resources to afford adequate nutrition without considerable sacrifice. In the words of one Aboriginal woman, 'I am very concerned about the cutbacks in health services. Is Health Canada trying to kill us? Do we not have the highest rate of diabetes of any group? As my doctor tells me, "You should do a talk show on how expensive it is to be a diabetic!" Supplies remain expensive. Proper food is expensive. Most of us live on limited incomes. How can we pay for it?' (Doyle-Bedwell, 2000, p. 27). A consideration of the equity consequences of health policy might direct policy makers to better understand the effects of health decisions and even lead to specific interventions in different population groups, especially those who are marginalized and vulnerable.

The issue of the extent of publicly funded hospital care provides another example where consideration of the equity implications of the location of the public/private boundary yields fruitful insights. For example, the decision by the British Columbia government to implement a reduction in the length of hospital stays for maternity patients in 1995 disproportionately affected women, especially Aboriginal women and those in rural areas, and their health through two avenues. First, maternal health was adversely affected by the reduction in professional care: maternal re-admissions increased substantially as a result of the policy change (Amporfu, 2004). Second, the policy shifted the burden of caring for new mothers and their infants from paid professional caregivers to unpaid non-market caregivers. Like other policies that treat caregiving as a private domestic responsibility, the early discharge policy for maternity patients, without appropriate supports, contributes to gender and racial discrimination and economic deprivation.

Any reduction in the scope of a public health insurance system will increase the importance of private health insurance coverage. Some insight into the consequences for equity of substantially reducing the scope of publicly provided health insurance can be gained by looking at patterns of private insurance in the United States. In that country, employer-provided health care policies play an important role in the private health insurance market: two-thirds of the non-elderly U.S. population is covered through employer-provided health insurance either directly or through dependent coverage (Baicker & Chandra, 2005). As a result of this tight linkage between employment and health insurance, patterns of inequity in the labour market are translated into patterns of inequity in access to health care coverage. Because full-time employees are much more likely to be covered by employer-provided health insurance plans, families who have no members working full time are much more likely to be uninsured and therefore to experience significant costs associated with illness and poor health. While 19 per cent of the U.S. non-elderly adult population were uninsured in 2003, over 41 per cent of poor women, 38 per cent of Latinas, and 37 per cent of women with less than a high school education were without any health insurance coverage (Kaiser Family Foundation, 2004). Moreover, of those women who were covered by employer-provided insurance, 39 per cent were covered as dependents, making them vulnerable to losing their coverage in the event of separation or divorce. Finally, a number of medical procedures that are important to women's health are less likely to be insured under employer-sponsored health insurance policies. For example, 87 per cent of these plans insure sterilization, and only 46 per cent insure abortion procedures (Kaiser Family Foundation, 2004).

Without doubt, public debate and rigorous and accountable policy decision-making leading to the fullest possible expression of societal values – namely social justice and equity – in public health care funding decisions requires (a) that the diverse implications of those decisions for all individuals in society be considered, and (b) that the trade-offs between different societal goals dictated by economic scarcity be clearly identified. In this process, researchers must come to recognize how persisting biases regarding gender/race/class hinder the research enterprise (Inhorn & Whittle, 2001, p.155). What gets funded in the public system and what does not clearly has implications for horizontal equity, including its gender and diversity dimensions. At a time when the public/private boundary is being redrawn within health care reform, equity considerations warrant particular attention. What is specifically required, as Hanson (1999) has argued, is 'a better understanding of the linkages between sex, gender and health ... in order to properly measure the burden of disease' (p.1). It also requires, however, that these linkages are examined in a wider context where a range of health determinants and other systems of inequality influence and shape all women's health. Understanding theses linkages will reduce errors and costly mistakes, and complete the base of evidence that is used for policy.

Conclusion

Weiss (1983) argued more than 20 years ago that 'every stage of the research process – from the formulation of the initial question to the development of conclusions – [is] punctuated with choices [and] ... resolved by applying value judgments' (p. 217). An explicit incorporation of an ethical perspective can reveal and make more transparent the way in which evidence is developed, counted, and evaluated. Incorporating a gender and diversity perspective into the research methodologies that support evidence-based health policy reveals that the current generation of economic costing studies are flawed in ways that echo some of the shortcomings of evidence-based medicine that have become better understood in recent years. The result of these flaws is that economic costing studies often obscure the contributions and burdens in the private sphere, particularly those that are 'hidden in the household.' Moreover, they tend to focus attention on narrow biomedical understanding of illness and disease. And, while prioritizing economic efficiency, these studies often make no significant contributions to our ability to assess health policy decisions from an ethical perspective.

As well as highlighting their shortcomings, approaching economic costing methodologies from an ethical perspective, with attention to gender and diversity, can lead us to constructive alternatives that advance our practice. First, it leads us to take explicit account of all the roles played by individuals, families, communities, and the public health care system in promoting health, treating disease and illness, and caring for those who are in poor health. This more holistic approach to understanding the costs, consequences, and trade-offs involved in different health policy decisions can ensure that *all* costs and benefits are accounted for, and that our measurements are not inherently biased. Second, by shifting the focus away from the state sector, we are reminded that the gendered work of parenting, educating, feeding, clothing, and caregiving done within households is a critical input into the production of health and the prevention of illness and disease. Labour market policy, child-care programs, income assistance, and other forms of social policy therefore are inextricably linked to health care costs; the data produced by COI studies can provide useful input into these other areas of policy making as well as within the health sector.

Finally, we are prompted to organize the data in all economic costing studies so as to facilitate an evaluation of the distributional consequences of health policy decisions as well as their efficiency. Tracking the incidence of costs across diverse groups of women within economic costing studies would allow these tools to serve the dual purposes of evaluating policies from the perspective of both equity and efficiency. Reporting the results of COI studies in this way could help us identify and document discrepancies in funding generosity across broad areas of health spending that may have important and overlooked implications when seen from an equity perspective. Reporting the results of CE studies in this way could allow us to compare the implications of specific interventions for different groups, and allow us to evaluate their consistency with societal values of social justice and equity, as well as their efficiency.

NOTES

1 The Cochrane Collaboration is an international not-for-profit and independent organization, dedicated to making up-to-date, accurate information about the effects of healthcare readily available worldwide. It produces and disseminates systematic reviews of healthcare interventions and promotes the search for evidence in the form of clinical trials and other studies of interventions. The international Campbell Collaboration (C2) is a non-profit organization that aims to help people make well-informed decisions about the effects of interventions in the social, behavioral and educational arenas. C2's objectives are to prepare, maintain and disseminate systematic reviews of studies of interventions.

2 According to Marks (2002), positivist realism requires researchers 'to make observations about objective reality, ensuring that error and bias are eliminated by isolating variables in order to be able to identify cause-effect relationships' (pp. 9–10).

3 In these studies, 'the association between a specific intervention and its outcomes is researched under within very strictly controlled conditions' (Ter Muelen & Dickenson, 2002, p. 231).

4 Economic evaluations can be defined as 'the comparative analysis of alternative courses of action in terms of both their costs and consequences' (Drummond et al., 1997 pp. 8–9). *Cost of illness* (COI) studies are partial evaluations since only costs are examined, whereas *cost-effectiveness analyses* (CEA) are full economic evaluations because both costs and alternatives are compared.

5 QALYs can be understood as 'collective scores that emerge from surveys that ask people to rank their preferred state of health in terms of the mobility and distress levels which affect normal daily life' (Davis, 1993, p. 129). DALYs are "composite measures of health status, which combine the time lost of premature mortality and the time lived with a disability" (Hanson, 1999, p. 4).

REFERENCES

Amporfu, E. (2004). The effect of hospital downsizing in British Columbia on the quality of care for maternity patients. Mimeo. Simon Fraser University, Vancouver.

Armstrong, P. (2001). Evidence-based health care reform: Women's issues. In P. Armstrong, H. Armstrong, & D. Coburn (Eds.), *Unhealthy Times: Political Economies Perspectives on Health and Care in Canada* (pp. 121–145). Toronto: Oxford University Press.

Baicker, K., & Chandra, A. (2005). The consequences of the growth of health insurance premiums.' *American Economic Review*, 95(2)(May), 214–218.

Barker, D.K. (1995). Economist, social reformers and prophets: A feminist critique of economic efficiency. *Feminist Economics*, 1(3).

Barker, D.K. & Kuiper, E. (2003). *Toward a Feminist Philosophy of Economics.* London and New York: Routledge.

Berg, M., Ter Meulen, R., & Van Den Burg, M. (2001). Guidelines for appropriate care: The importance of empirical normative analysis. *Health Care Analysis, 9*, 77–99.

Biller-Andorno, N., Reidar K.L., & Meulen, R.T. (2002). Evidence-based medicine as an instrument for rational health policy. *Health Care Analysis, 10*(3), 261–275.

Birch, S. (1997). As a matter of fact: Evidence-based decision-making unplugged. *Health Economics, 6*(6), 547–559.

Birmingham, C.L., Muller J.L., Palepu, A., Spinelli, J.J., & Anis, A.H. (1999).

The cost of obesity in Canada. *Canadian Medical Association Journal, 160*(4), 483–8.

Black, N. (2001). Evidence based policy: Proceed with care. *British Medical Journal, 323*(7307), 275–278.

Canadian Population Health Initiative. (2001). Retrieved 10 April 2005, from, http://secure.cihi.ca/cihiweb/dispPage.jsp?cw_page=cphi_aboutcphi_e.

Carr-Hill, R. (1994). Efficiency and equity implications of the health care reforms. *Social Science & Medicine, 49*(9), 1189–1202.

Carter, P., Sellers, S.L., and Squires, C. (2002). Reflections on race/ethnicity, class, and gender inclusive research. *African American Perspectives, 8*(1): 111–124.

Champagne, F., Lemieux-Charles, L., & McQuire, W. (2004). Introduction: Towards a broader understanding of the use of knowledge and evidence in health care. In L. Charles-Lemieux and F. Champagne (Eds.), *Using Knowledge and Evidence in Health Care: Multidisciplinary Approaches.* Toronto: University of Toronto Press.

Coast, J. (2004). Is economic evaluation in touch with society's health values? *British Medical Journal, 329*, 1233–1236.

Correa-de-Araujo, R. (2004). A wake-up call to advance women's health. *Women's Health Issues, 14*(2), 31–4.

Cox, E. (1993). The economics of mutual support: A feminist approach. In S. Rees, G. Rodley, and F. Stilwell (Eds), *Beyond the Market: Alternatives to Economic Rationalism.* Leichhardt, Australia: Pluto Press.

Crotty, M. (1998). The Foundations for Social Research. London: Sage.

Davis, A. (1993). Economising health. In S. Rees, G. Rodley, & F. Stilwell (Eds), *Beyond the Market: Alternatives to Economic Rationalism.* Leichhardt, Australia: Pluto Press.

Desjardins, S. (2004). Overview of Health Canada's COI Model. Presentation at the Gender Economic Costing Workshop, BC Centre of Excellence for Women's Health. 21 April, 2004. Vancouver.

Dickenson, D., & Vineis, P. (2002). Evidence-based medicine and quality of care. *Health Care Analysis, 10*(3), 243–259.

Djulbegovic, M., Morris, L., & Lyman, G. (2000). Evidentiary challenges to evidence-based medicine. *Journal of Evaluation in Clinical Practice, 6*(2), 99–109.

Dobrow, M.J., Vivek, G., & Upshur, R. (2004). Evidence-based health policy: Context and utilization. *Social Science & Medicine, 58*(1), 207–217.

Doyle-Bedwell, P. (2000). Speaking from the heart: Gender equity and Aboriginal women. In C. Amaratunga (Ed.), *Made to Measure: Women, Gender and Equity.* Vol. 1. Halifax: Maritime Centre of Excellence for Women's Health.

Drummond, M.F., O'Brien, B., Stoddart, G.L., & Torrance, G.W. (1997). *Methods for the Economic Evaluation of Health Programs.* 2nd ed. Oxford: Oxford University Press.

Egger, M., Davey Smith, G., & Altman, B.G. (2001). *Systematic Reviews in Health Care: Meta-Analysis in Context.* London: British Medical Journal Books.

Finkelstein, E., & Corso, P. (2003). Cost of illness analyses for policy making: A cautionary tale of use and misuse. *Expert Review of Pharmacoeconomics and Outcomes Research, 3*(4), 367–369.

Gray, J.A.M. (1997). *Evidence-Based Health Care: How to Make Health Policy and Management Decisions.* Edinburgh: Churchill Livingstone.

Greenhalgh, T. (2002). Intuition and evidence – uneasy bedfellows? *British Journal of General Practice, 52,* 395–400.

Hajdukowski-Ahmed, M., Denton M., O'Connor, M., and Zeytinoglu, I.U. (1999). Women's voices in health promotion: Theoretical and methodological implications. In M. Denton, M. Hajdukowski-Ahmed, M. O'Connor, & I. U. Zeytinoglu (Eds.), *Women's Voices in Health Promotion.* Toronto: Canadian Scholars' Press.

Hankivsky, O. (2004). *Caring and Social Policy.* Vancouver: University of British Columbia Press.

Hankivsky, O., Friesen J., Varcoe, C., McPhail, F., Greaves, L., & Spencer, C. (2004). Expanding economic costing in health care: Values, gender and diversity. *Canadian Public Policy, 30*(3), 257–282.

Hanson, K. (1999). *Measuring Up Gender, Burden of Diseases and Priority Setting Techniques in the Health Sector.* Working paper, Series no. 99.12. Cambridge: Harvard Centre for Population and Development Studies. Retrieved 25 June 2004, from http://www.hsph.harvard.edu/Organizations/healthnet/HUpapers/gender/hanson.html.

Harding, S. (1991). *Whose Science? Whose Knowledge? Thinking from Women's Lives.* Buckingham, UK: Open University Press.

Health Canada. (1999). *Health Canada's Women's Health Strategy 1999.* Retrieved 18 June 2004, from http://www.hc-sc.gc.ca/engligh/women/womenstrat.htm.

Health Canada. (2002a). *Economic Burden of Illness in Canada 1998.* Ottawa: Minister of Public Works and Government Services Canada.

Health Canada. (2002b). *Diabetes Among Aboriginal (First Nations, Inuit and Métis) People in Canada: The Evidence.* Retrieved 24 August 2004, from http://www.hc-sc.gc.ca/fnihb-dgspni/fnihb/cp/adi/publications/the_evidence.htm.

Hoffman, C., Stoykova B.A., Glanville, J.M. Misso, K., & Drummond M.F.

(2002). Do health care decision makers find economic evaluations useful? The findings of focus group research in UK health authorities. *Value in Health, 5*(2), 71–8.

Hunt, K., & Annandale, E. (1999). Relocating gender and morbidity: Examining men's and women's health in contemporary Western societies. Introduction to Special Issue on Gender and Health. *Social Science & Medicine, 48*(1), 1–5.

Inhorn, M., & Whittle, K.L. (2001). Rethinking difference: A feminist reframing of gender/race/class for the improvement of women's health research. *Social Construction of Health and Disease, 31*(1), 147–165.

Kaiser Family Foundation (2004). *Fact Sheet: Women's Health Policy Facts.* Retrieved 10 May 2005, from http://www.kff.org/womenshealth/6000-03.cfm.

Kaplan, R.M., & Groessl, E.J. (2002). Application of cost effectiveness in behavioural medicine. *Journal of Consulting and Clinical Psychology, 70*(3), 482–493.

Kelly, M.P., Speller, V., & Meyrick, J. (2004). *Getting Evidence into Practice in Public Health.* London: NHS Health Development Agency.

Knowler, W.C., Barrett-Connor, E., Fowler, S.E., Hamman, R.F., Lachin, J.M., Walker, E.A., & Nathan, D.M. (2002). Reduction in the incidence of type 2 diabetes with lifestyle intervention or metformin. *New England Journal of Medicine, 346*(6), 393–403.

Lin, V., & Gibson, B. (2003). *Evidence-based Health Policy: Problems and Possibilities.* Oxford: Oxford University Press.

MacMillan, J., MacMillan, A., Offord, D., & Dingle, J. (1996). Aboriginal health. *Canadian Medical Association Journal, 155,* 1569–1578.

Mankiw, G.N. (2003). *Principles of Microeconomics.* Scarborough, ON: Nelson Thomson Learning.

Marks, D.F. (2002). *Perspectives on Evidence-Based Practice.* HAD Contract no. 02/042, Project 00477. London: Health Development Agency, Public Health Evidence Steering Group.

McQueen, D., & Anderson, L. (2001). What counts as evidence: Issues and debates. In I. Rootman, M. Goodstadt, B. Hyndman, D. McQueen, L. Potvin, J. Springett, and E. Ziglio (Eds.), *Evaluations in Health Promotion: Principles and Perspectives.* Copenhagen: World Health Organization.

Mooney, G. (1999). *The Need to Establish the Value Base of Health Economics and Health Care.* Discussion paper no. 2/99 Sydney, Australia: Social and Public Health Economics Research Group.

Murray, C., & Lopez, A. (1996). *Global Burden of Disease and Injury Series: The*

Global Burden of Disease. Cambridge MA: Harvard School of Public Health for WHO and World Bank.

National Aboriginal Health Organization (2001). *Strategic Directions for an Evidence-Based Decision-Making Framework at NAHO*, 22 October.

National Health and Medical Research Council (NHMRC). (2000). *How to Use the Evidence: Assessment and Application of Scientific Evidence*. Canberra, Australia: National Health and Medical Research Council, AusInfo.

Niessen, L.W., Els, W.M., Grijseels, F., & Rutten, F.H. (2000). The evidence-based approach in health policy and health care delivery. *Social Science & Medicine, 51*(6), 859–869.

Noseworthy, T., & Watanabe, M. (1999). Health policy directions for evidence-based decision making in Canada. *Journal of Evaluation in Clinical Practice, 5*(2), 227–242.

Palmer, G., & Short, S. (2000). *Health Care and Public Policy: An Australian Analysis*. 3rd ed. South Yarra, Australia: Macmillan.

Raine, K.D (2004). *Overweight and Obesity in Canada: A Population Health Perspective*. Canadian Institute for Health Information. http://secure.cihi.ca/cihiweb/products/CPHIOverweightandObesityAugust2004_e.pdf

Rice, D.P. (2000). Cost of illness studies: What is good about them? *Injury Prevention, 6*, 177–179.

Robeyns, I. (2000). Is there a feminist economic methodology? Paper presented at the Workshop on Realism and Economics, University of Cambridge, 22 February 1999.

Rogers, W. (2004). Evidence-based medicine and women: Do the principles and practice of EBM further women's health? *Bioethics, 18*(1), 50.

Romanow Commission. (2002). *Building on Values: The Future of Health Care in Canada*. Saskatoon, SK: Commission on the Future of Health Care in Canada.

Ruzeck, S. (1999). Rethinking feminist ideologies and actions: Thoughts on the past and future of health reform. In A. Clarke & V. Olesen (Eds.), *Revision-ing Women, Health, and Healing: Feminist, Cultural, and Technoscience Perspectives* (pp. 303–323). New York: Routledge.

Ruzeck, S., Olesen, V., & Clarke, A. (Eds). (1997). *Women's Health: Complexities and Differences*. Columbus: Ohio State University Press.

Sackett, D.K., Rosenberg, W.M.C., & Gray, J.A.M. (1996). Evidence based medicine: What it is and what it isn't. *British Medical Journal, 312*(7023), 71–72.

Sassi F., Archard, L., & Le Grand, J. (2001). Equity and the economic evaluation of health care. *Health Technology Assessment, 5*(3), 5.

Sen, A. (2000). Economic progress and health. In D.A. Leon & G. Walt (Eds.),

Poverty, Inequality and Health: An International Perspective. Oxford: Oxford University Press.

Sherr, L. (2000). Women and clinical trials. In L. Sherr & J. Chichester (Eds.), *Women, Health and the Mind* (pp. 77–90). Chichester, UK: John Wiley & Sons.

Shiell, A. (1997). Health outcomes are about choices and values: An economic perspective on the health outcomes movement. *Health Policy, 30*, 5–15.

Sindall, C. (2003). Health policy and normative analysis: Ethics, evidence and politics. In V. Lin & B. Gibson (Eds.), *Evidence-Based Health Policy: Problems and Possibilities* (pp. 80–94). Oxford: Oxford University Press.

Stein, J.G. (2001). *The Cult of Efficiency.* Don Mills, ON: Anansi.

Tallacchini, M. (2002). Legalizing Science. *Health Care Analysis, 10*(4), 329–337.

Ter Meulen, R., & Dickenson, D. (2002) Into the hidden world behind evidence-based medicine. *Health Care Analysis, 10*, 231–241.

Thomas, B. (1991). Whose science? Sandra Harding's book nominated for award. *Update, 11*(3), 6.

Tremblay, M.S., Katzmarzyk, P.T., & Willms, J.D. (2002). Temporal trends in overweight and obesity in Canada, 1981–1996. *International Journal of Obesity, 26*(4), 538–43.

University of Sussex Institute of Development Studies (2005). *Gender and HIV/ AIDS: Challenging Stigma and Discrimination.* Retrieved 20 June 2005, from http://www.eldis.org/gender/dossiers/stigma.htm#consequences.

Vagero, D. (1994). Equity and efficiency in health reform: A European view. *Social Science & Medicine, 39*(9), 1203–1210.

Varmus, H. (2000). *Disease Specific Estimates of Direct and Indirect Costs of Illness and NIH Support.* Rev. ed. Washington, DC: National Institutes of Health.

Victora, C.G., Habicht, J-P., & Bryce, J. (2004). Evidence-based public health: Moving beyond randomized trials. *American Journal of Public Health, 94*(3), 400–405.

Walshe, K. (2001). Evidence based policy: Don't be timid. *British Medical Journal, 323*, 1187.

Weber, L., & Parra-Medina, D. (2003). Intersectionality and women's health: Charting a path to eliminating health disparities. *Gender Perspectives in Health and Medicine: Key Themes Advances in Gender Research, 7*, 181–230.

Weiss, C. (1983). Ideology, interests and information: The basis of policy positions. In D. Callahan & G. Jennings (Eds.), *Ethics, the Social Sciences and Policy Analysis.* New York: Plenum Press.

WHO. (1948). Preamble to the constitution of the World Health Organization as adopted by the International Health Conference, New York, 19–22 June 1946; signed on 22 July 1946 by representatives of 61 states (official records of the World Health Organization, no. 2, p. 100) and entered into force on 7 April 1948.

Willis, E., & White, K. (2003). Evidence-based medicine, The medical profession and health policy. In V. Lin & B. Gibson (Eds.), *Evidence-Based Health Policy: Problems and Possibilities* (pp. 33–43). Oxford: Oxford University Press.

Wyn, R., & Ojeda, V. (with Ranji, M.S. & Salganicoff, A.). (2003, April). *Women, Work, and Family Health: A Balancing Act*. Menlo Park, CA: Henry J. Kaiser Foundation.

PART THREE

The Social Determinants of Health

7 Women's Health and the Politics of Poverty and Exclusion

COLLEEN REID

Poverty and Women's Health: The State of Research and Theory

In Canada and internationally women are increasingly vulnerable to poverty, and poor people, who are disproportionately women, children, and people of colour, have more illnesses and die in greater numbers than people who are not poor (Ballantyne, 1999).

Despite critical feminist analyses of women's roles, experiences with paid and unpaid work, and occupational segregation, current measures of women's socioeconomic status and health rely on occupational measures derived primarily from male-centered experiences and understandings (Reid, 2002).

To date few health researchers adequately theorize the structural and ideological origins of social inequities, especially those based on gender, race, and class, and rarely are qualitative methods from a critical and interpretive paradigm applied (Reid, 2004).

Poverty and Women's Health: An International Perspective

About two thirds of the world's women live in countries where per capita income is low, life expectancy is relatively short, class and gender inequalities in income and wealth are great, and few health and welfare services are provided by the state (Doyal, 1995).

Most evidence suggests that the economic, social, and political conditions under which people live their lives are major factors that determine whether they develop illness and disease (Raphael, 2001).

Differences in life expectancies between countries can be explained in the first instance by differences in material wealth (GNP). After a certain threshold of material wealth and standard of living are achieved, there is a plateau effect such that differences in life expectancy and mortality rates can be explained by the relative differences in income between the wealthy and the poor (Wilkinson, 1992, 1996, 2000).

Overview

Ideologies of power, economic reward and exchange, and gender roles and relations are expressed through macro- and micro-level institutions and behaviours (Moss, 2002). In all developed countries, including Canada, these factors have increased income disparities and the rates and depths of poverty experienced by many, particularly single mothers, women with disabilities, Aboriginal women, and older women. Women's health, health promotion, and social epidemiology literatures suggest that poverty has a significant impact on women's health. In this chapter, the incidence of women's poverty and the relationship between poverty and women's health are reviewed from a critical feminist perspective. A qualitative case study then illustrates how poverty has its effects on women's health through both psychosocial and material pathways. The findings from the case study suggest that poverty and women's health need to be understood as social justice issues, and that fundamental changes in government policies and practices are required to enable all Canadians to equitably pursue good health.

What Is the Problem?

Women's Poverty in Canada

The decades between 1973 and 1993 marked a period of striking growth in income and wealth inequity in all developed nations. These increases in income inequality were attributable to a number of causes, including increases in differential wage rates for more and less skilled workers, devolution of publicly funded social services, tax policies favouring the rich, and the decline of labour unions (Moss, 2002). Rising income inequalities have been accompanied by an increase in the number of families living in poverty. In Canada there is a growing number of people living in poverty (see text box 7.1 for details). In Australia, the United Kingdom, the United States, and Canada, more than half of single-parent households with children have incomes below the poverty level; in the vast majority of cases, these single parents are women (United Nations Development Program [UNDP], 1999).

Text Box 7.1 Poverty in Canada

- In Canada, the number of people living at less than 50 per cent of the poverty line has grown dramatically in recent years, from 143,000 families and 287,000 unattached individuals in 1989 to 277,000 families and 456,000 unattached individuals in 1997 (National Council of Welfare, 2000b).
- For as long as poverty has been measured, lone mother families, older women, Aboriginal women, and women with disabilities have been consistently over-represented (Phipps 2003).
- Women suffer greater burdens of morbidity, distress, and disability (Doyal, 1995), including depression, stress overload, chronic conditions such as arthritis and osteoporosis, and injuries and death resulting from family violence; and women present more acute medical problems, are hospitalized at higher rates than men, use more prescriptive medications, and report feeling less healthy (Greaves et al., 1999)

Poverty is a normative concept that can be defined – in both absolute and relative terms – in relation to 'need,' 'standard of living,' 'limited resources,' 'lack of basic security,' 'lack of entitlement,' 'multiple deprivation,' 'exclusion,' 'inequality,' 'class,' 'dependency,' and 'unacceptable hardship' (Krieger, 2001). In Canada, the term *low income* refers to the low income cut-offs (LICOs) identified by Statistics Canada. These cut-offs define low income in relative terms, based on the percentage of income that individuals and families spend on the basic needs of food, clothing, and shelter in comparison with other Canadians. Families and unattached individuals with 'low incomes' usually spend more than 54.7 per cent of their income on food, shelter, and clothing (Health Canada, 1999). The LICO is a consistent and well-defined method that identifies those who are substantially worse off than the average. LICOs represent levels of income where people spend too much of their money for food, shelter, and clothing, based on their family size and where they live (Landucci, 2003).

Poverty and low income are gendered phenomena. Not only are more women than men likely to experience deprivation, but women experience poverty differently. The poverty rate for women is higher than for men in every age group, and disparity between socio-economic groups is growing (Health Canada, 1997). Currently, almost 19 per cent of adult women are living below the low-income cut-offs (Health Canada, 1997). Lone parent families headed by women have the highest incidence and depth of poverty for all family types, a situation that has improved very little over the past decade. In Canada, 15 per cent of all families are lone-parent, and more that five-sixths of them are headed by women (Health Canada, 1999). As well, older women are still more likely to be economically disadvantaged than their male counterparts. In 1997, 46 per cent of older women on their own were poor, and their average incomes were $3,000 below the poverty line (Townson, 2000). According to a Canadian Population Health Initiative report, lone mother families, older women, Aboriginal women, and women with disabilities have had remarkably consistent experiences of poverty for as long as data have been available (Phipps, 2003, p.8).

In Canada, the main causes of women's poverty are labour market inequities, domestic circumstances (marriage breakdown and motherhood), and welfare systems (National Council of Welfare, 2000a; Ruspini, 2001). While some evidence suggests that the wage gap between men and women is slowly closing, not all women have shared equally in these gains. Men still dominate higher-earnings groups and comprise a relatively small proportion of workers in the lowest-earnings categories (Townson, 2000). The majority of women remain in the lowest earnings categories, and some groups of women, such as young women, were worse off in 1994 than they were in 1984. Another factor that contributes to growing labour market inequities is that women are working increasingly in part-time, temporary, or contract employment (Townson, 2000). Such non-standard jobs offer little financial security, and few, if any, offer health care or disability benefits. When these non-standard jobs are considered when examining the wage gaps between women and men, the average earnings of women in 2000 were 63.9 per cent of men's, indicating a slightly widening gap from 64.8 per cent in 1997 (Jackson, 2003).

Additionally, the decline of the power of labour and trade unions, combined with the increase in contract and temporary labour, have diminished the status and rights of individual workers, many of whom are now isolated in space (as homeworkers) or in time, as employment tenure shortens (Moss, 2002). More recently, immigrant women have found employment as domestic servants, janitors, or low-wage workers in electronics and garment industries, work that is often isolating and demeaning, and offers no opportunity for advancement (Moss, 2002). Women consistently find themselves in low-status, low-paying jobs with few opportunities for advancement, and they are overrepresented among part-time workers and in the informal sector (United Nations Platform for Action Committee, 2004).

Many women are often 'one man away from welfare.' Women's poverty occurs as a consequence of the complex interplay of such factors as divorce and separation, as well as women's roles as mothers, homemakers, and caregivers (Townson, 2000). Women perform two-thirds of unpaid caregiving work in Canada. The enormous demands of unpaid work reduce many women's opportunities to participate fully in the workforce (United Nations Platform for Action Committee, 2004). This is compounded by the significant reduction in welfare payments in the last 10 years. For example in British Columbia, between 1995 and September 2003, welfare rolls have been reduced by 54.2 per cent, almost 34 per cent of which occurred from 2000 to 2003, mainly due to restrictions in eligibility (Ministry of Human Resources, 2003). In all provinces, welfare payments fall significantly short of the LICO. For instance, the total welfare income in 1998 for a single parent with one child ranged from a low of 50 per cent of the LICO in Alberta to a high of 69 per cent in Newfoundland (National Council of Welfare, 2000b).

Finally, measures of family income say little about the distribution of resources within the family unit. Male-female equity cannot be assumed in intra-household decision-making and allocation of resources (Moss, 2002). This may be particularly true in families where abuse occurs. Forms of economic abuse may include men forcing their wives to ask for money, giving them a set allowance, taking their money away, and not letting them know about or have access to family income (Townson, 2000).

Poverty and Women's Health

The growth in income and wealth inequity is paralleled by increasing socio-economic disparities in health (Moss, 2002). Health is powerfully affected by social position and by the scale of social and economic differences among the population (Raphael, 2001; Wilkinson, 1992, 1996, 2000). One of the most pervasive and enduring observations in public health is the 'gradient of health.' This gradient can be pictured as a line on a graph that remains consistent across gender, age groups, cultural groups, countries, and diseases. The gradient of health shows that people who have the lowest socio-economic status (SES) experience the highest rates of mortality and morbidity. As people move up the socio-economic gradient, their health improves relative to it (Deaton, 2002;

Reid, 2002). SES is 'a composite measure that typically incorporates economic status, measured by income; social status, measured by education; and work status, measured by occupation' (Adler et al., 1994, p. 15).

SES has its effect on health through material and psychosocial pathways. Exposure to low income and to health risks in the physical environment, as well as to psychosocial conditions such as stress, depression, low self-esteem, and anger, influence health and well-being (Brunner & Marmot, 2000; Raphael, 2001; Wilkinson, 1996, 2000). Research also suggests that more egalitarian societies, that is, societies with smaller differences in income between rich and poor, tend to have better health (Wilkinson, 1996). The social and economic structure of society, especially low income, income inequality, discrimination, and social exclusion, are seen as the ultimate determinants, the 'causes of the causes,' of disease and death (Deaton, 2002).

Generally, health improves with each increment in the social hierarchy, and this pattern holds for most causes of morbidity and mortality, although for women the trend is less consistent (Macintyre, 1998). In trying to understand the gradient of health, there appears to be a gender divide, such that work factors are considered for men and home factors are considered for women (Matthews & Power, 2002). For instance, current measures of socio-economic status rely on occupational measures derived primarily from a male-centred experience of work; understandings of women's SES have traditionally focused on women's roles within the home (Reid, 2002). Throughout life, the human experiences of birth, death, illness, and disability are embedded in social contexts. In any gender-dichotomized society, the fact that we are born biologically female or male means that our environments will be different, we will live different lives (Lorber, 1997), and we will have different experiences with health. All cultures characterize men and women differently and as suitable for different kinds of tasks and entitled to differing levels of economic, cultural, and political resources (Doyal, 1995). These differences determine differential exposure to risk; access to the benefits of technology, information, resources, and health care; and the realization of rights, all of which can influence health (World Health Organization, 1998). Indeed, women's everyday experiences must be understood within the context of the larger social organizational and ideological structures generated from outside experience (Anderson, 1987).

For decades mortality and morbidity rates have indicated that 'women are sicker but men die quicker' – women live longer, men die prematurely, and women experience more morbidity than do men. The life expectancy for Canadian women compared to Canadian men is almost seven years greater (Love, Jackson, Edwards, & Pederson, 1997). Generally, the data suggest that the same relationships exist for women from ethnically diverse groups, though causality is uncertain.[1] If one equates longevity with health, then women appear to be healthier than men (Reid, 2002). However, it is generally agreed that women suffer greater burdens of morbidity, distress, and disability (Doyal, 1995; see text box 7.1 for more details).

Research over the last decade suggests that gender differences in health are rooted in social roles against the backdrop of some male biological disadvantage. Standard explanations for why women report more ill health have included biological or genetic risks, risks acquired through social roles and behaviours (the burdens of domestic and female role responsibilities, such as child-rearing and housework), illness behaviour (women appear or act more sick), health-reporting behaviour (women are seen to be more verbal or 'complaining'), and differential health care access, treatment, and use (Hunt & Annandale, 1999; Macintyre, Ford, & Hunt, 1999; Reid, 2002).

Women's health researchers and advocates suggest that health promotion and disease-prevention activities must focus not only on diseases that are more common, more prevalent, or more serious among women, but also on priority health issues identified by women themselves, women's diversity, and the determinants of health (Cohen, 1998). Women's health is perceived as a continuum that extends throughout the life cycle and that is critically and intimately related to the conditions under which women live. Examinations of women's health require a social model of health that puts women's health needs at the centre of the analysis and focuses attention on the diversity of women's health needs over the life cycle (Ruzek, Clarke, & Olesen, 1997). The traditional oppression and disempowerment of women must also be addressed at both personal and societal levels, thus broadening the approach.

Case Study: The Wounds of Exclusion: Poverty, Women's Health, and Social Justice[2]

Research Context and Methods

The following case study is used to illuminate the link between poverty and women's health. For three years I worked with a collective organization in the greater Vancouver area named Women Organizing Activi-

Table 7.1 The Women's Socioeconomic Status[a] (n = 20)

Sources of financial support		Length of time living in poverty		Women's cited reasons for living in poverty	
Social assistance	8	1–3 years	4	Left abusive partner	2
Disability benefits I	2	4–6 years	7	Left drug-addicted partner	1
Disability benefits II	5	7–10 years	6	Left or was left by husband	4
Seniors pension	2	Lifetime	3	Disability or ill-health	6
Supporting husband	2			Cannot find a well-enough	
Ex-spousal support	1			paying job	5
				Have always been poor	2

[a] In 2000, on average, the women in this study lived on approximately $899.78 per month, or $10,797.39 per year. In 1995, the average annual income of Coquitlam households (in the Tri-City area) was $57,209. In that same year, the regional average income was $54,055 (Statistics Canada, 1996). The women thus lived in a relatively middle- to upper-income community.

ties for Women (WOAW). WOAW was a partnership between women on low income, community-service providers, and university-based researchers that aimed to examine and address poor women's health concerns and to improve their access to community services. Twenty of the more than 80 women on low income self-selected to participate in this study. The research participants were diverse in age (24 to 70), educational backgrounds, and previous work experiences. All identified themselves as 'poor,' most of them subsisted on B.C. Benefits, and 90 per cent identified as white. Tables 7.1 and 7.2 provide the women's demographic profiles.

The data set for this analysis included 32 interviews, 15 group research meetings, and ongoing participant observations and fieldnotes. The semi-structured, one-on-one interviews ranged in length from 45 minutes to two hours. Twenty women were interviewed in the first round, and 12 of the same women completed second interviews. The research meetings ranged in length between two and three hours, occurred every three to four weeks, and had an average of 11 women in attendance. The data were sorted, coded, and analysed with the qualitative data analysis program Atlas.ti 4.1. The coding was an iterative process; we went through the data several times, recalled codes, and reconfirmed the analysis. Through this process we recorded code and theory memos and operational notes concerning emerging conceptual and theoretical understandings (Denzin, 1994).

Table 7.2 The Women's Selected Demographic Characteristics (n = 20)

Education [a]		Race/Ethnicity [b]		Domestic status [c]	
Some elementary	1	White	15	Married	3
Some high school	3	White – French Canadian	1	Single, separated, or divorced	17
Grade 12 (high school) or GED equivalent	8	White – First Nations (children)	1	Mothers with dependent children	11
Some university	1	Asian	2	Mothers with grown children	6
University degree	1	African American	1	Women with no children	3
Data not collected	4			Married	3

[a] Of the women involved in this study, 80 per cent had at least completed high school, compared to the provincial average of 42% (Statistics Canada, 1996).
[b] According to the 1996 census data, 18 per cent of the population of British Columbia are 'visible minorities' (Statistics Canada, 1996). Of the women involved in my research study, 15% can be classified as visible minorities.
[c] Just over 5% of the total population of British Colombia receives income assistance. Of the entire income assistance caseload, 33.6% are single-parent families, 88.5% of which are led by females (Friends of Women and Children in B.C., 2002).

Research Findings

The case study with the women on low income revealed the multiple ways that living in poverty affected the women's health. Material deprivation affected both the women's access to health-promoting resources and nutritious foods. They also reported that they experienced a second tier of health care – one characterized by longer waits, discriminatory treatment, and difficulty accessing essential services and items. Finally, the women adopted unhealthy behaviours as a way of coping with and managing their shame, stress, and depression.

1 LIVING IN MATERIAL DEPRIVATION, AND THE COST OF ATTAINING GOOD HEALTH

In 2001, the research participants subsisted, on average, on $10,797.39 per year. In their locality, this was 18 per cent of the average household income (B.C. Ministry of Human Resources, 2002). All of the research participants spoke at length about their material deprivation and the challenges of budgeting and paying for food, housing, clothing, and transportation. After Elizabeth paid her rent, she said, at one research meeting: 'I get $359, and that's to cover everything.' The women's material deprivation was so severe that they were never able to pay all their bills. Kelly said, 'And it never stops, you're always thinking of how can I do this, how can I do that? Who can I not pay this month, who do I have to pay?'

Being materially deprived severely influenced the women's access to health essentials such as food, clothing, transportation, and child-rearing expenses. For instance, the women shared stories of sacrificing their own food so that their children could eat. At one research meeting Willow, appearing gaunt and thin, told us: 'There have been occasions where I have not had enough money to eat myself so that my children could ... Last month I lost almost 15 pounds.' At times the women could not afford enough food, and at others they could only afford less-nutritious and more filling food options for themselves and their families. As well as affecting aspects of their lives – where they lived, what they ate, and where the children went to school – living on a low income made it difficult to exercise control over family health. This echoes other findings that show that as a result of poverty the health needs of parents, particularly women, are often compromised in favour of their children (Shaw, Dorling, & Smith, 2000).

The women reported that for financial reasons they were unable to access services or resources that could improve or manage their health. Some, including food, health-promoting resources, and community recreation, were too costly; other services or resources were inaccessible due to transportation constraints. Isolation for financial reasons not only prevented the women from accessing community services, but also hampered their ability to meet friends and other people in their communities. Material deprivation causes those with lower incomes to have less access to health-enhancing resources and greater exposure to negative influences upon health than the income group above them (Raphael, 2001). Poverty imposes constraints on the material conditions of everyday life – by limiting access to the fundamental building blocks of health such as adequate housing, good nutrition, and opportunities to participate in society.

2 ACCESS TO THE HEALTH CARE SYSTEM AND
   HEALTH-PROMOTING RESOURCES

Although Canadian government rhetoric supports the notion of universal health care, the women studied reported significant barriers to accessing health care services. They suggested that the system was 'two-tiered' in three ways: in terms of access to and affordability of health-promoting resources; access to health care services, and discriminatory treatment by health care professionals. All of the women said they could not afford health-promoting 'extras,' such as physiotherapy, massage therapy, vitamins and supplements, eyeglasses, and non-generic medications. Seven women spoke of sacrificing essentials, such as food and paying their bills, to cover the cost of medications or therapies. Other women made the opposite choice and sacrificed their medications or therapies to buy food or pay essential bills. Susan, in an interview, explained her situation: 'This month I had to go off my supplements because I had to pay for other things. So I'm feeling it ... the supplements are very expensive. They're good quality and they're what I need. But it was a choice this month to not feel very good.'

Over half of the women felt that they had been treated inequitably by the health care system, specifically regarding length of stay in hospitals, consideration and respect from health care professionals, and access to dental care and homecare support. At one research meeting Katharine explained: 'Because we have no money, they don't keep us long. They are like, 'Next' .. But if you're rich you have a private room; then you can stay longer, the nurses treat you better, everybody treats you better.' And, according to Rene, some health care professionals acted as gatekeepers who effectively excluded low-income women from equitably accessing the health care system: 'It's like the foot specialist I went to who told me that if I lost weight and got off welfare I'd be okay. Now, what that had to do with the shin splints or the pain I was having I don't know.' Despite the rhetoric concerning Canadian universal health care system, the women's experiences are a revealing commentary on what looks more like two-tier health care. This group of poor women, who received the second-tier of health care services, was unable to access the same kinds of services that middle or upper-income people have to address their health.

3 BEING POOR: PSYCHOSOCIAL HEALTH PROBLEMS

Shaming stereotypes. As shown above, a prevailing finding from this study was the women's experience of being stereotyped – and shamed. The women suggested that the stereotype was rooted in the perception that welfare recipients choose to be on welfare. 'It's the biggest stereotype in the world to be a single mother on welfare ... So I'm a welfare bum who could get out if she wanted to, but she chooses to be there' (Willow, interview). The stereotype of the welfare recipient is predicated upon the notion that recipients do not have a valid reason for being on social assistance, that they choose to rely on the government for their financial support though they could easily find work and be financially self-reliant. The women spoke about being stereotyped as people who steal from society, abuse tax-payers' money, and are lazy and illegitimately disabled or sick.

The predominance of this stereotype led the women to evaluate themselves and each other negatively – as shameful and dependent clients of public charity. For instance, Elizabeth felt that she was 'less of a person' (interview), Katharine said she, as a poor woman, was the 'rots of society' (interview). Not only were the women's interactions with authorities shaming, but the very nature of the services that were meant to help them was humiliating. Community recreation's 'leisure access' cards, food banks, and other community services that labeled people as poor embarrassed many of the women.

In the psychological literature, shame, subordination, and being put down and disrespected are seen as extremely important, yet largely unrecognized, sources of stress and anxiety for everyone (Wilkinson, 2000, 1992, 1996). Shame is the primary emotion generated by constant monitoring of the self in relation to others (Scheff, Retzinger, & Ryan, 1989). Shame involves painful feelings that are not always identified as shame by the person experiencing them. Rather they are labeled with a wide variety of terms that disguise the experience of shame – being stressed and depressed, having low self-esteem, feeling inadequate, incompetent, vulnerable, angry, and helpless.[3] The research participants discussed these psychosocial health concerns at length, and often these terms were used interchangeably. As Kelly said, 'I'm just very low on the totem pole ... there's that stereotyping again. Like you're just a single, welfare mother ... If you feel like all your neighbors think you're a loser welfare bum, it's going to impact you (interview).

For six of the women, anger was a response to their shame and humiliation. Virginia Dawn said, 'At the time it used to really upset me when I was feeling it [stereotyped] more ... having that happen, you have a lot of anger. I used to be a very, very angry person' (interview). The women who reported struggling with anger felt that it was a consequence of being excluded and shamed. Scheff et al. (1989) contend that as humiliation increases, rage and hostility increase proportionally to defend against loss of self-esteem; and that hostility and anger can be viewed as an attempt to ward off feelings of humiliation and shame, and a lack of power to defend against insults.

While some women's shame was expressed as anger, others felt powerless and hopeless. Consistently encountering barriers, being stereotyped, and feeling invisible made some women feel helpless to change their situations: 'Once you get so low you can't see beyond. You just can't. I don't even know what I want to be when I grow up ... because there is no tomorrow' (Trina, interview). The deep feelings of shame that all the women reported had a significant influence on their psychosocial health.

Stress and Depression from Living in Poverty. As a consequence of their material deprivation the women reported that their lives were unpredictable and stressful. 'I know life has to have its ups and downs. But not continually having to worry 'is my hydro going to get cut off, or my cable, or my phone?' Having no food, that's a killer' (Elizabeth, interview). Budgeting was a major source of stress for all of the women – learning to juggle expenses, choosing which bills to pay and which to defer to the following month, and determining the exact amount of money needed to survive each month. For most of the women stress was ubiquitous and omnipresent: 'When I get stressed out, you tighten your muscles up, and you're constantly in a state of anxiety. It doesn't seem to ever leave me' (Martha, interview).

The mothers discussed the physical stress and fatigue of parenting; the worry concerning their ability to adequately provide for their children, having little support and security; and the uncompromising government stipulations that they find work as soon as their youngest child turns seven years of age.[4] The single mothers acknowledged that being solely responsible for their children, being exhausted, and wanting better for their children were major sources of stress. As well, all of the women reported that their unrelenting financial worries caused them stress and depression.[5] Poor women also experience more frequent, threatening, and uncontrollable life events than do members of the general population. Repetti and Wood (1997) cite that people living in poverty are likely to be exposed to multiple, persistent, uncontrollable demands, and to live in environments characterized by 'chronic burden[s].' For example, inadequate housing, dangerous neighborhoods, burdensome responsibilities, and financial uncertainties are commonplace, all of which are potent stressors (Belle, 1990). Chronic economic strain may 'grind away and deplete emotional reserves' (McLoyd & Wilson, 1991, cited in Repetti & Wood, 1997), possibly resulting in a diminished ability to reflect upon and develop a problem-focused plan of action. Poverty is among the chronic stressors that may require

constant coping in the short term – coping that is likely to be uninten-
tional and less action-oriented. Living in poverty does not allow time
for recuperation (Repetti & Wood, 1997).

3 HEALTH BEHAVIOURS

The research participants' material deprivation and psychosocial health
affected the range of health behaviours available to them. Significantly,
the women's material deprivation limited the positive health behaviours
at their disposal. For instance, most of the women had experienced
having insufficient money to buy food for themselves and their children, and times when they were undernourished and hungry. Some
could not afford nutritious foods and sacrificed healthy options for
cheaper options that would last longer and provide for more meals.
Trina spoke about the illusion of choice regarding healthy foods: 'You
watch on the news how wonderful it is that you should be eating all
these fruits and vegetables and it shows a handful of grapes and straw-
berries and stuff like that. You can't go out and buy that when you're on
assistance' (interview). All of the women spoke of the challenges of
participating in organized forms of physical activity because of prohibitive registration fees and costs associated with transportation, child
care, and clothing/equipment. Trina said, 'If you don't have any money,
you can't get there and you can't do anything if you don't have any
money. You have to have money. You need money to buy tickets. You
need money to have proper apparel' (interview). There is considerable
evidence for the relationship between physical activity and health (Reid
& Dyck, 2000). The women considered regular physical activity as a
means to address some major health problems such as heart disease
and diabetes, as a strategy for managing chronic health conditions such
as fibromyalgia and back problems, and as a way of meeting other
women in the community to socially integrate in a meaningful way. Yet,
all of the women faced material barriers to being regularly physically
active (Reid, 2004).

The women's shame and psychosocial health issues also influenced
their health behaviours. To some degree, eating comfort foods and
smoking are attempts to satisfy what may be partly social needs
(Wilkinson, 1996). Susan suggested that many women on low income
had disordered eating – they either under-ate or over-ate – and that
many used food for comfort and to manage chronic psychosocial health
problems: '[Poor women] have eating disorders ... Either they don't eat,

or they're bulimic, [or they] eat for comfort. And we do admit it, you know. So it's interesting how food does play a [part in] our emotional [health]' (research meeting). According to Walters, Lenton, & McKeary (1995), using food for comfort is an embedded social behaviour. From our earliest experiences, we learn that food is a source of comfort and it is used by women as a way of coping with their lack of control over their lives.

Three women reported that they consistently under-ate because of the stress of living in poverty, and two women reported that they struggled with anorexia and bulimia nervosa. Elizabeth suggested that low self-esteem was the primary reason for her disordered eating: 'I've never really felt that good about myself. So when my ex told me that the biggest two mistakes of his life – the first one was marrying me and the second one was having our son – so, you were like "What's wrong with me? There must be something wrong with me." And I think that was what started all my eating-type things' (interview). Contrary to common perceptions these poor women's eating behavior was not determined by a lack of knowledge; the women in this study were familiar with the basics of good nutrition.

Four of the research participants were regular smokers. Trina explained that the only indulgence she enjoyed was cigarettes. For her, smoking was comforting and a small luxury. 'The only thing I do is smoke cigarettes. I don't drink. I don't do drugs. I only smoke cigarettes. And I live in a co-op here. And there's nothing extra. Paid my taxes for my cigarettes that's for sure' (interview).[6]

For some women, cigarettes represent one of the few purchases directed solely towards their own pleasure and one of the few luxuries in their lives (Greaves, 1996). People facing difficulties often engage in behaviors that are short-term stress reducers but that entail risks to health (Health Canada, 1997). Smoking can be seen as a way of coping or maintaining 'equilibrium' (Calnan & Williams, 1991); some women smoke instead of expressing their anxiety and frustration with limited resources and decreased personal control (McDonough & Walters, 2001). The factors that predict smoking involve material circumstances, cultural deprivation, and indicators of stressful life events including marital, personal, and household circumstances (Jarvis & Wardle, 1999). Indeed, smokers are drawn disproportionately from those who are disadvantaged within their gender and class groups, and are concentrated among those who are most disadvantaged.

The social conditions under which health-damaging choices occur reflect material deprivation, efforts at stress management, and a minimal expression of power in the context of lives characterized by isolation, alienation, or excessive strain (Ruzek & Hill, 1986). Several research studies have found that, contrary to popular belief, women possess adequate knowledge, skills, and motivation to engage in health-enhancing behaviours, but that their unhealthy behaviours result from struggles to meet conflicting health priorities in the face of decreased resources (Anderson, Blue, Holbrook, & Ng, 1996) and from the psychosocial impact of living in poverty.

The Politics of Poverty and Exclusion: Women's Health as a Social Justice Issue

These case study findings reveal that poverty has an impact on women's health in multifaceted ways: that living in chronic material deprivation limits access to health promoting services and resources, and has a significant impact on the women's health behaviours; that it leads to struggles with shame, stress, and depression, both as a consequence of being stigmatized and stereotyped and as a result of living in material deprivation; that women living in poverty have a limited range of health resources at their disposal, and are often forced to compromise good health choices for bad ones, for financial reasons; and that at times they choose health behaviours such as over-eating and smoking in order to find comfort in their difficult day-to-day lives.

Health inequality researchers argue that the quality of social relations is a prime determinant of human welfare and quality of life, as is living in more egalitarian societies, in which deprivation does not diminish health standards; such societies also seem to be more socially cohesive (Wilkinson, 1996). Yet, in many societies people are systematically excluded from resources and opportunities.

While low-income people, particularly women, are subjected to increasingly punitive and restrictive welfare policies and practices, 'most governments are not yet prepared to address these problems seriously, nor are they prepared to ensure a reasonable level of support for low-income people either inside or outside of the paid labor force' (National Council of Welfare, 2000b, p.145). Doing something about poverty, discrimination, and inequitable access to resources involves notions of planned social and economic change (Becker, 1986). Addressing these larger issues turns the concept of health into a battleground over rights and resources (Rootman & Raeburn, 1994). While theory and research evidence support the link between poverty and ill-health, the extent to which any new program actually succeeds in empowering a community, and the ultimate impact this has on its collective health, remains to be demonstrated (Shiell & Hawe, 1996).

Health is widely recognized as a fundamental right of citizenship: 'The enjoyment of the highest attainable standard of health is one of the fundamental rights of every human being without distinction of race, religion, political belief, economics, or social condition' (WHO, 1948, cited in Hankivsky, 1999). In that vein, health is a social justice issue. Social justice concerns the degree to which a society supports the conditions necessary for all individuals to exercise capacities, express experiences, and participate in determining actions. Social justice requires not the melting away of difference, but the promotion and respect for group differences without oppression (Young, 1990). As shown in earlier chapters in this collection, numerous international platforms explicitly focus on women's right to health as an integral component of human rights protection and promotion.[7] International conventions, documents, and platforms obligate the global community, including Canada, to take concrete action to eliminate all forms of discrimination against women. Importantly, it is not enough to state or recognize human rights; rather, conditions must exist in which they can be exercised and realized (Hankivsky, 1999).

Health as a social justice issue is concerned with creating the opportunities for attaining full health potential and reducing health inequities (Hankivsky, 1999). Equity refers to conditions largely out of individuals' control that create unjust differentials in health. Lack of power at the individual, community, and societal levels is a major risk factor for poor health. Empowering the disadvantaged – or disempowering those who use their privilege to benefit themselves at the expense of the well-being of the community – is an important tool for health promotion. Protecting and restoring health involves a social justice ethic based on collective action and fair play that respects individual rights and experiences (Wallerstein & Freudenberg, 1998). Ultimately the decision all of us have to make is to choose between valuing human development and all its potentials, including good health and the avoidance of illness, or living within a society that excludes the poor and furthers inequities (Raphael, 2001).

NOTES

1 Differences in health status, health outcomes, and other health indicators that appear to correspond to race and ethnicity may mask the effects of socioeconomic status, diet, education, housing, and other factors (Jones, Snider, & Warren, 1996) Yet racial and ethnic differences should not be reduced to a question of social class. There is a complex relationship between social class and race that cannot be reduced to one or the other and that bears further investigation (Reid, 2002).

2 This case study is from *The Wounds of Exclusion: Poverty, Women's Health, and Social Justice* (Reid, 2004).

3 Lewis (1971) classified all of these terms as 'shame markers' because they occurred in a context that involved a perception of self as negatively evaluated by either oneself or someone else (cited in Scheff et al., 1989).

4 The liberal government was elected in BC in May 2001 and instituted new regulations for welfare recipients. Under the new laws, single mothers are now expected to return to work when their youngest child turns three years of age. In a conversation with several of the research participants in December 2001, they questioned how single mothers were expected to earn a living, pay for child care, and cover other living expenses. This was particularly troublesome since the minimum wage for untrained workers (presumably students, but this also applied to most of the single mothers in this study) was reduced to $6 per hour. With the new legislation, the women worried that single mothers with no previous work experience would be forced to leave their children unattended at home while working for this low wage.

5 All of the women said that stress was a health concern, 10 women reported depression, and 3 were diagnosed as clinically depressed.

6 It should be noted that Trina rolled her own cigarettes in order to save money.

7 According to the United Nations Social and Economic Council (1999): 'The realization by women of their right to the enjoyment of the highest attainable standard of physical and mental health is an integral part of the full realization by them of all human rights, and that the human rights of women and the girl child are an inalienable, integral, and indivisible part of universal human rights' (cited in Hankivsky, 1999).

REFERENCES

Adler, N.E., Boyce, T., Chesney, M.A., Cohen, S., Folkman, S., Kahn, R.L., & Syme, S.L. (1994). Socioeconomic status and health: The challenge of the gradient. *American Psychologist, 49*(1), 15–24.

Anderson, J.M. (1987). Migration and health: Perspectives on immigrant women. *Sociology of Health and Illness, 9*(4), 410–438.

Anderson, J.M., Blue, C., Holbrook, A., & Ng, M. (1996). On chronic illness: Immigrant women in Canada's work force – A feminist perspective. *Canadian Journal of Nursing Research, 25*(2), 7–22.

Ballantyne, P.J. (1999). The social determinants of health: A contribution to the analysis of gender differences in health and illness. *Scandinavian Journal of Public Health, 27*(4), 290–295.

B.C. Ministry of Human Resources (2002, 2 June). Income assistance rates. Retrieved 27 October 2004, from, http://www.mhr.gov.bc.ca/factsheets/2002/iarates.htm.

Becker, M.H. (1986). The tyranny of health promotion. *Public Health Review, 14*, 15–25.

Belle, D. (1990). Poverty and women's mental health. *American Psychologist, 45*(3), 385–389.

Brunner, E., & Marmot, M. (2000). Social organization, stress, and health. In M. Marmot & R.G. Wilkinson (Eds.), *Social Determinants of Health* (pp. 17–43). Oxford: Oxford University Press.

Calnan, M., & Williams, S. (1991). Style of life and the salience of health: An exploratory study of health related practises in households from differing socio-economic circumstances. *Sociology of Health and Illness, 13*(4), 506–529.

Cohen, M. (1998). Towards a framework for women's health. *Patient Education and Counselling, 33*, 187–196.

Deaton, A. (2002). Policy implications of the gradient of health and wealth. *Health Affairs, 21*(2), 1–9.

Denzin, N.K. (1994). The art and politics of interpretation. In N.K. Denzin & Y.S. Lincoln (Eds.), *Handbook of Qualitative Research* (pp. 500–515). Thousand Oaks, CA: Sage.

Doyal, L. (1995). What makes women sick: Gender and the political economy of health. London: Macmillan.

Friends of Women and Children in B.C. (2002, 15 July). *Report Card, 1*(4), 1–2.

Greaves, L. (1996). Smoke screen: Women's smoking and social control. Halifax: Fernwood and Scarlet Press.

Greaves, L., Hankivsky, O., Amaratunga, C., Ballem, P., Chow, D., De Konick, M., Grant, K., Lippman, A., Maclean, H., Maher, J., Messing, K., & Vissandjee, B. (2000). *C.I.H.R. 2000: Sex, Gender and Women's Health.* Vancouver: Centre of Excellence for Women's Health.

Hankivsky, O. (1999). Social justice and women's health: A Canadian perspective. Halifax, NS: Maritime Centre of Excellence for Women's Health. Retrieved 10 February 2000, from http://www.medicine.dal.ca/mcewh/oct-synthesis/hankivsky-justice.htm.

Health Canada. (1997). Final table June 26, 1997: Determinants and lifespan N.D.G. (Table). Ottawa: Health Canada.

Health Canada. (1999). *Statistical Report on the Health of Canadians*. Charlottetown, PEI: Federal, Provincial, and Territorial Advisory Committee on Population Health.

Hunt, K., & Annandale, E. (1999). Relocating gender and morbidity: Examining men's and women's health in contemporary Western societies. Introduction to special issue on gender and health. *Social Science & Medicine, 48,* 1–5.

Jackson, A. (2003). *Research Paper No. 22: Is Work Working for Women?* Ottawa: Canadian Labour Congress.

Jarvis, M.J., & Wardle, J. (1999). Social patterning of individual health behaviours: The case of cigarette smoking. In M. Marmot & R.G. Wilkinson (Eds.), *Social Determinants of Health* (pp. 240–255). Oxford: Oxford University Press.

Jones, W.K., Snider, D.E., & Warren, R.C. (1996). Deciphering the data: Race, ethnicity, and gender as critical variables. *Journal of American Medical Women's Association, 51*(4), 137–138.

Krieger, N. (2001). A glossary for social epidemiology. *Journal of Epidemiology and Community Health, 55*(October), 693–700.

Landucci, M. (2003). *Linking People to Food: Accessing Low and No-Cost Food in Surrey and White Rock*. Surrey, BC: Surrey Social Futures, Food for Kidz Coalition, Surrey Food Bank.

Lorber, J. (1997). *Gender and Social Construction of Illness*. Thousand Oaks, CA: Sage.

Love, R., Jackson, L., Edwards, R., & Pederson, A. (1997). *Gender and Its Relationship to Other Determinants of Health*. Toronto: Department of Behavioral Science, University of Toronto.

Macintyre, S. (1998). Social inequalities and health in the contemporary world: A comparative overview. In S. Strickland & P. Shetty (Eds.), *Human Biology and Social Inequality* (pp. 20–35). Cambridge: Cambridge University Press.

Macintyre, S., Ford, G., & Hunt, K. (1999). Do women 'over-report' morbidity? Men's and women's responses to structured prompting on a standard question on long standing illness. *Social Science & Medicine, 48,* 89–98.

Matthews, S., & Power, C. (2002). Socio-economic gradients in psychological distress: A focus on women, social roles and work-home characteristics. *Social Science & Medicine, 54*(5), 799–810.

McDonough, P., & Walters, V. (2001). Gender and health: Reassessing patterns and explanations. *Social Science & Medicine, 52,* 547–559.

Ministry of Human Resources. (2003). *Monthly Statistics – Support Clients by*

Family Type. Victoria: BC Statistics. Retrieved 27 October 2004, from www.bcstats.gov.bc.ca.

Moss, N.E. (2002). Gender equity and socioeconomic inequality: A framework for the patterning of women's health. *Social Science & Medicine, 54*(5), 649–661.

National Council of Welfare. (2000a). Justice and the Poor: A National Council of Welfare Publication. Ottawa: Minister of Public Works and Government Services Canada.

National Council of Welfare. (2000b). *Poverty Profile, 1998*. Ottawa: National Council of Welfare.

Phipps, S. (2003). *The Impact of Poverty on Health: A Scan of Research Literature*. Ottawa: Canadian Institute for Health Information.

Raphael, D. (2001). *Inequality Is Bad for Our Hearts: Why Low Income and Social Exclusion are Major Causes of Heart Disease in Canada*. Toronto: North York Heart Health Network.

Reid, C. (2002). *A Full Measure: Towards a Comprehensive Model for the Measurement of Women's Health*. Vancouver: B.C. Centre of Excellence for Women's Health.

Reid, C. (2004). *The Wounds of Exclusion: Poverty, Women's Health, and Social Justice*. Edmonton, AB: Qualitative Institute Press.

Reid, C., & Dyck, L. (2000). Implications: Future research, program and policy development. In C. Reid, L. Dyck, H. McKay, & W. Frisby (Eds.), *The Health Benefits of Physical Activity for Girls and Women: Literature Review and Recommendations for Future Research and Policy* (pp. 201–205). Vancouver: British Columbia Centre of Excellence for Women's Health.

Repetti, R.L., & Wood, J. (1997). Families accommodating to chronic stress: Unintended and unnoticed processes. In B.H. Gottlieb (Ed.), *Coping with Chronic Stress* (pp. 191–220). New York: Plenum.

Rootman, I., & Raeburn, J.M. (1994). The concept of health. In A. Pederson, M. O'Neill, & I. Rootman (Eds.), *Health Promotion in Canada: Provincial, National and International Perspectives* (pp. 56–71). Toronto: W.B. Saunders.

Ruspini, E. (2001). The study of women's deprivation: How to reveal the gender dimension of poverty. *International Journal of Social Research Methodology, 4*(2), 101–118.

Ruzek, S., & Hill, J. (1986). Promoting women's health: Redefining the knowledge base and strategies for change. *Health Promotion, 1*(3), 301–309.

Ruzek, S.B., Clarke, A.E., & Olesen, V.L. (1997). Social, biomedical, and feminist models of women's health. In S.B. Ruzek, A.E. Clarke & V.L. Olesen (Eds.), *Women's Health: Complexities and Differences* (pp. 11–28). Columbus: Ohio State University Press.

Scheff, T.J., Retzinger, S.M., & Ryan, M.T. (1989). Crime, violence, and self-esteem: Review and proposals. In A.M. Mecca, N.J. Smelser, & J. Vasconcellos (Eds.), *The Social Importance of Self-Esteem* (pp. 165–199). Berkeley: University of California Press.

Shaw, M., Dorling, D., & Smith, G.D. (2000). Poverty, social exclusion, and minorities. In M. Marmot & R.G. Wilkinson (Eds.), *Social Determinants of Health* (pp. 211–239). Oxford: Oxford University Press.

Shiell, A., & Hawe, P. (1996). Health promotion community development and the tyranny of individualism. *Health Economics, 5,* 241–247.

Statistics Canada. (1996). 1996 Census Nation Tables. Retrieved 20 July 2005, from, www.statscan.ca/english.

Townson, M. (2000). *A Report Card on Women and Poverty.* Ottawa: Canadian Centre for Policy Alternatives.

United Nations Development Program. (1999). *Human Development Report 1999.* New York: UNDP.

United Nations Platform for Action Committee. (2004). *Women and the Economy: A Project for UNPAC.* Winnipeg, MB: UNPAC.

Wall, N.B. (1993). The beautiful strength of my anger put to use. In L. Carty (Ed.), *And Still We Rise: Political Mobilizing in Contemporary Canada* (pp. 279–298). Toronto: Women's Press.

Wallerstein, N., & Freudenberg, N. (1998). Linking health promotion and social justice: A rationale and two case stories. *Health Education Research, 13*(3), 451–457.

Walters, V., Lenton, R., & Mckeary, M. (1995). Women's health in the context of women's lives. Report. Ottawa: Health Promotion Directorate, Health Canada.

Wilkinson, R.G. (1992). Income distribution and life expectancy. *British Medical Journal, 304*(6820), 165–168.

Wilkinson, R.G. (1996). *Unhealthy Societies: The Afflictions of Inequality.* London: Routledge.

Wilkinson, R.G. (2000). Putting the picture together: Prosperity, redistribution, health, and welfare. In M. Marmot & R.G. Wilkinson (Eds.), *Social Determinants of* Health (pp. 256–274). Oxford: Oxford University Press.

World Health Organization. (1998). *Gender and Health.* Technical paper. Geneva: WHO.

Young, I.M. (1990). *Justice and the Politics of Difference.* Princeton, NJ: Princeton University Press.

8 Women's Health at the Intersection of Gender and the Experience of International Migration

BILKIS VISSANDJÉE, WILFREDA THURSTON,
ALISHA APALE, AND KAMRUN NAHAR

As a composite of multiple biological and social dimensions, women's health and illness experiences are shaped by the resources and opportunities available to them as well as by health policies and practices. If based upon a multidisciplinary approach, health policies and practices will be attentive to the array of identities, practices, and visions that characterize Canadian women. Moreover, policies and practices which are sensitive to both gender and the experience of migration will better pertain to women as Canadians in a globalizing world.

While the multiple dimensions of women's health are outlined in gender-sensitive literature and advocated through various bodies of global governance and health, women's migration experiences have yet to be systematically acknowledged and incorporated as a determinant of health. Particular attention is required to understand the dynamics of migration and its subsequent gender-specific effects on the immigrant population's health. This pending issue has been identified as one of the major gaps in immigration health research (Dunn & Dyck, 2000; Hyman, 2001; Juteau, 1999; Kinnon, 1999; Spitzer, 2003). A growing, if nascent body of immigrant health research has established that gender and migration, and more particularly the dynamic imbrications between them, are determinants of health (Aroian, 2001; Boyd & Grieco, 2003; Des Meules et al., 2004; Iglesias et al., 2003; Meadows, Thurston, & Melton, 2001; Thurston & Vissandjee, 2005; Vissandjée et al., 2005; Vissandjée et al., 2001). Indeed, it can be argued that as a determinant of health, migration patterns the effects of other, generally acknowledged health determinants.[1] This premise is not, however, the fruit of a thematically unified corpus of literature and research findings; rather, it is a prologue based upon multiple isolated studies.

When health policy disengages from the core social institutions and infrastructures essential to immigrant women's health and well-being, it both reflects and perpetuates a culture of disadvantage that still persists for far too many women in Canada and around the world. In this post-millennium era, Canada continues to pride itself in having a multicultural identity, in leadership in population health, and in having a health care system that is available to all. Yet the recognition of this diverse demographic has not been fully translated into health care policies and services that comprise an integrated approach to the needs and interests of women experiencing migration.

As Margaret Somerville (1999) articulates, health care is never simply and only about health care. It is evident that health policy making and practice constitute a cultural, economic, legal, ethical, and political 'forum in which to work out the principles, attitudes, beliefs, myths and values [of health]' (p. xii). The definitions and determinants of healthiness for women indeed extend far beyond biology (Cohen & Maclean, 2003); in step with emerging health policy, research and care must not only embody a social determinant approach, but must also be sensitive to experiences of migration above and beyond the recognition of cultural diversity. This is a task which requires the interdisciplinary collaboration of multiple sectors committed towards enhancing Canadian health policy and delivery of services. Yet, initiatives such as these are up against some increasingly polarizing directions for both Canadian and international health policies, practices, and outcomes. At this juncture, one must reflect upon whether health care is a question of social rights and universal access or if it is a commoditized, albeit technologically sophisticated, biomedical response to disease (Farmer, 2003).

Through the advocacy of global human rights agendas, through such initiatives as the United Nations Millennium Development Goals and the Global Health Forum, the social dimensions of health are (re)gaining a platform; many health professionals and policy makers acknowledge that a purely biomedical approach to ill health translates into a health care mandate that often (arbitrarily) divides bodies into distinct compartments of illness or health. While specialized health research and technology is important, a purely biomedical approach to ill health often reinforces a health care lens that is focused on treating instead of preventing illness. Moreover, the profusion of a technologically and pharmaceutically driven scope in health research distorts ill health by minimizing or negating the strain of social ills, such as inequitable distributions of resources and opportunities and ensuing circumstances of social isolation, poverty, and insecurity. Social conditions such as these represent some of the most persistent challenges confronted by women and men experiencing migration (Anand, Peter, & Sen, 2004; Galabuzi & Labonte, 2002; Graham & Kelly, 2004; Marmot, 2005a; Wagstaff, 2002).

Throughout the twentieth century modern medicine has enjoyed extraordinary developments, and with these the means to attain and maintain health have greatly increased. Through the feminist movement and an emerging gender-sensitive health platform, the conceptualization and understanding of women's health, in both biological and social domains, have experienced promising advances. The social opportunities, resources, and conditions in the lives of many women in Canada have likewise improved significantly. Through the incorporation of a gender-lens in health research and care, it has been aptly demonstrated that gender is a salient determinant of social (in)equity and health. This is primarily due to the fact that the opportunities and resources to attain and maintain health are not evenly distributed between and among women and men (Côté, Kérisit, & Côté, 2003; 10/90 Global Forum for Health Research 2003–2004). In fact, according to the WHO Commission on the Social Determinants of Health, 'By far, the greatest share of health problems is attributable to broad social conditions' (Marmot, 2005a, p.1); concurrently we regard social investment as a critical vehicle to the health and well-being of *all* women in Canada.

The persistence of social inequities experienced by women have fuelled much of the motivation behind research endeavors that consider gender a complex, fluid construct. As such, emerging gender-sensitive health research has become attentive to the concept of intersectionality, where gender represents one of many 'forces' defining women's health experiences (Dyck & Mclaren, 2002; Spitzer, 2003). But there are others. For example, while women's experiences of migration were essentially 'invisible' in health and migration research throughout the 1960s and 1970s, recent research efforts are in the process of integrating migration – and within this, gendered experiences of migration – as yet another contributor to women's health where inequities may persist (Boyd & Grieco, 2003). Mapping migration and gender as intersecting social determinants of immigrant women's health, this chapter explores the experience of migration through a gender-lens; the integration of gender and migration as dimensions of immigrant women's health further contributes to evolving latitudes along which the conceptualizations and understanding of women's health continue to expand.

Integrating Migration and Gender into Women's Health

Migration

Immigration can be seen as voluntary, involuntary or a blend of both (CIC, 2005). The 'push-pull' factors in migration may include economic globalization and accompanying economic and educational needs and opportunities. Other factors, such as socio-political transition, family reunification, land reform, forced relocation, and/or persecution and ecological deterioration or disaster, may also be considered. Beyond these, there are multiple 'invisible elements' that shape the decision to migrate; for example, the degree of choice one has, the ability to act upon the decision to migrate, and the ability to do so in an informed and secure manner (Biidu, 2004). Following the decision and ability to migrate, immigrants are met with complex application, classification, and landing procedures (Hyman, 2001; Renaud et al., 2003). Overall, migration constitutes an experience of significant transition, offering new opportunities as well as many potential hardships. The immigration process – from the decision to migrate, to the journey itself, and through-out the settlement process – is a complicated affair, and the ability to meet immigration prerequisites is extraordinarily competitive.

Since 1990, Canada has typically accepted about 230,000 immigrants per year (Kessel, 1998). Currently, the top four regions of origin for Canada's most recent immigrants are Asia and the Pacific (54 per cent), Europe and the United Kingdom (18 per cent), Africa and the Middle East (18 per cent), and the United States, the Caribbean, and South and Central America (10 per cent) (Kinnon, 1999). Within Canadian perma-nent immigration policy, voluntary immigrants are classified into six categories: skilled workers, business class, provincial nomination, fam-ily class, international adoption, and Quebec-selected immigration (CIC, 2005). Involuntary immigration comprises two classes: namely, refugee resettlement or asylum seeker (CIC, 2005). While the majority of immi-grants integrate well into Canadian society (Kinnon, 1999), the new opportunities that may be associated with migration to Canada occur in tandem with the challenges of migration. As such, it is imperative that both the opportunities and challenges of migration are factored into the equation of immigrant health outcomes.

The relationship between migration and one's health outcomes var-ies with the impetus, experience, and outcomes of migration, as well as with the everyday processes of integration. For example, Kramer, Ivey,

& Ying (1999) explain that 'voluntary immigrants tend to have had more time to prepare both psychologically and practically and may come with resources and some level of English-language skill and have generally experienced less extreme stressors' (p.9). The protective factors maintained by voluntary immigrants, however, are typically absent from the experiences of involuntary immigrants. The latter often have pressing health care needs, not to mention the material and economic ones. For example, forced relocation due to political conflicts, natural disasters, or other related conflicts create significant vulnerabilities. Within this, exposure to multiple traumas such as rape, torture, socio-culturally sanctioned abuse, and domestic violence compose the backdrop against which the health care needs of many refugees and asylum seekers must be framed. Common to both voluntary and involuntary immigrants are the difficulties associated with uprooting, acculturation, and adaptation stressors and accompanying transformations in family dynamics and gender relations.

As a testimony to the complexity of immigration health, current research endeavours to span a broad range of interests, including population health studies and health care utilization, mortality differentials among recent immigrants, and the role of ethnicity and/or religion as factors in adaptation strategies and the rates of conjugal violence (see Kinnon, 1999). As research continues, directions of causality continue to be investigated; there are also debates on whether migration itself should be considered a health-risk factor. Certainly, the inclusion of migration as a determinant of health is seen as a significant advancement in Canadian health research (Kinnon, 1999; Vissandjée et al., 2001; Vissandjée et al., 2004). Yet, further research is needed to integrate gender and migration experiences into the equations of immigrant health, particularly as the push-pull factors that precipitate the decision to migrate vary between and among women and men (Boyd & Grieco, 2003).

Women and Migration

Since the 1960s, women have represented half of all international migrations (Zlotnick, 2003). Gender is thus a highly salient dimension within the context of migration, and the perceptions, norms, and performance of gender at an 'individual, familial, and social level' are responsive to the transforming events of migration at all stages (Boyd & Grieco, 2003). From the decision and the ability to migrate, to the policies and gendered expectations and norms in place in destination countries, female immigrants tend to be considered more vulnerable than male immigrants (Hampson, 2004; Kawar, 2004); this trend is well reflected in immigrant women's health outcomes.

Preliminary immigration health research has demonstrated that upon arrival in Canada, the health status of many recent immigrant women begins to deteriorate and continues to do so with the length of time spent in Canada, a phenomenon typically referred to as the 'healthy immigrant effect' (Dunn & Dyck, 2000; Hampson, 2004; Hyman, 2001; Noh & Kasper, 2003; Vissandjée et al., 2005). The gradual loss of health and well-being is related to multidimensional social factors, including isolation and loss of pre-existing support systems, language barriers, unemployment or work in employment ghettos with unsafe or unhealthy work conditions, and prolonged social insecurity and feelings of vulnerability arising through poverty, prejudice, and discrimination (Kawar, 2004). Likewise, remaining uninformed of existing services, as well as confronting barriers in accessing the health system and adapting to novel health care practices, represent significant challenges for many recent immigrants (Hyman, 2001; Spitzer, 2003; Vissandjée, et al., 2001).

While both women and men may be affected by such circumstances, declines in the originally optimal health status of recent immigrant women may also be explained with respect to gender. On a global scale, the distinct challenges experienced by female immigrants are noted in the persistent invisibility of women's interests and needs and corresponding gaps in a gender-sensitive management of migration. This may also be seen in the lack of protection extended specifically to female immigrants under national labour and human rights laws (Kawar, 2004). For example, more immigrant women than men are employed in the informal sectors of domestic services and the entertainment industry, most often without legal and social protection (Kawar, 2004). The risks of social disadvantage and exploitation are also differentially shaped by the gendered circumstances under which migration occurs. For example, women and children constitute the majority of refugees and externally or internally displaced persons; moreover, gender-based persecution is not universally included in the definition (and thus protection) of refugees (Biidu, 2004).

As discussed by Dyck and Mclaren (2002), while the distribution of responsibilities, information, opportunities, and rights throughout all phases of migration remain gendered, women's experiences of migration are closely related to the gendered distributions of 'local material conditions and social relations' (p. 5). How immigrant women's health is shaped by gender and migration is thus a function of multiple intersecting variables and may be operationalized through the framework of macro social conditions of particular relevance to the experience of migration, such as social integration, economic opportunity, and human security.

Social Integration and Inclusion

In the context of migration, social integration is frequently discussed in terms of acculturation and adaptation. However, these terms are repeatedly misunderstood. Integration is more than an exchange of 'old' traditions and relations for 'new' ones; rather, integration is better conceptualized as a 'sustained mutual interaction between newcomers and the societies that receive them' (Ray, 2002, October; Renaud et al., 2003; Spitzer, 2003; Vissandjée et al., 2005). As such, integration is a socially interactive process that may last for generations.

Being able to integrate into society in a way that enables women to fulfil their interests and potentials may be thought of as a three-way process. This sustained process depends upon immigrant women and men themselves having the abilities, interests, and commitment to such integration; immigrant women and men and their supporters having accessible and relevant resources and opportunities within civil society; and the existence of federally and institutionally guaranteed protections of women's rights and freedoms. Integration also depends heavily on the efforts of social institutions to foster the capacity for all women to bridge identities and experiences. Ongoing social support further facilitates the capacity that gives recent immigrant women the possibility of achieving their full potential and thus establishing themselves as citizens with a stake in Canada's future (Frith, 2003). Recognizing women's educational and professional qualifications, for example, would extend employment opportunities to recent immigrant women and establish some of the basic mechanisms through which women may build and live healthy, socially integrated lives.

Social support networks primarily involve various interpersonal relationships within families and local communities, including the emotional, instrumental, and informational support that is particularly relevant to health (Leppin & Schwarzer, 1990). The lack of social support experienced by many immigrant women may stem from joblessness, homelessness, or language deficits, and is considered a risk factor for ill health and mortality (Fuhrer & Stansfeld, 2002). For example, Donahue, Este, and Miller (2003) found that among the immigrant participants in their sample, 13 per cent were currently homeless and 87 per cent were considered at risk of becoming homeless; among the latter, over 50 per cent were women. This risk is accentuated by the fact that shelters and drop-in centres are often not accessible to immigrants and refugees due to linguistic barriers. Long delays for language programs such as ESL for English and COFI for French, and sustained difficulties in terms of culturally congruent approaches within health and social services likewise contribute to experiences of isolation (Bischoff et al., 2003; SCPI, 2005; Vergnaud, 2004; Vissandjee & Dupéré, 2000a).

While research demonstrates that immigrant women's well-being is strongly mediated by the extent to which their family members retain the cultural patterns of the country of origin, even with solid social networks, bonds may not necessarily be advantageous to immigrant women or their health needs (Choudhury et al., 2002; Lipson, Hosseini, Kabir, Omidian, & Edmonston, 1995; Meadows et al., 2001). For example, the marital relationship may be paradoxical. Marriage may improve economic and social support opportunities, but it also might reduce immigrant women's control over paid and/or unpaid work, particularly as most married women enter Canada as dependents (Fong, 1999). As important as it is to have social support and community, the nature of that support is likewise significant; social support systems not only generate some of the foundational opportunities for health, safety, and well-being, but also provide some means to protect against harmful relationships and unhealthy circumstances.

Overcoming Impoverishing Conditions: Economic Opportunities

Women's contributions are often economically un(der)recognized and/or un(der)valued; similarly, in the context of migration, research tends to look at the 'effects of migration on women' as opposed to the diverse ways that women, through migration, own, uphold, and mobilize resources for the welfare and well-being of their families (Biidu, 2004). The number of female migrants to developed countries outnumbers male migrants, and economic support offered by migrant women from abroad to their families and communities outweighs those made by men, an area for further research on the economic contributions made by women via migration (Biidu, 2004; Kawar, 2004; Zlotnik, 2003).

Immigrant women's participation in international labour markets is largely described in terms of two occupations: the sex-trade industry and domestic labour (Zlotnik, 2003). As part of globally gendered power dynamics embedded in one's socio-economic status, the large presence of women in risky and exploitative labours cannot be overlooked. While many recent immigrant women in Canada are also found among child-care workers, teachers, and nurses, there is a paucity of research on the full scope of the economic opportunities and challenges women encounter via migration. This is especially problematic, as recent immigrant women are often denied opportunities to employ their professional skills; instead they find their professional qualifications are devalued or go unrecognized (Kawar, 2004, p. 73).

It is estimated that 70 per cent of women in the world live in poverty (10/90 Global Forum for Health Research, 2003–2004). While this condition is not necessarily overcome or induced by migration, it is arguable that the structure of global immigration policies perpetuates conditions where poverty maintains a feminine face. As the resources and opportunities required to obtain recognized educational qualifications, meet language prerequisites, and offer professional and skilled labour are globally gendered, women are much more likely than men to depend on immigration via family-class sponsorships (Kawar, 2004). Ruddick (2003), Sweetman (2003), Li (2003a, 2003b), Pendakur & Pendakur (2002), Krieger (2000), Krieger & Gruskin (2001), and Reitz (2001) argue that if policies remain insensitive to the gendered conditions that limit women's access to resources and opportunities, female immigrants will continue to experience labour market inequities. This is likewise true with respect to Canadian immigration policies. For example, as Thobani (1999) argues, 'whereas men are defined as independent economic agents, women and children are defined only by their relation to the 'independent' male actors – as 'dependent' family members' (p. 12). Policies such as these further contribute to un(der)recognized and/or un(der)valued economic contributions made by women, including women experiencing migration.

Rather, migration should constitute an opportunity for women wherein the economic opportunities and accompanying labour rights and protections, as well as the social safety nets available to native-born Canadians, are extended to immigrant women as well (Galabuzi & Labonte, 2002; Graham & Kelly, 2004; Status of Women Canada, 2005–2006). Being paid an equitable wage, having the opportunity to apply and transfer previously acquired skills, as well as having access to programs to enhance or learn new skills, represent several reasonable expectations that most new immigrant women and men should encounter (Frith, 2003; Renaud et al., 2003). Yet, significant economic disparities and low levels of social mobility persist among recent immigrant women (Kawar, 2004). Particularly evident in the context of economic globalization, current distributions of the female labour force are continually marked by poorer and increasingly exploitative work conditions, part-time or irregular employment, lack of job security, or benefits and disproportionate incomes (Kawar, 2004). As such, the objectives of national policies must encompass gender gaps in access to economic resources, such as education, job training, and professional accreditation, as well as the ongoing challenges of overcoming the persistence of racism in Canada (Department of Canadian Heritage, 2005).

In spite of these challenges, Canada's recent immigrant women display incredible resilience, aptitude, and resourcefulness (Dyck & McLaren, 2002). The contributions made by women would be even better facilitated by the entrenchment of conditions wherein recent immigrant women might thrive socially and economically. Ensuring the extension of socio-economic protections to recent immigrant women would also contribute to the amelioration of the disproportionate embodiment of the healthy immigrant effect by women. Furthermore, ensuring a more equitable distribution of the socio-economic protections and advantages that facilitate enduring experiences of health and well-being for *all* Canadian women would contribute further to the ability of recent immigrant women to meet the many new opportunities and ambitions that may be enjoyed in Canada (Galabuzi & Labonte, 2002; Graham & Kelly, 2004; Status of Women Canada, 2005–2006).

Protecting Against Violence

Throughout the 1980s and 90s the public perception, awareness, and action against violence has changed considerably. As outlined in detail in Chapter 18 of this collection, while a gender-based perspective of violence in North America was primarily developed by second wave feminists in the 1980s, violence was constructed in terms of white women and their experiences of physical, emotional, or sexual violence (Rankin & Vickers, 2001). As part of the aftermath of the 6 December 1989 killings of 14 female engineering students in Montreal, the perception of gender-based violence changed; experiences of racism and other forms of discrimination were brought into the foreground in anti-violence discourse in Canada. Moreover, these shifts added to the expansion of understandings of 'the spectrum of violence' to include both personal and institutional violence (p. 40). It was in this context that the experiences of violence of immigrant women became more visible. Violence has since become one of the central points of focus in gender-based research conducted in the context of migration (Kinnon, 1999).

In its different shapes and forms, the prevalence of violence is now better understood as a horrific experience faced by an increasing number of immigrant women (Campbell et al., 2002; Muhajarine & D'Arcy, 1999; Smith, 2004). Research demonstrates that incidents of family conflict and violence may be exacerbated by the stresses bound in financial constraints, lack of permanent or stable housing, threats, and experiences of discrimination in civil society, and so on (Campbell et al., 2002; Cohen & MacLean, 2003; Muhajarine & D'Arcy, 1999). Efforts to protect against physical, sexual, or psychological abuse are often met with significant barriers in the mainstream host culture as well as risks of rejection from one's family and/or own culture (Agnew, 1998; CRI-VIFF, 2003). Similarly, efforts to redress institutional violence as well as violence as a product of social isolation and marginalization are met with significant challenges to entrench intolerance of violence and ensure the protection of all women at all levels of society.

How women respond to the many forms of violence that may accompany the experience of migration cannot be understood outside of the social factors that exonerate, perpetuate, and silence it. When the gendered conditions of social exclusion and impoverishment coalesce, women are unduly exposed to controlling, inequitable, and/or marginalizing circumstances. Further, in the context of migration, opportunities for recourse may be compromised, particularly when women are unable to benefit from legal protection. When socio-cultural stigmas, persistent language barriers, social isolation, and poverty frame the conditions under which violence occurs, social policies and the conditions that position recent immigrant women into vulnerable social and economic circumstances are implicated. It is therefore necessary for Canadian institutions, policies, civil society, and individual households to respond. Acknowledging the unnecessary obstacles experienced by recent immigrant women, including sexism, racism, and xenophobia, is the first step in ensuring the protection and promotion of rights and freedoms for all women in Canada (Agnew, 1996; Klein, 2001).

In the context of the post-9/11 era, human security is a mounting concern taking precedence over multiple areas of human rights, freedoms, and protections. Human security is likewise a significant concern for many women, including those experiencing migration. According to the Helsinky Process report (see Hampson, 2004), maintaining human security is deemed a socially collective action and is premised upon the empowering capacities encompassed within social conditions, such as socio-economic well-being. More specifically, according to a recent WHO report on violence, 'sustained, multi-sectoral responses' are the most effective means of protecting against violence. Protective factors include education, employment, housing, social safety, and justice when violence occurs (WHO, 2004).

According to Chen (2004), overall, health is deemed to be 'instrumental' to human security as it facilitates the capacity to contribute and enjoy a 'full range of human functioning' (p. 2). More specifically, the health problems that occur in the context of poverty and inequity are seen as most germane to human security. Yet, despite global advocacy for social investment as a means of insuring human security and health, the Canadian federal government is in the process of unravelling Canada's social safety nets (Status of Women Canada, 2005–2006). In the context of declining social transfer funds as a function of the 1990s political fixation on deficit-reduction and the increasing entrenchment of neo-liberal policies in health care and beyond research on the social dimensions of immigrant women's health is necessary to ramp up further support for health care policies and practices that best meet the needs and interests of all women in Canada. When conditions of inequity as embedded in experiences of social isolation and poverty continue to hamper opportunities for recent immigrant women to integrate and thrive in Canada, discourse on women's health in the context of migration must incorporate social (re)investment as a means to generate a climate of inclusivity, economic opportunity, security, and overall well-being for women in Canada.

Moving Health Policy and Practices Forward

While the twentieth century has enjoyed robust developments in health technology and science, according to Farmer (2003) it is in the twenty-first century that we will make our decisions about how these benefits are employed and dispersed. In this regard, Canada is at a crossroads. In the wake of significant biomedical advancement, will Canadian health policies promote a health care system of commodities or a system founded upon and in the protection of the social rights of all Canadians? As noted, Canada prides itself in having a multicultural identity and in maintaining a universally available health care system. However, health policies and services do not reflect Canada's diverse demographics and do not offer an integrated approach appropriate to the needs and interests of women experiencing migration. In this chapter, immigrant women's health is thus mapped at the intersection of gender and migration, dimensions which must be integrated into our conceptualization of women's health in Canada.

Responding to the social dimensions of immigrant women's health requires further social investment to accompany the advances in health care technology Canadian women already enjoy. As such, health policy and planning would engage the core social institutions and infrastructures essential to immigrant women's health and well-being in order to protect against the circumstances of disadvantage that persist for far too many women in Canada and around the world. More specifically, in an effort to abet the disadvantageous circumstances and conditions that may accompany women's experiences of migration, the discourse surrounding Canadian health policies and practices must further acknowledge and act in favour of sustained social investment as a critical imperative.

The resources and opportunities contained in basic social infrastructure, such as social integration, economic opportunity, and security are regarded as significant influences on one's health status and experiences (Farmer, 2003; Status of Women Canada, 2005–2006; 10/90 Global Forum for Health Research, 2003–2004; Walters, 2003). Unpacking these macro-conditions in the context of immigrant women's health is a work in progress that is best continued through integrated multi-tiered initiatives, particularly as the needs and interests of recent immigrants in Canada are diverse. At the crux lies a perspective of women's health that is informed by the evolving intersectionalities that constitute the meanings and experiences of being women, and being immigrant women. It is under the rubric of social (re)investment in Canada's core social institutions, including health care and education, that further recommendations, including those made by Status of Women Canada (2005–2006), Rankin & Vickers (2001), Hampson (2004), Scotland Executive, (2004), Vissandjée (2001), Vissandjée & Dupéré (2000a, 2000b), Vissandjée & DesMeules (2004), WHO (2004), Hyman (2001), and Smith (2004) are presented.

Recommendation 1: Build Upon the Voices of Immigrant Women

> Establish forums for immigrant women to voice their social, economic, political, and cultural concerns, interests, and needs. These forums should be built upon the use of inclusive language and be directly networked with health and social policy researchers. As such, the mechanisms adopted to integrate gender and migration into policy planning and implementation will be derived primarily from the voices of immigrant women.

The processes of integration into a new society are often lengthy and may take an entire lifetime and/or may involve several generations (Isajiw, 1999; Renaud et al., 2003). As such, the ongoing commitment of both recent immigrants and native-born Canadians is central to the development of a healthy and vibrant society. Language is one tool through which one expresses perceptions and shapes interactions with others. Within this, language is a significant factor in ensuring accuracy in communication and in building trust and respect (Bischoff et al., 2003; Vergnaud, 2004; Vissandjée & Dupéré, 2000a). Listening to immigrant women would involve active engagement with diverse groups of immigrant women throughout both the development and implementation of social programs for integration (Vissandjée, 2001; Vissandjée & Dupéré, 2000b). Yet for many recent immigrants, language barriers represent a fundamental challenge limiting their social interaction and the ability to develop relationships and build healthy social support systems, not to mention getting and keeping a job. While there are many programs available to help alleviate language barriers for immigrant women, using 'culturally attuned' language also must be among some of the fundamental issues addressed in every policy agenda.

Through further research on gender and migration in the context of women's health, Canadian health policy makers must provide forums in which further consultation with both recent immigrant women and those who have lived in Canada for a long time can take place. Herein, Canadian policy makers may gain the tools to actually employ 'languages' that reflect that, indeed, the voices of women experiencing migration are 'heard.' Moreover, by using inclusivity in health policy language and discourse, as well as reflexivity in research design and interdisciplinary health research teams, health policies can better integrate gender and migration as dimensions of immigrant women's health. Ensuring that women have access to the information to which al Canadian women are entitled, as well as the resources that enable women to contribute to and act upon this knowledge, must also be a policy priority.

Recommendation 2: Recognize Women's Diverse Contributions

Sustaining the capacity of recent immigrants for economic integration and fostering further economic opportunities for women requires a gender-sensitive strategy which may be operationalized through four broad areas:

- Strengthening government-supported access to further education and language training for employment and job retention
- Ensuring the extension of social assistance and protection to immigrant women in both the formal and informal spheres, as well as the dissemination of this information upon arrival
- Reducing institutional barriers to accreditation
- Fostering awareness in civil society through media campaigns concerning the social and economic contributions of recent immigrant women to the Canadian economy

Immigrants do not form a homogeneous group: they are differentiated by gender, ethnic origin, sexual orientation, ability, age, religious affiliation, profession, skills, and so on. As advocated by a recent Equality and Diversity Assessment Toolkit, the equality and diversity of immigrants must be processed together, for there is not 'equality of opportunity if difference is not recognized and valued' (Scotland Executive, 2004, p. 8). Women's experiences of migration thus may be analysed within the intersecting social, political, and economic contexts of both source and receiving countries, as well as women's identities as individuals and within a family (Boyd & Grieco, 2003). It is within this broad scope that women's economic contributions must be understood and facilitated. The various ways that women mobilize their skills and resources for the welfare of themselves and their families deserve much more recognition. Further efforts must be made to ensure that women working in informal sectors have access to the same social safety nets as do Canadians working in the formal sector. Moreover, anti-poverty strategies for recent immigrant women must be precise, targeting specific needs, skills, and interests into order to mirror the various experiences of migration, ranging from asylum-seekers to skilled workers, to family sponsorships, to business-persons and professionals.

Recommendation 3: Ensure the Security of All Women

- Promoting the security of immigrant women requires commitment at all levels of society. Anti-violence initiatives must operate along the full spectrum of individual and institutional violence and must be framed by gender-sensitive strategies.
- The participation of immigrant women in the dissemination and evaluation of multilingual media and literary publications must be insured, fostering awareness of the multiple forms of violence, including those embedded in social exclusion, poverty, and insecurity, for more inclusive and culturally appropriate anti-violence campaigns.
- Measures to ensure the protection of women from violence must also include guaranteed economic support, in terms of housing and health care, and including sponsored access to mental health and legal support.

In the absence of social protection, migration may be an experience of social inequality, powerlessness, isolation, and bewilderment. In the context of drastic cuts to social transfer funds as seen in the 1990s, there is risk of significant devastation in the programs critical to social integration of all Canadians. In this climate, how will Canadian immigration and refugee policies be affected in order to limit the potential social and gender-based inequities discussed above, and avoid contributing to conditions where the experience of migration to Canada constructs recent immigrants as 'people out of place'? Conditions of prolonged insecurity and the absence of protection and recourse against the violence of marginalization, discrimination, and exploitation strain health in all its dimensions, not to mention health behaviours. Yet, this does not have to be our direction.

Through the efforts of many dedicated contributors, Canada has already adopted several promising initiatives, such as the inclusion of gender-based persecution in the Refugee Protection Act (Kelson, 1999), an Anti-Racism Action Plan (Department of Canadian Heritage, 2005), and a national homeless initiative (SCPI, 2005). Moreover, the broadening emphasis of determining admissibility within Canadian immigration policy now includes education, language, and employability (Ray, 2002, May). In conjunction with such initiatives and with the collaboration of multiple contributors to women's health policies and practices in Canada, we support further efforts towards social investment, and, within this, the integration of gender and migration as dimensions of immigrant women's health. Our future as a healthy and vibrant Canadian society will be a reflection of the coordinated efforts and ambitions of all Canadians; as such, the interests and needs of all Canadians, including recent immigrant women, must be thoroughly integrated into a political, socio-economic, and cultural development of Canadian society.

NOTE

1 Health Canada has identified 12 such determinants: income and social status; employment; education; social environments; physical environments; healthy child development; personal health practices and coping skills; health services; social support networks; biology and genetic endowment; gender; and culture. See Health Canada (1999), p. 13.

REFERENCES

Agnew, V. (1996). *Resisting Discrimination : Women from Asia, Africa, and the Caribbean and the Women's Movement in Canada.* Toronto: University of Toronto Press.

Agnew, V. (1998). *In Search of a Safe Place: Abused Women and Culturally Sensitive Services.* Toronto: University of Toronto Press.

Anand, S., Peter, F., & Sen, A. (2004). *Public Health, Ethics and Equity.* Oxford: Oxford University Press.

Aroian, K. (2001). Immigrant women and their health. *Annual Review of Nursing Research, 19,* 179–226.

Beiser, M., Hou, F., Hyman, I., & Tousignant, M. (2002). Poverty and mental health among immigrant and non-immigrant children. *American Journal of Public Health*, 92(2), 220–227.

Biidu, D.G. (2004). The gender dimension of the Hague Declaration on the Future of Refugee and Migration Policy. In F. Reysoo & C. Verchuur. *Femmes en movement: Genre, migrations et nouvelle divisions internationale du travail.* Berne, Switzerland: Commission Suisse pour L'Unesco. www.iued.unige.ch.

Bischoff, A., Bovier, P.A., Rrustemi, I., Gariazzo, F., Eylan, A., & Loutan, L. (2003). Language barriers between nurses and asylum seekers: Their impact on symptom reporting and referral. *Social Science & Medicine*, 57(3), 503–512.

Boyd, M., & Grieco, E. (2003, March). Migration fundamentals – women and migration: Incorporating gender into international migration theory. *Migration Information Source.* Retrieved April 2005, from http://www.migrationinformation.org/Feature/display.cfm?ID=106.

Campbell, D.W., Sharps, P.W., Gary, F., Campbell, J.C., & Lopez, L.M. (2002, January). Intimate partner violence in African American women. *Online Journal of Issues in Nursing*, 7(1).

Chen, L. (2004). Health as a human security priority for the 21st century. The Helsinki process. Paper prepared for *Human Security* Track III. Helsinki, Finland: Finnish Ministry for Foreign Affairs.

Citizenship and Immigration Canada. (2005). Immigrating to Canada. Retrieved April 2005, from http://www.cic.gc.ca/english/immigrate/index.html.

CRI-VIFF. (2003). Le Centre de recherche interdisciplinaire sur la violence familiale
et la violence faite aux femmes. Retrieved April 2005, from http://www.criviff.qc.ca/accueil.asp.

Choudhury, U.K., Jandu, S., Mahal, J., Singh, R., Sohi-Pabla, H., & Mutta, B. (2002). Health promotion and participatory action research with South Asian women. *Journal of Nursing Scholarship*, 34(1), 75–81.

Cohen, M., and MacLean, H. (2003). Violence against Canadian women. In M. DesMeules, D. Stewart, H. Maclean, J. Payne, A. Kazanjian, and B. Vissandjée (Eds.). *The Canadian Women's Health Surveillance Report: Canadian Public Health Initiative – Health Canada.* Retrieved 19 July 2005, from http://secure.cihi.ca/cihiweb/products/WHSR_Chap_21_e.pdf.

Côté, A., Kérisit, M., & Côté, M. (2003, November). *Sponsorship ... For Better or for Worse: The Impact of Sponsorship on the Equality Rights of Immigrant Women.* Status of Women Canada. Retrieved 19 July 2005, from http://www.swc-cfc.gc.ca/pubs/pubspr/0662296427/200103_0662296427_e.pdf.

Department of Canadian Heritage. (2005). *A Canada for All: Canada's Action Plan Against Racim – an Overview.* Retrieved April 2005, from www.multiculturalism.pch.gc.ca.

DesMeules, M., Gold, J., Kazanjian, A., Manuel, D., Payne, J., Vissandjée, B., McDermott, S., & Mao, Y. (2004). New approaches to immigrant health assessment. *Canadian Journal of Public Health, 95*(3), I22–I26.

Donahue, P., Este, D., & Miller, P. (2003). *Diversity Among the Homeless and Those at Risk.* Executive summary. Calgary: Heritage Canada.

Dunn, J.R., & Dyck, I. (2000). Social determinants of health in Canada's immigrant population: Results from the National Population Health Survey. *Social Science & Medicine, 51*, 1573–1593.

Dyck, I., & McLaren, A. (2002, March). *Becoming Canadian? Girls, Home and School and Renegotiating Feminine Identity.* Working Paper. Series No. 02-08. Vancouver: Vancouver Centre of Excellence. Research on Immigration and Integration in the Metropolis.

Farmer, P. (2003). *Pathologies of Power: Health, Human Rights and the New War on the Poor.* Berkeley: University of California Press.

Fong, J. (1999). Where do they belong? The 'fate' of Chinese immigrant women. *Canadian Women's Studies: Immigrant and Refugee Women, 19*(3), 64–68.

Frith, R. (2003). Integration. *Canadian Issues* (April), 35–36.

Fuhrer, R., & Stansfeld, S.A. (2002). How gender affects patterns of social relations and their impact on health: A comparison of one or multiple sources of support from 'close persons.' *Social Science & Medicine, 54*(5), 811–825.

Galabuzi, G.E., & Labonte, R. (2002, November). *Social Inclusion as a Determinant of Health.* Paper presented at the Social Determinants of Health Across the Life-Span Conference, Toronto.

Graham, H., & Kelly, M.P. (2004). *Health Inequalities: Concepts, Frameworks and Policy.* London: Health Development Agency. Retrieved April 2005, from http://www.hda.nhs.uk/Documents/health_inequalities_concepts.pdf.

Health Canada. (1999). *Strategies for Women's Health.* Ottawa: Minister of Public Works and Government Services.

Hyman, I. (2001). *Health Policy Working Paper Series: Immigration and Health.* Applied Research and Analysis Directorate. Ottawa: Minister of Public Works and Government Services. Retrieved April 2005, from http://www.hc-sc.gc.ca/iacb-dgiac/arad-draa/english/rmdd/wpapers/Immigration.pdf.

Hyndman, J. (1999). Gender and Canadian immigration policy: A current snapshot. *Canadian Women's Studies: Immigrant and Refugee Women, 19*(3), 6–10.

Iglesias, E., Robertson, E., Johnsson, S.E., Engfeldt, P., & Sundquist, J. (2003). Women, international migration and self-reported health: A population-based study of women of reproductive age. *Social Science & Medicine, 56,* 111–124.

Isajiw, W.W. (1999). *Understanding Diversity: Ethnicity and Race in the Canadian Context.* Toronto: Thompson Educational.

Juteau, D. (1999). *L'ethnicité et ses frontière.* Montréal: Presses de l'Université de Montréal.

Kawar, M. (2004). Gender and migration: Why are women more vulnerable? In F. Reysoo & C. Verchuur (Eds.), *Femmes en movement: Genre, migrations et nouvelle divisions internationale du travail.* Berne, Switzerland. www.iued.unige.ch.

Kelson, G. (1999). Recognizing gender-based persecution in Canada: Are Canada's gender guidelines being used consistently? *Canadian Women's Studies: Immigrant and Refugee Women, 19*(3), 149–153.

Kessel, G.C.J. (1998). The Canadian immigration system. In I. Hyman (2001), *Health Policy Working Paper Series: Immigration and Health.* Applied Research and Analysis Directorate. Ottawa: Minister of Public Works and Government Services. Retrieved April 2005, from http://www.hc-sc.gc.ca/iacb-dgiac/arad-draa/english/rmdd/wpapers/Immigration.pdf.

Kinnon, D. (1999). *Canadian Research on Immigration and Health: An Overview.* Metropolis Project, Health Canada. Retrieved April 2005, from http://dsp-psd.communication.gc.ca/Collection/H21-149-1999E.pdf.

Klein, A. (2001). *HIV/AIDS and Immigration Final Report: Canadian Strategy on HIV/AIDS.* Toronto: Canadian HIV/AIDS Legal Network.

Kramer, E., Ivey, S., &Ying, Y. (Eds.). (1999). *Immigrant Women's Health: Problems and Solutions.* San Francisco: Jossey-Bass.

Krieger, N. (2000). Discrimination and health. In L. Berkman & I. Kawachi (Eds.), *Social Epidemiologist* (pp. 36–75). Oxford: Oxford University Press.

Krieger, N., & Gruskin, S. (2001). Frameworks matter: Ecosocial and health and human rights perspectives on disparities in women's health – The case of Tuberculosis. *Journal of the American Medical Women's Association, 56*(4), 137–142.

Leppin, A., & Schwarzer, R. (1990). Social support and physical health: An updated Meta-Analysis. In L.R. Schmidt, P. Schwenkmezger, J. Weinmans, & S. Maes (Eds.), *Theoretical and Applied Aspects of Health Psychology.* London: Harwood Academic.

Li, P.S. (2003a). *Destination Canada: Immigration Debates and Issues.* Toronto: Oxford University Press.

Li, P.S. (2003b). Understanding economic performance of immigrants. *Canadian Issues* (April), 25–26.

Lipson, J.G., Hosseini, T., Kabir, S., Omidian, P.A., & Edmonston, F. (1995). Health issues among Afghan women in California. *Health Care for Women International, 16*, 279–286.

Marmot, M. (2005a). Social determinants of health inequalities. *The Lancet, 365*, 1099–1104.

Marmot, M. (2005b). *Commission on Social Determinants of Health: Questions and Answers*. World Health Organization. http://www.who.int/social_determinants/en/.

Meadows, L.M., Thurston, W.E., & Melton, C. (2001). Immigrant woman's health. *Social Science & Medicine, 52(9)*, 1451–1458.

Muhajarine, N., & D'Arcy, C. (1999). Physical abuse during pregnancy: Prevalence and risk factors. *Candian Medical Association Journal, 160*, 1007–1011.

Noh, S., & Kasper, V. (2003). Diversity and immigrant health. In P. Anisef & M. Lanphier (Eds.), *The World in a City* (pp. 316–353). Toronto: University of Toronto Press.

Pendakur, K., & Pendakur, R. (2002). Colour my world: Has the minority-majority earnings gap changed over time? *Canadian Public Policy, 28(4)*, 489–511.

Rankin, P., & Vickers, J. (2001). *Women's Movements and State Feminism: Integrating Diversity into Public Policy*. Ottawa: Status of Women Canada.

Ray, B. (2002, May). *Country Profiles; Canada: Policy Legacies, New Directions, and Future Challenges*. Retrieved April 2005, from http://www.migrationinformation.org/feature/display.cfm?ID=20.

Ray, B. (2002, October). *Migration Fundamentals – Immigrant Integration: Building to Opportunities*. Retrieved April 2005, from http://www.migrationinformation.org/feature/display.cfm?ID=57.

Reitz, J.G. (2001). Immigrant skill utilization in the Canadian labour market: Implications of human capital research. *Journal of International Migration and Integration, 2(3)*, 347–378.

Renaud, J., Gingras, L., Vachon, S., Blaser, C., Godin, J.F., & Gangé, B. (2003). Ils sont maintenant d'ici! *Les publications du Québec, Centre d'études ethniques*. Montreal: Université de Montréal.

Ruddick, E. (2003). Immigrant economic performance: A new paradigm in a changing labour market. *Canadian Issues* (April), 16–17.

Scotland Executive. (2004). *Equality and Diversity Impact Assessment Toolkit: Patient Focus and Public Involvement Fair for All; The Wider Challenge*. Edingburgh, Scotland. http://www.scotland.gov.uk/library5/health/eqdiat.pdf.

Sen, G., Germain, A., & Chen, L. (1994). Reconsidering population policies: Ethics, development, and strategies for change. In G. Sen, A. Germain, & L. Chen (Eds.), *Population Policies Reconsidered: Health, Empowerment, and*

Rights (pp. 3–11) (Harvard series on Population and International Health). Cambridge: Harvard University Press.

Smith, E. (2004). *Nowhere to Turn? Responding to Partner Violence against Immigrant and Visible Minority Women*. Ottawa: Canadian Council on Social Development. Retrieved April 2005, from http://www.ccsd.ca/pubs/2004/nowhere/.

Somerville, M. (Ed.). (1999). *Do We Care? Renewing Canada's Commitment to Health*. Montreal: McGill-Queen's University Press.

Spitzer, D.L. (2003). *What's Sex and Gender Got to Do With It? Integrating Sex and Gender into Health Research*. Ottawa: Institute for Gender and Health, Canadian Institutes for Health Research, Health Canada.

Spitzer, D.L. (2004). *Gender and Health Disparities*. Ottawa: Institute for Gender and Health, Canadian Institutes for Health Research, Health Canada.

Status of Women Canada. (2005–2006). *Strategic Outcome: Gender Equality and the Full Participation of Women in the Economic, Social, Cultural and Political Life of Canada*. Report on plans and priorities. http://www.tbs-sct.gc.ca/est-pre/20052006/SWC-CFC/SWC-CFCr5601_e.asp#section2_1_1.

Sweetman, A. (2003). Immigration and the 'New Economy.' *Canadian Issues* (April), 21–22.

Sundquist, J., Behmen-Vincevic, A., & Johnsson, S.E. (1998). Poor quality of life and health in young to middle aged Bosnian female war refugees: A population-based study. *Public Health, 112,* 21–26.

SCPI (Supporting Communities Partnership Initiative). (2005). *The National Homelessness Initiative*. Government of Canada. Retrieved April 2005, from http://www.homelessness.gc.ca/initiative/scpi_e.asp.

10/90 Global Forum for Health Research. (2003–2004). *Helping Correct the 10/90 Gap*. Retrieved April 2005, from www.globalforumhealth.org.

Thobani, S. (1999). Sponsoring immigrant women's inequalities. *Canadian Women's Studies: Immigrant and Refugee Women, 19*(3), 11–16.

Thurston, W.E., & Vissandjée, B. (2005). An ecological model for understanding culture as a determinant of health. *Critical Public Health, 15*(3), 229–242.

Vergnaud, G. (2004). Compétence et conceptualisation. *Revue ARSI, 70*(9), 4–15.

Vissandjée, B. (2001). The consequences of cultural diversity. Canadian Women's Health Network. *Network Magazine, 4*(2) (Spring).

Vissandjée, B., & DesMeules, M. (2004). Gender, ethnicity and the migration experience: Social determinants of health. In *A Canadian Snapshot of Fields of Study and Innovative Approaches to Understanding and Addressing Health Issues*. Halifax: Atlantic Health Promotion Research Centre.

Vissandjée, B., & Dupéré, S. (2000a). Culture, migration et enquête: Défis

incontournables. *Journal of International Migration and Integration, 1*(4),
477–492.

Vissandjée, B., & Dupéré, S. (2000b). La communication interculturelle en
contexte clinique: Une question de partenariat. *Revue canadienne de recherche
en sciences infirmières, 32*(1), 99–113.

Vissandjée, B., DesMeules, M., Cao, Z., Abdool, S., & Kazanjian, A. (2004).
Integrating ethnicity and migration as determinants of Canadian women's
health. *BMC Women's Health.* Retrieved April 2005, from http://www.
biomedcentral.com/qc/1472-6874/4/S1/S32.

Vissandjée, B., Hyman, I., Spitzer, D., Schotsman, A., & Kamrun, N. (2005).
*Understanding Gender, Race and Ethnicity in the Context of Migration Determi-
nants of Women's Health: A Meta-Analysis.* IGH-CIHR report.

Vissandjee, B., Kantiebo, M., Levine, A., & N'Dejuru, R. (2003). The cultural
context of gender identity: Female genital excision and infibulation. *Health
Care for Women International, 24,* 115–124.

Vissandjée, B., Weinfeld, M., Dupéré, S., & Abdool, S. (2001). Sex, gender,
ethnicity, and access to health care services: Research and policy challenges
for immigrant women in Canada. *Journal of International Migration and
Integration, 2*(1), 55–75.

Wagstaff, A. (2002). Poverty and health sector inequalities: Policy and practice. Theme Papers. *Bulletin of the World Health Organization, 80*(2).

Walters, V. (2003). The social context of women's health. In M. Des Meules,
D. Stewart, A. Kazanjian, H. Maclean, J. Payne, & B. Vissandjée (Eds.),
Canadian Women's Health Surveillance Report. Ottawa: Canadian Public
Health Initiative, Health Canada.

World Health Organization. (2004). *Preventing Violence. A Guide to Implementing the Recommendations of the World Report on Violence and Health.* Retrieved
April 2005, from http://whqlibdoc.who.int/publications/2004/
9241592079.pdf.

Zlotnick, H. (2003, March). Migration fundamentals – The global dimensions
of female migration. *Migration Information Source.* Retrieved April 2005,
from http://www.migrationinformation.org/feature/display.cfm?ID=57.

9 Cultures of Dis/ability: From Being Stigmatized to Doing Disability

LISA DIEDRICH

As the editors note at the outset of their introduction to this volume, '"health" is an evolving concept,' not some essential quality that can be easily measured and quantified. In this chapter, I consider some of the ways that 'disability' is also a concept in the making that expands and complicates how we understand the relationship between health and illness. There is perhaps a danger in discussing disability within the context of 'women's health,' especially if the term *women's health* maintains the hierarchical health/illness binary, a binary that disability scholars and activists find problematic.[1] Within such a binary logic, disability is understood as lack, something to be fixed, just as illness is understood within this binary frame as lacking health. The experiences of disability and disabling chronic illnesses challenge this simplistic either/or dichotomy between health and illness and between ability and disability.[2] By writing dis/ability with a slash, as I do in my title, I want to signal not only this binary logic that structures much of our thinking about disability, but also the possibility of undermining or taking apart that logic.

In order both to understand this structuring binary logic and to create methods for deconstructing it, I explore some of the key concepts and explanatory models that emerge with an analysis of disability as not only an *embodied and relational experience* but also a *socio-cultural and political event* (see Text Box 1). First, I consider a key concept – stigma – that has contributed to, perhaps paradoxically, the emergence of disability studies and disability rights activism. I say 'perhaps paradoxically' because, of course, the stigma often associated with disability is not usually understood as a desirable characteristic for an individual or group to have. And yet, the experience of stigmatization has meant that

---

Text Box 9.1 Dis/ability Key Concepts

Stigma   Medical Model of Disability   Social Model of Disability
Post-structural Models of Disability   'Experience'   Genealogy
Antiscience

---

people with disabilities often have a unique view of the world, as well as a unique view of stigmatization as a cultural practice that might be taken apart, analysed, and challenged. After delineating this particular concept, I discuss the historical emergence of disability as a category of identity, and explore in detail some poststructural theories and methodologies – in particular genealogy and science studies – that I think offer the most promise as explanatory models of disability. Like gender as a category of analysis for feminist scholars, disability as a category of analysis is best approached through an interdisciplinary methodology. The study of the experiences and events of disability brings together numerous fields: biology, medicine, history, politics, sociology, and psychology, to name just a few. Rosemarie Garland-Thomson, who has been at the forefront of attempts to demonstrate the various ways that feminist theory and disability studies have and might continue to influence and challenge each other, has argued that if we integrate disability into feminist theory and activism, we will transform that theory and activism in necessary ways. In her important essay 'Integrating Disability, Transforming Feminist Theory,' Garland-Thomson (2002) discusses four domains of feminist theory 'that can be deepened by a disability analysis': representation, the body, identity, and activism (p. 6). As Garland-Thomson's four domains suggests, not only feminist theories but also feminist movements, along with other social movements, have influenced the rhetoric and practices of the disability rights movement. Disability is not simply something that happens to a person; it is something that one does and continues to do, in multiple and always changing ways. I conclude this chapter, then, with a brief discussion of 'doing' disability in the Canadian context.

Stigma and Stigmatization

An important early work that would influence later theories of disability is Canadian sociologist Erving Goffman's classic study *Stigma: Notes on the Management of Spoiled Identity*, first published in 1963. All of Goffman's work, including *Stigma*, diagnoses the self in relation to particular others and to society and social norms in general. As Eliot Freidson (1983) noted in a celebration of Goffman's work just after his death, Goffman 'focused on the individual self, in a world that at once creates and oppresses it.' Freidson also insisted that, 'Goffman's work is intensely moral in character, marked by a passionate defense of the self against society' (p. 359). In *Stigma*, Goffman gathers together diverse materials as evidence for his account of the personal experience of stigma and the social practice of stigmatization. His sources include autobiographical accounts of stigmatized individuals, and clinical and sociological studies of stigmatized groups. Goffman looks at autobiographical accounts because he is interested in what he calls 'social information,' which he describes in his preface as 'the information the individual directly conveys about himself' (n.p.). Autobiography, as I will discuss in more detail below, will become an important tool and resource for understanding and challenging the stigma associated with disability.

Goffman, in his preface, defines stigma as 'the situation of the individual who is disqualified from full social acceptance' (n.p.). Although one is stigmatized because of an attribute that is deeply discrediting, Goffman explains, what we need in order to understand how stigma works is not a language of attributes but a language of relationships. Goffman does not offer an essentialist theory of stigma. For him, stigma is not based on certain fixed qualities that remain the same across time and cultures; rather, it is based on historical categorizations of difference. We will hear echoes of Goffman's anti-essentialist understanding of stigma when I turn to the poststructural models of disability below.

Stigma opens with a letter to 'Miss Lonelyhearts' from a 16-year-old girl, who signs her letter 'Desperate,' and explains that she was born without a nose. The letter writer is desperate because she has come to the realization that her appearance 'scares people,' even herself, and that 'no boy will take me' (n.p.). When she asks her father what she did 'to deserve such a terrible bad fate,' he admits he doesn't know, but says that perhaps she did something in the 'other world before [she] was born or that maybe [she] was being punished for his sins.' 'Desperate's' letter demonstrates how stigma works, not as the consequence of a fixed attribute – a face without a nose – but as a consequence of social relations – the girl without a nose in relation to others. As a young girl, 'Desperate' adjusts relatively well to her situation, but when she reaches adolescence, as it becomes more important for her to fit an ideal of femininity, her stigma becomes more difficult for her to bear. She learns by the reactions of others to her appearance that the ideal of femininity does not include facial disfigurement. It is only at adolescence, then, that she becomes, as Goffman would say, disqualified from full social acceptance. Her father's explanations for why she might deserve to be disqualified from full social acceptance are what Goffman calls 'stigma theories,' which are ideologies that rationalize the practices of stigmatization (p. 5); and her father's theory of divine retribution is one of the oldest and most enduring stigma theories. Even in more secular times and cultures, the possibility that one might be literally marked by one's sins or perceived immorality continues to have cultural force as an explanation for the stigmatization of an individual or group.

For Goffman, the experience of stigma and the social and cultural practices of stigmatization reveal the ways in which all identity is relational. To clarify this crucial theoretical point, he distinguishes between 'virtual social identity' and 'actual social identity'; that is, between the normative expectations or assumptions made about a person's identity by others and the actual attributes that person possesses (p. 2). Not all stigmas are visible; some of the hidden stigmas that Goffman discusses include homosexuality, a history of mental illness, and a criminal past. Goffman explains that there is a difference between the plight of the discredited, those whose stigmas are immediately perceived by others, and the discreditable, those whose stigmas are hidden in the present but are potentially perceivable in the future (p. 4). This distinction remains crucial when we try to understand the multiple experiences and events of disability, some of which are invisible in certain circumstances, including learning and developmental disabilities, deafness, and chronic and remitting conditions such as chronic fatigue syndrome, multiple sclerosis, or HIV/AIDS. Others, on the other hand, are visible or even hypervisible, including those that require what we might think of as bodily extensions: white canes or guide dogs for persons who are blind or wheelchairs for persons with mobility impairments.[3]

Although Goffman's work is sometimes read as enforcing normalization because he describes in detail the socialization process through which the stigmatized individual 'learns and incorporates the standpoint of the normal' (p. 32), I contend that *Stigma* points towards a proto-political critique of normalization through his discussion of the creation of 'action groups' that challenge stigmatization via the publication of counter-narratives 'that give voice to shared feelings' and which help to 'consolidate belief in the stigma as a basis for self-conception' (p. 27). Moreover, Goffman suggests that a stigmatized person is often more conscious of her particular situatedness than are so-called normals. Indeed, Goffman maintains that the stigmatized person often becomes 'a critic of the social scene, an observer of human relations' (p. 111). The stigmatized individual is a phenomenologist[4] of sorts, who, Goffman argues, 'can become "situation conscious" while normals present are spontaneously involved *within* the situation, the situation itself constituting for these normals a background of unattended matters. This extension of consciousness on the part of the stigmatized persons is reinforced ... by his special aliveness to the contingencies of acceptance and disclosure, contingencies to which normals will be less alive' (p. 111). This notion of the stigmatized person's 'special aliveness' will become key to the articulation of dis/ability consciousness that emerges in the late twentieth century, and suggests in particular the importance of the perceptions and experiences of persons with disabilities in the formulation of an ethics and politics of women's health. As Susan Wendell (1996) notes in her insightful feminist philosophical inquiry into disability, *The Rejected Body*, 'The experiences and interests of both people with disabilities and those who care for people with disabilities are vitally relevant to central philosophical concerns of feminist ethics and to feminist ethical approaches to practical matters such as abortion, euthanasia, and health care reform' (p. 139).

Dis/ability and 'Experience'[5]

As Lennard Davis (1997) notes in his introduction to *The Disability Studies Reader*, disability, as a representative category of human identity, has only recently emerged in conjunction with those other identity categories: race, class, gender, and sexuality. Only in the last 20 years, according to Davis, have people with disabilities seen themselves as a 'single, allied, united physical minority,' and this perception of unity has brought both the struggle for civil rights through the disability rights movement and the struggle for a new discourse on the experiences of disability through disability studies (p. 3).

Not surprisingly, with the emphasis on disability as a category of identity, much of the early focus in the disability rights movement and disability studies has emphasized an identity-based politics and forms of activism over and often against what is perceived of as exclusively theoretical work. Some recent work in disability studies perhaps signals the beginning of a shift in emphasis from identity politics to a critique that might be understood as 'postmodern' or poststructuralist, and it is this critique that I think affords the most promise for both disability studies and activism (see, for example, Mitchell & Snyder, 1997; Corker & Shakespeare, 2002; Shildrick, 2002; and Davis, 2002). In their important volume on the uses of a 'postmodern approach' for disability studies, Marian Corker and Tom Shakespeare (2002) assert in their introduction that 'It is our contention that disability studies, particularly in Britain, has suffered from a theoretical deficit, and has been reluctant to take advantage of this [post-structuralist][6] scholarship' (p. 1). Like Sandra Harding (1991), who considers three stages in the development of feminist epistemology, including feminist empiricism, feminist standpoint epistemologies, and feminist postmodernism (see also Maynard, 1994), Corker and Shakespeare (2002) investigate poststructuralism as an alternative epistemological framework for disability studies. Poststructuralism, according to Corker and Shakespeare, challenges both the medical models of disability, 'which perceive and classify disability in terms of a meta-narrative of deviance, lack and tragedy, and assume it to be logically separate from and inferior to "normalcy"' (p. 2), and the social model of disability, which has 'roots in historical materialism' and understands disability as 'socially ... constructed on top of impairment' (p. 3). Although Corker and Shakespeare understand that accessibility, in terms of the built environment and social structures, as well as in terms of language, is a crucial focus of the disability rights movement, they are also concerned that a dismissal of poststructuralism on the grounds that it is often inaccessible to those untutored in its particular language and practices is not a prudent move for either disability studies in the academy or the disability rights movement. They insist that many poststructuralist theories and methods are useful for both disability studies and the disability rights movement because they offer 'a different view of the subject, arguing that subjects are not autonomous creators of themselves or their social worlds. Rather, subjects are embedded in a complex network of social relations' (p. 3), which is also of course one of the theses of Goffman's earlier work.

I agree with Corker and Shakespeare that poststructuralism in general offers many useful tools for disability studies and the disability rights movement. One such useful tool is genealogy, which I will delineate as a method and in relation to disability in more detail below. However, as I hope my opening discussion of Goffman's theorization of stigma and the practices of stigmatization indicates, I wouldn't necessarily argue that disability studies in its current form suffers from a 'theoretical deficit.'[7] Instead, I would argue that disability studies has for the most part not yet adequately problematized the category of experience. It seems to me that the general current trend in the disability rights movement and disability studies is to make visible experiences of disability that have been previously hidden from history and not addressed politically. While this approach brings to light alternative modes of being and alternative spaces that more conventional history and politics fail to acknowledge or even see, it does not necessarily reveal the ways that experience itself is a category of representation that emerges and operates within a particular socio-cultural and historical milieu. In her essay on the use of experience as historical evidence, feminist historian Joan Scott (1992) challenges the notion of 'writing as reproduction, transmission[, or] the communication of knowledge gained through (visual, visceral) experience' (p. 24). Rather than relying on 'experience as the origin of knowledge' of the individual subject, Scott prefers to emphasize 'the constructed nature of experience' (p. 25). She is interested, therefore, in the 'categories of representation' and how these categories operate within given ideological systems; and one such system is what Garland-Thomson (2002) has called the 'ability/disability system' (p. 3). 'Experience' itself is an explanatory category, Scott asserts, and reinforces her point by placing it in quotes (p. 26).[8]

Scott (1992) begins and ends her influential discussion of 'experience' as historical evidence with readings of Samuel Delany's (1988) memoir, *The Motion of Light in Water: Sex and Science Fiction Writing in the East Village*, about being homosexual in New York in the early 1960s. According to Scott, Delany's memoir is evidence of alternative modes of being (homosexual) and alternative spaces (for the practices of homosexual sex and community) that are not recorded in conventional histories. Yet, Scott also understands Delany's memoir as an example of a text that 'drastically raises the problem of writing the history of difference, the history, that is, of the designation of 'other,' of the attribution of characteristics that distinguish categories of people from some presumed (and usually unstated) norm' (p. 22). What is important about the rendering of 'experience,' according to Scott, is not simply to make visible experiences previously invisible, but rather to reveal the ways that 'experience' is not a reliable or self-evident source of knowledge, and that certain discursive regimes allow certain 'experiences' to emerge in history while others get covered over, or denied.

Scott's assertions about 'the problem of writing the history of difference,' and her analysis of Delany's memoir as an exemplary case of this
problem, are useful in considering the particular (and multiple) histories of difference that disability studies seeks to write, especially because, as David T. Mitchell and Sharon L. Snyder (1997) note in the
introduction to the edited volume *The Body and Physical Difference: Discourses of Disability*, the 'discourse of disability has been largely defined
by the genre of autobiography' (p. 9). Because of this, disability is often
perceived as an essentially private and individual experience which
other disabled and able-bodied individuals can have insight into through
the medium of personal narrative. According to Mitchell and Snyder,
while these narratives provide 'an understanding of disability on an
individual level,' they are less likely to give the reader a sense of the
social and political structures that bring the disability category into
being (p. 9).

Dis/ability and Genealogy

I am interested here, then, in the ways that specific 'experiences' of
disability come into being and are articulated within specific cultures,
institutions, and practices. It is my view that genealogy, as Foucault
(1977, 2003b) delineated it, is an especially useful methodology for
disability studies and activism, and I also believe that, conversely, the
multiple experiences, events, and practices of disability provide new
understanding of what it means – theoretically and practically – to 'do'
genealogy. In *Disability/Postmodernity*, Corker and Shakespeare (2002)
acknowledge that Foucault's work and his genealogical method provide resources for understanding disability. According to Corker and
Shakespeare, '[a] Foucauldian perspective on disability might argue ...
that a proliferation of discourses on impairment give rise to the category "disability." Though these discourses were originally scientific
and medical classificatory devices, they subsequently gained currency
in judicial and psychiatric fields of knowledge. "Disabled people" did
not exist before this classification although impairment and impair-
ment-related practices certainly did. Thus Foucault shows us that social
identities are effects of the ways in which knowledge is organized, but
his work is also significant for its explication of the links between
knowledge and power' (pp. 7–8). And in another essay in the Corker
and Shakespeare volume, Shelley Tremain (2002) states that '[t]heorists
and researchers in disability studies should adopt ... [a] genealogical

approach to their work' (p. 33); and she herself provides a genealogical analysis of 'the emergence of impairment as an object of knowledge/ power' (p. 34) through various disciplinary domains, including the disciplinary domain of disability studies itself.[9]

Similarly, although they do not necessarily use the term *genealogy* to describe their methodology, many scholars in disability studies have done important work that I would maintain is genealogical. Several focus on the relationship between the normal and the pathological or abnormal that Foucault following Canguilhem sought to diagnose. For example, Lennard Davis's *Enforcing Normalcy* (1995) offers a genealogical account of the emergence of the concept of the norm in the nineteenth century, and Rosemarie Garland Thomson's important work on the representation of disability in literature and culture, *Extraordinary Bodies* (1997), denaturalizes the normal by inventing the term *normate*. According to Garland-Thomson, 'This neologism names the veiled subject position of cultural self, the figure outlined by the array of deviant others whose marked bodies shore up the normate's boundaries. The term *normate* usefully designates the social figure through which people can represent themselves as definitive human beings' (p. 8). Several scholars of Deaf culture, moreover, have delineated competing discourses of deafness, and have historicized the changing 'experience' of deafness in Western cultures from the eighteenth to the twentieth centuries (see, for example, Davis, 1995, 1997; Harlan Lane, 1984, 1997; Oliver Sacks, 1989; & Douglas Baynton, 1997). And, finally, in *The Disabled State*, Deborah Stone (1984) diagnoses the emergence of the disability category in the social policy and laws of several Western nations, including the United States, Britain, and Germany. In her genealogical investigation, Stone explores 'how the concept of disability came to be associated with clinical medicine and clinical reasoning' (pp. 27–28).

In order to demonstrate further what I take to be an intimate relationship between disability and genealogy, I want to introduce several key terms in Foucault's work – *antisciences, descent,* and *emergence* – that I believe will help clarify why I think genealogy is such a promising methodology for understanding the experiences and events of disability. Although I focus on disability here, I believe genealogy is also a useful methodology for approaching health in general and women's health in particular. Much of Foucault's own work was on the historical category of health, and other scholars have utilized a Foucaultian framework to analyse the practices and institutions of health (see, for example, Diprose, 1994; Rose, 1994, 1996). By approaching disability through the framework of genealogy and genealogy through the framework of disability, I am interested in demonstrating an interdisciplinary methodology, as well as diagnosing the moments of arising, of forces and figures of disability within history. I not only believe genealogy helps to locate some of the lost events of disability, even or especially those events covered over by the emergence of disability studies and the disability rights movement in its current form, but I also believe genealogy gives us a mode in which to imagine other domains, practices, and figures of disability. Finally, I will also consider how a shift from an analysis of the forms of being disabled and the methods of knowing disability to an analysis of *how disability is done* – through multiple and often divergent practices and by several doers at once – allows us to understand how disability is enacted in various domains, not just in the past but in the present as well.

Antisciences

In his recently published lectures at the Collège de France presented in 1975–1976 and entitled 'Society Must Be Defended,' Foucault (2003b) provides one of his clearest delineations of what he means by the term *genealogy*. In his first lecture in this course, which would introduce such concepts as 'disciplinary power' and 'normalizing society,' Foucault describes one of the effects of the various social movements of the 1960s and early 1970s as 'the insurrection of subjugated knowledges' (p. 7). For Foucault, this insurrection of subjugated knowledges is both a return of historical knowledges that have been repressed or buried, and the emergence of 'a whole series of knowledges that have been disqualified as nonconceptual knowledges, as insufficiently elaborated knowledges: naive knowledges, hierarchically inferior knowledges, knowledges that are below the required level of erudition or scientificity' (p. 7). These buried and disqualified knowledges are knowledges first and foremost of struggles, struggles that have been covered over by the tyranny of totalizing discourses, and especially the totalizing discourses of science. What is most interesting for my purposes here is that Foucault explicitly 'give[s] the name "genealogy" to this coupling together of scholarly erudition and local memories, which allows us to constitute a historical knowledge of struggles and to make use of that knowledge in contemporary tactics' (p. 8). For Foucault, 'genealogies are, quite specifically, antisciences' (p. 9). This notion of *an antiscience born from struggle* resonates, it seems to me, with the projects of disability studies and the disability rights movement. The tactics utilized by both projects challenge the expert knowledges of scientific institutions, and in particular the institution of medicine.

The biomedical model of disability approaches disability as a problem that science and medicine can and must fix; disabled people must be normalized through the disciplinary practices of medicine. Disability studies scholars and disability rights activists have sought to replace, or at least supplement, the biomedical model of disability with a social model of disability (Davis, 1997; Oliver, 1990, 1996; Shakespeare, 1998; Wendell, 1996), or more recently, as discussed above, with a postmodern model of disability (Corker & Shakespeare, 2002; Shildrick, 2002). These antiscience models of disability that are opposed to the biomedical model consider the ways in which social attitudes, conventions, and physical surroundings disable individuals, and work to deconstruct normative attitudes and conventions and reconstruct the material world to better enable the full social participation of people with disabilities. Investigating disability allows us to ask big questions, questions that science often claims to be best positioned to answer, including: What makes humans human? What is the relationship between thought and language? How do we articulate experiences of the body? What is considered normal and abnormal within a particular culture?

As Foucault (2003b) makes clear, genealogies are not a celebration of 'the lyrical right of the ignorant' nor 'some immediate experience that has yet to be captured by knowledge'; nor, for that matter, do they reject 'the contents, methods, or concepts of a science' (p. 9). Rather, genealogies oppose the 'centralizing power-effects that are bound up with the institutionalization and workings of any scientific discourse' (p. 9). This challenge to the 'rise of power that is bound up with scientific knowledge' is a challenge to disciplinary power, and thus Foucault believes we must struggle for a new right that is 'both *anti*disciplinary and emancipated from the principle of sovereignty' (pp. 39-40). Disability studies is, in its marginal position in the university and its struggle to bring a new object of study into being through multiple and sometimes conflicting perspectives, necessarily *inter*disciplinary. But, perhaps it is more useful to think of it as antidisciplinary, which, in Foucault's formulation, brings into being a method that is inventive and always unfinished, and necessarily on the outside of the institutionalization of scientific discourses.

Foucault's opposition to the principle of sovereignty might also be understood in relation to disability. Because the 'experiences' of disability are so varied (the concept covers physical and mental disabilities; visible and invisible disabilities; congenital, sudden, or progressive disabilities; permanent or temporary disabilities), and because most of us will, at some point in our lives, become disabled, investigating the 'experiences' of disability gives us insight into the complicated and changing relationship between selves, bodies, and worlds. Selves and bodies in the world are not autonomous and sovereign, but always come into being in relation to others, are often vulnerable, and fail to fit the norm in one way or another at one time or another. In their essay entitled 'Bodies Together: Touch, Ethics and Disability,' Janet Price and Margrit Shildrick (2002) explore what they understand as 'the permeability between bodies and between embodied subjects' (p. 62). They do so both by writing together (as Janet and Margrit) and by scrutinizing critically their experiences as a woman with MS (Price) who has 'deceased sensation across large areas of her body' (p. 69), and as a woman who does not have decreased sensation (Shildrick), but who nonetheless wonders why her own hand suddenly feels clumsy when it holds Janet's hand, which cannot press back in return (p. 72). For Shildrick and Price, 'the instability of the disabled body is but an extreme instance of the instability of all bodies' (p. 72). By recognizing the relational aspect of embodiment, they begin to posit an alternative ethics not based on the principle of sovereignty, but one in which responsibility lies 'in the uncertainty and risk of response to the unknowable other' (p. 74).[10]

Descent

Genealogy, in Foucault's formulation, is not only an antiscience, but we also might think of it as articulating an antihistory, or at least an antihistoricist history. In his analysis of the genealogical method as it emerges in the work of Nietzsche, Foucault (1977) notes first that genealogy 'opposes itself to the search for "origins"' (p. 140). A genealogist is not interested in discovering the origins of things, or their continuous, linear development from a locatable historical origin; rather, the genealogist seeks to discover moments of 'the dissension of other things' (p. 142). What is important for the genealogist is not the essence of things, but the fabrication of essences 'in a piecemeal fashion from alien forms' (p. 142). What are the accidents that become essences, and how does this historical process happen? What other things, relations, and struggles are lost in the pursuit and founding of historical origins? A genealogist of disability would look, for example, for the invention not the essence of the concepts of the normal and the abnormal, and their relationship to the categories disabled and able-bodied. And, of equal importance, the genealogist of disability would look for what Foucault (2003a) called 'the invention of positive technologies of power' – the 'positive technique[s] of intervention and transformation' (pp. 48, 49) – that emerge with the idea of the norm, or bring that idea into being through practices. As Davis (1995, 2002) does, a genealogist of disability might thus describe the invention of the norm (along with that which is determined to be outside the norm) through various technologies and practices, including, for example, statistics, which Davis characterizes as a technology of industrialization. At the same time, the genealogist will listen for those 'fleeting articulations that the discourse [of the origin, of the normal] has obscured and finally lost' (Foucault 1977, p. 143). What alien forms have been covered over by the forms that we now take to be familiar? What singular events have been lost in the telling of a progressive history? What experiences of the body – 'its conditions of weakness and strength, its breakdown and resistances,' as Foucault would say (p. 144) – might the genealogist be able to discern underneath or from within the 'distant ideality of the origin' (p. 145)?

While the historicist examines and instantiates origins, the genealogist traces lines of descent in all their complexities. The genealogist looks for discontinuities, but also, paradoxically, surprising continuities, those echoes of counter-narratives that reverberate across time and space, if only we could hear them. Such an examination requires that the genealogist 'identify the accidents, the minute deviations – or, conversely, the complete reversals – the errors, the false appraisals, and the faulty calculations that gave birth to those things that continue to exist and have value for us; it is to discover that truth or being do not lie at the root of what we know and what we are, but the exteriority of accidents' (Foucault, 1977, p. 146). Disability, often linked quite literally as well as metaphorically, to accidents, illuminates Foucault's shift of emphasis from some interior truth of identity to the exteriority of accidents. As John Hockenberry (1995) explains in his memoir *Moving Violations*, about his life marked by a car accident when he was 19 that left him paralyzed from the waist down, 'From the beginning, disability taught that life could be reinvented' (p. 79). 'In fact,' he continues, 'such an outlook was required. The physical dimensions of life could be created, like poetry; they were not imposed by some celestial landlord.

Life was more than renting some protoplasm to walk around in. It was more than being a winner or a loser. To have invented a way to move about without legs was to invent walking. This was a task reserved for gods, and to perform it was deeply satisfying. None of that was apparent to the people who stared. To them, I was just in a wheelchair. To me, I was inventing a new life' (p. 79).

The genealogist of disability is concerned, then, not with discovering the truth or being that lies at the root of what we know of disability and what we are as disabled, but with demonstrating the heterogeneity and multiplicity of the experiences, events, and practices of disability. By attempting to show the multiple lines of descent, the genealogist acknowledges that the experiences, events, and practices of disability – and the disabled body – have a history and a geography, and that disability and the disabled body – and all human existence and embodiment – may yet be thought otherwise, may yet be reinvented.

The genealogist, according to Foucault (1977), must articulate a history of the body, in particular a history of the body as it is inscribed by events, manifests 'desires, failings and errors,' and becomes debilitated (p. 148). Foucault's interest in the body inscribed by history connects with disability scholars and activists who assert that able-bodiedness is always a temporary condition. In *Extraordinary Bodies*, Thomson (1997) notes that because anyone can become disabled at any time, disability is 'more fluid, and perhaps more threatening, to those who identify themselves as normates than such seemingly more stable marginal identities as femaleness, blackness, or nondominant ethnic identities' (p. 14). Foucault emphasized this, too, asserting that, theoretically and methodologically, the diagnosis of descent rather than the fixing of an origin brings the body 'and everything that touches it' into view (p. 148).

Emergence

Along with descent, the genealogist is concerned with the emergence, the moment of arising, of forces and figures in history. Like the practice of tracing descent, the concept of emergence challenges the notion of history as a record of continuity and progress, and acknowledges discontinuity in history and as an aspect of 'our very being' (Foucault, 1977, p. 154). The genealogist of disability might consider the moment of arising of disability activism in the public sphere and of disability studies in the academic sphere, and attempt to articulate the confrontation between these two emergent figures: the disability activist and the disability studies scholar. In his introduction to *The Disability Studies*

Reader, Davis (1997) describes such a moment of arising when he writes, '[T]here have been people with disabilities throughout history, but it has only been in the last twenty years that one-armed people, quadriplegics, the blind, people with chronic diseases, and so on, have seen themselves as a single, allied, united physical minority. Linked to this political movement, which is detailed in Joseph Shapiro's (1994) *No Pity: People with Disabilities Forging a New Civil Rights Movement*, David Hevey's *(1992) The Creatures Time Forgot: Photography and Disability Imagery*, and Oliver Sacks's (1989) *Seeing Voices*, among other works, has been the political victory of the passage of the Americans with Disabilities Act (ADA) of 1990, which guarantees the civil rights of people with disabilities' (Davis, 1997, p. 3).

Besides the disability rights activist and the disability studies scholar, there are countless other figures of disability: the grotesque, the freak, the monster, the poster child, the crip, the supercrip, the Not Dead Yet activist, the person with AIDS (PWA), the AIDS activist, the long-term care patient (at home and in a care facility), the disabled person who is heroic, overcoming, or embittered, the disabled person who, like the late Christopher Reeve, is determined to walk again, and the disabled person who does not care if she walks again, the wheelchair athlete, and so on. Besides the disability rights movement and disability studies, there are also multiple domains of disability: the rehabilitation clinic and other domains within and alongside the institution of medicine, the long-term care facility, the deaf school that trains students to sign and the deaf school that is oralist in approach and doesn't allow signing, the special education class, the paralympics, the special olympics, the telethon, the law before and after the Americans with Disabilities Act, and so on. Disability is multiple; it is *enacted* between multiple figures and across multiple domains. Genealogy as theory and method recognizes this multiplicity, and is interested in understanding this multiplicity not in order to fix (in both senses: to repair and to fasten or make stable) disability once and for all, but to open up disability as a myriad of experiences, events, and practices that tell us something about what it means to be human, embodied, and the relationship between bodies, selves, and worlds.

Doing Disability after Foucault

Although I have focused primarily on Foucault's work in order to demonstrate what genealogy might do for disability studies and what disability does for genealogy, I want to briefly consider an approach that is clearly inspired by Foucault's genealogical work, but also attends to work in science studies and feminist science studies developed after Foucault. Exploring the conjunction between science studies and disability studies has only just begun, and I hope to encourage further borrowings and minglings between these fields of inquiry. It appears that there has been some resistance to science studies within disability studies, and this may be because of the attempt in disability studies and activism to understand and analyse disability from outside of the biomedical model. Yet, science studies, as formulated by Latour and others (see, for example, Latour & Woolgar, 1986; Latour, 1987, 1993; Haraway, 1991, 1997) is indeed, in Foucauldian terms, an anti-scientific study of science. Rather than conceiving of science as engaging in some pure practice of discerning facts about things apart from 'interest, justice, and power,' science studies demonstrates that the knowledge of things and human politics and forms of power cannot be separated from each other (Latour 1993, p. 3). In science studies, according to Latour, 'we are always attempting to retie the Gordian knot by crisscrossing, as often as we have to, the divide that separates exact knowledge and the exercise of power – let us say nature and culture' (p. 3). Disability studies clearly attempts to retie this knot, too, by criss-crossing multiple domains of nature and culture, or nature/culture.

Because Foucault's own work was always historical, and because he explicitly cautioned about the difficulties of diagnosing one's own archive, his genealogical method on the surface seems less adequate at discerning contemporary discursive regimes and their enactment in practices.[11] Yet, recent work in science studies has begun to attempt to bring into view these contemporary discursive regimes, and the modes of ordering that create supposed unities, such as, for example, 'the medical profession,' 'Western medicine,' 'present-day medicine,' and 'science' (Berg & Mol 1998). What happens when we disaggregate a concept, event, or experience we have formerly understood as unified? This is what Annemarie Mol (1998, 2002) attempts to do in her work when she demonstrates the ways in which a particular disease, atherosclerosis, is never just one thing, but multiple things. In her book *The Body Multiple*, Mol (2002) is concerned not with how medicine knows a particular disease, or how a patient knows her illness, but rather how that disease is enacted through practices. Mol calls her work 'empirical philosophy,' though it is also a genealogy of atherosclerosis that 'foregrounds practicalities, materialities, *events*' (pp. 12–13). Illness, for Mol, 'is something being done to you, the patient. And something that, as a patient, you do' (p. 20). I find this approach very useful for understanding disability. How do we do disability? This is a question we must continue to ask, while recognizing that there can be no definitive answer. The exploration of *the doing of disability* is what matters, and this is also what matters if we are to better understand the concepts and practices that enact women's health.

Doing Disability in Canada

Briefly, then, I want to consider some examples of doing disability within the Canadian context. As this volume shows, context matters. The experiences and events of disability in the Canadian context in the twenty-first century are not necessarily the same as the experiences and events of disability south of the Canada-U.S. border or further south in Mexico, to name just two out of a multiplicity of other possible contexts. The United Nations declared 1981 the International Year of the Disabled, and adopted the World Programme of Action Concerning Disabled Persons the following year. The goals of the World Programme are: '(i) to support the full and effective participation of persons with disabilities in social life and development; (ii) to advance the rights and protect the dignity of persons with disabilities; and (iii) to promote equal access to employment, education, information, goods and services' (www.un.org/esa/socdev/enable/). The World Programme and the United Nations' definitions of impairment, disability, and handicap (see Text Box 2) indicate that the UN has adopted the social model of disability. The UN definitions distinguish between a physical or psychological impairment, which is not in itself necessarily disabling, and the built environment and social conventions and attitudes that may disable or handicap a person from 'normal' functioning. In *The Rejected Body*, Susan Wendell (1996) appreciates the UN definitions because they explicitly recognize 'the possibility that the primary causes of a disabled person's inability to do certain things may be social; they may be lack of opportunities, lack of accessibility, lack of services, poverty or discrimination, and they often are' (p. 13). However, she is also critical of the UN definitions because they 'seem to imply that there is some universal, biologically or medically describable standard of structure, function, and human physical ability' (p. 14). Wendell worries that by emphasizing that one becomes disabled or handicapped only when one is limited or prevented from fulfilling 'a role that is normal, depending

---

Text Box 9.2 United Nations Definitions

Impairment: Any loss or abnormality of psychological, physiological, or anatomical structure or function;

Disability: Any restriction or lack (resulting from an impairment) of ability to perform an activity in the manner or within the range considered normal for a human being and;

Handicap: A disadvantage for a given individual, resulting from an impairment or disability, that, limits or prevents the fulfilment of a role that is norma, depending on age sex, social and cultural factors, for that individual. (www. un.org/esa/socdev/enable/)

---

on age, sex, social and cultural factors,' as the UN's definitions suggest, the concept of disability gets narrowed such that it doesn't even include the disabling conditions of the 'normal' aging process.

Although the United Nations has recognized the need to oppose discrimination that people with disabilities face worldwide, the experiences and events of disability differ from context to context because of widely varying laws and policies on disability and entitlements for the disabled enacted by governments throughout the world. In Canada, people with disabilities are protected from discrimination under Section 15 of the Canadian Charter of Rights and Freedoms (see Text Box 3), as well as under both federal and provincial human rights legislation, and through case law. In particular, the Canada Human Rights Act of 1985 states that its purpose is to guarantee 'the principle that all individuals should have an opportunity equal with other individuals to make for themselves the lives that they are able and wish to have and to have their needs accommodated, consistent with their duties and obligations as members of society, without being hindered in or prevented from doing so by discriminatory practices based on race, national or ethnic origin, colour, religion, age, sex, sexual orientation, marital status, family status, disability or conviction for an offence for which a pardon has been granted' (http://laws.justice.gc.ca/en/H-6/).

What Canada does not have, perhaps because it does not need it in light of the provisions in the Canadian Charter and the Canada Human Rights Act, is legislation that deals exclusively with disability, like the

Test Box 9.3 Federal Disability Policy in Canada

Section 15 of the Canadian Charter of Rights and Freedoms, which states:
15.(1) Every individual is equal before and under the law and has the right to the equal protection and equal benefit of the law without discrimination and, in particular, without discrimination based on race, national or ethnic origin, colour, religion, sex, age, or mental or physical disability.
(2) Subsection (1) does not preclude any law, program or activity that has as its object the amelioration of conditions of disadvantaged individuals or groups including those that are disadvantaged because of race, national or thnic origin, colour, religion, sex, age or mental or physical disability.
(http://laws.justice.gc.ca/en/charter/)

Americans with Disabilities Act enacted by the U.S. Congress in 1990. Geographer Vera Chouinard (1999), for one, argues that such an act would 'build upon the legal protection from discrimination provided in the Canadian Charter of Rights and Freedoms' (p. 283). She believes this is especially important in a time of neoliberalization signaled by '[r]ecent changes in state policy towards the disabled at the federal level of the Canadian state and at the provincial level in Ontario [that] suggest the emergence of a regulatory regime characterized by the dismantling of programmes to assist the disabled, exclusion of the disabled from the policy process, resistance to proactive legislation to protect the rights of the disabled, reductions in social assistance, and disciplinary measures and incentives aimed at reducing the numbers of disabled persons receiving welfare benefits' (p. 282). As Chouinard shows quite convincingly, the situation for people with disabilities in Canada is at best difficult and at worst 'depressing' (p. 270). As many disability scholars and activists have noted, one of the most difficult aspects of life for most disabled people is finding work to support themselves (see, for example, Wendell, 1996; Mairs, 1996; Longmore, 2003). Because making a living is difficult for many disabled people, they must struggle simply to survive, which, as Chouinard also notes, means they are less able to advocate for their rights locally, nationally, and globally.

Kim England's (2003) recent study of disability, gender, and employment in the Canadian banking industry in particular demonstrates the
difficulties people with disabilities in general have of avoiding poverty,
despite attempts by the Canadian government through the Employment Equity Act to create equity for groups underrepresented historically and still today in various employment sectors (the groups include
women, visible minorities, and Aboriginals, as well as persons with
disabilities). As England notes, citing work by Gail Fawcett (2000) and
statistical evidence from the 1986 and 1991 Health and Activity Limita-
tion Survey (HALS), disabilities 'double the likelihood of living in
poverty' (2003, p. 431). England argues that the ableist attitudes of
employers, the inaccessibility of the built environment in and around
places of work, and misperceptions about what kinds of accommodation people with disabilities might require (pp. 432–433) are the major
barriers to meaningful employment for people with disabilities, all of
which contributes to their social exclusion. England mentions the political work of Canada's DisAbled Women's Network (DAWN) to expose
the obstacles disabled people, and especially disabled women, face in
their struggle for full equality and citizenship.

Through research, education, information sharing, and political protests that range from lobbying for an Ontarians with Disabilities Act to
direct action, DAWN is an organization that offers a progressive, feminist critique of those structures – state, economic, and environmental –
that have shaped the experiences and events of disability in Canada in
the late twentieth and early twenty-first centuries (see Text Box 4). They
seek to transform those structures that limit the ability of people, and
especially women, with disabilities from fully participating in the public and political spheres, and also to transform the attitudes about what
it means to be disabled and to do disability. This is no small task, and
DAWN's resources, if not their determination, are limited. Despite the
many 'socio-spatial barriers to disabled women's activism' in Canada
that Chouinard (1999) catalogues, it is clear that DAWN has struggled
to bring about an 'insurrection of subjugated knowledges' in Foucaultian
terms (Foucault 2003a, p. 7). This is apparent if we look at one particular
case in which they and other disability rights groups in Canada brought
the subjugated knowledges of people with disabilities into the public
domains of Canadian law and bioethics. DAWN had intervener status
in the much-publicized case of Robert Latimer, who was convicted of
killing his 12-year-old daughter Tracy, who was born with severe cere-
bral palsy and reportedly suffered from extreme pain because her

---

Text Box 9.4 Disabled Women's Network (DAWN) Ontario Mission Statement

"DAWN Ontario is a progressive, volunteer-driven, feminist organization promoting social justice, human rights and the advancement of equality rights through education, research, advocacy, coalition-building, resource development, and information.

Our mission is to generate knowledge, information and skills to secure the inclusion, citizenship, human rights and equality of women and girls with disabilities.

We work to illuminate the causes and multidimensional consequences of the growing inequality of wealth, income, power and opportunity in Canada; and to move this critical national problem on to the front burner of Canadian politics and public discourse.' (http://dawn.thot.net/)

'muscles were so tightly contracted that they twisted her body' (Schneider, 1998, p. 6; see also Enns, 1999; Michalko, 2002).

Robert Latimer killed Tracy on 23 October 1993, and the case has been prominent in the media and the consciousness of many Canadians ever since. Latimer's defense was that he killed his daughter because she was in extreme and persistent pain because of her condition; killing her, he maintains to this day, was an act of mercy to end her suffering. A majority of the public seems to have agreed that Latimer's act was merciful, and many have found his life sentence with no parole for 10 years an unduly harsh punishment. Disabled activists, including members of DAWN, have been outspoken in their opposition to this interpretation of Latimer's actions, and the Supreme Court of Canada ruled unanimously in 2001: 'We cannot find that any aspect of the particular circumstances in this case or the offender diminishes the degree of criminal responsibility borne by Mr. Latimer ... In summary, the minimum mandatory sentence is not grossly disproportionate in this case' (cited in Tibbetts, 2001, p. A1).

In an interview about the case in 1994 and in a speech at a vigil for Tracy Latimer in 1995, Catherine Frazee, who is a former chief commissioner of the Ontario Human Rights Commission and current co-director of the Ryerson-RBC Institute for Disability Studies Research and Education, spoke about why the Latimer case makes people with disabilities fear for their lives, and forces them to find the 'courage to confront the insidious stereotypes which underlie public sympathy for Robert Latimer' (http://dawn.thot.net/frazee1.html). Frazee (1994) calls the Latimer case a 'powerful wake up call for many in the disabled community' because it suggests that many Canadians 'feel confident that Tracy Latimer's life has far less value than a nondisabled life.' Disability studies scholars and disabled activists offer an important perspective on controversial bioethical issues like euthanasia, abortion, and genetic testing, although their position is often not sought in controversial cases (see, e.g., Mairs, 1996; Hubbard, 1997). In the Latimer case, Frazee (1994) states emphatically: 'The nondisabled population in this case is most guilty of a colossal failure of the imagination. People ... often say to a disabled person, "I can't imagine how you cope." The inability to imagine what the disability experience is all about is translated into a kind of collective mythology that a person with a disability lives a tragic life, marked by deprivation and suffering. This is simply not so and we have a responsibility to communicate that more and more daringly' (p. 1).

I end this chapter with a snapshot of political activism and its link to the imagination and daring forms of communication, because despite many obstacles, and what Chouinard (1999) says is a depressing situation for many disabled people, people with disabilities still struggle to transform the world that they live in. DAWN and other groups show that there are many ways of doing disability, and that we cannot understand disability as a state of being. This shift from being stigmatized to doing dis/ability is why disability studies and the disability rights movement is an example of genealogy, or the 'coupling together of scholarly erudition and local memories, which allows us to constitute a historical knowledge of struggles and to make use of that knowledge in contemporary tactics' (Foucault 2003a, p. 8).

NOTES

1 Interestingly, a recent collection of essays that offers a fascinating comparative and historical approach to women's health in the Canadian and U.S. contexts does not include any essays explicitly on disability (Feldberg et al. 2005).

2 Arthur W. Frank (1995) argues that in postmodernity, partly because of the success of Western medicine to keep people alive, many illnesses have become chronic in character. Frank says that we, in the West at least, now live in a 'remission society,' with many people living lives that are somewhere in between the categories of healthy and ill.

3 In her book *The Rejected Body*, Susan Wendell (1996) discusses the ways that having chronic fatigue syndrome or myalgic encephalomyelitis (ME) has shaped her understanding of disability. Wendell writes, 'Perhaps the type of disability I have also influences my appreciation of diversity in disability politics. Because my disability is no longer readily apparent, and because it is an illness whose symptoms vary greatly from day to day, I live between the world of the disabled and the world of the non-disabled' (p. 76).

4 For a discussion of people with disabilities as phenomenologists, see my essay 'Breaking down: A phenomenology of disability' (Diedrich, 2001).

5 This section and the next on genealogy is adapted with permission from my (2005) Introduction: Genealogies of 'disability,' *Cultural Studies*, 19(6), 649–666. http://www.tandf.co.uk/journals.

6 Corker and Shakespeare (2002) do acknowledge the problem of the conflation of 'poststructuralism' with 'postmodernism,' and admit that many of the theorists who they categorize as poststructuralist, including Foucault, refuse this label for their work.

7 This criticism is often levelled against Women's Studies and Black Studies and other interdisciplinary minority studies. While I certainly think there is a tension between theory and activism in all of these interdisciplinary fields of study (which relates to a tension between theory and empirical work in these interdisciplinary fields as well as in more traditional disciplines, such as sociology, political science, history, and literature), I find it interesting that these interdisciplinary fields of study are often perceived from the outside as untheoretical, and also, relatedly, lacking in rigor. It is true that sometimes theory is critiqued from within as well, but in both instances – in the case of the critique from the inside as well as the critique from the outside – such a critique can only be made by ignoring or covering over a long history of theoretical work.

8 Paul K. Longmore and Lauri Umansky's (2001) impressive volume *The New Disability History: American Perspectives* offers examples of both of the historical approaches that Scott delineates: making visible and deconstructing 'experience' as a category of analysis. Douglas Baynton (2001), for example, investigates not simply the hidden history of the disabled in United States history, but 'the *concept* of disability' and the

ways it 'has been used to justify discrimination against other groups by attributing disability to them' (p. 33).

9 Tremain (2005) has also edited a recent volume of essays that utilize Foucault's work in general, not only his genealogical method, to think about disability.

10 In her discussion of the biopolitics of immunity, Donna Haraway also articulates an ethics of vulnerability. According to Haraway (1991), 'Life is a window of vulnerability. It seems a mistake to close it. The perfection of the fully defended, "victorious" self is a chilling fantasy ... whether located in the abstract spaces of national discourse, or in the equally abstract spaces of our interior bodies' (p. 224).

11 Foucault (1972) believed that it is impossible to describe one's own 'archive,' or 'the general system of the formation and transformation of statements' (p. 130), precisely because one is within it. The archive, in other words, is that which delimits what one can and cannot say; there is no thought from the outside of one's own archive. And yet, Foucault (2002) also submits, in the introduction to *The Archaeology of Knowledge*: 'I have tried to define this blank space from which I speak, and which is slowly taking shape in discourse that I still feel to be so precarious and so unsure' (p. 17).

REFERENCES

Baynton, D. (1997). A silent exile on this earth: The metaphoric construction of deafness in the nineteenth century. In L. Davis (Ed.), *The Disability Studies Reader* (pp. 128–50). New York: Routledge.

Baynton, D. (2001). Disability and justification of inequality in American history. In P.K. Longmore and L. Umansky (Eds.), *The New Disability History: American Perspectives* (pp. 33–57). New York: New York University Press.

Berg, M., & Mol, A. (1998). Difference in medicine: An introduction. In M. Berg & A. Mol (Eds.), *Differences in Medicine: Unraveling Practices, Techniques, and Bodies* (pp. 1–12). Durham and London: Duke University Press.

Canguilhem, G. (1989). *The Normal and the Pathological*. C.R. Fawcett (Trans.). New York: Zone Books.

Chouinard, V. (1999) Body polictics: Disabled women's activism in Canada and beyond. In R. Butler & H. Parr. (Eds.), *Mind and Body Spaces: Geographies of Illness, Impairment, and Disability* (pp. 269–294). London and New York: Routledge.

Corker, M., & Shakespeare, I. (2002). Mapping the terrain. In M. Corker & T. Shakespeare (Eds.), *Disability/Postmodernity* (pp. 1–17). London and New York: Continuum.

Davis, L. (1995). *Enforcing Normalcy: Disability, Deafness, and the Body*. New York: Verso.

Davis, L. (2002). *Bending Over Backwards: Disability, Dismodernism and Other Difficult Positions*. New York and London: New York University Press.

Davis, L. (Ed.). (1997). *The Disability Studies Reader*. New York: Routledge.

Delany, S. (1988). *The Motion of Light in Water: Sex and Science Fiction Writing in the East Village*. Minneapolis: University of Minnesota Press.

Diedrich, L. (2001). Breaking down: A phenomenology of disability. *Literature and Medicine*, 20(2), 209–230.

Diedrich, L. (2005). An ethics of failure: Anti-heroic cancer narratives. In M. Shildrick & R. Mykitiuk (Eds.), *Ethnics of Body: Postconventional Challenges* (pp. 135–152). Boston: MIT Press.

Diedrich, L. (2005). Introduction: Genealogies of disability. *Cultural Studies*, 19(6), 649–666.

Diprose, R. (1994). *The Bodies of Women: Ethnics, Embodiment and Sexual Difference*. London and New York: Routledge.

England, K. (2003). Disabilities, gender and employment: Social exclusion, employment equity and Canadian banking. *The Canadian Geographer/Le Geographe Canadien*, 47(4), 429–450.

Enns, R. (1999). *A Voice Unheard: The Latimer Case and People with Disabilities*. Halifax: Fernwood.

Fawcett, G. (2000). *Bringing Down the Barriers: The Labour Market and Women with Disabilities in Canada*. Ottawa: Canadian Council on Social Development.

Fedberg, G., Ladd-Taylor, M., Li, A., & McPherson, K. (Eds.). (2003). *Women, Health, and Nation: Canada and the United States since 1945*. Montreal and Kingston: McGill-Queen's University Press.

Foucault, M. (1972). *The Archaeology of Knowledge and the Discourse on Language*. A.M. Sheridan Smith. (Trans.) New York: Pantheon.

Foucault, M. (1977). *Language, Counter-memory, Practice: Selected Essays and Interviews*. D. Bouchard & S. Simon (Trans.). Ithaca, NY: Cornell University Press.

Foucault, M. (2003a). *Abnormal: Lectures at the Collége de France 1974-1975*. Graham Burchell (Trans.). New York: Picador.

Foucault, M. (2003b). *'Society Must Be Defended': Lectures at the Collége de France 1975–1976*. M. Bertani & A. Fontana (Eds.). D. Macey (Trans.). New York: Picador.

Frank, A.W. (1995). *The Wounded Storyteller: Body, Illness, and Ethnics*. Chicago and London: University of Chicago Press.

Frazee, C. (1994). A wake up call: An interview with Catharine Frazee. Why is the Latimer case important? http://dawn.thot.net/frazee1.html.

Freidson, E. (1983). Celebrating Erving Goffman, 1983. *Contemporary Sociology, 12*(4), 359–362.

Garland-Thomson, R. (2002). Intergrating disability, transforming feminist theory. *National Women's Studies Association Journal, 14*(3), 1–32.

Goffman, E. (1963). *Stigma: Notes on the Management of Spoiled Identity*. New York: Simon & Schuster.

Haraway, D. (1991). *Simians, Cyborgs, and Women: The Reinvention of Nature*. New York: Routledge.

Haraway, D. (1997). *Modest_Witness@Second_Millenium.Female_Man©_Meets_Oncomouse™. Feminism and Technoscience*. New York: Routledge.

Harding, S. (1991). *Whose Science? Whose Knowledge: Thinking from Women's Lives*. Ithaca: NY: Cornell University Press.

Hevey, D. (1992). *The Creatures Time Forgot: Photography and Disability Imagery*. New York: Routledge.

Hockenberry, J. (1995). *Moving Violations: War Zones, Wheelchairs, and Declarations of Independence*. New York: Hyperion.

Hubbard, R. (1997). Abortion and disability. In Lennard Davis (Ed.), *The Disability Studies Reader* (pp. 187–200). New York: Routledge.

Lane, H. (1984). *When the Mind Hears: A History of the Deaf*. New York: Random House.

Lane, H. (1997). Constructions of deafness. In L. Davis (Ed.), *The Disability Studies Reader* (pp. 153–171). New York: Routledge.

Latour, B. (1987). *Science in Action: How to Follow Scientists and Engineers through Society*. Milton Keynes, UK: Open University Press.

Latour, B. (1993). *We Have Never Been Modern*. Catherine Porter (Trans.). Cambridge: Harvard University Press.

Latour, B., & Woolgar S. (1986). *Laboratory Life: The Construction of Scientific Facts*. 2nd ed. Princeton: Princeton University Press.

Law, J. (1994). *Organizing Modernity*. Oxford: Blackwell.

Law, J., & Mol, A. (2002). Complexities: An introduction. In J. Law & A. Mol (Eds.), *Complexities: Social Studies of Knowledge Practices* (pp. 1–22). Durham and London: Duke University Press.

Longmore, P.K. (2003). *Why I Burned My Book and Other Essays on Disability*. Philadelphia: Temple University Press.

Longmore, P.K., & Umansky, L. (2001). *The New Disability History: American Perspectives*. New York: New York University Press.

Mairs, N. (1996). *Waist-High in the World: A Life Among the Nondisabled*. Boston: Beacon Press.

Maynard, M. (1994). Methods, practice and epistemology: The debate about feminism and research. In M. Maynard & J. Purvis (Eds.), *Researching Women's Lives from a Feminist Perspective* (pp. 10–26). London: Taylor & Francis.

Michalko, R. (2002). *The Difference Disability Makes*. Philadelphia: Temple University Press.

Mitchell, D.T., & Snyder, S.L. (1997). Introduction. Disability studies and the double blind of representation. In D.T. Mitchell & L. Snyder (Eds.), *The Body and Physical Difference: Discourses of Disability* (pp. 1–31). Ann Arbor: University of Michigan Press.

Mol, A. (1998). Missing links, making links: The performance of some atheroscleroses. In M. Berg & A. Mol (Eds.), *Differences in Medicine: Unraveling Practices, Techniques, and Bodies* (pp. 144–165). Durham and London: Duke University Press.

Mol. A. (2002). *The Body Multiple: Ontology in Medical Practice*. Durham and London: Duke University Press.

Oliver, M. (1990). *Understanding Disability: From Theory to Practice*. London: Macmillan.

Price, J., & Shildrick, M. (2002). Bodies together: Touch, ethics and disability. In M. Corker & T. Shakespeare (Eds.), *Disability/Postmodernity* (pp. 62–75). London and New York: Continuum.

Rose, N. (1994). Medicine, history and the present. In C. Jones & R. Porter (Eds.), *Reassessing Foucault: Power, Medicine, and the Body* (pp. 48–72). London and New York: Routledge.

Rose, N. (1996). Identity, genealogy, history. In S. Hall & P. Du Gay (Eds.), *Question of Cultural Identity* (pp. 128–150). London: Sage.

Sacks, O. (1989). *Seeing Voices: A Journey into the World of the Deaf*. Berkeley: University of California Press.

Schneider, C.E. (1998). Hard cases. *Hastings Center Report, 28*(2), 6.

Scott J.W. (1992). Experience. In J. Butler & J.W. Scott (Eds.), *Feminists Theorize the Political* (pp. 22–40). New York and London: Routledge.

Shakespeare, T. (Ed.). (1998). *The Disability Reader: Social Science Perspectives*. New York: Cassell.

Shapiro, J. (1994). *No Pity: People with Disabilities Forging a New Civil Rights Movement*. New York: Three Rivers Press.

Shildrick, M. (1997). *Leaky Bodies and Boundaries: Feminism, Postmodernism and (Bio)Ethics*. New York: Routledge.

Shildrick, M. (2002). *Embodying the Monster: Encounters with the Vulnerable Self*. London: Sage.

Stone, D. (1984). *The Disabled State*. Philadelphia: Temple University Press.

Thomson, R.G. (1997). *Extraordinary Bodies: Figuring Physical Disability in American Culture and Literature*. New York: Columbia University Press.

Thomson, R.G. (Ed.). (1996). *Freakery: Cultural Spectacles of the Extraordinary Body*. New York: New York University Press.

Tibbetts, J. (2001). 'Royal Mercy' Latimer's only hope. *Ottawa Citizen, 19* (January), A1.

Tremain, S. (2002). On the subject of impairment. In M. Corker & T. Shakespeare (Eds.), *Disability/Postmodernity* (pp. 32–47). London and New York: Continuum.

Tremain, S. (Ed.). (2005). *Foucault and the Government of Disability*. Ann Arbor: University of Michigan Press.

Wendell, S. (1996). *The Rejected Body: Feminist Philosophical Reflections on Disability*. New York: Routledge.

10 Negotiating Sexualities in Women's Health Care

CYNTHIA MATHIESON

There's some overlap [between lesbian and heterosexual women] ... but lesbian women have to deal with things like invisibility, discrimination ... I don't see how keeping a whole part of yourself secret with either everyone or with some people at certain times could not affect your health. (Mathieson, 1998, p. 1637)

I don't think that my doctor understood that it [sexual orientation] had a lot to do with my life ... no understanding of how that particular issue impacts on my life as a woman ... the most striking thing to me was ... lack of acknowledgment of what it meant to be a lesbian and how it affected my health or my life. (Bailey, Gurevich, & Mathieson, 2000, p. 16)

There are no illnesses unique to lesbians and bisexual women, yet women who identify as such face specific challenges, as the above citations suggest. Not being able to be open about sexuality has implications for health and health care, as does the impact of disclosure of identities that challenge normative expectations. The health care setting can be viewed as one arena where a woman must negotiate her identity, and the health concerns of women who challenge these expectations with their sexual identities can only be understood by acknowledging up front the negative attitudes held by individuals, institutions, and society.

Women who openly claim identities as lesbians, or bisexuals, confront long-held societal assumptions.[1,2] These are (a) sexual identity is preordained by biology and that it is static – an essentialist view (Fuss, 1989); (b) an individual can be attracted to only a male or a female – a monosexist view (Nagle, 1995); and (c) individuals are normally attracted to the opposite gender – a heterosexist view. In this normative framework, sexual identity is also conceptualized as the attribute of an individual in isolation from her socio-political context (Firestein, 1996). When the context is health care, there is a real problem in ascribing behaviours and outcomes to women based solely on their self-identification. From this alone, no assumptions can be made about one's personal history, current relationship status, or future sexual attractions. More to the point, no conclusions can be drawn about health status and health histories.

Unfortunately, as the research indicates, health care providers often make assumptions, a situation that can place clients at risk. Traditional medical knowledge and medical providers play a crucial role in the enforcement of norms and behaviours (Sherwin, 1992). As clients, women face systemic barriers that construct lesbians and bisexual women as 'errors of classification' within 'juridico-medical discourses' (Butler, 1991, p.303). The communication between health care providers and their lesbian, and bisexual, clients is a critical juncture where sexual identity, not just health care needs, are therefore negotiated. These individuals add their voices, sometimes at a personal cost, to the continuing discourse about what it is to be non-heterosexual in our society. Their narratives hold the potential for new discourses that explain how sexuality, culture, and the socio-political context intersects and shapes women's health (Brown & Syme, 2002).

Vulnerability is amplified when the experience of being lesbian or bisexual is compounded by multiple discrimination incurred as a result of other identities based on minority status. In the case of lesbians and bisexuals, individuals 'who have both same and other-gender attractions come from many racial, ethnic, religious, and social class backgrounds' (Rust, 1996, p. 53). These backgrounds cannot automatically be subsumed by sexual identity. Claiming any sexual identity is always done within the context of an individual's history and culture. Gender, ethnic, and class oppression are all political factors affecting health, illness, and medical care, and each factor – alone and together – influences views of health and health care.

Overview

Why privilege sexual identity in a view of health in the first place? Quite simply, sexual identity matters; it has profound ramifications for a woman's health care in a heterosexist and homophobic[3] society. The

United Nations Commission on Human Rights (2005) recognizes the existence of discrimination based on sexual orientation, including discriminatory experiences affecting health (see text box 10.1). The Women's Health Policy of the Public Health Association of Australia (PHAA) (2004) affirms sexual identity as a determinant of health. It further recommends that federal and state policy prioritize the needs of lesbian and bisexual women to address systemic discrimination (see text box 10.1). Health Canada (2002) clearly acknowledges sexual orientation as a factor affecting experiences in the health system. This chapter poses the question: If gender and sexual identity are 'determinants' of health, what exactly does this mean? How do lesbian and bisexual women 'do' gender in the health care context, which is only one of many venues in which a woman may disclose her sexual identity? Indeed, a woman's health and health care may depend on this disclosure.

While the overall theoretical framework of this chapter is feminist, it is also grounded in the understanding that sexualities are constructed through discourse (Kitzinger & Wilkinson, 1995). In addition to integrating personal experiences, the production of accounts is a dynamic discourse that enhances visibility of sexualities. The process of challenging theories and beliefs about sexuality is therefore facilitated by the accounts that are available (Mathieson & Endicott, 1998). Before 1990, lesbians – much less bisexual women – were basically invisible in health research. In their historical analysis of the medical construction of lesbianism, Stevens and Hall (1991) argued that the contemporary health care experience of lesbian clients should be viewed in the historical context of how medical ideologies are constructed. In brief, these ideologies have pathologized lesbianism (a) through moral condemnation, (b) through medicalization of lesbianism as a disease, and (c) through specific targeting of lesbians. The authors point out: 'Many medical descriptions legitimated dreadful stereotypes of lesbian women': schizophrenic, psychopathic, aggressive, hostile, man-haters, sadistic, to name a few (p. 297). It was the emergence of the gay and lesbian movement in the 1950s that started a resistance to this deviance model. Still, the empirical evidence from the United States, the United Kingdom, and Canada overwhelmingly points to a history of discriminatory attitudes towards gays, lesbians, and bisexuals on the part of health care providers. A study by Druzin, Shrier, Yacowar, & Rossignol (1998) also documents discrimination against gay, lesbian, and bisexual family physicians by patients.

Transgender health, or trans-health, is a newly emerging field that

Text Box 10.1 International Initiatives

The United Nations Commission on Human Rights (CHR) (2005) recognizes discrimination based on sexual orientation. In 2004, a special report dealt with sexual orientation and health. Ongoing efforts by the CHR represent worldwide advocacy on behalf of Lesbian/Gay/Bisexual/Transgendered/Intersex (LGBTI) persons.

In the United States, the Strategic Plan 2004–07 of the Gay and Lesbian Medical Association (GLMA, 2004) advances an agenda for across-the-board health system competence around health issues of LGBT individuals. There is a special Trans Health Care Committee.

The Public Health Association of Australia (PHAA, 2004) currently affirms sexual identity as a social determinant of health, noting special health risks and issues incurred by lesbians and bisexual women. PHAA recommends that federal and state policy prioritize the needs of lesbians and bisexual women to address systemic discrimination.

The International Gay and Lesbian Association (IGLA, 1999) focuses public and government attention on cases of discrimination against lesbians, gay men, bisexuals, and transgendered persons, including cases related to health. The IGLA works with international organization and the international media.

The Department of Constitutional Affairs (2004) in the United Kingdom is developing a federal government strategy for transsexual people in the context of family, social, and health policies.

will create additional challenges. If lesbianism and bisexuality by their very existence confront normative assumptions about sexualities, the challenge is even greater with transgenderism. Transgendered persons open themselves to extreme discrimination in a health care system which is entrenched in 'heteropolarity' and 'heteronormativity' (Wilton, 1996). Some transgendered persons may seek medical intervention for gender reassignment surgery, in which case the gender transition decisions involve physical, legal, and psychosocial changes. The diagnosis of 'gender identity disorder' as a clinical disorder in the *Diagnostic and Statistical Manual – IV – TR* (2000) is noted by Golden (2000) as problematic and suspect. The diagnosis, used as an assessment tool for deciding who is an acceptable candidate for surgical intervention, inherently pathologizes transgenderism. The criteria for diagnosis are premised on either/or categories: male versus female, with a fundamental assertion that one's sex must match one's gender. Bornstein (1994) argues that the 'myth' of being trapped in the wrong body is a powerful metaphor that relies on and sustains these restrictive binary categories. According to Gamson (1998), 'The presence of visibly transgendered people, people who do not quite fit, potentially subverts the notion of two naturally fixed genders; the presence of people with ambiguous sexual desires potentially subverts the notion of naturally fixed sexual orientation' (p. 596).

Although this chapter focuses on research as it pertains to lesbian and bisexual women, it is recognized that the need for more research and analysis of transgendered women's experiences are critical. That is, the experiences of lesbian and bisexual women cannot be made to stand in for the diverse health care needs of the transgender population.

Reviewing the lesbian health care literature from 1970 to 1990, Stevens (1992) identified 28 U.S. studies. In general, these studies indicated that health care providers held negative attitudes towards lesbian and gay clients; these attitudes negatively affected quality of care and health outcomes. Assumptions of heterosexuality by health care providers acted as a barrier to care, and the negative impact of disclosing one's sexual orientation was singled out as particularly problematic. Lesbians did not pursue traditional health care for routine medical concerns because of a sense of marginalization; that is, of not being part of mainstream society. Faced with negative attitudes, lesbians and bisexual participants in these studies often said or implied that they made decisions not to seek care.

In 1993, Simkin had a pioneer article published in Canada entitled 'Unique Health Care Concerns of Lesbians.' Ramsay's (1994) review article a year later in *Canadian Woman Studies* stated that as far as Canadian data was concerned, there was 'virtually no existing information on lesbian health or health care needs' (p. 22). By 1996, in *Canadian Family Physician*, Moran reported on lesbian health care needs in a Canadian sample. My own work on lesbian and bisexual health sprung directly from Ramsay's alert about the lack of empirical research in the Canadian context.

Text Box 10.2 Canadian Update: Sexual Identity and Health

Canadian research on lesbian and bisexual health has emerged within the last 10 years.

The Women's Health Strategy recognizes diversity among women. Sexual orientation is noted as one facet of this diversity that can affect women's experience in the health system (Health Canada, 2002).

Health issues of particular concern for lesbians and bisexual women include: the risk of breast and cervical cancer; the risk of sexually transmitted infections during woman-to-woman sex and exposure to high-risk factors for HIV/AIDs; factors involved in mental health, including domestic violence.

Lesbian and bisexual women need to negotiate their sexual identities in the health care setting because societal attitudes are grounded in heterosexist and homophobic attitudes. Some women report that they do not feel comfortable enough to disclose to health providers and that they do not seek care because of this.

Women report negative impacts of disclosure and inappropriate advice from providers as a direct result of their sexual identity.

Current research calls for systemic changes in the health care interaction to address barriers to care. Fear and lack of knowledge on the part of providers needs to be addressed.

To date, local and provincial initiatives provide some important resources for lesbian and bisexual women, for health care providers, and policy makers.

Trans-health is a newly emerging field that will require strong advocacy.

In sum, research about lesbian/bisexual health and health care is really very new, about a decade old, and, as such, there is no definitive body of research on lesbian or bisexual health. Boehmer (2002) reviewed 3,777 articles published in English – the public health research from 1980 to 1999 – to determine the inclusion of lesbian, gay, bisexual, and transgender (LGBT) populations. This publication confirmed that LGBT issues have been seriously neglected by health researchers. In a review paper, Bernhard (2001) refers to several factors concerning why lesbians are less likely than other women to seek health care: homophobic attitudes of health care professionals, limited access to care, and expected or actual negative interactions with health care providers. In the recent Canadian research, women are still reporting barriers to health care as a direct result of their sexual identity: heterosexist assumptions on the part of health care providers, negative impacts of disclosure, and inappropriate health advice (Mathieson, 1998; Simkin, 1998). Anderson, Healy, Herringer, Isaac, and Perry (2001) report on the ramifications of the anti-lesbian/anti-gay social climate in northern British Columbia, highlighting barriers to accessible health care for lesbians. The question posed at the outset of this section – Why privilege sexual identity in our view of health? – calls up the wider implications of all of the research findings thus far. 'Lesbian and bisexual women are receiving less than optimum health care in a Canadian system that prides itself on equal access' (Mathieson, 1998, p. 1639). Why?

Disclosure

> I actually don't go, I don't take care of certain parts of my health because I haven't found doctors that I trust ... And if I don't have a choice, like if it's a specialist and I've waited ... six to seven weeks to get to see this person, I'm not going to say, 'No, I'm not going to take the appointment,' but I'm going to choose what parts of my life I'm going to bring into that discussion. (Mathieson, 1996)

Lesbians and bisexuals live in environments that range from hostile to friendly, making them aware of subtleties in language and behaviours that indicate, on a daily basis, safety or danger (Deevy, 1990, p. 37). Disclosing is a risk; there is inevitably a psychological cost that is associated with both revealing and concealing one's sexual identity (Mathieson & Gurevich, 1997). The dominant ideologies of mainstream culture and of medical discourse both sustain a situation where lesbian and bisexual health needs may go unnoticed. Unequal power relations are inherent in mainstream health care to begin with. Over and above this, physicians may not even know who their lesbian or bisexual patients are, a fact likely to undermine adequate health care because lesbianism and bisexuality are invisible within it. In seeking any type of professional help, lesbian and bisexual women face continual, ongoing decisions about disclosing their sexual identities. If they choose not to disclose, they will not be able to discuss their health needs within the context of their entire life, which is the basis of continuity of care. There have been U.S. legal cases where lesbians or bisexual women were not allowed to participate in the medical care of their partners because providers did not realize their sexual identities (Kendall, 1995). Disclosure may be a greater problem for bisexual women because bisexuality is understood even less than lesbianism (Gruskin, 1999, p. 73). And the problem may be greater for poor women and women of colour because of asymmetrical power relationships with their health care providers (Stevens, 1995).

Do women feel safe enough in the health care system to disclose? Lesbian and bisexual women have reported that disclosure of their sexual orientation affects care; negative experiences include demeaning comments and insults, avoidance of physical contact, breaches of confidentiality (Brogan, 1997; Rose & Platzer, 1993; Stevens & Hall, 1990). In one of my studies (Mathieson, 1998), over 80 per cent of the 98 participants spontaneously reported that needing to feel safe was the major criterion for disclosing to physicians. Half of the sample said that they had foregone seeking health care of one type or another at least once due to sexual orientation. A third of the sample said they had forgone seeking routine care, such as annual check-ups, and approximately the same proportion said that they did not go for regular breast screening and Papanicolao (Pap) tests. The noted barriers to care were heterosexist assumptions, physicians' negative responses to disclosure of sexual orientation, and an implicit responsibility for patients to educate their health care providers. Canadian nurses and physicians to whom this information was presented in seminars found these data a serious cause for concern, especially the items about screening. In another study with 254 Canadian lesbian women, Bergeron and Senn (2003) concluded that being more open about one's sexuality was related to increased disclosure to health providers. The more comfortable women were with their providers, the more likely they were to seek preventative care. Davis (2000), in an Ontario study, reported that about half of lesbian clients did not come out to their providers despite the fact that 91 per cent thought this knowledge was important for providers to have. In brief, feeling safe enough to disclose to one's health provider is associated with regular care seeking (Diamant,

Schuster, & Lever, 2000) and better use of health care services (White & Dull, 1998).

Fear and lack of knowledge on the part of health care providers may lead to substandard care (Lee, 2000). More specifically, heterosexist assumptions interfere with effective therapeutic communication with clients and as such act as a barrier to care. Stevens (1995) believes that the impact is twofold, on both a structural and interpersonal level; that is, the structure of health care is obstructive to health care delivery, and health care providers' heterosexist assumptions prohibit supportive interactions with clients. In the Canadian study cited earlier (Mathieson, 1998), more than two-thirds of the participants reported being *always* aware of heterosexist assumptions (e.g., during the health history, restrictive titles or categories on health care forms, the clinic or waiting room environment).

If a provider holds negative views of their clients' sexual identities, the disclosure poses risks for the client. Stevens (1994b) described a study in the United States with a sample of 45 economically and racially diverse lesbians in 332 health care interactions. Seventy-seven per cent of these interactions were evaluated negatively. Participants frequently mentioned the term *vulnerable* to describe how they felt in the health care setting. They also communicated the experience of 'compounded vulnerability ... Their sense of unprotectedness seemed to be added to in geometric proportions with each identity that did not match the male, heterosexual, Euro-American, middle-class able-bodied norm' (p. 220). In one of my studies (Mathieson, 1998), participants were asked how their physicians responded to disclosure. Of 98 women, 15 reported being told their sexuality was pathological, and some were referred to psychiatric services. Seven women felt that they had 'rough' internal examinations after disclosure, and four women reported they were refused care. Logically, one result from these negative experiences is that women activate protective strategies. They may choose not to disclose, they may try to educate their providers, they may overtly challenge mistreatment, or they may stop seeking health care or fail to initiate it.

Negotiating Identities in the Health Care Context

A heterosexual woman does not have to decide whether or not to disclose her sexual orientation to a health care provider; it is assumed that she is heterosexual. It is virtually impossible to imagine an instance where she would need to say to her physician, 'By the way, I am heterosexual,' in order to frame her questions or concerns. A heterosexual woman may have to disclose that she is abused, or that she has a sexually transmitted infection, or that she is an addict, but sexual identity will never become a separate issue in that encounter. The way heterosexist assumptions play out in health care often places major responsibility on the client – first for initiating disclosure, and then for educating the provider if necessary. A common health history story describes physicians asking, 'Do you have a boyfriend? or 'Are you married?' to start the sexual history. Another variation is, 'Are you sexually active?' followed by the assumption that the partner is a man. This question-answer exchange may be followed by inappropriate birth control advice. Such conversations actually place the client in a doubly vulnerable position: she is forced to disclose in order to correct misinterpretations; the provider may not understand the disclosure; and even then there may be continued risk afterwards.

In previous research I reported that bisexual women represented a distinctive voice, as they feel that the whole idea of bisexuality poses a conceptual problem for providers, who seem to focus on the client's relationships with men to the exclusion of women partners (Mathieson, 1998). At the very least, this focus could seriously skew the health history and may lead to misinformation about health risks.

Every time a woman comes out to her provider, she adds her voice to the discourse about what it is to claim a lesbian or bisexual identity. Thus, such conversations go beyond the general discussion of health needs by challenging the assumptions that underlie constraining definitions of sexualities. Openly claiming these identities in the health care setting has the power to destabilize assumptions that arise when providers interpret the identities as self-explanatory labels.

Heath care professionals can implement pragmatic changes to instigate positive change. In dealing with clients, staff need to start by adopting a more inclusive language (e.g., 'partner' instead of 'spouse') and by improving sensitivity and communication skills. By asking heterosexist questions in the health history, providers perpetuate the idea that heterosexuality is normative. It is paramount to ask about a woman's sexual orientation in a non-judgemental fashion. What the health care provider should be asking is, 'What do I need to know about your life and relationships that will help me to best meet your health needs?' thereby opening the door for disclosure. Likewise, the key question to ask about sexual activity is, 'Are you having unprotected sex with men, with women, or with both?' Also, waiting rooms and clinic areas need to signal a lesbian-positive environment, whether it be through customized brochures or posters on the wall. Simkin (1998) recommends that health care providers post a sign in their waiting room that says, 'We do not discriminate on the basis of race, sex or sexual orientation.' Ramsay (1994) emphasized that responses to disclosure can be unintentionally value-laden, and, as such, professionals should not respond to disclosure by saying, 'It doesn't matter to me.' (p. 26). Disclosure obviously does matter; otherwise it would not be privileged within the health care interaction. Better responses are, 'Thanks for telling me,' or 'I don't know a lot about lesbians/bisexuals, but perhaps we can both work together in dealing with your health concerns.' All of these small practical changes are actually significant political acts because they allow for the entrance of lesbian/bisexual issues into the health care system (Bailey, Gurevich, & Mathieson, 2000).

Health Behaviours and Risk

Like the general population, lesbians and bisexual women engage in behaviours that place them at risk for health problems (e.g., smoking, drinking, risky sex) and positive ones that are preventative (e.g., screening for cancer). Simply identifying these behaviours does not explain motivation. Health promotion models often assume that given the circumstances, individuals are able to avail themselves of the best course of action, which is not always true. Population-based U.S. studies are instructive for a very general comparison of lesbians/bisexual women to heterosexual women on the topic of health behaviours and risk.[4] These studies do not imply that lesbian and bisexual health concerns gain legitimacy only through comparison against a heterosexual group; rather, such data should serve as a prompt to assess if lesbians/bisexual women are at an increased risk for poor health outcomes and why.

Data was recently analysed from 93,311 participants in the Women Health Initiative in the U.S. (Valanis et al., 2000). Heterosexual and non-heterosexual post-menopausal women aged 50 to 79 years old were compared on a variety of factors: demographics, psychosocial risk, screening practices, and health-related behaviours. Despite higher socio-economic status, lesbian and bisexual women used alcohol and cigarettes more often than their heterosexual counterparts, exhibited risk factors for cardiovascular disease and for reproductive cancers, and scored lower on assessment of mental health and social support. Other data from this study indicated lower recommended rates of Pap testing and mammography screening services for non-heterosexual women.

Similar findings are reported by Aaron et al. (2001) in a cross-sectional community survey of 1,010 self-identified lesbians in the United States. Compared with the general population of women, lesbians reported more cigarette, alcohol, and heavy alcohol use; lesbians were less likely to report having had a Pap test within the past two years but more likely to report ever having had a mammogram. Diamant, Wold, Spritzer, & Gelberg (2000) analysed data from 4,697 participants in a Los Angeles County Health Survey. Lesbian and bisexual women were statistically more likely than heterosexual women to have poor health behaviours (e.g., alcohol consumption, smoking) and worse access to health care. During the preceding two years, lesbians, but not bisexual women, were less likely than heterosexual women to have had a Pap test and a clinical breast examination.

Data is equivocal on the issue of whether lesbians are less likely to seek routine gynecological care, especially Pap tests (Ferris, Batish, Wright, Cushing, & Scott, 1996). In the Boston Lesbian Health Project, Roberts and Sorensen (1999) found that annual Pap test screening within the two-year duration of the project was reported by lesbians at a rate similar to that of the general population. The authors conclude that lesbians do not differ in terms of cancer screening and physical examination; this conclusion is in contrast to the study by Diamant et al. (2000). There is also a general sense among both health care providers and lesbians themselves that lesbians do not require Pap smears because they are not at risk for cervical cancer (Price, Easton, Telljohann, & Wallace, 1996).

Health Issues

Lesbians and bisexual women may perceive themselves less at risk than the rest of the population for a variety of illnesses, and, as such, fail to take preventative measures. Even when risk is known or suspected, women may not be able to access appropriate health care support due to discrimination in the health care system (Stevens & Hall, 2001). In either case, there are health issues particular to lesbians and bisexual women that reinforce the case for disclosure of their sexual identity in the health setting in order to ensure appropriate care. Some examples are discussed below.

Breast Cancer

Bernhard (2001) points out that there are no longitudinal, prospective studies that investigate whether lesbians are at higher risk for breast cancer (and this same absence of research applies to the case for cervical cancer), although estimates have been proposed up to triple that of heterosexual women (Rosser, 1992). Still, several epidemiological factors have been identified that support an increased risk of breast cancer for lesbians: fewer pregnancies, having children later in life, higher body mass index, and less access to prevention and treatment (Solarz, 1999). Failure to have regular check-ups, already mentioned, has a direct impact on risk because delayed diagnoses increase mortality for all cancers.

Sexually Transmitted Infections (STIs)

The definition of 'lesbian' as a woman who has sex with other women and not men contributes to the myth of lesbian invulnerability to sexually transmitted infections, including HIV/AIDS. Sex between women lacks the legitimate status of real sex within the context of the dominant discourses about sexual activity (Gurevich, 1997). While women in general have occupied a 'precarious location within the politics of HIV,' (Gurevich, Mathieson, Bower, & Dhayanandhan, 2007), it has not helped that lesbianism has been invisible throughout the HIV/AIDS discourse. Women who have sex with women have been excluded form HIV/AIDS and safer sex health promotion campaigns (Cole & Cooper, 1991; Stevens, 1993), and, to date, there has been little biological or epidemiological research focusing on the risk of STIs during female sexual contact. Research exploring the safe sex practices of lesbians and bisexual women indicates that lesbians believe they are at low risk for contracting HIV/AIDS, although their behavior indicates otherwise (Gruskin, 1999, p. 89). Some studies report that STIs are less common in lesbians than in heterosexual women (Simkin, 1993; White & Levinson, 1995), but lesbians and bisexual women are still at risk. Also, like the general population, lesbians and bisexual women may be exposed to any number of high-risk factors for HIV/AIDS: for example, they may share needles for injection drug use; they may have unprotected sex with infected male or female partners. STIs such as chlamydia and herpes – and, more rarely, syphilis and gonorrhea – can be transmitted by woman-to-woman contact (O'Hanlan, 1995; Richardson, 1994; White & Levinson, 1995).

About a decade ago, AIDS Vancouver Women's Programs published a report in which Brabazon (1994) noted: 'Without clear information about risks for women who have sex with women, safer sex becomes a matter of discretion, rather than an informed choice. We cannot identify a distinct community that includes all women who have sex with women that share a common culture, language, or tradition. Differences in ethnicity, social class, and sexual practices create distinct groups of lesbians, bisexual women, and others who do not identify with these labels. Socialization may occur between or among members of these groups to varying degrees. Other women who have sex with women may not identify with any group, whether they are in a relationship with a woman, a man, or not in a relationship at all' (pp. 6–7). This report challenged the mythology that lesbians do not have sex with men (also see Diamant, Schuster, McGuigan & Lever, 1999). It demonstrated the consistency – and inconsistency – between women's assessment of risk of various sexual activities (e.g., sharing sex toys) when compared with the Canadian AIDS Society Guidelines, pointing to the need for current and accurate information about risky sexual behaviours. It also concluded that perceived risk, even when accurate, did not necessarily predict behaviour change.

Providers are often ill informed about HIV/AIDS and lesbians, resulting in misinformation or no information at all. Lesbians and bisexual women have reported that they do not have good information from providers or from available resources about what constitutes 'risk' in woman-to-woman sex, and that they did not need, or were advised that they did not need, pelvic exams or screening because as lesbians they were not at risk for cervical cancer or sexually transmitted infections (Mathieson, Bailey, & Gurevich, 2002). Yet there is enough empirical evidence around issues of safer sex and HIV to expect providers to incorporate this information into their practice and teaching (Goldstein, 1995; Stevens, 1993; Stevens 1994a). In sum, several factors seem to combine as a stumbling block to vaginal health for lesbians: under-screening, providers' heterosexist assumptions, and misinformation on all sides.

Mental Health

Mays and Cochran (2001) cite both day-to-day and lifetime discrimination attributed to sexual orientation as the underlying correlate of mental health for gays and lesbians. Some hypotheses for overuse of tobacco, alcohol, and drugs point to the role of lesbian bars for a social life, the use of drugs to cope with stress, and the lack of appropriate treatment centres for this population. 'Straying from the heterosexual ideal can result in the lesbian or bisexual woman being arrested, killed or verbally harassed, losing employment and housing, losing the support of family or loved ones, or losing her children. She often internalizes negative feelings about homosexuality, resulting in self-destructive behaviour such as alcohol use, depression, or even suicide' (Gruskin, 1999, p. 29).

Hughes, Haas, and Avery (1997) compared the mental health of lesbians with heterosexual women by analysing data from the Chicago Women's Health Survey. They found that lesbians had therapy more often and had a higher rate of suicide attempts. Yet both groups had similar histories of clinical depression, considered a predisposing factor for suicide. At the same time, the researchers also found that lesbians had lower rates of alcohol and drug abuse. If the lesbians in the study used drugs and alcohol less often and were not more clinically depressed than the heterosexual women, what is to account for their more frequent use of therapy and increased suicide attempts? Special stressors faced by non-heterosexual women come into play: decisions about disclosure, hiding one's sexual orientation, lack of support for one's sexual identity, lack of relationships, absence of role models, heterosexism, and homophobia. Lack of appropriate therapeutic support may also be an issue. In a different U.S. study (Bernhard & Applegate, 1999) about mental health, lesbians and heterosexual women reported similar levels of stress and comparable mental health status, although the components of stress differed: heterosexual women reported stress related to family issues, and lesbians, stress due to sexual identity.

In the U.S. National Lesbian Health Care Survey: Implications for Mental Health, Bradford, Ryan, and Rothblum (1994) took a broad view of experiences that have an impact on the mental health of lesbians. Their survey investigated suicide, physical abuse, rape, incest, tobacco and alcohol use, counselling, social support, and coming out. The authors concluded that this sample showed a distressingly high prevalence of life events and behaviours related to mental health problems; for example, 37 per cent had been physically abused and 32 per cent had been raped or sexually attacked. Factors of age, race, and class seemed to have interactive effects. In general, lesbians who were older, who earned less, and who were not white reported higher levels of abuse, mental distress, and reliance upon professional help. Worry about money was the primary concern for lesbians in the survey, and was greatest for African American lesbians and those aged 54 and younger. The authors conclude with an important implication for intervention: mental health delivery requires an assessment of psychological resources and adaptability of lesbians when surviving in a hostile environment. Implicit in the discussion was the importance of social support networks – mainly through lesbian friends and lesbian community activities – as an important buffer against stress.

As part of a larger Canadian study looking at health care experiences, we (Mathieson, Bailey, & Gurevich, 2002) tried to tease out participants' views of physical and mental health care by asking about typical health needs. Ninety-eight lesbian/bisexual participants were asked to identify by checking Yes or No whether certain health services were important to them. Then the participants were asked to rank their top three most desired services. Physical examination and psychological counselling were the two categories chosen most often in the first-, second-, and third-ranked choices. Because this checklist was part of a larger interview in which we collected individual's health care stories, we heard participants say that the importance attributed to certain health care services reflected the fact that they are not necessarily able to access them. As we noted, 'This may be less a matter of geographical accessibility than of protective strategy' (p. 18), since throughout the interview women reported avoiding health care to protect themselves from homophobic providers. The importance of psychological counselling signals that mental health requires more attention, but it also suggests a host of related factors that affect health, including: battering/domestic violence, substance abuse, alcohol problems, and childbearing issues, among others (Gentry, 1992; Hall, 1993; Kenney & Tash, 1993, Morrow, 1994).

Alcohol use, depression, and suicide may be a result of loneliness and extreme psychosocial stress brought on by daily interactions in hostile contexts. Sometimes these contexts exist within the personal space of the lesbian or bisexual women and are not necessarily the result of heterosexism. In this light, Morrow (1994) singles out lesbian domestic violence: 'The abuse of women in relationships was viewed as a direct result of sex roles in our patriarchal society ... It is difficult for everyone, including the lesbian community, to acknowledge that women hurt other women' (p 19-20). Elliot (1996) notes that the percentage of lesbian women reporting abuse is comparable to that of heterosexual women, although, until recently, the issue of same-sex domestic violence has been invisible. The implications for health care providers is this: 'being' lesbian or bisexual does not protect one from domestic violence or battering.

In summary, there are no illnesses unique to lesbians or bisexual women. There is evidence, however, that some health issues have particular significance, especially because providers lack understanding about the context of the lesbian or bisexual client's life and/or the information to properly evaluate risk. Attitudes by providers and experiences within society and the health care system may exacerbate negative outcomes, creating barriers rather than equal access to quality of care.

Moving Forward

This chapter calls for systemic change in health care for lesbians and bisexual women. A review of the pertinent literature points to unique health issues and assumptions that act as barriers to care. Nonetheless, there is some good news in the Canadian context. There are indications of a growing awareness on the part of health care providers of the importance of acknowledging and understanding the health needs of lesbians and bisexual women, including ways to make medical school curricula more inclusive (see Gibson & Saunders, 1994; Robb, 1996; Robinson & Cohen, 1996). One national goal should be a Canadian agenda much like that promoted in the United States by the Gay and Lesbian Medical Association (2004), whose current Strategic Plan advances a program for across-the-board health system competence around lesbian, gay, bisexual, and transgendered health issues.

Local Canadian initiatives contribute to the national resource base for lesbian and bisexual women. For example, the Women's Creative Network explored the experiences of 150 self-identified 'lesbians, dykes and queer women' in Victoria, BC in areas of health, legal rights, education, and income security. The objective was to inform federal policy and academic discourse about the issues important to the lesbian and gay communities (Lightwater & Rabinovitch, 2001). This study grounds health care as one of several equally important themes in the general well-being of lesbians, including the need for increased access to appropriate health care, especially mental health services and the need for training for health care providers. The Women's Health Bureau of Health Canada, in conjunction with the former BC Ministry of Health and Ministry Responsible for Seniors, and the BC Centre for Excellence in

Women's Health, released *Caring for Lesbian Health: A Resource for Canadian Health Care Providers, Policy Makers and Planners* (Hudspith, 1999). This work identified the health care concerns of lesbians and provided information about what can be done to improve access to quality care. More recently the Transgender Health Program in Vancouver, BC (Vancouver Coastal Health, 2003) created an internet site for transgendered persons, their social support network, and health care personnel. The scope of the program reflects the health needs of transgendered persons: information about clinical and trans-specialty services (endocrinology, surgical, and post-surgical care); general information resources; materials for specific sub-populations (age-appropriate materials); medical settings (trans-sensitive intake, assessment, and charting); trans-mental health; child and youth issues; drug and alcohol use; human rights. Education, for both clients and providers, and advocacy are highlighted. The program's advocacy role is especially important as an aid for transgendered persons to navigate the systemic barriers that prevent them from gaining access to health services which can be quite specialized. This program contributes distinctly because it is fashioning a public conversation about guidelines for transgender health, and, by doing so, is helping to make that sexual identity a visible one (also see Ryan, Brotman, & Rowe, 2000). Most recently, the program has focused upon planning education regarding transgendered health for health care providers.

Research to date has certainly enumerated the problems in health care for lesbian and bisexual women. Health research that is inclusive of sexual identities has the power to enhance understanding of those identities. Even more important, though, is that the discourse that takes place during disclosure in the health care setting acts as a site of resistance to mainstream medical thinking and practice. Lesbianism, bisexuality, transgenderism – these are all boundary-disrupting phenomena. Disclosures have the power to 'take on the more directly political': the regulatory institutions such as medicine that continue to enforce gendered boundaries (Gamson, 1998, p. 597). Gavey (1989) notes: 'Individuals ... are active and have a "choice" when positioning themselves in relation to various discourses ... women can identify with and conform to traditional discursive constructions ... or they can resist, reject, and challenge them' (p. 464). To create that 'choice' to which Gavey refers, the barriers need to be confronted by those responsible for health care delivery: our federal and provincial governments, health care organizations, and individual providers.

Firestein (1996) refers to an emerging LesBiGay/Transgender (LBGT) paradigm that can account for the diversity of ways in which individuals experience and express their sexual attractions, behaviour, and relationships. Ongoing efforts by the United Nations Commission on Human Rights (2005) represent worldwide advocacy on behalf of LBGT persons, so the notion of such a paradigm is active on an international level. Canadian investigators, with proper allocation of resources, need to do more research, on both a national and a local level within communities. Work at the community level is particularly important, since further data is not very helpful unless the knowledge that is translated into workable recommendations, the 'uptake,' is backed by empirical evidence. Ongoing research at the interface of sexualities and health needs to aim for making a LBGT paradigm the gold standard of health research and health care. Adopting this framework in the Canadian health system might seem radical, as it surely would have sweeping ramifications for clients, individual providers, and for national policy, but it is necessary to ensure inclusion and quality of care, free from discrimination. Hopefully, some day this paradigm will not be radical at all.

NOTES

1 There is often disagreement about definitions of lesbianism and bisexuality. In this chapter, these terms are viewed from the perspectives of the individuals who consciously choose to adopt that label for themselves. This view contrasts with the social ascription of homosexual, heterosexual, or bisexual purely as a result of the gender(s) to which one is primarily attracted (see Wilton, 1998, 2000, for discussion). For example, some women who partner with other women may not identify as lesbians. Women also use diverse terms to self-identify: lesbian, dyke, gay, queer. Some women may reject labels entirely.
2 The term *transgender* (or *trans*) 'refers to a person with a gender identity that is different from her or his birth sex or who express gender in ways that contravene societal expectations of the range of possibilities for men and women. The umbrella term may include cross-dressers, drag kings/queens, transsexuals, people who are androgynous, two-spirit people, and people who are bi-gendered or multi-gendered.' (Vancouver Coastal Health, 2003). Native people developed the term *two-spirit* to recognize the

existence of individuals whose spirits are both masculine and feminine, accepting them as having special spiritual qualities (see Firestein, 1996).
3 Homophobia is the fear or hatred of homosexuals and of homosexuality.
4 The researchers discussed in this section often reach conclusions based on statistical significance with large sample size and probabilities; generalized research, however, cannot be used to predict an individual's behaviour within unique contexts.

REFERENCES

Aaron, D., Markovic, N., Danielson, M., Hannold, J., Janosky, J., & Smith, N. (2001). Behavioral risk factors for disease and preventative health practices among lesbians. *American Journal of Public Health, 91*, 972–975.

American Psychiatric Association. (2000). *Diagnostic and Statistical Manual of Mental Disorders IV-TR*. Washington, DC: APA.

Anderson, L., Healy, T., Herringer, B., Isaac, B., & Perry, Y. (2001). *Out in the Cold: The Contradictory Context of Health and Wellness for Lesbians in Northern Communities*. Vancouver: British Columbia Centre of Excellence for Women's Health.

Bailey, N., Gurevich, M., & Mathieson, C.M. (2000). Invoking community: Rethinking the health of lesbian and bisexual women. *Feminist Voices*, (10).

Bergeron, S., & Senn, C. (2003). Health care utilization in a sample of Canadian lesbian women: Predictors of risk and resilience. *Women and Health, 37*, 19–35.

Bernhard, L. (2001). Lesbian health and health care. *Annals of Nursing Research, 19*, 145–177.

Bernhard, L., & Applegate, J.M. (1999). Comparison of stress and stress management strategies between lesbian and heterosexual women. *Health Care for Women International, 20*, 335–347.

Boehmer, U. (2002). Twenty years of public health research: Inclusion of lesbian, gay, bisexual, and transgender populations. *American Journal of Public Health, 92*, 1125–1130.

Bornstein, K. (1994). *Gender Outlaw: On Men, Women and the Rest of Us*. New York: Routledge.

Brabazon, C. (1994). *Acknowledging diversity: Questioning authority*. Report on the findings of the women who have sex with women survey. Vancouver: AIDS Vancouver Women's Programs.

Bradford, J., Ryan, C., & Rothblum, E.D. (1994). National lesbian health care

292   Cynthia Mathieson

survey: Implications for mental health. *Journal of Consulting and Clinical Psychology, 62*, 228–242.

Brogan, M. (1997). Healthcare for lesbians: Attitudes and experiences. *Nursing Standard, 11*, 39–42.

Brown, A., & Syme, V. (2002). A post-colonial analysis of health care discourses addressing aboriginal women. *Nurse Researcher, 9*, 28–41.

Butler, J. (1991). *Inside/Out: Lesbian Theories, Gay Theories*. New York: Routledge.

Cole, R., & Cooper, S. (1991). Lesbian exclusion from HIV/AIDS education: Ten years of low-risk identity and high risk behavior. *Sexuality Information and Education Council of the United States (SIECUS) Report* (January), 18–23.

Davis, V. (with Social and Sexual Issues Committee). (2000). Lesbian health guidelines: Policy statement approved by the council of the Society of Obstetricians and Gynecologists. *Journal SOGC Canada, 22*, 202–205.

Deevy, S. (1990). Older lesbian women: An invisible minority. *Journal of Gerontology Nursing,16*, 35–37.

Department for Constitutional Affairs. *Government Policy Concerning Transgender People* (2004). Retrieved 5 March 2005, from http://www.dca.gov.uk.

Diamant, A.L., Schuster, M.A., & Lever, J. (2000). Receipt of preventative health services by lesbians. *American Journal of Preventive Medicine, 19*, 141–148.

Diamant, A.L., Schuster, M.A., McGuigan, K., & Lever, J. (1999). Lesbian's sexual history with men. *Archives of Internal Medicine, 159*, 2730–2736.

Diamant, A.L., Wold, C., Spritzer, K., & Gelberg, L. (2000). Health behaviors, health status, and access to and use of health care. *Archives of Family Medicine, 9*, 1043–1051.

Druzin, P., Shrier, I., Yacowar, M., & Rossignol, M. (1998). Discrimination against gay, lesbian and bisexual family physicians by patients. *Canadian Medical Association, 158*, 593–597.

Elliot, P. (1996). Shattering illusions: Same-sex domestic violence. In C.M. Renzetti & C.H. Miley (Eds.), *Violence in Gay and Lesbian Domestic Partnerships* (pp 1–8). Birmingham, NY: Harrington Press.

Ferris, D., Batish, S., Wright, T., Cushing, C., & Scott, E. (1996). A neglected lesbian health care concern: Cervical neoplasia. *Journal of Family Practice, 43*, 581–584.

Firestein, B. (1996). *Bisexuality: The Psychology and Politics of an Invisible Minority*. Thousand Oaks, CA: Sage.

Fuss, D. (1989). *Essentially Speaking*. London: Rouledge, Chapman & Hall.

Gamson, J. (1998). Must identity movements self destruct? A queer dilemma.

In P. Nardi & B. Schneider (Eds.), *Social Perspectives in Lesbian and Gay Studies: A Reader* (pp 589–604). New York: Routledge.

Gavey, N. (1989. Feminist poststructuralism and discourse analysis: Contributions to feminist psychology. *Psychology of Women Quarterly, 13*, 459–475.

Gay and Lesbian Medical Association (GLMA). (2004). *Strategic Plan 2004–2007*. Retrieved 1 March 2005, from http://www.glma.org.

Gentry, S. (1992). Caring for lesbians in a homophobic society. *Health Care for Women International, 13*, 173–180.

Gibson, G., & Saunders, D.E. (1994). Gay patients. *Canadian Family Physician, 40*, 721–725.

Golden, C. (2000). The intersexed and the transgendered. In J. Chrisler, C. Golden, & P. Rozee (Eds.), *Lectures on the Psychology of Women* (2nd ed., pp. 80–95). Boston: McGraw Hill.

Goldstein, N. (1995). Lesbians and the medical profession: HIV/AIDS and the pursuit of visibility. *Women's Studies, 24*, 531–552.

Gruskin, E.P. (1999). *Treating Lesbians and Bisexual Women: Challenges and Strategies for Health Professionals*. Thousand Oaks, CA: Sage.

Gurevich, M. (1997). *Missing Bodies: Lesbian and Bisexual Women in the HIV Pandemic*. Paper presented at the 58th annual conference of the Canadian Psychological Association, Toronto.

Gurevich, M., Mathieson, C.M., Bower, J., & Dhayanandhan, B. (2007). Disciplining desires, bodies and subjectivities: Sexualities in HIV positive women. *Feminism and Psychology, 17*, 9–38.

Hall, J.M. (1993). An exploration of lesbians' images of recovery from alcohol problems. In P.N. Stern (Ed.), *Lesbian Health* (pp. 91–108). Washington, DC: Taylor & Francis.

Health Canada. (2002). *Women's Health Strategy*. Women's Health Bureau. Retrieved 25 February 2005, from http://hc-sc.gc./English/women/womenstrat.htm.

Hudspith, M. (1999). *Caring for Lesbian Health: A Resource for Canadian Health Care Providers, Policy Makers and Planners*. Health Canada/Women's Health Bureau, the B.C. Ministry of Health & Ministry Responsible for Seniors, and the B.C. Centre for Excellence in Women's Health. Retrieved 5 January 2005, from http://www.hc-gc.ca/english/women/facts.

Hughes, T.L., Hass, A.P., & Avery, L. (1997). Lesbians and mental health: Preliminary results from the Chicago Women's Health Survey. *Journal of the Gay and Lesbian Medical Association, 1*, 137–148.

International Gay and Lesbian Association (IGLA). (1999). Home page and overview. Retrieved 6 March 2005, from http://www.igla.info.

Kendall, K. (1995). Legal issues pertinent to gays and lesbians. Lecture presented to lesbian, gay, bisexual, and transgender health and culture course, School of Public Health, University of California, Berkeley.

Kenney, J.W., & Tash, D.T. (1993). Lesbian childbearing couples' dilemmas and decisions. In P.N. Stern (Ed.), *Lesbian Health* (pp. 119–130). Washington, DC: Taylor & Francis.

Kitzinger, C., & Wilkinson, S. (1995). Transitions from heterosexuality to lesbianism: The discursive production of lesbian identities. *Developmental Psychology, 30,* 95–104.

Lee, R. (2000). Health care problems of lesbian, gay, bisexual and transgender clients. *Western Journal of Medicine, 172,* 403–408.

Lightwater, J., & Rabinovitch, J. (2001). *Lesbian Issues in Canada: A Profile of Victoria.* Victoria, BC: Women's Creative Network.

Mathieson, C.M. (1996). Interview material for *A Descriptive Study of Lesbian Health Care Issues.* Unpublished manuscript.

Mathieson, C.M. (1998). Lesbian/bisexual health care: Straight talk about experiences with physicians. *Canadian Family Physician, 44,* 1634–1640.

Mathieson, C.M., & Endicott, L. (1998). Lesbian and bisexual identity: Discourse of difference. *Atlantis, 23,* 38–47.

Mathieson, C.M., & Gurevich, M. (1997). Revealing and concealing: Theorizing the impact of disclosure on women's health. Paper presented at the 105th APA Convention, Chicago.

Mathieson, C.M., Bailey, N., & Gurevich, M. (2002). Health care services for lesbian and bisexual women: Canadian data. *Health Care for Women International, 23,* 185–196.

Mays, V., & Cochran, S. (2001). Mental health correlates of perceived discrimination among lesbian, gay, and bisexual adults in the United States. *American Journal of Public Health, 91,* 1869–1876.

Moran, N. (1996). Lesbian health care needs. *Canadian Family Physician, 42,* 879–884.

Morrow, J. (1994). Identifying and treating battered lesbians. *San Francisco Medicine* (17 April), 20–21.

Nagle, J. (1995). Framing radical bisexuality: Toward a gender agenda. In N. Tucker (Ed.), *Bisexual Politics: Theories, Queries and Visions* (pp. 305–314). New York: Haworth Press.

O'Hanlan, K.A (1995). Lesbian health and homophobia: Perspectives for the treating obstetrician/gynecologist. *Current Problems in Obstetrics, Gynecology & Fertility* (July/August), 97–133.

Price, J., Easton, A., Telljohann, S., & Wallace, P. (1996). Perceptions of cervical cancer and pap smear screening behavior by women's sexual orientation. *Journal of Community Health, 21,* 89–105.

Public Health Association of Australia (PHAA). (2004). Lesbian and Bisexual Health Policy. Retrieved 1 March 2005, from http://www.phaa.net.au.

Ramsay, H. (1994). Lesbians and the health care system: Invisibility, isolation and ignorance – You say you're a what? *Canadian Woman Studies, 14*, 22–28.

Richardson, D. (1994). Inclusions and exclusions: Lesbians, HIV and AIDS. In L. Doyal, J. Nadoo, & T. Wilton (Eds.), *AIDS: Setting a feminist agenda* (pp. 159–170). London: Taylor & Francis.

Robb, N. (1996). Medical schools seek to overcome 'invisibility' of gay patients, gay issues in curriculum. *Canadian Medical Association Journal, 155*, 765–770.

Roberts, S., & Sorenson, L. (1999). Health related behaviors and cancer screening of lesbians: Results from the Boston Lesbian Health Project. *Women and Health, 28*, 1–12.

Robinson, G., & Cohen, M. (1996). Gay, lesbian and bisexual health care issues and medical curricula. *Canadian Medical Association, 155*, 709–711.

Rose, P., & Platzer, H. (1993). Confronting prejudice. *Nursing Times, 89*, 52–54.

Rosser, S. (1992). Ignored, overlooked or subsumed: Research on lesbian health and health care. *National Women's Studies Association Journal, 5*, 183–203.

Rust, P. (1996). Managing multiple identities: Diversity among bisexual women and men. In B. Firestein (Ed.), *Bisexuality: The Psychology and Politics of an Invisible Minority* (pp. 53–83). Thousand Oaks, CA: Sage.

Ryan, B., Brotman, S., & Rowe, B. (2000). *Access to Care: Exploring the Well-Being of Gay, Lesbian, Bisexual and Two-Spirited People in Canada.* Montreal: McGill University Press.

Sherwin, S. (1992). *No Longer Patient: Feminist Ethics and Health Care.* Philadelphia: Temple University Press.

Simkin, R. (1993). Unique health care concerns of lesbians. *Canadian Journal of Ob/Gyn and Women's Health Care, 5*, 516–522.

Simkin, R. (1998). Not all your patients are straight. *Canadian Medical Association Journal, 159*, 370–375.

Solarz, A. (1999). *Lesbian Health: Current Assessments and Directions for the Future.* Washington, DC: Institute of Medicine.

Stevens, P. (1992). Lesbian health care research: A review of the literature from 1970 to 1990. *Health Care for Women International, 13*, 91–120.

Stevens, P. (1993). Lesbians and HIV: Clinical research and policy issues. *American Journal of Orthopsychiatry, 63*, 289–294.

Stevens, P. (1994a). HIV prevention education for lesbians and bisexual women: A cultural analysis of a community intervention. *Social Science & Medicine, 39*, 1565–1578.

Stevens, P. (1994b). Lesbians' health-related experiences of care and noncare. *Western Journal of Nursing Research, 16*, 639–659.

Stevens, P. (1995). Structural and interpersonal impact of heterosexual assumptions on lesbian health care clients. *Nursing Research, 44*, 25–30.

Stevens, P.E., & Hall, J.M. (1990). Abusive health care interactions experienced by lesbians: A case of institutional violence in the treatment of women. *Response to the Victimization of Women and Children, 13*, 23–27.

Stevens, P., & Hall, J.M. (1991). A critical historical analysis of the medical construction of lesbianism. *International Journal of Health Services, 21*, 291–307.

Stevens, P., & Hall, J.M. (2001). Sexuality and safer sex: The issue for lesbian and bisexual women. *Journal of Obstetric, Gynecologic and Neonatal Nursing, 30*, 439–447.

United Nations Commission on Human Rights. (2005). Sexual rights and sexual orientation. Retrieved 10 March 2005, from http://www.iglhrc.org.

Valanis, B., Bowen, D., Bassford, T., Whitlock, E., Charney, P., & Carter, R. (2000). Sexual orientation and health: Comparisons in the Women's Health Initiative Sample. *Archives of Family Medicine, 9*, 843–853.

Vancouver Coastal Health. (2003). Transgender Health Program. Retrieved 9 September 2005, from http://www.vch.ca.

White, J.C., & Dull, V.T. (1998). Room for improvement: Communication between lesbians and primary care providers. *Journal of Lesbian Studies, 2*, 95–110.

White, J.C., & Levinson, W. (1995). Lesbian health care: What a primary care physician needs to know. *Western Journal of Medicine, 162*, 463–466.

Wilton, T. (1996). Which one's the man? The heterosexualisation of lesbian sex. In D. Richardson (Ed.). (1994). *Theorizing Heterosexuality/Telling it Straight* (pp. 125–142). Buckingham, UK: Open University Press.

Wilton, T. (1998). Gender, sexuality and healthcare: Improving services. In L. Doyal (Ed.), *Women and Health Service: An Agenda for Change* (pp. 147–162). Buckingham, UK: Open University Press.

Wilton, T. (2000). *Sexualities in Health and Social Care*. Buckingham, UK: Open University Press.

11 Mothering and Women's Health

COLLEEN VARCOE AND GWENETH HARTRICK DOANE

In order for all women to have real choices all along the line, we need fully to understand the power and powerlessness embodied in motherhood in patriarchal culture. (Rich, 1976, p. 67)

This lawyer that I got is just a blessing. He was the [child protection] ministry's lawyer so he knew how the ministry worked, he understood exactly what was going to happen every step of the way. He knew what they were going to do to me. And then he sat me down and he said, 'Be prepared to work like hell because they're going to make you. You're not going to get your kid back just like that. It doesn't matter, you know, how innocent you may look on the sidelines where your son was taken from his father. They're still going to make you out to be a bad mother. So you've gotta to do everything you can to show them that you are a good mother.' (Daisy, interview, 2003)

Mothering is a social experience that is constructed and shaped by structural conditions and intertwined with competing and conflicting social discourses that have significant implications for the health of women. Mothering affects women's health in diverse ways. Because mothering requires material, economic, and social investments that are not usually compensated in material or economic ways, through mothering women are made more vulnerable to a variety of health risks, especially overwhelming workloads, poverty, and violence. At the same time, the experience of mothering may have a positive impact on women's health. In this chapter we explore these conditions, discourses, and implications. We draw upon intersectional analyses to illustrate that understanding mothering in relation to women's health is well served by attention to the diversity of women's experiences as they are shaped by multiple structural and social conditions, and to the resources and capacities women bring to mothering roles. While we draw predominantly on women's experiences in the Canadian context, the experiences of women in Canada share similarities with those of women in other industrialized Western countries. Reading mothering with a critical awareness of the impact of these structural conditions and intersecting discourses promises to contribute a deeper understanding of diverse women's experiences, their health, and the influences that shape their health and health experiences. We argue that such analyses are critical for the development of policies and practices that promote women's health.

Mothering: Looking with Fresh Eyes

Mothering. What images does that word conjure up for you? A beautiful woman with Ivory Soap skin tranquilly rocking a baby? Children romping at a park while their smiling mother looks on? Or is it a kitchen scene where mom and the kids are baking cookies? While you may not actually imagine mothering in these stereotypical ways, it is probably fair to say that if you have grown up in North America and watched television or even looked at the cover of a parenting magazine you have been surrounded by such imagery. Yet your own personal experience of being mothered or of mothering may be at odds with these images. For many women the experience of mothering is not so 'picture perfect.' And, the disjuncture may be great between what mothering is 'supposed' to look and feel like according to dominant societal messages and how women actually live and experience mothering in today's contemporary world.

Mothering: A Social Construction

Although we tend to think of mothering as a domestic or personal affair, how women become mothers and live mothering is greatly determined by larger public/contextual forces. In particular, mothering is shaped by gendered Western ideals and the realities of late neo-liberal capitalism. Issues of racism, classism, heterosexism, ageism, and ableism are embedded within these ideals and realities and serve to generate a range of unstated 'norms' that profoundly shape the experiences of women/mothers. Within this social and economic context, mothering experiences are shaped by various ideologies and discourses, and evaluated against the 'gold standard' of mothering within a two-parent family with primary attention to the children (Ford-Gilboe, 2000).

As a social construction, mothering is also experienced and evaluated against a range of idealized images that are reflected and promoted in popular media, and, too often, in professional practices and academic research. Within the Canadian context, researchers have advanced critical analyses of how mothering is shaped by discourses enacted in policy and practice in areas such as substance use (S.C. Boyd, 1999, 2004), violence (Irwin, Thorne, & Varcoe, 2002), child custody (S.B. Boyd, 1996, 2003) and child welfare (Swift, 1995; 1998) as well as across these themes (e.g., Greaves, Pederson, et al., 2004; Greaves, Varcoe, et al., 2002) and within the context of the lives of women facing particularly challenging circumstances, such as women who immigrate to Canada (e.g., McLaren & Dyck, 2004) and Aboriginal women (e.g., Fiske, 1992, 1993; MacDonald, 2002). Subsequently, to understand mothering and its relationship to women's health, and to understand how women negotiate these contexts and experiences, requires an understanding of the socially constructed process of mothering, including the material realities and the discourses within which mothering experiences are embedded.

Mothering: A Nexus of Discourses

A range of 'mothering' discourses (good and bad mothering, chief among them) operate within wider social discourses. Fundamental to mothering discourses are two competing views: first, that women are natural mothers by virtue of their biology (biological essentialism); and second, that women fulfil the social role of mothering because of their gendered social positions of disadvantage. As Bobel (2002) outlines and illustrates, the essentialist position has guided maternalist discourses in their pivotal role in moral reform movements throughout the past several centuries in the Western world. As Bobel explains, the idea that there are essential differences between women and men, with women being morally superior due to their reproductive abilities, has been used in various ways to promote the interests of some women. Most recently, maternalist discourses are flourishing with the rise of neoliberalism in tandem with religious fundamentalism – women as mothers are central to the doctrines of the fundamentalist forms of a range of religions (Kissling & Sippel, 2001/2002). However, while these maternalist discourses achieved some gains for some women (in the West, predominantly white, middle-class women), they rest on accommodation of patriarchal understandings of men and women and thus do not challenge the gendered division of labour, the gendered division between public and private spheres, or the preeminence of biology as a determinant of social life (Bobel, 2002). The second view, because of its emphasis on social disadvantage, tends to draw attention to diversity and inequities among women and between groups of women.

Mothering discourses have been the subject of considerable feminist scholarship. Adrienne Rich is considered to be the originator of modern feminist interest in motherhood, with her book *Of Woman Born: Motherhood as Experience and Institution* (Rich, 1976) offering a complex analysis of the experience of motherhood in relation to the politics of feminism. Interestingly, feminist analyses have taken up varied positions on mothering, including both the essentialist and the social disadvantage positions. Some feminists have used biological essentialism and motherhood to argue the value of women, whereas others have critiqued essentialist positions, especially for their failure to challenge patriarchal ideologies.

For example, the essentialist view of women as 'natural' mothers is contested by Weiss (1998) as 'prejudiced against women interested in pursuing a life in which children are not the raison d'être of the women or their exclusive focus of attention' (p. 89). Focusing upon the notions of bonding (constructed as a natural process of connection between parent and child) and 'motherly love' (constructed as a natural disposition), Weiss posits that these are modern notions that serve 'to resurrect old justifications for certain social practices in a new scientific rhetoric. For bonding is, perhaps first and foremost, a theory that lends legitimacy to the notion that women are the only appropriate attendants for children. It is ... an ideological justification for keeping women in the home with their children, hence perpetuating their inequality in the labor market' (p. 88). Weiss offers a skilful refutation of bonding and motherly love as 'natural,' using the example of parents of 'appearance impaired' children (children with externally visible problems such as cleft palate or spina bifida) to show that maternal (or indeed parental) bonding is a social, rather than biological phenomenon. Parents abandoned most (68.4 per cent) of the 250 appearance-impaired children in her study, regardless of any functional impairment; but tended not to abandon (7 per cent of) the 100 children without appearance impairment, despite serious functional problems. Despite such critiques, biological essentialism underlies much 'everyday' thinking about mothers in the Western world. In this view, good mothers are 'natural,' bond with their children, and display motherly love.

What Is a 'Good' Mother? Living within the Discourses

The ideals of 'good mothering' are situated within a wide range of influential discourses that are contradictory and fluctuating. Today, the 'norm' of mothering within a dual-parent heterosexual couple exerts a particularly powerful influence on the discourse of good mothering. This mothering discourse outlines specific and select options for how women should become and live out the life of mother. Weedon (1987) used the example of the inadequacies felt by new mothers to illustrate these dynamics. Discourses tell the new mother that 'she is supposed to meet all the child's needs single-handed, to care for and stimulate the child's physical, emotional and mental development and to feel fulfilled in doing so' (p. 34). The language and discourse surrounding the social institution of motherhood serve to shape, constrain, coerce, and potentiate a mother's experience, the meanings she assigns to the experience, to her child's behavior, and to herself, and the action in which she engages as a mother (Davies & Harre, 1990).

One of the most significant features of mothering discourse is the way that discursive ideas and practices operate to obscure and gloss over the existence of multiple and varying forms of mothering. Forms of mothering that do not fit the normative discourse of biological, two-parent family such as stepmothering, mothering within a lesbian couple, mothering by very young women, mothering within a communal household, grandmothers as primary caregivers, and non-custodial mothering are marginalized, and in some ways demonized (think evil stepmother) and stigmatized (think 'welfare mother', 'teen mother'). For example, Eicher-Catt (2004) illustrates how non-custodial mothering is so far outside the normalized discourse as to present a confounding cultural paradox. She shows how difficult it is against the backdrop of idealized discourses of normal and natural motherhood for women to live and be seen simultaneously as competent and non-custodial.

As a fundamental Western ideology, liberal individualism (see the Introduction, this collection) also exerts its influence by intersecting with motherhood discourse. The valuing of economic independence intertwined with the realities of neoliberal restructuring of Canada means that mothers increasingly are expected to work outside the home

(Statistics Canada, 2000). As of 1999, 61 per cent of women with children under the age of three were employed, a figure that doubled over the preceding two decades. Further, rates of separation and divorce (entangled with escalating rates of violence against women) mean that women are increasingly lone parents, often living below the poverty line and often on social assistance (Statistics Canada, 2000b). At least partly due to gender economics, many children are not being raised by their mothers. For example, the 2001 Canadian Census reported that 56,790 grandchildren under the age of 18 were living with their grandparents without parents in the home (Statistics Canada, 2001). Based on federal and provincial/territorial reports from 2000, Farris-Manning and Zandstra (2004) estimated that approximately 76,000 children in Canada were in the care of state child protection services across the country. These trends, juxtaposed against other discourses and ideals of good mothering, have produced new discourses such as those of the 'working mother' and the 'welfare mom.'

These new discourses rely upon the often invisible but powerful ideal of 'exclusive' mothering. That is to say, the idea that women devote themselves to mothering exclusively, foregoing labour force participation. Paradoxically, exclusive mothering implies economic dependence. Yet, the economic and social conditions do not exist for most women to care for children without also participating in waged work. In Canada, the 'typical' mother is working outside the home, and is often the lone head of a household and/or living under or near the poverty line (see Text Box 11.1). Indeed, as Canadian statistics illustrate, social policy increasingly forces women with dependant children into waged labour, even when the work available is not adequate to cover the costs of safe child care. At the same time neoliberal policies such as cuts to minimum wage levels have the effect of deepening women's poverty even as they attempt to participate in the waged labour force (Morrow, Hankivsky, & Varcoe, 2004; Ricciutelli, Larkin, & O'Neill, 1998).

Women's Participation in the Discourses of Mothering

Against these social discourses and inferred norms, women simultaneously participate in the construction of themselves and of one another as 'persons' and as 'good mothers.' Chodorow (1978) and Rabuzzi (1988) have argued that the expression of 'self' is a particularly difficult psychological issue for women who are mothers. Whereas liberalist discourses about what constitutes a healthy, mature adult stress the importance of autonomy, differentiation, and separation of the indi-

Text Box 11.1 Mothers in Canada

Mothers in Canada are increasingly lone heads of households
- From 1961 to 1996, female-headed lone-parent families increased from 9% of all families with children, to 18.5%; male-headed lone-parent families increased from 2.5% to 3.8% (Statistics Canada, 2000b).
- As of the last available census data (1996), 83% of lone-parent families were female-headed (Statistics Canada, 2000b).

Lone mothers tend to be poor
- In 1997, 56% of all families headed by lone-parent mothers had incomes which fell below the low-income cut-offs (Statistics Canada, 2000b).

Mothers in Canada increasingly work outside the home
- The employment rate of women with children has grown particularly sharply in the past two decades, especially for those with preschool-aged children. By 1999, 61% of women with children younger than age 3 were employed, more than double the figure in 1976 (Statistics Canada, 2000a).

Even when employed outside the home, mothers do the majority of child care and domestic work
- Even when employed, women are still largely responsible for looking after their homes and families. In 1998, women employed full time with a spouse and at least one child under age 19 at home spent 4.9 hours per day on unpaid work activities, an hour and a half more per day than their male counterparts (Statistics Canada, 2000a).

Mothers fare poorly economically following separation
- Revenue Canada income tax returns show that in the year of separation, women experience a median loss of 38% of adjusted family income; in comparison, men see an immediate 11% net gain.
- On separation, women are usually the custodial parent, and, in the year of separation, only 35% of women receive support payments from their former spouse.
- In the year following separation, women's net family income loss is 23%, while men experience a 10% net gain in income (Ministry of Women's Equality, 2000).

vidual from others, throughout the life cycle, discourses around mothering in Western culture often emphasize women's abnegation of themselves (Oakley, 1981), selflessness (Lemkau & Landau, 1986) and self-sacrifice (Davies & Harre, 1990). For women who are mothers these conflicting discourses offer confusing and contradictory edicts about self-definition and action (Hartrick, 1996). How does one 'take oneself up as a mother' amidst such conflicting discourses and contrasting identities? Moreover, what is the toll on women as they attempt to meet the overwhelming edicts and/or feel competent and able as women/ mothers?

As women live within these discourses and edicts the discourses also begin to shape their experiences and relations with one another. Blackford (2004) offers an example of how women exert influence on one another in line with ideologies of good mothers. Using Foucault's conception of the panopticon, Blackford studied mothers in suburban playgrounds, showing how on the playground the mothers became a 'community that gazed at the children only to ultimately gaze at one another, seeing reflected in the children the parenting abilities of one another' (p. 223). The mothers were occupied by etiquette rules and competition with one another, keeping one another in line with larger suburban child-centred ideologies.

In sum, discourses tell us that *good* mothers are exclusively devoted to their children, which requires economic dependence, *and* are economically independent, a conundrum that is resolved within heterosexual patriarchal relations when women are economically dependent on a male partner within an economic family unit. Good mothers are simultaneously selfless and dependent, *and* autonomous and independent. Women who fail to meet these contradictory expectations are positioned within a deficit discourse (Standing, 1999).

Mothering at the Intersections, or Discourses in Action

Of course, the difficulty of negotiating the competing discourses of mothering varies with the conditions of women's lives. Another significant feature of the discourses is the way they gloss over differences between particular mothers; that is, as Standing (1999) notes, dominant discourses ignore the fact that 'not all mothers operate within the same structural, cultural and discursive contexts' (p. 59). Yet, experiences of mothering and the discourses that shape those experiences vary with women's diverse social locations as they intersect, particularly along the lines of race, class, religion, sexuality, ability, and culture. For example, McLaren and Dyck (2004) show how human capital, a central tenet of liberalism, shapes the experiences of mothers who are also immigrants. The basic idea of human capital is that people acquire assets in the form of education and skills through legitimate means, and, as independent economic actors, trade these assets for wages. McLaren and Dyck describe how, within these neoliberal discourses and within shifting immigration policies, immigrant mothers in Canada were constructed as deficient in comparison with the 'ideal immigrant.' Studying mothers and daughters who had recently arrived in Canada from a variety of source countries (including Taiwan, Hong Kong, Korea, and Iran) and settled in an outer suburb of Vancouver, British Columbia, they illustrate how the women who immigrated to Canada as 'dependents' and were mothers, were particularly marginalized and devalued in the face of 'national narratives of citizenship that valorized independence located in the labour market' (p. 52). Within neoliberal discourses their 'belonging' (in Canada and to Canadian society) was contingent on this economic independence and contribution, and their mothering work discounted.

As the discourses of 'belonging' had particular salience for the immigrant women in McLaren and Dyck's (2004) study, other discourses have particular bearing for women in different circumstances in relation to the dominant discourses. For example, women who can acquire the assets necessary to be deemed worthy according to liberalist discourses, such as women/mothers who have the opportunity to pursue a career, do not fair well within the mothering discourse that calls for self-abnegation. Such women often face the social stigma of 'putting themselves and/or their careers ahead of their children' (Hartrick, 1996). Thus, women who do not participate in paid labour can be seen as inadequate as workers and citizens, and their mothering discounted, while those who do paid work can be seen as inadequate as mothers.

Particularly pernicious discourses operate at the confluence of the contradictory discourses of exclusive mothering and economic independence. Women who require state resources for exclusive mothering are rendered inadequate through the discourse of 'welfare mom.' S.C. Boyd (2004) points out that in the present throes of neoliberalism, welfare is no longer about helping the poor, but is about ending 'welfare dependency,' a political construct that ignores the employment history of women. And, Boyd argues, 'the restructuring of welfare falls on women with children ... with "poor bashing" becoming "a national sport of which single mothers are the target"' (p. 143). Similarly, very young women (perhaps unless they have the advantage of material wealth and a heterosexual relationship) are labelled and evaluated within the discourse of 'teen mother,' a discourse that often intersects with 'welfare mom' and 'unfit mother.' Importantly, the 'teen mother' discourse is reflective of certain privileges and Eurocentric values. For example, the disparaging connotations of 'teen mother' may not reconcile with values in some Aboriginal communities where young mothers may be valued differently than in dominant Canadian culture.

These discourses have performative functions; the circulation of discourses accomplishes changes in status and/or actively creates entities. Calling a woman a 'welfare mom,' a 'stay at home mom,' a 'working mother,' a 'single mother,' and 'unfit mother,' and so on, invokes certain norms and ideas. 'Welfare mom' implies (undesirable) economic dependence, 'working mother' implies comparison with the (more ideal) 'stay at home mom,' 'stay at home mom' implies (undesirable) non-participation in the paid labour force, 'single mother' implies contrast with the (preferable) married, heterosexual mother, and 'unfit mother' implies something altogether unnatural. Assigning status in these ways creates a certain subject to be treated in certain ways. For example, Cleeton (2003) studied an American city's response to an elevated infant mortality rate among the babies of African American, urban, impoverished women. Cleeton shows how the 'good mother/bad mother' discourse and the obstetrics discourse of the frail female body interacted and transformed the women 'from single mothers who could not begin prenatal care before the second trimester because too few physicians will treat Medicaid patients, into sexually immoral, illegal-drug-using women who deliberately harmed their babies' (p.41). Cleeton analysed an education campaign poster depicting the women as undisciplined, ignorant, irresponsible mothers who use drugs that kill their babies. Through these discourses, 'the everyday experience of urban minority impoverished women doing the work of mothering was transformed into evidence of their "natural" maternal inadequacy' (p. 41). In Canada, Tait (2000) offers a similar critique of public awareness campaigns that portray fetal alcohol syndrome as an Aboriginal health problem. While motherhood may be construed as 'natural' elsewhere, racism and classism configure these particular women as *naturally inadequate*. Viewing women as 'natural mothers' and/or as 'naturally inadequate' as mothers has profound influences for their experiences, and their health.

An Example: Aboriginal Mothering at the Intersections

Without question, in Canada, the group most effected by the destructive confluence of the discourses and material actualities of mothering are Aboriginal people. Along with significant losses of rights and marginalization from the labour force for Aboriginal women, the dynamics of colonialism include pernicious constructions of Aboriginal women (Fiske, 2006; Fiske & Browne, 2006), the colonization of childbirth (Fiske, 1992, 1993, 1995; Jasen, 1997; Kaufert & O'Neil, 1993) and the widespread removal of Aboriginal children from their parent's care through the residential school system, forced adoption, and child welfare policies (Fournier & Grey, 1997; Royal Commission on Aboriginal Peoples, 1998). Jasen argues that the ideology of the natural, 'wild' woman was particularly active in European colonization of Aboriginal women's childbirth experiences. 'As part of its "civilizing mission," the Canadian government adopted an interventionist policy which led, in recent decades, to the practice of evacuating pregnant women to distant hospitals' (Jasen, 1997, p. 383), a practice that dominates today. Indeed, despite evidence of good birthing outcomes in rural settings (e.g., Thommasen, Klein, Mackenzie, & Grzybowski, 2005a; Thommasen et al., 2005b) and costs associated with evacuation (e.g., Kornelsen & Grzybowski, 2005) the practice of evacuation, particularly for Aboriginal women, is increasingly commonplace. Further, as Benoit and her colleagues (Chapter 19, this collection) show, Aboriginal women residing in both non-urban and urban areas have greater difficulties than their non-Aboriginal counterparts accessing health care for themselves and their newborns. Writing specifically with reference to Inuit women, Kaufert and O'Neil (1993) show how discourses of risk function to keep such practices and inequities in place, discourses that intersect with other mothering discourses.

Removal of Aboriginal children from their parents' care was also part of the 'civilizing mission' by European settlers (Furniss, 1995, 1999). The incarceration of multiple generations of children, and the well-documented abuses suffered by those children, has had deep and destructive effects on entire communities, and on mothers in particular. Although the last residential schools closed in the 1960s, discourses that constructed Aboriginal women as irresponsible and negligent fostered what Fiske (1993) calls the 'inferiorization of Aboriginal motherhood' (p. 20). These discourses supported a new form of removal of Aboriginal children from their families and communities, and the children were sent to various countries and placed in non-Aboriginal foster homes throughout the 1960s and 1970s (Fiske 1993; Fournier & Grey, 1997). Under current child welfare policies, discourses of 'unfit' mothers and children 'at risk' have supported the continued removal of Aboriginal children from the care of their parents and communities. For example, in 2001 in British Columbia, approximately 45 per cent of the children in state care were Aboriginal, and few of these children were placed in Aboriginal foster homes (Government of British Columbia, 2001). In addition, and perhaps partially as a buffer to these dynamics, many Aboriginal women provide primary care to their grandchildren, adding to their mothering work. Through these historic and ongoing acts of colonization and racism supported by various discourses of mothering, loss of language, culture, dignity, and parenting skills have undermined mothering, and continue to do so.

Mothering, Women's Health, and Health Care Discourses

Another complicating factor for women/mothers is the way in which mothering discourses interface with health care discourses. Many psychological and medical discourses present unquestioned sources of knowledge that are embedded within patriarchal liberalist society (Caplin, 1990; Cushman, 1995). Moreover, this unquestioned knowledge is often taken up by health care practitioners in ways that are undermining and detrimental to women/mothers. One of the most extreme examples is the intersection of the psychological discourse surrounding mothers and child development. Harris (1998) describes how during the latter half of the twentieth century there was a dramatic shift in thinking about the role of mothers in the psychological development of children. According to Harris, within psychological discourse, mothers began to be held accountable for all that was good, bad, and pathological in their children. Subsequently, the influence and culpability of mothers in child development have become deeply embedded, normative beliefs (Harris, 1998). Hoskins and Lam (2001) illustrate the impact of this psychological discourse on the health of mothers with daughters experiencing anorexia. Their research highlights the deleterious effect the impossible task of being 'the perfect mother' has on the health of these women/mothers: 'Through nothing more than their maternal roles, etiological descriptors position mothers into a sharply polarized struggle between being too ambivalent and being too over-protective ... mothers, as stand-ins for families are scripted as being on the one hand, "too protective, controlling, connected, enmeshed or on the other hand, lacking in support, commitment, individuation, and affiliation"' (p. 166).

Two other examples of problematic health discourses that intersect with mothering include infertility and mental illness. The assumption that all women want to be mothers, and the expectation that all women will be mothers, has lent authority to the idea that infertility (encompassing various reasons, including biological reasons for involuntary childlessness) is a problem to be rectified. Letherby (2002) argues that these dominant discourses regarding expectations of women, the value of biological identity, and medical science support each other towards seeking biomedical solutions to the social state of involuntary childlessness (child-freeness). Ulrich and Weatherall (2000) studied women who wanted children, but could not easily have biological children. The women's reasons for wanting children included the idea that motherhood is 'natural instinct,' is 'a stage in the development of a relationship,' and is a 'social expectation.' The women constructed motherhood as physical, psychological, and social completeness and fulfilment and experienced infertility as guilt, inadequacy, and failure. As in the case of mothers' presumed causal role in their daughters' anorexia, it is possible to see how expectations placed on women potentially have negative impacts on their health and well-being.

Discourses regarding mental illness and mothering also intersect in ways that are extremely oppressive for women. Savvidou, Bozikas, Hatzigeleki, and Karavatos (2003) illustrate how such discourses construct mothers with mental illnesses as violent and as incapable of mothering. Women with mental illnesses felt they were the victims of societal attitudes even before they became pregnant. Indeed, although involuntary sterilization now supposedly is illegal in Canada, debates regarding birth control for women with mental illness continue, reflecting the assumption that such women are incapable of caring for their children (Morrow & Chappell, 1999). In a study of policy discourse on mothering in Canada, women with mental illness were depicted in media and social policy and practices as dangerous to their children (Greaves et al., 2002; 2004). Media analysis showed that newspaper writers, often using myth and fairy tale genres, constructed women with mental illnesses as dangerous and incapable mothers.

Mothering and Women's Health

Overall, the experiences of mothering and the discourses that shape those experiences have significant effects on women's well-being – encompassing social, economic, physical, and mental well-being. The discourses of mothering have impact on women whether or not they are 'mothers' in any of the possible senses. Letherby (2002) notes that 'as motherhood is valued rhetorically (even though it has little material and social status) non-motherhood is defined as "lesser." Non-mothers or women who achieve motherhood in unconventional ways are defined in lay, medical, and even some social science and feminist literature as "problematic," "unnatural," "abnormal"' (p. 285). Girls and women are influenced by ideologies of motherhood and these complex and competing discourses, whether or not they can or do become mothers in any way. For example, McLaren (1996) showed how young women in school understood the competing ideals of mothering and waged work in ways that were congruent with the dominant discourse of exclusive mothering, and understood the desirability of employment in ways that reflected the fact that alternatives to exclusive mothering lacked social legitimacy and institutional support.

Mothering affects women's health in multiple interacting ways. Mothering requires a material, economic, and social investment, but usually is not compensated in material or economic ways. This means that women are made more vulnerable to a variety of health risks, especially overwhelming workloads, poverty, and violence, by motherhood. At the same time, the experience of mothering may have a positive impact on women's health. We offer examples of each below.

Mothering Work and Women's Health

One of the most significant ways that mothering impacts women's health is in terms of workload. In Canada, studies consistently show that women, particularly those with children, do a much greater proportion of non-labour force work in comparison with their male counterparts, regardless of whether or not they are also participating in the paid labour force (Marshall, 1993; Baines, Evans, & Neysmith, 1998; Statistics Canada, 2000b). The work of mothering in addition to other forms of work means that the workloads of women who are mothers are higher than those of women who are child-free, or men, regardless of whether or not those men have children. And, these workloads can have a detrimental impact on women's health. For example, one of the most significant facets of mothering work is its location within the broader framework of reproductive work (Hartrick, 2002). The reproductive work of mothering extends far beyond the biological bearing of children and includes the daily activities necessary to sustain the physical and emotional well-being of significant others and of society in general. The gendered division of labour sanctifies women's responsibility for the reproductive work of society and this responsibility is further promoted through socially structured arrangements that foster the expectation that women take up the responsibility for nurturing and sustaining their family and/or significant others. The sheer volume of women's domestic and reproductive labour has major implications for women's health (Doyal, 1995). In poorer countries women literally 'work themselves to death,' and in more affluent countries women's reproductive work is associated with an increased incidence of depression and other illness (Doyal, 1995).

Of particular importance when thinking of women's health is how policy makers and health care practitioners often fail to recognize the time, energy, and material resources women expend in their daily 're-productive work' and the impact this has on their health (Messias et al., 1997). Paradoxically, women's health is often subsumed within the larger topic of family health – as though the two go together (Hartrick, 2002). While there is little recognition of the detrimental impact of reproductive labour, as is shown elsewhere throughout this book, women's 'health care' is often narrowly associated with women's reproductive work in the form of childbearing.

Mothering is not only the work of reproduction, nor is it confined to the business of socializing the young to society. In the early development of her alternative sociology, Canadian Dorothy Smith (1987) illustrated how mothers do the work of larger social organizations in multiple ways. For example, Smith argued that although sociological literature analyses what mothers do in relation to schools so that it does not appear as work, mothers' work is integral to the work of schools. She shows how mothers' work with children's social processes, communication skills, reading skills, work habits, and so on, is necessary for the work of schools. However, as Smith points out, the 'notions of good mothering practices take no account of the actual material and social conditions of mothering work' (p. 168). So, the expectation that mothers teach children how to read or draw presupposes the time and the materials with which to do so. This analysis has since been echoed and expanded by others. For example, Standing (1998, 1999) argues that similar dynamics operate in the United Kingdom. Both policy makers and educational theorists propose parental involvement as a solution to falling educational standards but present such involvement as 'ungendered, with no recognition that the work required of mothers is difficult to do under conditions of sole supporting mothering and low income' (1999, p. 57). Similarly, in some situations the gender neutral term *parenting* is employed regardless of who is actually doing the work. Thus, good mothering is shaped and constrained by gendered material and social conditions, yet judged against class assumptions that presume a certain (and far from common) standard of living. And, multiple competing discourses obscure the work and gendered nature of mothering.

Mothering, Poverty, and Women's Health

As noted earlier, many mothers in Canada are lone heads of their households and many are living under or near the poverty line. That mothering is accompanied by increased exposure to health risks, particularly poverty, is clearly borne out by the differential incomes of mothers in Canada. Women's incomes decline as they take on the work of mothering. Lone mothers in particular are poor, in Canada as well as in other countries such as Sweden and Britain (Baker & North, 1999; Weitoft, Haglund, & Rosen, 2000; Whitehead, Burström, & Diderichsen, 2000). Women who are partnered and separate from those partners experience significant declines in income. Revenue Canada income tax returns show that in the year of separation, women experience a median loss of 38 per cent of adjusted family income; in comparison, men see an immediate 11 per cent net gain. On separation, women are usually the custodial parent, and, in the year of separation, only 35 per cent of women receive support payments from their former spouse. In the year following separation, women's net family income loss is 23 per cent, while men experience a 10 per cent net gain in income (Ministry of Women's Equality, 2000).

Poverty has particular impacts on the health of lone mothers and their children. As described by Reid (Chapter 7, this collection), poverty and material deprivation have significant impacts for women, and especially mothers, including hunger and malnutrition and the consequences of both, and higher morbidity and mortality. For example, in Atlantic Canada, McIntyre et al. (2003) studied lone mothers, finding that 78 per cent reported household food insecurity during one study month and 96.5 per cent reported household food insecurity over a year. The research found that mothers compromised their own nutritional intake in order to preserve the adequacy of their children's diets. Child hunger was similar to maternal hunger over the one-month study period (23 per cent); however, it was lower than maternal hunger over the preceding year (McIntyre et al., 2002).

Studies also suggest higher mortality rates for lone mothers, but poverty alone does not explain the relative disadvantage. In Britain and Sweden, higher mortality rates have been found for lone mothers compared to the rest of the population. For example, in Sweden lone mothers showed an almost 70 per cent higher premature risk of death than mothers with partners (Weitoft et al., 2000). A study in Britain (Whitehead et al., 2000) found that about 50 per cent of the health disadvantage of lone mothers was accounted for by poverty and joblessness, whereas in Sweden these factors only accounted for between 3 per cent and 13 per cent of the health gap. However, employment does not mean better health for lone mothers (Baker & North, 1999). These studies suggest that lone mothering effects health beyond the effects of poverty, and that neoliberal policies to promote 'welfare to work' will not improve health.

The dynamics of poverty and mothering, particularly lone mothering, are deeply entwined with violence against women. First, mothering is an area in which abusive partners can exert power and control (Hardesty, 2002; McFarlane, Parker, Soeken, Silva, & Reed, 1999; Varcoe & Irwin, 2004). Second, economic independence is the greatest factor in women's decisions to enter, remain in, or leave abusive relationships (Barnett, 2000; Lambert & Firestone, 2000). Third, women's concerns about their children influence such decisions; women both stay in and leave abusive relationships partly because of what they believe is best for their children (Henderson, 1990; Hilton, 1992; Humphreys, 1995a, 1995b; Irwin, Thorne, & Varcoe, 2002; Varcoe & Irwin, 2004). Fourth, whether women leave or stay with abusive partners, through their children they are exposed to those partners at least as long as the children are dependent (Varcoe & Irwin, 2004). Finally, women also experience violence from their children (Jackson, 2003). The effects of violence on the health of women are multiple and enduring (see Chapter 18, this collection), and exposure to violence is exacerbated by the dynamics of mothering.

In sum, women's health is effected by mothering, with issues of workload, poverty, and violence having particularly detrimental impacts. However, despite the conditions under which many women mother, and despite the actual and potential negative impacts of mothering on women's health, many women also find significant reward in and draw strength from mothering.

Mothering and the Positive Impact on Health

Rather than being an 'expectation,' or a 'sacrifice,' mothering can have a positive effect on health, be a strategy for survival, and a source of strength. Motherhood is often cited as a positive factor for women's physical health, with, for example, considerable evidence that childbearing, and, to a less well-known extent, breastfeeding, are protective against breast cancer (Collaborative Group on Hormonal Factors in Breast Cancer, 2002). Mothering may also promote women's health in other ways. For example, mothering may act as a buffer against intimate partner violence (Irwin et al., 2002). In a study regarding policy related to mothering, women with mental illnesses, or women who used substances or experienced violence, commonly saw 'the advent of a pregnancy or the birth of a child as a significant life event where positive decisions can be made about someone else's welfare and [saw] an opportunity ... for redirecting their goals and will ... [Mothers who used substances] remarked that their children were the best motivation for change, and the women who were experiencing violence expressed that often their key motivator was their child's safety' (Greaves et al., 2002, p. 96). Similarly, although lone mothers have been viewed primarily through a deficiency lens (Ford-Gilboe, 2000; Wuest, Ford-Gilboe, Merritt-Gray, & Berman, 2003), Ford-Gilboe found that families headed by a lone mother had similar strengths in comparison with two-parent families, but that the single-parent families had some unique ways of operating that reflected their daily lives. She suggested that perhaps single-parent families expressed more optimism and pride because they faced more chronic challenges.

Similarly, Hartrick's (1996) study, exploring the process of self-definition for women who were actively engaged in mothering, highlighted the potential of the mothering experience for women's own self-development. The women who participated in the study described how they had developed new knowledge and clarity about themselves through their mothering experiences. One example was a participant who described learning 'the lesson of loving her children so much that she would give up herself.' Through that experience she learned about the depth of her ability to care for and give to another human being, about her own value as a person, and how 'important it is to not give myself up even in the name of caring' (Hartrick, 1994, pp. 141–142).

Mothering can also be seen as a significant asset to communities. Indeed, in recent research (Smith, Varcoe, & Edwards, 2005), two different Aboriginal communities saw birth and child-rearing as central to healing the devastating inter-generational effects of residential schools. Similarly, Fiske (1992) described how for Carrier women, motherhood is not thought of as confined to the nurturing of children, but, rather, women integrate their social and political community involvement, merging domestic authority and public leadership to take responsibility for adult children and the community more broadly. And, these women have drawn upon their special responsibilities and attachment to children and communities to further their claims for political equity.

Implications for Policy and Practice

Understanding mothering as a socially constructed experience that is shaped by structural conditions and intertwined with competing and conflicting social discourses: (a) reveals the complex nature of the mothering experience; (b) draws attention to the diverse experiences of women; and (c) enables critical examination of the effects of mothering on women's health. Such analyses suggest implications for both policy and practice.

First, given the power of discourses in shaping women's experiences of mothering it is vital that practitioners pay attention to discourses. This 'paying attention' involves listening for what and how discourses are shaping the experiences of particular women in their particular situations and locations. In addition, paying attention to discourse involves carefully scrutinizing how the intersecting discourses are shaping and ultimately limiting the choices and resources available to women, including how practitioners themselves are drawing on different discourses as they interpret and respond to women. Furthermore, it requires that special attention is paid to the ways in which discourses are shaping the larger contexts within which women live and access health care. Countering the detrimental effects of constructing and responding to women as 'welfare moms,' 'working moms,' 'bad mothers,' 'crack moms,' and 'unfit mothers' needs to be accompanied by the use of more constructive capacity-promoting language, ideas, and responses. At the same time, however, countering and commandeering discourses is not sufficient – for example, Fiske (1993) has shown that motherhood discourses have failed to alter Aboriginal women's political subordination in the absence of change to the women's material and political power. Thus, the impact of mothering on the material, economic, and political concerns of women remains critical.

Second, therefore, the work of mothering needs to be acknowledged in the development of social policy and the implementation of such policy. For example, social welfare policies need to take into account rather than ignore the work of mothering, such as is the case in policies such as those in British Columbia that require women to seek full time employment when their youngest child turns three years of age.

Finally, policies and practices in social services and health care need to be filtered through a complex, gendered, and intersectional understanding of mothering. To this end, Greaves et al. (2002) offer a policy filter within a mothering framework that they suggest ought to be applied to all policy and legislation. Among the questions they suggest are those regarding the extent to which any policy recognizes the influence of gender, race, and class, as well as questions that can enhance recognition of the interrelatedness of multiple health determinants (such as poverty) and health issues (such as mental illness, violence, and substance use). The importance of understanding policy through such a filter is underscored by the issue of a national child-care program. After decades of lobbying by feminists, and a decade of promises by successive Liberal governments, the promise of such a program was briefly on the table in 2005 only to be replaced by a federal program to provide families with a child-care allowance of $1, 200 per child, per year. As critics point out, such a program will not increase child-care spaces or quality and will not significantly assist those who most need it. However, for the most part the public debate focuses on child care decontextualized from the wider issues of inequality, women's poverty, women's health, and the cuts to social programs that have characterized the preceding decades of government policy. As Yalnizyan (2005) notes, over the recent decades the economic security of families has rested increasingly on the degree to which women in households are willing to increase or engage in paid work. And, even as the need for more supports for child care has grown, budget cutbacks have meant a 'freeze or even a reduction in the available supply of regulated and/or subsidized child care' (p. 16). In the absence of a contextual understanding of the need for child care, rhetoric purporting that a national child-care program will 'disadvantage' families in which mothers 'choose' to provide care at home flourishes, overlooking the fact that only very privileged families can make such choices, and putting at risk the possibility of providing some relief to those who are most disadvantaged.

Overall, using intersectional analyses and understanding mothering as a social construction emphasizes the importance of using a capacity lens to identify and build upon the strength and resources women already possess and employ in their mothering. Taking an intersectional lens to understanding motherhood turns attention to both the contradictory discourses and the material conditions within which motherhood is enacted. It turns attention not only to the ways in which women construct themselves and are constructed in relation to motherhood (whether they bear and/or provide care for children or not) and the conditions under which they construct themselves and enact mothering work, but also to the complex relations among these influences. Using a capacity lens to understand these complexities offers opportunities to find ways to promote health within and through motherhood. Such an approach suggests that the material conditions of mothering in interaction with the ways of understanding motherhood simultaneously must be enhanced. In this way, beginning with an awareness of and intentionally enlisting capacity strengthens the potential of women for mothering and for promoting women's health.

REFERENCES

Baines, C.T., Evans, P.M., & Neysmith, S.M. (1998). Women's caring: Work expanding, state contracting. In C.T. Baines, P.M. Evans, & S.M. Neysmith (Eds.), *Women's Caring: Feminist Perspectives on Social welfare* (2nd ed., pp. 3–22). Toronto: Oxford University Press.

Baker, D., & North, K. (1999). Does employment improve the health of lone mothers? *Social Science & Medicine, 49*(1), 121–131.

Barnett, O.W. (2000). Why battered women do not leave. Part 1: External inhibiting factors within society. *Trauma, Violence, and Abuse, 1*(4), 343–372.

Blackford, H. (2004). Playground panopticism: Ring-around-the-children, a pocketful of women. *Childhood, 11*(2), 227–249.

Bobel, C. (2002). *The Paradox of Natural Mothering*. Philadelphia: Temple University.

Boyd, S.B. (1996). Is there an ideology of motherhood in (post) modern child custody law? *Social & Legal Studies, 5*(4), 495–521.

Boyd, S.B. (2003). *Child Custody, Law and Women's work.* Don Mills, ON: Oxford University.

Boyd, S.C (1999). *Mothers and Illicit Drugs: Transcending the Myths.* Toronto: University of Toronto Press.

Boyd, S.C. (2004). *From Witches to Crack Moms: Women, Drug Law and Policy.* Durham, NC: Carolina Academic Press.

Caplin, R.S. (1990). *Don't Blame Mothers: Mending the Mother Daughter Relationship.* New York: Harper & Row.

Chodorow, N. (1978). *The Reproduction of Mothering: Psychoanalysis and the Sociology of Gender.* Berkeley: University of California.

Cleeton, E.R. (2003). Are you beginning to see a pattern here? Family and medical discourses shape the story of black infant mortality. *Journal of Sociology and Social Welfare, 30*(1), 41–64.

Collaborative Group on Hormonal Factors in Breast Cancer. (2002). Breast cancer and breastfeeding: Collaborative reanalysis of individual data from 47 epidemiological studies in 30 countries, including 50,302 women with breast cancer and 96,973 women without the disease. *Lancet, 360,* 187.

Cushman, P. (1995). *Constructing the Self, Constructing America: A Cultural History of Psychotherapy.* New York: Perseus.

Davies, B., & Harre, R. (1990). Positioning: Conversation and the production of selves. *Journal for the Theory of Social Behaviour, 20,* 43–63.

Doyal, L. (1995). *What Makes Women Sick: Gender and Political Economy of Health.* New Brunswick, NJ: Rutgers University Press.

Eicher-Catt, D. (2004). Noncustodial mothering. *Journal of Contemporary Ethnography, 33*(1), 72–108.

Farris-Manning, C., & Zandstra, M. (2004). *Children in Care in Canada: A Summary of Current Issues and Trends with Recommendations for Future Research.* Ottawa: Child Welfare League of Canada and Foster LIFE Inc.

Fiske, J.-A. (1992). Carrier women and the politics of mothering. In G. Crees & V. Strong-Boag (Eds.), *British Columbia Reconsidered: Essays on Women.* Vancouver: Press Gang.

Fiske, J.-A. (1993). Child of the state, mother of the nation: Aboriginal women and the ideology of motherhood. *Culture, 13*(1), 17–35.

Fiske, J.-A. (1995). Political status of Native Indian women: Contradictory implications of Canadian state policy. *American Indian Culture and Research Journal, 19*(2), 1–30.

Fiske, J.-A. (2000). By, for, or about? Shifting directions in the representation of Aboriginal women. *Atlantis, 25*(1), 11–27.

Fiske, J.-A. (2005). Boundary crossings: Power and marginalisation in the formation of Canadian Aboriginal women's identities. *Gender & Development*, *14*(2), 247–258.

Fiske, J.-A., & Browne, A. (2006). Aboriginal citizen, discredited medical subject: Paradoxical constructions of Aboriginal women's subjectivity in Canadian health care policies. *Policy Sciences*, *39*(1), 91–111.

Ford-Gilboe, M. (2000). Dispelling myths and creating opportunity: A comparison of the strengths of single-parent and two-parent families. *Advances in Nursing Science*, *23*(1), 41–58.

Fournier, S., & Grey, E. (1997). *Stolen from Our Embrace: The Abduction of First Nations Children and the Restoration of Aboriginal Communities*. Vancouver: Douglas & MacIntyre.

Furniss, E.M. (1995). *Victims of benevolence: The Dark Legacy of the Williams Lake Residential School*. Vancouver: Arsenal Pulp Press.

Furniss, E.M. (1999). *The Burden of History: Colonialism and the Frontier Myth in a Rural Canadian Community*. Vancouver: University of British Columbia Press.

Government of British Columbia. (2001). *British Columbia Children's Commission Annual Report*. Victoria, BC: Government of British Columbia.

Greaves, L., Pederson, A., Varcoe, C., Poole, N., Morrow, M., Johnson, J., & Irwin, L. (2004). Mothering under duress: Women caught in a web of discourses. *Journal of the Association for Research on Mothering*, *6*(1), 16–27.

Greaves, L., Varcoe, C., Poole, N., Morrow, M., Johnson, J., Pederson, A., et al. (2002). *A Motherhood Issue: Discourses on Mothering under Duress*. Ottawa: Status of Women Canada.

Hardesty, J.L. (2002). Separation assault in the context of post divorce parenting: An integrative review of the literature. *Violence Against Women*, *8*(5), 597–626.

Harris, J.R. (1998) The nurture assumption. Why children turn out the way they do. New York: Free Press.

Hartrick, G.A. (1994). Women Who are Mothers: Experiences of Self-definition. Unpublished dissertation. Victoria, BC.

Hartrick, G.A. (1996). The experience of self for women who are mothers: Implications for the unfolding of health. *Journal of Holistic Nursing*, *14*(4), 316–331.

Hartrick, G.A. (2002). Women's reproductive work: A precarious obligation. In B.S. Bolaria & H. Dickinson (Eds.), *Health, Illness and Health Care in Canada* (3rd ed., pp. 231–246). Scarborough, ON: Nelson.

Henderson, A. (1990). Children of abused wives: Their influence on their mothers' decisions. *Canada's Mental Health*, *38*(2–3), 10–13.

Hilton, N.Z. (1992). Battered women's concerns about their children witnessing wife assault. *Journal of Interpersonal Violence, 7,* 77–86.

Hoskins, M.C., & Lam, E. (2001). The impact of daughters' eating disorders on mothers' sense of self: Contextualizing mothering experiences. *Canadian Journal of Counselling, 35*(2), 157–175.

Humphreys, J. (1995a). Dependent-care by battered women: Protecting their children. *Health Care for Women International, 16,* 9–20.

Humphreys, J. (1995b). The work of worrying: Battered women and their children. *Scholarly Inquiry for Nursing Practice: An International Journal, 9*(2), 127–145.

Irwin, L., Thorne, S., & Varcoe, C. (2002). Strength in adversity: Motherhood for women who have been battered. *Canadian Journal of Nursing Research, 34*(4), 47–57.

Jackson, D. (2003). Broadening constructions of family violence: Mothers' perspectives of aggression from their children. *Child and Family Social Work, 8*(4), 321.

Jasen, P. (1997). Race, culture and the colonization of childbirth in northern Canada. *Social History of Medicine, 10*(03), 383–400.

Kaufert, P.A., & O'Neil, J. (1993). Analysis of a dialogue on risks in childbirth: Clinicians, epidemiologists and Inuit women. In S. Lindenbaum & M. Lock (Eds.), *Knowledge, Power and Practice: The Anthropology of Medicine in Everyday Life* (pp. 32–54). Los Angeles: University of California Press.

Kissling, F., & Sippel, S. (2001/2002). Women under oppressive regimes: Women and religious fundamentalisms. *Conscience* (Winter).

Kornelsen, J., & Grzybowski, S. (2005). The costs of separation: The birth experiences of women in isolated and remote communities in British Columbia. *Canadian Women's Studies, 24*(1), 75–80.

Lambert, L., & Firestone, J.M. (2000). Economic context and multiple abuse techniques. *Violence Against Women, 6*(1), 49–67.

Lemkau, J.P., & Landau, C. (1986). The selfless syndrome: Assessment and treatment considerations. *Psychotherapy, 23,* 227–232.

Letherby, G. (2002). Challenging dominant discourses: Identity and change and the experience of 'infertility' and 'involuntary childlessness.' *Journal of Gender Studies, 11*(3), 277–288.

MacDonald, K. (2002). *Missing Voices: Aboriginal Mothers Who Have Been at Risk of or Who Have Had Their Children Removed from Their Care.* Vancouver: Law Foundation of British Columbia.

Marshall, K. (1993). *Employed Parents and the Division of Housework: Perspectives on Labour and Income.* Ottawa: Statistics Canada.

McFarlane, J., Parker, B., Soeken, K., Silva, C., & Reed, S. (1999). Research exchange: Severity of abuse before and during pregnancy for African American, Hispanic, and Anglo women. *Journal of Nurse Midwifery, 44*(2), 139–144.

McIntyre, L., Glanville, N., Officer, S., Anderson, B., Raine, K., & Dayle, J. (2002). Food insecurity of low-income lone mothers and their children in Atlantic Canada. *Canadian Journal of Public Health, 93*(6), 411–415.

McIntyre, L., Glanville, N., Raine, K., Dayle, J., Anderson, B., & Battaglia, N. (2003). Do low-income lone mothers compromise their nutrition to feed their children? *Canadian Medical Association Journal, 168*(6), 686–691.

McLaren, A.T. (1996). Coercive invitations: How young women in school make sense of mothering and waged labour. *British Journal of Sociology of Education, 17*, 279–299.

McLaren, A.T., & Dyck, I. (2004). Mothering, human capital, and the 'ideal immigrant.' *Women's Studies International Forum, 27*(1), 41–54.

Messias, D., Regev, H., Im, E., Spiers, J., Van, P., & Meleis, A.I. (1997). Expanding the visibility of women's work: Policy implications. *Nursing Outlook, 45*, 258–264.

Ministry of Women's Equality. (2000). *Women Count 2000: A Statistical Profile of Women in British Columbia*. Victoria: Government of British Columbia.

Morrow, M., & Chappell, M. (1999). *Hearing Women's Voices: Mental Health Care for Women*. Vancouver: British Columbia Centre of Excellence for Women's Health.

Morrow, M., Hankivsky, O., & Varcoe, C. (2004). Women and violence: The effects of dismantling the welfare state. *Critical Social Policy, 24*(2), 358–384.

Oakley, A. (1981). Interviewing women: A contradiction in terms. In H. Roberts (Ed.), *Doing Feminist Research* (pp. 30–61). London: Routledge & Kegan Paul.

Rabuzzi, K.A. (1988). *Motherself: A Mythic Analysis of Motherhood*. Bloomington: Indiana University Press.

Ricciutelli, L., Larkin, J., & O'Neill, E. (1998). *Confronting the Cuts: A Sourcebook for Women in Ontario*. Toronto: Inanna.

Rich, A. (1976). *Of Woman Born. Motherhood as Experience and Institution*. London: Virago.

Royal Commission on Aboriginal Peoples. (1998). *Report of the Royal Commission on Aboriginal Peoples*. Ottawa: Canada Communications Group.

Savvidou, I., Bozikas, V.P., Hatzigeleki, S., & Karavatos, A. (2003). Narratives about their children by mothers hospitalized on a psychiatric unit. *Family Process, 42*(3), 391–403.

Smith, D., Varcoe, C., & Edwards, N. (2005). Turning around the intergenerational impact of residential schools on Aboriginal people: Implications for health policy and practice. *Canadian Journal of Nursing Research, 37*(4), 39–60.

Smith, D.E. (1987). *The Everyday World as Problematic: A Feminist Sociology.* Toronto: University of Toronto Press.

Standing, K. (1998). Writing the voices of the less powerful: Research on lone mothers. In J. Ribbens & R. Edwards (Eds.), *Feminist Dilemmas in Qualitative Research: Public Knowledge and Private Lives* (pp. 24–38). London: Sage.

Standing, K. (1999). Lone mothers' involvement in their children's schooling: Towards a new typology of maternal involvement. *Gender and Education, 11,* 57–73.

Statistics Canada. (2000a). *Statistics Canada – The Daily: Women in Canada.* Ottawa: Statistics Canada.

Statistics Canada. (2000b). *Women in Canada: A Gender-Based Statistical Report.* Ottawa: Statistics Canada.

Statistics Canada. (2001). *Census of Population.* Ottawa: Statistics Canada.

Swift, K.J. (1995). *Manufacturing 'Bad' Mothers: A Critical Perspective on Child Neglect.* Toronto: University of Toronto Press.

Swift, K.J. (1998). Contradictions in child welfare: Neglect and responsibility. In C.T. Baines, P.M. Evans, & S.M. Neysmith (Eds.), *Women's Caring: Feminist Perspectives on Social Welfare* (2nd ed., pp. 160–190). Toronto: Oxford University Press.

Tait, C. (2000). Aboriginal identity and the construction of fetal alcohol syndrome. In L. J. Kirmayer, M.E. Macdonald, & G.M. Brass (Eds.), *The Mental Health of Indigenous Peoples* (pp. 95–111). Montreal: McGill University Culture and Mental Health Research Unit.

Thommasen, H.V., Klein, M.C., Mackenzie, T., & Grzybowski, S. (2005a). Perinatal outcomes at Bella Coola General Hospital: 1940 to 2001. *Canadian Journal of Rural Medicine, 10*(1), 22–28.

Thommasen, H.V., Klein, M.C., Mackenzie, T., Lynch, N., Reyes, R., & Grzybowski, S. (2005b). Obstetric maternal outcomes at Bella Coola General Hospital: 1940 to 2001. *Canadian Journal of Rural Medicine, 10*(1), 13–21.

Ulrich, M., & Weatherall, A. (2000). Motherhood and infertility: Viewing motherhood through the lens of infertility. *Feminism & Psychology, 10*(3), 323–337.

Varcoe, C., & Irwin, L. (2004). 'If I killed you, I'd get the kids': Women's survival and protection work with child custody and access in the context of woman abuse. *Qualitative Sociology, 27*(1), 77–99.

Weedon, C. (1987). *Feminist Practice and Poststructuralist theory*. New York: Basil Blackwell.

Weiss, M. (1998). Conditions of mothering: The bio-politics of falling in love with your child. *Social Science Journal, 35*, 87–106.

Weitoft, G., Haglund, B., & Rosen, M. (2000). Mortality among lone mothers in Sweden: A population study. *Lancet, 355*(9211), 1215–1219.

Whitehead, M., Burström, B., & Diderichsen, F. (2000). Social policies and the pathways to inequalities in health: A comparative analysis of lone mothers in Britain and Sweden. *Social Science & Medicine, 50*(2), 255–270.

Wuest, J., Ford-Gilboe, M., Merritt-Gray, M., & Berman, H. (2003). Intrusion: The central problem for family health promotion among children and single mothers after leaving an abusive partner. *Qualitative Health Research, 13*(5), 597–622.

Yalnizyan, A. (2005). *Canada's Commitment to Equality: A Gender Analysis of the Last Ten Federal Budgets (1995 – 2004)*. Ottawa: Canadian Feminist Alliance for International Action (FAFIA).

PART FOUR

Key Issues in Women's Health

12 Women, Drug Regulation, and Maternal/State Conflicts[1]

SUSAN C. BOYD

This chapter provides a brief overview of ways in which women suspected of using illegal drugs are regulated in North America. Canada and the United States share a border and a common language as well as a history of being former British [and French] colonies. However, even though there are some historical similarities, the regulation of women in Canada is not identical to that in the United States. This chapter explores the regulation of women who use illegal drugs in North America in the criminal justice, medical, and social service systems. The regulation of women's bodies, reproduction, and the war on drugs all intersect. Women's bodies are viewed as the newest terrain on which to advance the war on drugs. However, drug prohibition is a failure. It contributes to the criminalization and marginalization of the poor. It perpetuates race, class, and gender oppression. More recently it has become a tool to once again limit women's reproductive autonomy and independence. By providing an overview of relevant developments over time, as well as key examples and landmark cases, this chapter also attempts to show how women's health related to drug use is shaped by criminal justice, social service, and medical policies and practices. Similarities and differences in policy and practice as well as the global 'Americanization of criminal law and drug policy' are examined.

The Americanization of international law has significance for Canada and other nations throughout the world, especially since the invasion of Afghanistan and Iraq and the enactment of anti-terrorist laws following the terrorist attack on the Twin Towers in New York in 2001. In the past, feminist writers have pointed out that militarization is a key source of violence against women. I assert that criminal justice, drug policy, and militarization converge and legitimize the use of force and violence against domestic populations and other nations and increase the regulation of women, especially women suspected of using illegal drugs.

Prior to the 1980s, there was little feminist research about women who used illegal drugs. When women were included in conventional research studies, they were constructed as more sexually permissive, immoral, pathological, and criminal than their male counterparts. Women's transgressions of the law were viewed as doubly deviant, for not only had they broken the law, but they had also challenged middle-class norms about feminine behavior. Feminist health writers and activists challenged conventional research about women who used illegal drugs. They called for more women-friendly drug treatment centres and sought to restructure 12-step programs to better serve women. They also brought attention to the legal use of prescribed drugs and to the pharmaceutical industry. However, like their conventional counterparts, early activists did not challenge the basic premise of the disease model of addiction underlying drug treatment, the effects of maternal drug use, and drug law. Too often, they mistook the effects of poverty for the effects of drugs.

A shift occurred in 1981 when Marsha Rosenbaum's ethnographic study was published. Her book *Women on Heroin* led the way for a sociological feminist analysis of illegal drug use. Since then, there has been a small explosion of feminist research on women and illegal drugs. This new body of research gives voice to women's experience and demonstrates that men are not subject to the same gendered forms of regulation that women are (Campbell, 2000; Humphries, 1999; Maher, 1995; Martin, 1993; Murphy & Rosenbaum, 1999; Taylor, 1993). Social factors such as race, class, and gender inequality shape women's drug use. My own work has contributed to this field by examining how women are vulnerable to interlocking spheres of informal and formal regulation. Women's drug use is shaped and regulated by drug law and the criminal justice system as well as by family law, social service and medical policy, and non-state agencies such as Narcotics Anonymous (NA). The regulation of women who are suspected of illegal drug use centers on double standards of morality, sexuality, pregnancy, birth, and mothering. However, not all women are treated the same. Poor women and women of colour are viewed as more deviant than other women (Boyd, 1999, 2004).

Since the 1980s, the war against drugs and the war on abortion and women's reproductive rights have intersected. Feminist researchers refer to this struggle as maternal/state conflicts. Both the state and a host of non-state moral reformers consider a pregnant woman to be a danger to her foetus. In the United States, women have been criminally charged for harming the foetus. Some U.S. prosecutors see women's wombs as the new battlefield for expanding the war on drugs (Logli, 1990, p. 23). Women who are suspected of using illegal drugs during pregnancy have been charged with homicide, trafficking to the foetus, and child endangerment.

A Feminist Perspective

A sociological feminist perspective illuminates how women's drug use is shaped by social, cultural, and political concerns. It also allows us to move away from male-centred and individualistic psychological theorizing about women and drug use. In North America, there is significant regulation by state agencies and criminal laws of women and men suspected of illegal drug use. The fields of medicine, social work, and psychiatry have developed new knowledges and techniques to identify, categorize, manage, and discipline illegal drug users. These professions compete and overlap with each other in their surveillance of women who use illegal drugs. Medical discourse, technology, and interventions have advanced foetal rights and maternal/state conflicts. However, legal discourse 'sets itself above other knowledges' (Smart, 1989, p. 10), and harsh drug laws legitimize punitive social service and medical policy. By examining the historical roots of drug prohibition, we can see the role that women have played in these events and how drug laws are gendered, racialized, and class-based. We can also see how drug laws shape health and social service policy and practice.

Historical Precedent

People have used plants and drugs for healing and spiritual use since time began. However, contemporary drug users in Western nations are more familiar with recreational and therapeutic drug use. The rise of the modern pharmaceutical industry, or what is referred to as the psycho-pharmaceutical revolution of the 1950s, has changed the face of drug use in Western nations. Hundreds of synthetic drugs are now available, and prescription drugs such as Valium and Prozac are household names. For example, according to the National Institute for Health Care Management (NIHCM) and the National Centre for Policy Management

(NCPA), in 1965 only 300 prescription drugs were on the market compared to 9,500 in 2002 (NIHCM, 2002; NCPA, 2002). Pharmaceutical companies favor synthetic drugs over natural drugs such as coca leaves, opium, and marijuana, because natural drugs cannot be patented as easily as synthetic drugs, thus their potential for profit is limited. Natural drugs have become associated with colonized and racialized peoples. Drugs that are domestic to Third World nations are seen as unscientific and dangerous (Boyd, 1991). Western nations tend to demonize drugs and plants that originate from outside their borders, even when domestic production is occurring within their own borders. Nevertheless, there is little worldwide consensus about which drugs are dangerous. Western nations tend to favor the legalization of alcohol and tobacco – our most toxic drugs – and the criminalization of drugs such as opium, cocaine, and marijuana.[2] However, due to the failure of drug prohibition, a number of Western nations have been at the forefront of drug reform. Drug researchers and activists have contributed to a wide array of work that criticizes the war on drugs and explores the roots of prohibition and alternatives to punitive drug laws and policy.

Exploring a few of the earliest documented drug scares in Western history provides us with some understanding of the historical roots of contemporary drug regulation and punishment. It also lends some understanding to the myths and concerns that shape drug policy today, especially in relation to women. In the following section I draw from my earlier work in order to provide a context for the current war on drugs. Ever since the witch hunts of the Middle Ages, women suspected of using plants and drugs condemned by religious authorities and the state have been portrayed as dangerous, immoral, and sexually promiscuous. The witch hunts, the gin craze, and the anti-opiate and alcohol prohibition movements provide us with some insight into the regulation of women.

The Witch Hunts

Researchers have written that pagan believers honoured Mother Earth, diversity, and the spiritual importance of women. Their beliefs conflicted with the rise of the Roman Catholic Church; however, it was not until the twelfth century that the Roman Catholic Church emerged as the first patriarchal centralized authority with the military, political, and religious power to construct, identify, and persecute 'pagan believers' and to subordinate women (Bianchi, 1994; Faith, 1993). Christian patriarchal practices of retribution replaced reconciliation, and by the thirteenth century the Inquisition emerged as a tool the Roman Catholic Church used to identify and discipline those identified as witches. During the witch hunts people were charged with the crimes of heresy and witchcraft. The majority of those people were poor women living outside of urban areas. Often these women were the midwives and healers of their communities; some were political dissenters. What is striking about the witch hunts is their gendered nature – women comprised about 80 to 85 per cent of condemned witches (Ehrenreich & English 1973, p. 8).

The church believed that witches had supernatural powers and that these powers were aided by the use of specific plants for healing and pagan rituals. *The Malleus Maleficarum* (The Witches' Hammer) was written in 1484 by two Dominican monks. It served as a tool to identify and punish women suspected of witchcraft and was used as a guide for church and secular authorities. *The Malleus Maleficarum* condemned women who possessed healing knowledge. Women who knew how to use plants to heal were viewed as a threat to the Church because healing was considered the domain of God, not of lay people. They were especially critical of healers and midwives who aided women during pregnancy and birth (Kramer & Sprenger, 1971). Healers and midwives were constructed as witches who were non-Christian, unscientific, and dangerous. Central to the witch hunts was the control of female sexuality, reproduction, and women's independence. All women were seen as sexually immoral, but Christian authorities claimed that witches were even more so because they interfered with male virility and reproduction, and consorted with the devil. Up until the eighteenth century, throughout Europe, torture and trials accompanied the witch hunts. As many as one million to nine million people were sentenced to death; the majority of these were women (Ehrenreich & English, 1973; Pfohl, 1994).

A number of historical factors led to the end of the witch hunts, including the Protestant Reformation of the sixteenth century and the writings of the Enlightenment thinkers which contributed to more diverse Christian religious and political beliefs in Europe (Pfohl, 1994). Middle-class people protested against public executions and voiced their growing concern about their own vulnerability. Reform movements to curtail corporal punishment, combined with a lack of consensus about who was believed to be deviant, also contributed to a shift in practice.

The Gin Craze

As early as the 1700s, secular and religious authorities were targeting a new group of women as immoral consumers of drugs. In 1736 – the same year that Britain dropped witchcraft as a statutory offence – one of the most 'infamous' gin laws was enacted (Warner, 2002). During the early 1700s the process for producing distilled gin changed; it became cheaper to make, and thus more available to poor consumers. Gin became very popular, so this era became known as the 'gin craze.' Historian Jessica Warner (2002) notes that gin became the 'first modern drug.' Wealthy moral reformers, many of whom were members of the College of Physicians in London, viewed gin consumption by the poor as contributing to social decay and the root cause of immorality and poverty. It is interesting to note that they did not condemn gin consumption of the rich or beer consumption – which was the drug of choice for women, men, and children in Britain, partially because it was cheap, and clean drinking water was not readily available to the urban poor.

Gin was perceived as especially harmful to women, who were depicted as losing their maternal instincts and fleeing their maternal duties when they drank it. The survival of the family and the nation was linked to their gin consumption (Musto, 2002; Warner, 2002). Rather than examine the terrible living conditions poor women suffered during this era, gin and women were viewed as the cause of social and private problems – in much the same way as witches and their drug use had been perceived.

During both of these early drug scares, women were seen as more deviant and sexually immoral than men; moreover, maternal fitness became an issue linked to the survival of the nation. Similar concerns continued to shape later drug scares and the prohibition of specific drugs. In contemporary times, just as back then, women's illegal drug use continues to be seen as a sign of 'social decay' and 'deviance' (Campbell, 2000), especially public displays of inebriation by poor women. However, historically, there has been little public condemnation of the drugs that the wealthy consume.

The Anti-opiate and Alcohol Prohibition Movements

The colonization of what is now known as North America – Canada and the United States – occurred during the same era as did the witch hunts and the gin craze. Western law, imperialism, Christianity, white supremacy, and eugenics theory informed colonial practices. The condemnation of drugs associated with Indigenous peoples – and later, people of colour – have shaped drug prohibition history on that continent. Alcohol and liquid opiates, the drugs of choice of the colonizer, were rarely scrutinized. During the colonization of North America, settlers consumed patent medicines which contained opiates, marijuana, and cocaine. Right up until the early 1900s it was believed that women, as the caretakers of their families, should always have these remedies on hand to help heal their children and other family members. This was especially true for poor women, who could not afford the services of a doctor, and rural women, who lived far away from the nearest doctor. In Canada, the United States, and elsewhere, opiate use was acceptable in society during the 1700s and early 1800s (Berridge & Edwards, 1981; Kandall, 1996; Mitchinson, 2002). Women's aliments, including reproductive problems, were treated with opiates and other patent medicines. Prior to the nineteenth century, the opiate user in Canada and the U.S. was a law-abiding white middle- and upper-class woman (or man) (Gray, 1999). Her use was considered to be a personal rather than a legal matter.

However, by the late 1800s the anti-opium movement emerged and prevailing ideas and practices began to shift. In fact, many physicians and moral reformers active in the anti-opium movement were also involved in the temperance movement. Both movements argued that moderate use of opiates and alcohol was impossible; thus they supported prohibition of these substances. The focus of the anti-opium movement centred on the opium trade. However, later domestic concerns by moral entrepreneurs brought attention to opium smoking by Chinese laborers in Canada and the United States. Opium smoking was seen as a deviant activity by foreign 'Others' – those labeled *outsiders* to the nation state. In the early 1900s, moral reformers (many of whom were women such as Emily Murphy in Canada and Sara Graham-Mulhall in the U.S.) in both nations 'educated' white Christian citizens about devious and immoral men of colour seducing white moral women and leading them into sexual slavery, crime, and addiction. Black and Chinese men were constructed as sexual menaces, and fears about the 'mixing of the races,' white women's sexual immorality, economic concerns, and the breakdown of the family and the nation led to the criminalization of specific drugs associated with racialized groups (Boyd, 1991; Comack, 1986; Nelson, 2002). By the early 1900s, opium smoking, and later cocaine and marijuana, were criminalized in both nations.

Initially, there was little criticism of the copious amounts of liquid opium that white Canadians and U.S. citizens consumed. During the 1700s and early 1800s there was no distinction between medical and non-medical use of liquid opiates. However, the rise in power of the medical profession, combined with class tensions, culminated in a concern about patent medicines that contained opiates, cocaine, and marijuana. There was concern about self-medication, 'infant doping' (self-medicating infants to soothe them and to calm stomach aliments), and recreational use of these drugs. There was also concern about improper labelling of substances in patent medicines. Overdose and poisoning became central concerns of moral reformers, physicians, and politicians.

In Britain, the Ladies' Sanitary Association criticized working-class and poor women for leaving their children in the care of others while they worked. It was believed that the nurses who cared for the infants drugged them so that they slept while their mothers were away. Working-class mothers came under scrutiny and attention; their perceived employment outside the home was seen as the root of the problem. No attention was given to middle- and upper-class infant doping, or to the fact that most working-class women were domestic workers. No attention was given to the fact that opiates provided relief to infant gastrointestinal problems, which were exacerbated by poor housing, sanitation, and poverty. Historians Berridge and Edwards (1981) noted that poverty and gastrointestinal problems caused more infant deaths than opiates. As it does today, focus on the use of opium by mothers deflected attention away from the social and economic conditions of poor and working-class women's lives (Ibid.). These drugs also came under regulation in Canada, the United States, and a host of other Western nations during the early 1900s.

Alcohol-prohibition movements also emerged during this time. Unlike the earlier gin craze, the prohibition of all alcoholic substances began to be advanced. Women were at the forefront of the alcohol prohibition movement. Lacking the vote and formal political participation in most Western nations, women emerged as moral reformers who sought to transform 'immoral' people and campaigned against all alcohol use (Hannah-Moffat, 2001). Alcohol-prohibitionist women viewed alcohol as a threat to the home and family and campaigned successfully for criminalization in the United States and Canada. Religious fervor (predominantly Protestant), sobriety and self-control, morality, and abstinence were central to their concerns (Levine, 1992). Alcohol was seen as the root of domestic violence, poverty, criminality, and the breakdown of the family. Unlike earlier views advanced about women, moral reformers believed that women were the protectors of home and family and more moral than men (Rose, 1996). Alcohol prohibition came into law in 1919 in the U.S. and it wasn't repealed there until 1933. In Canada, federal prohibition only lasted a year, although several provinces maintained prohibition longer.

Sociologist Craig Reinarman notes that drug scares have always been a popular media creation in the United States. Often drug scares are fueled by moral entrepreneurs or vocal 'claims-makers' who take ownership of a social problem by identifying and defining it and by producing knowledge about it (Reinarman, 2000; Best, 1995, 1999). During the twentieth century, more and more drugs were added to the federal list of prohibited drugs in Canada and the U.S. Drug laws became more punitive, even though there was no evidence to suggest that criminalized drugs were more dangerous than many legal drugs. Nor was there any substantial evidence, regardless of the propaganda, that the people who used illegal drugs were dangerous (Musto, 1987).

Reinarman (2000) notes that the United States is attached to prohibitionist ideology and practice. Drug scares there have become a way of life. Since the mid-1980s, many feminist activists have noted that the war on drugs has become a war on women (Bloom, Chesney-Lind, & Owen, 1994).

Criminal Justice Surveillance

In North America today, a host of myths and ideologies shape drug discourse which in turn shape social responses. These myths and ideologies also play a significant role in the regulation of women. Historically, drug laws have been linked to the regulation of women's morality and the loss of control over their own sexuality and reproduction. Myths about unfit mothers and dangerousness to children inform drug policy and the regulation of women. Myths about the dangerousness of some drugs and the people who use them also fuel the war on drugs. Everyday, mainstream media, state representatives (politicians and the police), and moral reformers claim that more regulation and bigger budgets are needed to protect society from ruthless drug traffickers and dangerous drugs. However, our legal drugs, tobacco and alcohol, are our most toxic drugs – more toxic than cannabis, our most benign illegal drug, and heroin and cocaine (Alexander, 1990; Boyd, 1991). In addition, state officials rarely arrest major drug traffickers. The majority of drug arrests are for drug possession rather than drug trafficking, and it is the visible, low-level drug dealer/user that is most vulnerable to arrest, rather than the 'drug kingpin.' In the United States and Canada, cannabis offences surpass any other illegal drug category. In addition, in 2002, 80 per cent of all drug arrests in the U.S were for possession, and, in the same year, 66 per cent of all drug offences in Canada were for possession (Desjardins & Hotton, 2004, p. 3; Dorsey, 2003).

Almost seven million people were under criminal justice surveillance in 2001 in the United States – two million in prison and the remaining on probation and parole (Bureau of Justice Statistics, 2002, p. 1). The increase in criminal justice regulation over the last 30 years is directly related to the war on drugs and more recently to the war against terrorists. The Bush Jr. administration has publicly sought to link domestic illegal drug use with terrorist groups and the proposed Vital Interdiction of Criminal Terrorist Organizations (VICTORY) Act of 2003 further erodes civil liberties and expands state power to identify and punish drug traffickers suspected of funding terrorist groups.

In the United States and Canada, women make up 11 per cent and 14 per cent of all those charged with drug offences. Even though there are more men in prison for drug offences than women, the percentage of women in prison convicted for drug offences is significantly higher than their male counterparts. For example, in 2002, 30 per cent of female federal prisoners in Canada were serving time for a drug offence compared to 22 per cent of men (Boe, Nafekh, Vuong, Sinclair, & Cousineau, 2003). Interestingly, drug use surveys demonstrate that in both nations, women use almost half the amount of illegal drugs than men use, and women are less likely to be involved in the drug trade (Canadian Centre on Substance Abuse, 2004; Single, Van Truong, Adalf, & Ialomiteanu, 1999). Nevertheless, the female prison population has increased since the 1970s. In the U.S. 'the number of women in state and federal prisons increased nearly eightfold between 1980 and 2001' (Covington & Bloom, 2003, p. 3). The increase in imprisoned women does not correspond to an increase in women's criminality or violent behaviour; rather, it is directly related to the war on drugs (Covington & Bloom, 2003, p. 3; U.S. Federal Bureau of Prisons, 2002).

Canada is often seen as a proponent of liberal drug policy, and in recent years the legalization of medical marijuana and the opening of a safe-injection site in 2003 in Vancouver, BC, lends some credibility to this argument. However, Canada's drug laws are quite harsh, and the possession of small amounts of marijuana is illegal even though numerous government commissions have advocated decriminalization. In fact, the latest report of the 2002 Senate Special Committee on Illegal Drugs recommended the legalization of marijuana possession. Even though the majority of the Canadian population favours marijuana reform, successive Canadian governments have failed to enact new laws to decriminalize/and or legalize marijuana (Nolan, 2003).

Since 2002, over one million women are moving through the U.S. criminal justice system in federal, state, county, and city jails and on probation and parole (U.S. Federal Bureau of Prisons, 2002, p. 52). Only recently has the war on drugs led to increased prison sentencing for women in Canada. Since 1997, the proportion of women in federal prison serving time for a drug offence has increased by 20 per cent (Correctional Service Canada 2002–2003). Increased prison sentencing for drug convictions in Canada may reflect the overall increase in drug offences since 1981, primarily due to possession and cannabis charges (Dell, Sinclair, & Boe, 2001, p. 60; Desjardins & Hotton, 2004, pp.1–3). Outside of their vast numbers what is most striking about women and men in prison for drug charges in both the United States and Canada is the overrepresentation of poor people and people of colour. In the United States, Black and Hispanic women are overrepresented in prison, while in Canada Black and First Nations women are overrepresented. In the U.S., criminal charges against women suspected of using illegal and legal drugs during pregnancy also shapes drug policy and practice. These women have overwhelmingly been poor and women of colour.

Maternal/State Conflicts

Women's bodies and reproductive autonomy continue to be a contested area in Canada, the United States, and other nations. The struggle for women's reproductive autonomy is well-documented by critical and feminist activists and scholars. The contemporary women's health movement in Canada and the U.S. has championed women's reproductive rights.

Historically, the realm of reproduction was women-centred. However, the witch hunts and the rise and consolidation of power by the male-dominated medical profession during the nineteenth and early twentieth centuries were instrumental in wresting control of pregnancy and birth from women. The newly established medical profession strengthened its fragile position by redefining pregnancy and birth and by portraying women as ignorant about pregnancy, childbirth, and child care. Medical surveillance and regulation were deemed necessary by the profession (Arnup, 1994; Oakley, 1984). Thus, they appropriated control of pregnancy and birth, taking it away from women and those who helped them deliver children (midwives and healers).

Prior to the nineteenth century, a woman in Canada could legally obtain birth control and an abortion before quickening (when the first movements of the unborn child are felt). Abortion and birth control were criminalized in Canada during the nineteenth century (McLaren, 1978). Since then, the medical pursuit of more knowledge about the foetus in utero has become a significant aspect of the medical profession's claim to legitimacy. Today, knowledge about the foetus is obtained through technological means such as ultrasound, rather than using the mother as intermediary, thus displacing her as the primary information source.

The medicalization of women's bodies and the regulation of drug use are intertwined. Both the anti-abortion movement and the war on drugs draw from earlier assumptions about women's role in society. Maternal/state conflicts emerged in the 1960s and early 1970s as many women in Canada, the United States – and elsewhere – challenged gender roles and sought equality, not only in the home but also in the workplace and in politics. In the 1960s, women once again demanded more control over their bodies and reproduction. The discovery and use of oral contraceptives and the decriminalization of abortion in 1969 were accompanied by medical discourse which portrayed the foetus as separate from the pregnant woman.

In Canada, the 1988 landmark decision in *Morgentaler v. The Queen* made it clear that the Canadian Supreme Court justices were committed to 'state interest in the foetus ... if not full legal personality' (Brodie, Gavigan, & Jenson, 1992, p. 127). The foetal rights movement in North America also gained momentum after the legalization of birth control and abortion by representing the foetus as a person with legal rights.

Foetal personhood has become a symbol for the anti-choice movement. Medical, legal, and anti-choice discourse and practice have contributed to the erosion of women's reproductive rights. In fact, pregnant women are seen as adversaries to the foetus. Feminist researchers note that legal and medical discourses about the foetus legitimize punitive practices towards women, and contribute to the ideology of mothering in which women are viewed as self-sacrificing givers of life, powerful in their maternal love. All those mothers who do not conform to this ideology are perceived as incapable of nurturing and parenting their children (Murphy & Rosenbaum, 1999; Boyd, 1999; Humphries, 1999; Roth, 2000). Problems related to poverty, marginalization, lack of medical care, gender inequality, and racism are ignored in favour of an individualistic ideology that portrays mothers as solely responsible for their health, pregnancies, maternal outcomes, and parenting.

Although physicians in the 1700s and 1800s showed some concern about maternal drug use, contemporary medical interest and regulation of women who used narcotics during pregnancy did not emerge until the 1960s. Researcher Elizabeth Armstrong discusses the irony of the 'discovery' of foetal alcohol syndrome (FAS) in 1973. This discovery was followed by the first reports of neonatal abstinence syndrome (NAS) in 1979, when guidelines for care were then developed. Armstrong (1998) notes that most often a new syndrome is the 'result of determined investigation and scientific entrepreneurship. In the case of FAS, moral fervor powered the discovery as much as medical curiosity' (p. 2025). A similar analysis can be applied to the diagnosis of NAS. The medical profession and a host of other professions (including those in the fields of criminal justice and social work) saw maternal drug use as a new, exciting, and expanding field of research and practice.

In Canada, a number of legal cases made the headlines in the 1980s and 1990s when social services attempted to detain pregnant women suspected of using drugs during pregnancy, highlighting attempts to extend legal personhood to the foetus. Social workers in Canada have continued to extend their regulation through the surveillance of maternal drug use. Legal cases demonstrate that they are also concerned about maternal drug use, and have attempted to 'apprehend the foetus' in order to protect it from legal and illegal drug use by pregnant women.

Controversies over court-ordered interventions, including caesareans, foetal rights, foetal apprehension, and legal personhood are being explored by a growing number of feminist researchers. As early as 1992, Maier's study on 'Baby R' in Vancouver, BC, explored 'reproductive violation' (Maier, 1992). The following year, the 1993 Royal Commission on New Reproductive Technologies in Canada expressed concern about criminal and civil interventions in pregnancy because interventions contravened women's Charter rights. More recently, Canadian researcher Lorna Turnbull (2001) provided a thorough overview of many cases in her book, *Double Jeopardy: Motherwork and the Law.*

What is significant about these cases is the attempt to regulate women's behaviour during pregnancy and to apprehend a child that is not yet born. The foetus cannot become a ward of the court because the term *child* under family and child service acts such as that of Manitoba (1995) refers to infants that have been delivered. Thus, these cases challenge the legal definition of the term child and open it up to debate and redefinition.

These cases rest on the assumption that the foetus is in need of protection from the mother and that the mother is unfit. Women in both the United States and Canada have been subject to forced medical interventions in order to 'save' the foetus. Forced obstetrical interventions, including caesarian sections, have occurred in both nations when women disagree with medical professionals about risk and the necessity of such treatment (Kolder, Gallagher, & Parsons, 1987; Roth, 2000; Turnbull, 2001).

Discourse is shaped by myths about mothering, the dangerousness of certain drugs, and welfare moms who drain limited economic and social supports. Furthermore, myths about the dangerousness of certain drugs and the perceived immorality of women who use illegal drugs have justified welfare cutbacks and denial of aid. It is assumed that women who use illegal drugs are promiscuous and have multiple children in order to claim welfare support. It is believed that they endanger the developing foetus and are unfit to parent. Welfare policy (including risk assessment tools) reflects these assumptions and thus women suspected of drug use are vulnerable to state surveillance and child apprehension.

One of the most famous cases in Canada involved solvent use during pregnancy. In 1996, Winnipeg Child and Family Services brought forward an application to have the court force a young First Nations woman who was pregnant to enter drug treatment. They claimed that she was using solvents and that they were a danger to the foetus. The Manitoba Court of Queen's Bench ordered the young women into drug treatment until the child was born. The Canadian media portrayed the woman as an unfit mother who already had two other children damaged beyond repair by her solvent use during her pregnancies. It was assumed by the media and social service agencies that there is a link between solvent use and foetal damage during pregnancy. In fact, a clear and definable foetal solvent syndrome has not been discovered (Addiction Research Foundation, 1997, p. 2; Medrano, 1996). On appeal, the Supreme Court of Canada agreed to hear the case. Meanwhile, the young women in question gave birth to a healthy infant.

In October 1997, the Supreme Court of Canada ruling on the case stated that the courts cannot force pregnant women into drug treatment in order to protect the unborn foetus. In addition, the court ruled that Canadian law does not recognize the unborn child as a legal person (Boyd, 1999, p. 24). Since this groundbreaking ruling, unlike in the United States, Canadian policy and practice has not shifted despite several legal challenges to women's reproductive autonomy, and despite welfare cutbacks and denial of economic and social supports to some women. For example, former Ontario premier Mike Harris justified welfare cutbacks and intrusive interventions by claiming that women on welfare were drug users. He did not provide any evidence (Etsten, 2000, p. 8). Social service agencies in Canada view illegal drug use as a significant variable related to harms to children (such as FAS, NAS, abuse, and neglect) (British Columbia Ministry of Children and Family Development, 2003). In 2002, then Canadian Alliance MP Keith Martin (currently a Liberal) introduced a private members' bill, Bill-C-233, an act to amend the Criminal Code (protection of child before birth). The bill would amend the Criminal Code to extend legal personhood to the foetus. It would make it an offence for a woman who is pregnant to consume a substance harmful to a foetus that she does not have a fixed intention to abort. The bill seeks to provide legal protection of the health of the foetus before it is born. It also 'authorizes' the courts to make orders to confine women in treatment facilities during their pregnancy and to report to physicians weekly upon their release in order to protect the foetus. Bill C-233 was not ratified. Nevertheless, poor women and women of colour suspected of illegal drug use in Canada continue to be vulnerable to intervention and child apprehension by the state.

The most disturbing shifts in relation to the regulation of women who use illegal drugs occurred in the United States in the 1980s. Concerns about crack cocaine led to draconian drug legislation that was race- and class-based (harsher penalties are imposed for crack cocaine than for powder cocaine, used by more affluent people), and which culminated in harsh sentencing, rigid mandatory minimums, two- and three-strikes-out legislation, little judicial discretion, the elimination of parole for federal drug offences, and the expansion of the prison industrial complex.

These early policy changes occurred under the leadership of conservative politicians such as Ronald Reagan and George Bush Sr. Conservative policy opened the way for a more conventional view of family values and the role of women. Women who did not subscribe to conventional and conservative family values were seen as a threat. Single mothers, in particular, were depicted as draining already strained social and economic supports. Illegal drug users, especially if they were single-parent mothers, were increasingly depicted by moral reformers as threats to the moral fabric of society and family breakdown. Women's 'compulsion' to use illegal drugs was perceived as overriding their maternal instincts. Moral reformers representing medical, social service, and legal fields generated fears that women who used illegal drugs during pregnancy did damage to the developing foetus. Politicians and mainstream media also contributed to the moral panic generated about maternal illegal drug use. Little attention was given to the actual lived realities of the women who used illegal drugs. The impact of poverty, race and gender oppression, lack of medical services, housing, and services was ignored. Women were increasingly blamed as individuals for failing as mothers and for endangering their born and unborn children. As in the past, it was poor mothers – especially women of colour – who were represented as being the most neglectful and dangerous.

Moral panic about maternal drug use deflects attention away from the one social factor that is known to have a negative influence on pregnancy. This social factor is poverty. World heath advocates have continually pointed out that poverty in itself has a damaging impact on pregnancy and maternal outcomes. In the United States and Canada, the numbers of poor women have been growing as social and economic supports decrease. Today more children live in poverty in both countries than 20 years ago (Bashevkin, 2002), but few politicians and moral reformers are crying out about poverty and its impact on pregnancy. Rather, fears related to a woman's reproductive autonomy and her perceived endangerment of the foetus have now culminated in a modern-day witch hunt in the U.S., and prosecutors are at the forefront of this attack on women. If maternal drug use is suspected, women are even more vulnerable to criminal sanctions. A woman's behavior during pregnancy (including whether she seeks 'proper' medical attention, is physically present at a drug production site, obeys her doctor's orders, drinks alcohol, or uses illegal drugs) is under scrutiny, and she is increasingly seen as criminally culpable.

The case of Regina McKnight is but one of the many cases that have not had a favorable outcome in the United States. Regina is a young Black woman who suffered a stillbirth when she lived in South Carolina in 1999. Following her delivery she was asked to provide a urine sample, which tested positive for drugs. At the time she was not informed that she might be subject to legal sanctions depending on the outcome of the urine test. She was later arrested and convicted of homicide in 2001, and sentenced to 20 years in prison (with an 8-year suspended sentence).

Her conviction rested solely on the 'evidence' that at delivery her daughter tested positive for benzoylecgonine, a breakdown product in the metabolism of cocaine. However, the autopsy also revealed that two other factors possibly contributed to the infant's death – the diseases choriomnionitis and funisitis. These diseases are not directly related to maternal cocaine use; women who do not use illegal drugs can develop both of these diseases. The state ignored this rationale, and, instead, contended that the cause of death by these diseases was 'undetermined.' Therefore, it must have been the cocaine that killed the infant. They also argued that if it had not been for the cocaine, the stillborn foetus would have been viable at the time of its birth (at seven to eight months gestation), and able to live outside the mother's body after the birth (*State of South Carolina v. Regina D. McKnight,* 2001).

Foetal viability is an important element in many of these criminal cases for several reasons. Most criminal statutes do not extend to the foetus, and thus establishing whether the foetus would have been viable is significant to the prosecutor. If it can be established that the foetus could have lived outside of the mother's body, the possibility of its being granted the same legal status as a live child is greater (Boyd, 2004).

In 1973, the U.S. Supreme Court noted in *Roe v. Wade* that the state has a compelling interest when the foetus is deemed viable (able to live outside the mother's body). Foetal viability has taken on greater significance since then, as reproductive technology advances and as the anti-abortion and foetal rights movement grows in power in the United States. Increasingly, the foetus and the mother are represented as separate from one another, and the relationship is seen as adversarial – the mother being a danger to the developing foetus.

The term *viability* has also become significant. In the United States, it has become the watershed word in the battle over women's reproductive rights. As foetal viability extends, women's reproductive rights have diminished and come under attack. Anti-abortion and foetal rights advocates have been pressing for the foetus to be granted legal rights. They view 'legal personhood' as an important strategy towards criminalizing abortion and regulating women's activities during pregnancy and birth. The argument for legal personhood put forward by moral reformers and anti-abortion and foetal rights advocates has fuelled the regulation of all pregnant women – and especially those women suspected of using illegal drugs and alcohol.

Feminist activists state that such advances in foetal rights have resulted in a situation in the U.S. where women's bodies and rights are under attack. Unsubstantiated fears about maternal drug use have culminated in increased social service, legal, and medical surveillance over the last 20 years. However, feminist activists and researchers assert that maternal/state conflicts are not just about abortion rights. They are also about the regulation of all women and their reproduction rights. They are about who gets to reproduce and who has the right to keep and raise their children. They are about health and women's bodies and women's independence and rights.

Women in the United States have plenty to worry about. Since the mid-1980s, over 300 women have been arrested and charged because of their behaviour during pregnancy, most of these arrests due to suspicions related to maternal drug use. Women have been arrested for child endangerment, trafficking to the foetus, manslaughter, homicide, and assault with a deadly weapon. Thirty states have foetal homicide laws. The majority of the women arrested have been poor and women of colour (Center for Reproductive Law and Policy, 1996; Taylor, 2004). In addition, thousands of women in the U.S. are impacted by state laws that equate illegal drug use with child abuse. Moreover, 18 states have civil child-welfare laws that regulate maternal drug use (Paltrow, Cohen, & Carey, 2000).

It is mistakenly assumed that maternal drug use is the sole factor bringing about negative pregnancy and maternal outcomes. Furthermore, illegal drug use while parenting is viewed as placing the child at risk, and thus state apprehension of the child is justified even though there is little voluntary drug treatment for mothers and pregnant women. It is believed that the drive to use drugs supersedes the parenting role. Women who use illegal drugs are seen as out of control and a danger not only to their developing foetus but also to their live children.

These negative portrayals of mothers ignore the abundance of research that demonstrates that women who use illegal drugs can be adequate parents. In addition, when non-judgemental prenatal care and social and economic supports are provided, maternal outcomes improve (Boyd, 1999; Colten, 1980; Hepburn, 1993; Murphy & Rosenbaum, 1999). In fact, when these supports are in place, illegal drug-using women have had the same maternal outcomes as non-drug-using women (Hepburn, 1993, 2002). Midwives have been at the forefront of providing maternal supports to women who use illegal drugs in Scotland and England. They and other medical professionals claim that while maternal drug use is a risk, it is a manageable risk.

Illegal drug use is just one variable among many that effect pregnancy and maternal outcomes. Poor pregnancy outcomes are associated with social and economic deprivation. Poverty and violence, as well as lack of housing, social and economic support, health care, and prenatal and antenatal care – all are risk factors that negatively shape women's pregnancies and maternal outcomes.

Recently, 27 leading medical doctors and scientists in the United States urged the media to cease perpetuating myths about babies exposed to maternal cocaine use. They asked the media to stop using the terms 'crack baby' and 'meth baby' because these terms stigmatize infants and lack scientific validity. In their letter, they state, 'Throughout almost 20 years of research, none of us has identified a recognizable condition, syndrome or disorder that should be termed "crack baby."' They also state: 'By definition, babies cannot be "addicted" to crack or anything else' (Arendt, Behnke, Black, Brown, Chasnott, & Chaukin, 2004).

It has not escaped the attention of feminist researchers that maternal/ state conflicts in the United States and Canada arose in the late 1960s and early 1970s, at the same time that women challenged gender roles and fought for more rights. As noted earlier, alcohol researcher Elizabeth Armstrong states that the 'discovery' of foetal alcohol syndrome (FAS) – and I would include the discovery of neonatal abstinence syndrome (NAS) in the late 1970s – emerged against the backdrop of women's quest for reproductive autonomy (Armstrong, 1998). Today in the U.S., maternal/state conflicts have culminated in the arrest, imprisonment, and punishment of women suspected of using illegal drugs during pregnancy and/or when parenting, resulting in separation due to prison time and/or state apprehension of their children due to allegations of child abuse.

For poor women, women of colour, and women on social assistance, drug testing when they give birth has become routine. Social workers and medical professionals work hand in hand with the criminal justice system (Boyd, 2004; Paltrow, 2004). Feminist researcher Dorothy Roberts states that the foster-care system in the United States has become an 'apartheid institution,' for it is Black children who make up the majority of children in care. Foster-care rates have tripled in some U.S. cities since the 1980s, and the increase is directly related to civil and criminal child abuse statutes that equate illegal drug use with child abuse (Roberts, 2002).

Women's reproductive autonomy has been under further attack by President Bush Jr. since 2000. He publicly acknowledges that his Christian fundamentalist beliefs shape his political actions. Recent legislation supported and signed by Bush Jr. grants the foetus new rights. Late-term – also called partial-birth – abortions were criminalized in 2003. The legislation criminalizes 'intact dilation and extraction' after the first trimester.

The developing foetus has been eligible for health care in the United States under the State Children's Health Insurance Program since 2002, though the alternative of granting universal health care to poor women or pregnant women has not. The Senate passed and Bush Jr. signed the Unborn Victims of Violence Act in 2004, which creates a separate federal offence for any individual who during the commission of specific crimes causes death or bodily harm to a 'child in utero.' Thus, the new act defines the foetus – anything from a zygote to a foetus – as an independent victim of crime with legal rights that are separate from the mother's. Critics note that the act does not make it an offence to attack pregnant women. Rather the act serves as a vehicle to extend the legal rights of the foetus and to further erode women's reproductive rights. In 2005, in response to a United Nations commission which reaffirmed support for the Beijing Conference on the Status of Women 10 years ago, the Bush Jr. administration urged the United Nations to renounce abortion rights. The administration refused to reaffirm the declarations if they included the right to abortion.

However, it is not all bad news in the United States. A 2004 ruling in New York involving allegations of maternal alcohol consumption was dismissed in court. Stacey Gilligan was arrested and charged in September 2003 with two counts of child endangering based on allegations that she had consumed alcohol in her 35th week of pregnancy. The prosecutor argued that she had delivered alcohol to her infant through the umbilical cord right after it was born. The court ruled that New York child endangerment laws were not intended to apply to a pregnant woman and her foetus, and the prosecutor's claim that she delivered alcohol through the umbilical cord to the infant at birth was rejected (Taylor, 2004). The American Civil Liberties Union, the National Advocates for Pregnant Women, and numerous medical, public health, family organizations, and individuals opposed the prosecution of women arrested for maternal drug use. Their hard work has culminated in some victories for women.

On 25 April 2004, the March for Women's Lives took place in Washington, DC. A million women gathered to support women's health and reproductive rights. They also gathered to demonstrate their opposition to Bush Jr. and his administration's policies related to women's health and reproductive autonomy. The rally was the largest in U.S. history (Hurman, 2004, p. A9). The March for Women's Lives represents the effort of many women's organizations, health advocates, civil liberty groups, and individuals.

The Future

The focus on pregnant women's behavior deflects attention from the race, class, and gender bias of legal, medical, and social service policy that seeks to regulate women during pregnancy. There is an assumption that these punitive policies will provide healthier pregnancies and maternal outcomes. This is not in fact the case. Punitive policies have deterred pregnant women from accessing services, making them more vulnerable to negative health problems (Goldberg, Abrahamson, & Waldman, 1999). This focus also deflects our attention away from the fact that the United States does not provide universal medical care that would enable women to have healthier pregnancies. Welfare cutbacks and the denial of services and financial aid to mothers suspected of illegal drug use and convicted of drug offences have set up a dire situation for American women and their children (Boyd, 2004; Hirsch, 1999). This focus on women's behavior also deflects attention away from the fact that corporate interests and the wealthy are enjoying increased tax breaks and incentives, especially since President Bush Jr. and the Republican Party took office. Corporate welfare and incentives for the rich are ignored while single mothers, especially those who are suspected of using illegal drugs, are vilified.

Further, U.S. drug laws and drug policies have been instrumental in punishing poor women and mothers, who face insurmountable obstacles to providing for themselves and their children. Faced with the prison industrial complex, welfare and housing cutbacks, a lack of universal health care, and draconian laws that disenfranchise felony drug offenders and deprive them of welfare and housing benefits, women struggle to maintain themselves and their families. Their plight is further burdened by the following factors: maternal/state conflicts; conservative and narrow views of women's rights; and President Bush Jr.'s religious convictions about women's role in the family and society, as well as his personal quest to limit women's reproductive rights.

Women in other nations should attempt to follow what is going on in the United States. Critics of drug policy note that American military, economic, and social support is usually accompanied by the Americanization of criminal law, including drug law (Nadelmann, 1993). In order to be eligible for U.S. trade and financial incentives, nations thus have to adopt drug laws that comply with U.S. law. Since 2001, the United States has been more forceful in its request that other nations adopt similar drug and anti-terrorist laws to mirror its own. However, the adoption of an American model of law and enforcement has done little to bring peace or safety to the world.

U.S. drug law has little to offer women. Increased military and criminal justice regulation cannot address social issues or abolish the root causes of negative drug use and terrorism. Recent history attests that drug prohibition in the United States is a failure. Only history can tell us about the ultimate impacts of hastily enacted anti-terrorism laws following in the wake of the 11 September 2001 terrorist attacks on the World Trade Center and the Pentagon. However, terrorist acts have not stopped since 2001, while civil liberties and rights have been curtailed and ethnic and religious profiling has increased. It is here that we might learn a lesson from Western drug prohibition. More laws, harsh sentencing and punishment, and the prison industrial complex have not curtailed illegal drug use in the United States. The Americanization of drug law has instead contributed to social problems and increased militarization at home and in other nations.

In Canada, we seem to swing between implementing draconian drug law, policy, and practice, and striving for more humane drug policy. Cutbacks in health care, housing, and social services have done little to aid Canadian women and their families. Nevertheless, since the 1970s Canadians have overwhelmingly indicated that they would like to see a change in drug policy. Yet, the current Conservative government plans to push forward more punitive drug legislation.

Programs such as Fir Square at B.C. Women's Hospital in Vancouver represent a change in attitude and health policy towards pregnant women who use illegal drugs. At Fir Square, medical and social service professionals strive to work with pregnant women to create an environment where family unification rather than child apprehension is the goal. Pregnant women who wish to withdraw from drugs or to stabilize their drug use (through methadone maintenance, for example) are welcome at Fir Square. Maternal drug use is viewed as a risk, but not as the sole factor determining pregnancy outcomes or parenting skills. Unlike some American women entering hospital programs, Canadian women entering Fir Square are not at risk of arrest.

This chapter has presented a brief overview of some of the issues relevant to women in Canada and the United States in relation to the regulation of women who are suspected of using illegal drugs. More work is needed in this area, especially feminist cross-cultural research that will expand the perimeters of women's health research by addressing the overlapping and competing spheres of legal, medical, and social service regulation of women who use illegal drugs. In looking at drug regulation domestically and around the world, it becomes apparent that regulation rarely has anything to do with women's health or with the dangerousness of a specific drug. It has much more to do with political and social factors.The war on drugs is a women's health issue. It is time for a radical change in drug policy. It is time for the women's health movement to challenge drug prohibition in Canada and the United States.

NOTES

1 Sections of this chapter appeared in *Psychotropes*, *10* (3–4, 2004), 153–172.
2 There are many health problems associated with heavy use of tobacco and alcohol, some of which are irreversible. Outside of constipation, there are no organic or long-term health problems related to opium. Rather, due to the criminalization of some narcotics, health-related problems such as overdose deaths due to unknown potency and quantity and the transmission of blood-borne diseases increase (Stevenson et al. 1956). See David Shewan and Phil Dalgarno (2005), pp. 1–17, for a fuller discussion concerning widely held assumptions about heroin use and addiction.

REFERENCES

Addiction Research Foundation. (1997). Solvent's effect on fetus unproven. *The Journal*, *26*(1), 2.
Alexander, B. (1990). *Peaceful measures: Canada's way out of the 'war on drugs.'* Toronto: University of Toronto Press.

Arendt, R., Behnke, M., Black, M., Brown, E., Chasnoff, I.J., Chavkin, W., et al. (2004, 25 February). Top medical doctors and scientists urge major media outlets to stop perpetuating 'crack baby' myth. Retrieved 20 April 2004, from http://www.jointogether.org/sa/files/pdf/sciencenotstigma.pdf.

Armstrong, E. (1998). Diagnosing moral disorder: The discovery and evolution of foetal alcohol syndrome. *Social Science & Medicine, 47*(12), 2025–2042.

Arnup, K. (1994). *Education for Motherhood: Advice for Mothers in Twentieth-Century Canada.* Toronto: University of Toronto Press.

Bashevkin, S. (2002). *Welfare Hot Buttons: Women, Work, and Social Policy Reform.* Toronto: University of Toronto Press.

Berridge, V., & Edwards, G. (1981). *Opium and the People: Opiate Use in Nineteenth Century England.* London: Allan Lane.

Best, J. (1995). Typification and social problems construction. In J. Best (Ed.), *Images of Issues: Typifying Contemporary Social Problems* (2nd ed., pp. 3–10). New York: Aldine de Gruyter.

Best, J. (1999). *Random Violence: How We Talk about New Crimes and New Victims.* Berkeley: University of California Press.

Bianchi, H. (1994). *Justice as Sanctuary.* Bloomington: Indiana University Press.

Bloom, B., Chesney-Lind, M., & Owen, B. (1994). Women in California prisons: Hidden victims of the war on drugs. In The Drug Policy Foundation (Ed.), *The Crucial Next Stage: Health Care and Human Rights* (Section G: 1–10). Washington, DC: Author.

Boe, R., Nafekh, M., Vuong, B., Sinclair, R., & Cousineau, C. (2003). *The Changing Population of the Federal Inmate Population: 1997 and 2002.* Ottawa: Research Branch. Correctional Service of Canada.

Boyd, N. (1991). *High Society: Legal and Illegal Drugs in Canada.* Toronto: Key West Books.

Boyd, S. (1999). *Mothers and Illicit Drugs: Transcending the Myths.* Toronto: University of Toronto Press.

Boyd, S. (2004). *From Witches to Crack Moms: Women, Drug Law, and Policy.* Durham, NC: Carolina Academic Press.

British Columbia Ministry of Children and Family Development. (2003). *Protocol Framework and Working Guidelines Between Child Protection and Alcohol and Drug services.* Victoria, BC: Ministry of Children and Family Development. Retrieved 20 June 2003, from http://www.mct.gov.bc.ca/publications/privacy_charter/pfwg_toc.htm.

Brodie, J., Gavigan, S., & Jenson, J. (1992). *The Politics of Abortion.* Toronto: Oxford University Press.

Bureau of Justice Statistics. (2002). *Probation and Parole Statistics*. Retrieved 18 April 2003, from http://www.ojp.usdoj.gov/bjs/pandp.htm.

Campbell, N. (2000). *Using Women: Gender, Drug Policy, and Social Justice*. New York: Routledge.

Canadian Centre on Substance Abuse. (2004). Highlights: Canadian Addiction Survey. Ottawa: Author.

Center for Reproductive Law and Policy. (1996, February). *Punishing Women for Their Behavior During Pregnancy*. Fact sheet. New York: Author.

Colten, M. (1980). A comparison of heroin-addicted and non-addicted mothers: Their attitudes, beliefs, and parenting experiences. In *Heroin-Addicted Parents and Their Children: Two Reports*. National Institute on Drug Abuse Services Research Report, pp. 1–18. Washington, DC: U.S. Department of Health and Human Services; Public Health Service; Alcohol, Drug Abuse, and Mental Health Administration.

Comack, E. (1986). 'We will get some good out of this riot yet': The Canadian state, drug legislation and class. In S. Brickey and E. Comack (Eds.), *The Social Basis of Law: Critical Readings in the Sociology of Law* (pp. 67–89). Toronto: Garamond Press.

Correctional Service Canada. (2002–2003). *Departmental Performance Report* (2002–2003). Retrieved 10 June 2005, from http://www.csc-scc.gc.ca/text/pblct/dpr/2003/section_3_overview_of_changes_e.shtml.

Covington, S., & Bloom, B. (2003). Gendered justice: Women in the criminal justice system. In B. Bloom (Ed.), *Gendered Justice: Addressing Female Offenders* (pp. 3–23). Durham, NC: Carolina Academic Press.

Dell, C., Sinclair, R., & Boe, R. (2001). *Canadian Federally Incarcerated Adult Women Profiles: Trends from 1981 to 1998*. Ottawa: Research Branch. Correctional Service of Canada.

Desjardins, N., & Hotton, T. (2004). Trends in drug offences and the role of alcohol and drugs in crime. *Juristat, 24*(1), 1–24.

Dorsey, T. (Ed.). (2003). *Drugs and Crime Facts: Enforcement*. U.S. Department of Justice. Bureau of Justice Statistics. Retrieved 25 April 2004, from http://www.ojp.gov/bjs/pub/pdf/dcf.pdf.

Ehrenreich, B., & English, D. (1973). *Witches, Midwives, and Nurses*. New York: Feminist Press.

Etsten, D. (2000). Controversial proposed legislation heightens stigma. *Journal of Addiction and Mental Health, 3*(6), 8.

Faith, K. (1993). *Unruly Women: The Politics of Confinement and Resistance*. Vancouver: Press Gang.

Goldberg, D., Abrahamson, D., & Waldman, A. (1999). *Amici Curiae. Ferguson V. The City of Charleston, South Carolina*, No. 99-936, U.S. Supreme Court, 1–30.

Gray, M. (1999). Long day's journey into night. *Drug Policy Letter, 39*, 12–14.

Hannah-Moffat, K. (2001). *Punishment in Disguise.* Toronto: University of Toronto Press.

Hepburn, M. (1993). Drug use in pregnancy. *British Journal of Hospital Medicine, 49*(1), 51–55.

Hepburn, M. (2002). Providing care for pregnant women who use drugs: The Glasgow Women's Reproductive Health Service. In H. Klee, M. Jackson, & S. Lewis (Eds.), *Drug Misuse and Motherhood* (pp. 250–260). London: Routledge.

Hirsch, A. (1999). *Some Days Are Harder than Hard: Welfare Reform and Women with Drug Convictions in Pennsylvania.* New York: Center for Law and Social Policy.

Humphries, D. (1999). Crack mothers: Pregnancy, drugs, and the media. Columbus: Ohio State University Press.

Hurman, T. (2004, 26 April). Protesters defend abortion rights. *Globe and Mail,* A9.

Kandall, S. (1996). *Substance and Shadow: Women and Addiction in the United States.* Cambridge, MA: Harvard University Press.

Kolder, V., Gallagher, J., & Parsons, M. (1987). Court-ordered obstetrical interventions. *New England Journal of Medicine. 316*(19), 1192–1196.

Kramer H., & Sprenger, J. (1971). *The Malleus Maleficarum.* New York: Dove Publications.

Levine, H.G. (1992). Temperance cultures: Concern about alcohol problems in Nordic and English-speaking cultures. In M. Lader, G. Edwards, & C. Drummond (Eds.), *The Nature of Alcohol and Drug Related Problems* (pp. 16–36). New York: Oxford University Press.

Logli, P. (1990). Drugs in the womb: The newest battlefield in the war on drugs. *Criminal Justice Ethics, 9*(1), 23–39.

Maher, L. (1995). *Dope Girls: Gender, Race and Class in the Drug Economy.* Unpublished doctoral dissertation. Rutgers, State University of New Jersey (New Brunswick, NJ).

Maier, K. (1992). Forced cesarean section as reproductive control and violence: A feminist social work perspective on the 'Baby R' case. Unpublished master's thesis, Simon Fraser University, Burnaby, BC.

Manitoba Government. (1995). *The Child and Family Services Act.* Winnipeg, MB.

Martin, D. (1993). Casualties of the criminal justice system: Women and justice under the war on drugs. *Canadian Journal of Women and the Law, 6*(2), 305–327.

McLaren, A. (1978). Birth control and abortion in Canada 1870–1920. *Canadian Historical Review, 59*(3), 319–340.

Medrano, M. (1996). Does a discrete fetal solvent syndrome exist? *Alcoholism Treatment Quarterly, 14*(3), 59–76.

Mitchinson, W. (2002). *Giving Birth in Canada 1900–1950*. Toronto: University of Toronto Press.

Murphy, S., & Rosenbaum, M. (1999). *Pregnant Women on Drugs: Combating Stereotypes and Stigma*. New Brunswick, NJ: Rutgers University Press.

Musto, D. (1987). *The American Disease: Origins of Narcotic Control*. Expanded ed. New York: Oxford University Press.

Musto, D. (Ed.). (2002). *Drugs in America: A Documentary History*. New York: Routledge.

Nadelmann, E. (1993). *Cops Across Borders: The Internationalization of U.S. Criminal Law Enforcement*. University Park: Pennsylvania State University Press.

National Center for Policy Analysis (NCPA). (2002). *Idea House. Pharmaceutical Use*. Retrieved 24 May 2002, from http://www.ncpa.org/health/pdh/mar98.html.

National Institute for Health Care Management (NIHCM). (2002). *Prescription Drug Expenditures in 2001: Another Year of Escalating Costs*. Rev. ed. Washington, DC: National Institute for Health Care Management, Research and Educational Foundation.

Nelson, J. (2002). 'A strange revolution in the manners of the country': Aboriginal-settler intermarriage in nineteenth-century British Columbia. In J. McLaren, R. Menzies, & D. Chunn (Eds.), *Regulating Lives: Historical Essays on the State, Society, the Individual and the Law* (pp. 23–62). Vancouver: University of British Columbia Press.

Nolan, P. (2003). *Cannabis: Report of the Senate Special Committee on Illegal Drugs*. Toronto: University of Toronto Press.

Oakley, A. (1984). *The Captured Womb*. Oxford: Basil Blackwell.

Paltrow, L. (2004). Do pregnant women have rights? *Alternet*. Retrieved 22 April 2004, from http://www.alternet.org/story.html?StoryID=18493.

Paltrow, L., Cohen, D., & Carey, C. (2000). Governmental responses to pregnant women who use alcohol and other drugs: Year 2000 overview. Retrieved 12 March 2003, from http://www.advocatesforpregnantwomen.org/articles/gov_response_review.pdf.

Pfohl, S. (1994). *Images of Deviance and Social Control: A Sociological History*. 2nd ed. New York: McGraw-Hill.

Reinarman, C. (2000). The social impact of drugs and the war on drugs: The social construction of drug scares. In S. Tree (Ed.), *The War on Drugs: Addicted to Failure* (pp. 58–65). Washington, DC: Institute for Policy Studies.

Roberts, D. (2002). *Shattered Bonds: The Colour of Child Welfare*. New York: Basic Civitas Books.

Rose, K. (1996). *American Women and the Repeal of Prohibition*. New York: New York University Press.

Rosenbaum, M. (1981). *Women on Heroin*. 2nd ed. New Brunswick, NJ: Rutgers University Press.

Roth, R. (2000). *Making Women Pay: The Hidden Costs of Foetal Rights*. London: Cornell University Press.

Shewan, D., & Dalgarno, P. (2005). Low levels of negative health and social outcomes among non-treatment heroin users in Glasgow (Scotland): Evidence for controlled heroin use? *British Journal of Psychology, 10*, 1–17.

Single, E., Van Truong, M., Adlaf, E., & Ialomiteanu, A. (1999). *Canadian Profile: Alcohol, Tobacco and Other Drugs*. Toronto: Canadian Centre on Substance Abuse and Centre for Addiction and Mental Health.

Smart, C. (1989). *Feminism and the Power of the Law*. London: Routledge.

State of South Carolina v. Regina D. McKnight. (2001). No. 00-GS-26-0432, 00-GS-26-3330, S.D. Court of General Sessions (14–16 May 2001).

Stevenson, G., Lingley, L., Trasov, G., & Stansfield, H. (1956). *Drug Addiction in British Columbia: A Research Survey*. Unpublished manuscript, University of British Columbia, Vancouver.

Taylor, A. (1993). *Women Drug Users*. Oxford: Clarendon Press.

Taylor, D. (2004). Does a foetus have more rights than its mother? *The Guardian*. Retrieved 23 April 2004, from http://www.guardian.co.uk/women/story/0,3604,1201291,00html.

Turnbull, L. (2001). *Double Jeopardy: Motherhood and the Law*. Toronto: Sumach Press.

U.S. Federal Bureau of Prisons. (2002). *Statistical Data*. U.S. Department of Justice. Retrieved 17 February 2003, from http://www.bop.gov.

Warner, J. (2002). *Craze: Gin and Debauchery in an Age of Reason*. New York: Four Walls Eight Windows.

13 Women's Voices Matter: Creating Women-Centred Mental Health Policy

MARINA MORROW

In Canada, despite government commitments to health and mental health promotion[1] and to supporting citizen engagement, the degree to which mechanisms have been developed to support the meaningful involvement of people in health care policy decision-making varies greatly from province to province and region to region. The discrimination and stigma associated with mental illness[2] and the enduring belief that people with mental illness cannot make competent decisions means that the engagement of mental health care recipients[3] has lagged in comparison with other populations. This engagement has come with the evolving belief that people with mental illness can make meaningful contributions to policy and service delivery decision-making. It is also the result of contestation by anti-psychiatry activists, the psychiatric survivor movement,[4] and some feminists who have argued that involving psychiatric survivors in decision-making is a right of citizenship (e.g., Chamberlin, 1978). These groups have been pivotal in putting forth recovery models that support the involvement of people with mental illness not only in policy decision-making but in a wide range of active community roles (e.g., Everett et al., 2003).

This chapter begins with a discussion of women's mental health and then goes on to critically explore citizen engagement mechanisms for the involvement of mental health care recipients, the participation barriers faced by women, and the implications for women-responsive mental health policy and program development. Additionally, the ways in which women have pressured the system from outside formal mechanisms will also be explored in order to assess how these tactics have succeeded in pushing for changes in mental health care and in opening up more space for women's participation.

The arguments in this chapter are supported by information drawn from a three-year comparative study (2000–2003) of mental health reforms in the provinces of British Columbia, Ontario, and Quebec.[5] These three provinces were chosen for study because, although each encompasses some of Canada's major urban centres, each has developed mental health policy in its own unique way.

Women and Mental Health

In order to apprehend the importance of public participation mechanisms for women's involvement in mental health policy decision-making one must, as Barnes and Bowl (2001) assert, understand mental health as a 'gendered concept.' That is, our very notions of 'mental health,' 'mental illness,' and 'madness' arise from discursive practices that have positioned women as more vulnerable to mental instability.

So when we then ask, why are the concerns of women with mental health problems unique in comparison with men's? And, why is it necessary to actively attend to involving women in participation mechanisms? The answer to these questions comes in understanding the historical role that medical science, and psychiatry in particular, has played with respect to understanding women's mental health. In Foucault's (1965) historical study of the experience of madness he illustrates how one of the key surviving discourses about mental illness emerges during the Renaissance – that is, that 'madness' is to be juxtaposed against reason. As Barnes and Bowl (2001) argue, 'In a society in which the scientific rationality of enlightenment thinking provides the key point of reference, the irrationality of the insane presents a profound threat to social order as well as to personal integrity' (p. 9). Given that women have historically been understood as located on the 'irrational' or 'nature' side of the nature/culture binary, it is not surprising that in Western thinking, women more than men have come to be understood as mentally unstable. Indeed, the classic example of the nineteenth-century belief that hysteria was tied to women's reproductive organs (a wandering uterus) provides evidence of this. The dominance of men in medical science combined with sexist beliefs solidified this understanding of women, and henceforth psychiatry and psychology continued to view women through the lens of mental instability.

For most of the nineteenth century, a woman's mental state was tied explicitly to her anatomy – that is, being a woman made you more susceptible to madness. Later, with the study of psychology, women who did not adhere to traditional gender roles were often deemed mentally ill (Astbury, 1996; Caplan, 1987a; Chesler, 1972; Ripa, 1990). Broverman et al. (1970) in their now famous study in which they examined sex-role stereotyping in clinical judgments of men and women discovered that the healthy ideal to which psychologists and psychiatrists adhered in mental health reflected characteristics associated more with traditional male gender-roles than with female roles. The result was a double bind, which meant that with respect to mental health if a woman conformed to her gender role (for example, by being passive) she was seen as unhealthy as an adult, but if she did not (for example, by being assertive) she was deemed unhealthy as a woman (Broverman, Broverman, Clarkson, Rosencrantz, & Vogel, 1970; Kimball, 1975). What this research suggested was that the traditional female sex role had negative mental health consequences for women (Woolsey, 1977). These studies also raised important questions about the validity of diagnostic practices, and stimulated critiques of the ways in which the *Diagnostic and Statistical Manual of Mental Disorders (DSM)*[6] reflects deeply held sexist and racist beliefs (Caplan, 1987b, 1995, 2005; Pavkov, Lewis, & Lyons, 1989).

Critiques were also developed regarding the ways in which psychiatry and psychology position women, and how the systems ostensibly set up to help women in fact function as systems of social control (e.g., Chan, Chunn, & Menzies, 2005). Historically, examples abound of how women suffering violence at the hands of male partners and/or trauma as a result of early childhood sexual abuse were disbelieved or diagnosed as mentally ill (Rush, 1980). Lesbians, in particular, were pathologized and 'treatment' in both of these instances often consisted of exhortations to women to take up roles associated with heterosexual femininity with more enthusiasm (Blackbridge & Gilhooly, 1985).

Debates about the relevance of diagnostic categories notwithstanding, contemporarily the evidence within the fields of psychiatry and psychology shows that although men and women do not vary in the overall prevalence of mental illness, sex and gender differences do exist in the types of diagnoses, the development and course of mental illness, treatment practices,[7] and in the access and utilization of mental health services.

Gender differences exist in the rates of specific mental health problems (Gold, 1998; Prior, 1999). Women are about twice as likely as men to be diagnosed with depression (Health Statistics Division, 1998) and anxiety (Howell, Brawman-Mintzer, Monnier, & Yonkers, 2001), while men are about four times more likely than women to be diagnosed with substance use problems or antisocial behaviours. Data from the National Population Health Survey also reveals that women are more likely to experience recurring depressive episodes, and that 72 per cent of people who reported a depressive episode were women (Health Statistics Division, 1998). Women are more likely than men to be diagnosed with seasonal affective disorder, eating disorders, panic disorders, and phobias. Women also attempt suicide more often than men. Men have a higher incidence of completed suicide, substance abuse, antisocial personality disorder, and early-onset schizophrenia than women do. Obsessive-compulsive disorder, schizophrenia, and bipolar disorder appear to be diagnosed equally among men and women (Federal Provincial and Territorial Advisory Committee on Population Health, 1996), although the onset of schizophrenia tends to be later in women.

With respect to mental health care utilization, many studies have found that women are more likely than men to use services for mental health care reasons (Lefebvre, Lesage, Cyr, Toupin, & Fournier, 1998; Rhodes, Goering, To, & Williams, 2002). Interestingly, data collected for the 2003 Canadian Community Health Survey, shows that overall, women are 2.9 times more likely to use primary health care services for mental health complaints, yet are also more likely to report that their mental health care needs are unmet (Statistics Canada, 2003).

Attention to the diversity among women has not been as well developed. However, although the literature on the experiences of Aboriginal, racialized, and immigrant women is in its nascent stages, increasingly, the impact of colonization on the mental health of women in Aboriginal communities is being explored, especially with respect to the intersections between mental health and experiences of violence (den Heyer, Wien, Knockwood, & Virick, 2001; Farley, Lynne, & Cotton, 2005; Health Canada, 2003; Kirmayer, Brass, & Tait, 2001; Roberts, Roberts, & Chen, 1997). The specific concerns of women of colour and immigrant women who come into contact with the mental health system are also receiving more attention with examinations of the effects of acculturation and racism on women's mental health (Boyer, Ku, & Shakir, 1997; Canadian Task Force on Mental Health Issues Affecting Immigrants and Refugees, 1988; Chui, Morrow, Clark, & Ganeson, 2005; Health Canada, 2003; Morrow, Smith, Lai, Jaswal, forthcoming).

Research demonstrates that the differing rates of mental illness and substance use problems between and among men and women are the result of an interaction between biological and psychosocial factors across the lifespan (see Chapter 2, this collection). However, research and treatment has tended to focus more on biological factors, leading to a biomedically biased mental health system (Morrow & Chappell, 1999).

Psychosocial explanations examine the ways in which women are more vulnerable to poorer mental health as the result of socialization into the female gender role (e.g., how socialization may result in lower self-esteem and greater vulnerability to depression) and the ways in which particular social roles and experiences may be associated with poorer mental health.

Poverty and social inequality are also key factors in mental health, factors which disproportionately affect women and especially Aboriginal and elderly women (e.g., CPHI National Roundtable, 2003; Ross, 2003; Saraceno & Barbui, 1997; Wilton, 2003). For women with mental illness, poverty is often associated with increased risk of violence and abuse (Anderson & Chiocchio, 1997). Research has also shown a strong connection between poverty, violence, mental illness, and addictions (Harris, 1997, 1998).

Other possible social explanations of mental illnesses in women include the adverse effects of inferior social status, impaired self-esteem, disproportionate burden of family caregiving, sexual abuse and sexual discrimination, economic inequities, and constricted educational and occupational opportunities.

In addition to gender, social differences which effect people's status and access to resources such as race, ethnicity, sexual orientation, gender identity, and class are important for understanding the development of mental health problems, their subsequent progression, and the supports needed to ameliorate the effects for different population groups. Applying an intersectional analysis to the study of differences between and among men and women is therefore a necessary tool for improving knowledge about diverse populations. That is, analyses of mental health must recognize that gender inequality is a feature in all populations, while not losing sight of the importance of race, ethnicity, class, and other social dimensions.

The established knowledge base regarding the differences between men's and women's mental health concerns and the evidence of systemic sexism within psychology and psychiatry provide a powerful rationale for actively engaging women in public participation mechanisms on issues related to mental health policy and service delivery.

Citizen Engagement, the Mental Health System, and Women

Barnes and Bowl (2001) assert that 'ideology, power and practice have contributed to the disempowerment of people who have been diagnosed with mental illness' (p. x). In particular, the tension in psychiatry between social control and care and treatment of people is an ongoing controversy with concrete implications for the civil rights of people with mental illness diagnoses, and therefore for their full participation in the community (Barnes & Bowl, 2001).

Citizenship is not just about having citizenship rights (e.g., legal or civil rights, political rights, or social and economic rights), it is also about the capacity to 'practice as citizens.' As Barnes and Bowl (2001) point out, 'In terms of the relationship between the individual and the state this can mean, in practice, the extent to which people are able to contribute to the creation of public services which are often the form through which this relationship is mediated' (p. 15). That is, citizenship is integrally tied to political participation. Indeed, a key campaign of psychiatric survivors has been to petition for a voice in their own treatment and in the development of mental health policy.

Women historically were excluded from the rights and responsibilities of citizenship, and thus feminists have argued for women's equal representation in formal politics and have shown the ways in which women's traditional roles as caregivers have presented obstacles to the practice of citizenship. For feminists, democratic ideals had to be put into practice in the form of participatory democracy. Indeed, as Vogel (1994) indicates, the ideal of radical democratic citizenship was the idea that women's citizenship 'would evolve from praxis and the self-organization of women and from the dialogue between autonomous groups' (p. 87).

The struggle of women with mental illness to be accepted as full citizens in their communities, and as being able to make valuable contributions to social and cultural life, has been hampered by stigma and discriminatory practices which keep these individuals from being able to gain and maintain employment and other active community roles. Thus, the experiences of women with mental illness underscores the importance of seeing citizenship as a combination of having individual rights and the ability to meaningfully participate in society and its political decision making processes (Lister, 2003).

Institutions and state and social practices shape the experience of citizenship for women with mental illness. For example, the practice of involuntary committal, where women lose the right to determine their own treatment, and the experience of many women with mental illness who are mothers, who lose the right to have contact with their children (Greaves et al., 2004), are both illustrative of the ways in which women's experience of citizenship is constrained by state practices. Citizenship for people with mental illness involves mechanisms that would foster their participation in decision making about their lives, and about the practices and polices that impact them. This involvement must include attention to the ways in which social and power differences among people with mental illness may constrain, in particular, the engagement of women and racialized groups.

Citizen engagement must be understood within the broader context of service delivery and policy development in mental health care in Canada. In Canada, mental health policy development generally falls under provincial jurisdiction, and the delivery of services and management of mental health budgets are handled regionally in most provinces and territories (Ontario is the exception). The federal government plays a peripheral role by guiding policy direction through the development of federal initiatives and by facilitating communication between the federal, provincial, and territorial levels. However, the federal government has an important role to play in ensuring that mental health receives funding on par with other forms of health spending. Indeed, one of the oft-levelled criticisms is that mental health care is given an inadequate share of the federal health care budget (Romanow, 2002). Others have argued that a national body is needed to oversee mental health care and for information exchange (Kirby, 2006).

Although the federal government has released a number of important documents pertaining to mental health over the last decade (e.g., *Mental Health for Canadians: Striking a Balance* (National Health and Welfare Canada, 1989), followed by the two-phase study by the Federal/Provincial/Territorial Advisory Network on Mental Health (1997) aimed at making recommendations regarding an integrated system of care for the seriously mentally ill), these reports have not incorporated an analysis of the ways in which mental illness affects women and men differently. Partly out of this concern a federal/territorial/provincial committee was struck to look at women's mental health, and this committee released its report in 1993 (Federal/Provincial/Territorial Working Group on Women's Health, 1993). As of 2005 this was the last federally supported document on women's mental health that has been produced in Canada. Indeed, the more recently released report from Senator Michael Kirby (2006), which is otherwise comprehensive in its review of the Canadian mental health system, virtually ignores the specific concerns of women (Ad Hoc Working Group on Women, 2006). Thus, national reports, the federal government, and organizations have paid limited attention to mental health generally, and less attention to the concerns specific to women.

Commitments to involving mental health care recipients and their families in policy and treatment decision-making processes emerged in formal policy statements and mental health plans in the late 1980s, and mechanisms to enact this involvement were established. Currently, these involvement mechanisms vary, and are dependent in part on how vibrant the psychiatric survivor movements are in each locale, the role of women within these movements, and the degree to which mechanisms for participation have been formally built into mental health structures. Mechanisms can include things like the establishment of committees that formally consult and advise policy makers, strategies designed to facilitate the leadership of mental health care recipients in service delivery development, and other initiatives that facilitate the participation of people with mental illness in the larger community.

The degree to which the mental health system is responsive to women can therefore be assessed through an examination of (1) the degree to which governments have made explicit commitments to women's mental health, including resources to support those commitments; and (2) the degree to which women who are or have been recipients of mental health care are supported in citizen engagement mechanisms for influencing mental health policy and practice. These two components are integrally linked. That is, generally women and women's advocates have pressured governments to make explicit policy commitments to women, and these commitments in turn have often facilitated women's participation. It should be noted that initiatives vary with respect to their perspectives on the practices of psychiatry, and evidence of initiatives is not necessarily synonymous with critical/progressive practice vis-à-vis women.

Examples from the provinces of Ontario, Quebec, and British Columbia illuminate the differences in approaches and highlight the degree to which each province is responsive to women's mental health concerns.

Women and Mental Health Policy in Ontario, Quebec and British Columbia

Each of these provinces have different histories with respect to the development of initiatives on women's mental health. These initiatives, in turn, are influenced by the overall policy context and the degree to which the governments in each jurisdiction have actively engaged psychiatric survivor groups, women's movement organizations, and community-based mental health services.

Ontario

In Ontario, there is a strong and radical movement of psychiatric survivors that have had a direct impact on the direction of policy. This combined with sympathetic support from some politicians, bureaucrats, and academics has resulted in the development of some important user-directed initiatives, for example, the Ontario Consumer Development Initiatives, which supported mental health care recipients in peer-directed projects (Trainor, Shepherd, Boydell, Leff, & Crawford, 1997), and economic development models that have acted outside of the mental health system (Church, 1997, 2001).

The psychiatric survivor movement in Ontario has been characterized by a high degree of interaction between participants in the movement, other activists, and mental health professionals. This activity peaked in the late 80s and early 90s with the Canadian Mental Health Association initiative, *Building a Framework of Support*, which was the first attempt in Canada to put into policy a consultative framework that would bring psychiatric survivors together with policy makers and mental health care providers (Trainor, Pomeroy, & Pape, 1993). This framework has recently been re-released and some user-directed initiatives continue to flourish (Trainor, Pomeroy, & Pape, 2004).

Although many of the activists in this movement were women, few allied themselves directly with the feminist movement and therefore links with community-based women's organizations, and an analysis of the specific mental health needs of women were not consistently developed as part of the psychiatric survivor movement in Ontario (see Burstow, 2005, for a discussion of this relationship).

Of the provinces studied, Ontario had the widest range of hospital-based specialized programs for women's mental health. Indeed, Ontario appears to have moved beyond government policy commitments to women's mental health into funding for actual programs. The bulk of these programs are concentrated in Toronto (e.g., the Women's Therapy Centre). Further, the University of Toronto has a Women's Mental Health Program in the Department of Psychiatry. At the time of the research the department had identified women's mental health as a priority. The result of this program has been more research in the area of women's mental health and more education for psychiatry residents on women's mental health. The Women's Mental Health and Addiction Research Section at the Centre for Addiction and Mental Health (one of Canada's leading addiction and mental health teaching hospitals) is active in professional training, education, and public forums, and in maintaining community partnerships.

Ontario, especially in the urban centre of Toronto has a well-developed women's movement and a community-based women's service sector (e.g., women's centres, shelters, rape crisis centres, and so on) and a well-developed hospital-based support system for women, and some links between the two domains are evident in programming and practice. Toronto should also be noted for its well-developed ethno-specific service sector, which includes some programming specific to racialized women and immigrant and refugee women, both at hospital and community-based levels. Formal provincial mechanisms to involve women diagnosed with mental illness in policy making processes, however, are not consistent.

Quebec

Several developments in Quebec are important with respect to raising the specific concerns of women at policy and program levels. The first is the work of psychiatric survivors and the second is the role of the women's movement and the women's service sector. Quebec has a particularly vibrant and politicized community-service sector that includes representation from mental health organizations and women's groups. Through the work of psychiatric survivors and other mental health advocates, the community-service sector has managed to keep mental health visible at the provincial policy level. The role of the women's movement is more complex. Fractures within the women's movement and especially the 'uneasy' relationship between francophone women's organizations and organizations in the diverse ethnic communities[8] that make up Québec, has limited the ability of women's groups to respond to a wider constituency of women. Nevertheless, women's groups in Quebec have come together at certain points historically to effectively draw the government's attention to women's mental health issues. As in the Ontario case, alliances between community-based organizations and academics has also proved fruitful for advancing certain policy strategies, and, in the case of Quebec, alternative approaches to mental health treatment.

Two key consumer/advocacy groups were formed in Quebec in the

1980s. Le regroupement des ressources alternatives en santé mental du Québec, established in 1983, is composed of a variety of community organizations that deal with mental health and promote alternatives to psychiatry. Le regroupement is closely aligned with researchers in Quebec who are interested in alternative mental health models, issues related to culture and mental health, and the evaluation of mental health services based on the concept of 'empowerment.'

Agitation by a provincial association of consumers in Quebec City in the 1980s resulted in the establishment, in 1990, of L'association des groupes d'intervention en défense de droits en santé mentale du Québec (l'AGIDD-SMQ), which is an umbrella organization that oversees consumer advocacy groups throughout the province.[9] L'AGIDD is state-funded and its advocacy function is acknowledged and built into Quebec's 1989 Mental Health Policy.

White (1996) refers to the relationship between these groups and the government as 'conflictual collaboration,' or 'contradictory participation,' to describe the ways in which their autonomy is constrained through the demands arising from government funding. Indeed, although these groups have been able to lobby for the rights of individual mental health care recipients, their ability to affect systemic change has been limited.

L'AGIDD is part of larger coalitions (regroupement), some of which are sectoral (mental health) and some of which are intersectoral (youth, poverty, women, different ethnic groups). These groups are organized at the local level, the regional level, and the provincial level. Individual groups provide services, and the coalitions address larger systemic issues. Mental health groups have historically played a very strong role on these coalitions and have been at the forefront of both developing and critiquing partnerships with government. L'AGIDD also played an active role in critiquing the first official mental health policy released in 1989.

Early feminist critiques of the Quebec 1989 mental health policy focused on how the policy gave only 'lip service' to women's concerns, and argued that it avoided in depth discussion about sex differences in mental health and how traditional gender roles might influence mental health (Guberman, 1990). Although the links between organizations like l'AGIDD and women's groups have not always been strong, the women's sector has played a role in influencing mental health policy. For example, in 1995 Action Autonomie (a group under the l'AGIDD umbrella) instituted a feminist committee that was well linked with other women's organizations in the community (e.g., Herstreet, a service for homeless women, and a broader association of groups working with people on the street). During the years 1993 to 1996, they developed *Le plan d'action en matière des condition feminine*, which resulted in the Ministry of Health and Social Services announcing in 1994 that it was committed to integrating women's issues into mental health. Shortly after this announced commitment Le regroupement des resources alternatives en santé mental du Québec formed a women's committee and undertook a review of their own services. The result has been an ongoing committee that documents women's experiences, develops educational material for mental health groups on women, and fosters collaboration with women's organizations in the community.

In 1997, *Ècoute-moi quand je parle!* was released. The report recommended that 'the Quebec mental health policy recognizes that the sex of a person is a determining and major factor in mental health, at all ages' and 'The Policy [i.e., Quebec's 1989 Mental Health Policy] must institute an analysis that takes into account not only the data concerning each sex, but also the nature of the relationships between men and women, the social and economic realities of the two groups, their expectations and their life conditions' (p. 22). Further, the report foregrounded the social context of women's lives (e.g., single motherhood, violence, and so on) and the social measures of support that are needed to improve women's mental health. The government responded by setting up a committee to monitor issues related to women's mental health.

In 1998, a mental health plan based on models in British Columbia, Ontario, and Alberta was developed in Quebec, and for the first time introduced a focus on people with serious mental illness.[10] Women's groups resisted this focus, in part because they felt that it meant that the mental health concerns of women (which include those related to experiences of violence and trauma and do not always result in diagnoses of serious mental illness) would not be adequately addressed, and, specifically, that this policy shift would mean more psychiatric services over community-based supports.

In 2000, the Ministry of Social Services and Health organized a forum on mental health to mobilize forces in the implementation of the 1998 provisions. Consumer groups were actively involved in the review and a consortium of women's organizations – Table des groupes de femmes de Montréal, in conjunction with the Groupe d'appui à la transformation des services de santé mentale au Québec – produced a report titled *Pour une analyse féministe de la transformation des services de santé mentale au Québec*. This report focused on an analysis of services and on how services could better respond to women with mental health problems.

At the time of my comparative research, a 'partnership' policy was being developed that would outline the relationship between government and community-based groups. The community sector was seeking stronger funding and more autonomy. It was hoped that this would strengthen and further politicize the community sector, and that for mental health this might mean more support for alternatives to psychiatry.

In 2003, a conference (Women, Psychiatry, and Secondary Victimization: Towards a Change in Socio-cultural Perspectives) sponsored by a l'AGIDD member organization was convened to focus on women's mental health and survivors of secondary trauma caused by certain practices in psychiatry. It was the first conference of its kind in Quebec, and it signalled another concrete step on the part of consumer organizations to integrate the concerns of women.[11] Despite this, specialized services for women with mental health problems are few, and the knowledge transfer between women's organizations and mental health orginizations is still relatively infrequent.

British Columbia

The situation in BC differs from that of Ontario and Quebec in that at the time of my study BC had the least formalized consumer survivor movement, which meant that psychiatric survivors had not historically had a strong political voice. Although BC has been part of some important women's mental health initiatives, it has had less activity than Quebec with respect to bringing women's mental health concerns to the forefront of provincial policy. Like Ontario, BC also has some specialized services for women, some of which are located in hospital settings.

BC's health system was regionalized beginning in the 1990s, and in 1998 the BC Mental Health Plan was released. This plan has remained the template for reform, and subsequent governments have focused on commitments to implement it. Under the NDP government (1996–2000) a number of innovative recommendations were implemented, including, the establishment of the BC Mental Health Advocate, whose job it was to track systemic problems in the mental health care system. Further, BC succeeded in having a separate funding envelope for mental health services (i.e., money from the health budget reserved for mental health). Both of these distinct features were lost in the change to the Liberal government in 2001.[12]

During my study of the three provinces, BC had been undergoing dramatic health care restructuring, including the rapid amalgamation of 52 regional health authorities into 6 and the removal of addictions from under the jurisdiction of Ministry of Children and Families to the Ministry of Health Services. The amalgamation of addictions and mental health has been given high priority on the policy agenda in recent years, with subsequent planning and development focused on policy statements and service development that reflect this new structure. Further, cuts and changes to the social welfare system, particularly changes to eligibility requirements for income assistance and disability benefits and the lack of affordable housing – especially in the provinces urban centre of Vancouver, have had especially negative effects on people with mental illness (Morrow, 2006).

As mentioned, the consumer survivor movement in BC has been less organized than in Quebec and Ontario. Key activists have come forward to critique the system and lobby for change, but no sustained movement has occurred. In part this is because the government has not invested money in consumer leadership and involvement, and instead has left this to non-profit organizations. Prior to 1998, there was a strong consumer advisory committee that was supported by the NDP government, and from 1998 to 2001 there was a provincial mental health steering committee (The Mental Health Population Health Advisory Committee), but it did not consistently involve mental health care recipients. The current BC Mental Health Monitoring Coalition is made up primarily of established organizations that represent mental health care recipients and is not psychiatric survivor-driven. Non-profit mental health advocacy organizations are pulled into consultation in a variety of different but inconsistent ways across the province. The priorities of the region appeared to dictate, resulting in some regions that have strong consumer involvement (e.g., Vancouver Coastal Health Authority and the Northern Health Authority) and others where this involvement is minimal.

There was evidence in the community-based mental health sector of some specialized programs for women, and, in some instances, of a feminist analysis of mental health issues. For example, the Vancouver/Richmond Mental Health Network, a consumer-run organization that provides alternatives to psychiatry, had a strong group of feminists in the 1990s who instituted women-only groups and began developing the idea of a safe house. The Motivation, Power and Achievement Society (formerly the Mental Patients' Association[13]) has developed specialized housing for single mothers with mental illness and their children. There is also one transition house for women with mental illness in Vancouver, (Peggy's Place) and, at the time of the research, at least one drop-in/ advocacy organization had women-only space (the Kettle Friendship Society).

In 1998, shortly after the mental health plan was released, a group of individuals came together at the invitation of the BC Centre of Excellence for Women's Health (BCCEWH) to discuss the ways in which the plan did not comprehensively address women's mental health. Subsequent to this, the provincial government funded a province-wide study that examined the experiences of women with serious mental illness within the mental health system. The resulting report, *Hearing Women's Voices: Mental Health Care for Women* was released in 1999 and was the starting place for subsequent research at the BCCEWH on issues particular to women's mental health (Morrow, 2002a, 2003a; Morrow & Chappell, 1999); and a long-standing Women's Mental Health Discussion Group, which brought together mental health care practitioners, psychiatric survivors, researchers, and policy makers.

During this time, the Ministry's Advisory Council on Women's Health, which had a sub-committee on mental health, supported the work of the BCCEWH at both research and policy levels. The provincial Women's Health Bureau funded the Ministry's Advisory Council on Women's Health, and its role was to advise the provincial government.[14]

In 2003, the BCCEWH hosted an interdisciplinary, cross-sectoral national symposium on women's mental health to develop priorities for a national research agenda (Morrow, 2002c). A unique feature of this symposium was the involvement of community-based researchers and psychiatric survivors. Subsequent to this meeting, the BCCEWH released a policy brief on creating a national strategy on women's mental health (Morrow, 2003b) that was meant to feed into national activities on mental health, involving, at the time, the Canadian Alliance on Mental Health and Mental Illness and the Canadian Mental Health Association, both of which have agitated for a national mental health strategy. More recently, much of the activity at the BCCEWH has focused on examining the intersections between violence, mental health, and substance use and the cross-training of mental health workers and women's advocates on these issues. Further, the BCCEWH has joined with feminist activists and academics to raise awareness of women's mental health concerns leading up to and following the release of the Kirby Report (Ad Hoc Working Group on Women, Mental Health, Mental Illness & Addiction, 2006).

Although research on women's mental health and policy development is strong, and there is evidence to suggest that mental health care recipients have been involved in some of these initiatives, very little concrete change has occurred at the service level. BC does have some specialized programs for women (e.g., Reproductive Mental Health, at BC Women's Hospital, individual workers on mental health teams that work on issues related to women and trauma, a transition house for women with mental illness), but at the government level, initiatives and planning are still frequently carried out without consulting women's groups and specialists in women's mental health.

Discussion

A review of provincial policy demonstrates broad philosophical consistency across provinces. All jurisdictions have committed to improving access to mental health services, improving coordination of the mental health system, decentralizing administration and service delivery, promoting opportunities for 'self-help,' preventing unnecessary hospitalization, and increasing community (consumer and family) participation in the decision-making process (McNaughton, 1992; Morrow, 2002b). However, this review also makes it clear that mental health policy continues to be guided by frameworks that are gender-neutral and do not take into account relations of race, class, and other forms of social difference. Even the few women-specific supports that have been developed rarely employ an intersectional analysis that understands gender as bound together with relations of class, race, age, sexual orientation, and ability.

Although a gender analysis is largely absent from the documents reviewed in each province, there is an acknowledgement that mental health care recipients and their needs are not homogeneous, and a wide range of services is therefore required. In most provinces stakeholder participation in policy making is now institutionalized, involving committees or councils with representation from mental health consumers, family members or caregivers, service providers, and other community members. This participatory policy structure theoretically gives marginalized groups of women access to the policy-making process, although, as evidenced, the degree to which this actually occurs is variable. Specifically, there is little institutionalized space for the critique of psychiatric practices.

In reviewing evidence from each of these three provinces, what is striking is the degree to which women's mental health programming, both at the hospital and community level, has developed in the absence of consistent government commitments to women's mental health. Indeed, policy statements about women's mental health are generally brief in provincial mental health plans and they are rarely accompanied by specific strategies for fostering women's mental health care.

Mechanisms that foster the participation of mental health care recipients are evident in several provinces in the form of advisory committees, and, perhaps more meaningfully, in the form of user-directed initiatives.

However, the only evidence of avenues for women's engagement was at the non-governmental organization (NGO) level and most often through community-based mental health services, the women's movement, and the women's service sector. The most common form of participation was in the form of consultation – sometimes government-initiated, but more often initiated by groups concerned about women's mental health. User-directed initiatives do not always directly influence policy but in several evaluations they have been found to foster the capacity and skills needed to more fully participate in decision-making processes.

Finally, although there was evidence in each province of interactions between the women's movement (usually through service-providing organizations), women's mental health is not currently a key issue for the Canadian women's movement. This finding is consistent with the work of others (e.g., Burstow, 2005) who argue that feminist involvement in mental health is critical in order to maintain a critique of the practices of psychiatry that might be damaging to women.

Women-Centred Mental Health Care: Fostering Meaningful Participation for Women

The ability to foster women's meaningful participation in the policies and practices of mental health is dependent on the strength of collaborations between psychiatric survivor organizations, women's movement organizations, and community-based mental health services. Further, the adoption of women-centred care principles in mental health more generally might facilitate both a better understanding of women's specific mental health needs and help develop mechanisms that actively engage women in decision-making. In turn, women's engagement would allow a space for the critique/evaluation of practices that are harmful to women.

Women-centred care models, which originally emerged in the women's health movement over concerns that the health care system did not adequately address the unique needs and concerns of women, are comprised of the following key elements: a focus on women, involvement and participation of women, empowerment, respect, and safety (Doyal, 1998). Further, services that are women-centred should address the complexities of women's lives, be inclusive of diversity, provide integrated service delivery, and information and education (Barnett, White, & Horne, 2002).

Although the development of women-centred models has been primarily focused on the development and delivery of services to women, women-centred principles have also been extended to discussions about health policy development. The most obvious examples of this are the development of gender-based analysis tools (see Chapter 5, this collection) to review health policies for their potentially differential impact on men and women. The other ways in which the concept of women-centred mental health care is advanced in policy is through reports focused specifically on the concerns of women (e.g., Federal/Provincial/Territorial Working Group on Women's Health, 1993; Gawthier, Leclerc, & Roberge, 1997; Memoire de L'R des centres de femmes du Quebec, 1997; Morrow, 2003b) and through government consultations and participation mechanisms that involve women.

The consistency with which these principles are applied varies, however, and governments have been hesitant to put political will behind their stated commitments to women's mental health. Thus, the most progressive work on women and mental health is occurring outside of institutional settings and (although to a limited degree) in the women's movement and in the community.

An important marker of citizenship is the degree to which individuals in a society have access to forms of political participation, including the ability to influence public policy. Given that people's experiences of citizenship are marked by gender and other forms of social difference, it follows that gender neutral understandings of mental health and mental illness will not suffice in the development of participatory mechanisms. For women's voices to matter they must be heard, and this requires action on behalf of governments, policy makers, and providers to ensure the establishment of mechanisms that support women's participation.

NOTES

1 Health Canada has a Mental Health Promotion Division. See http://www.
   hc-sc.gc.ca/hppb/mentalhealth/mhp/index.html.

2 In this chapter, the term *mental illness* is understood as a contest concept
   and is used with this awareness. That is, as will be outlined, debates exist
   about the scientific validity of diagnostic labels of mental illness. Despite
   this, however, it is also recognized that many people suffer from real
   disabling conditions that affect their mental health.

3 A wide range of terms exist to describe people who have used the mental
   health system. Most of these terms reflect differing perspectives on the
   treatment of people in the context of psychiatry. For example, the terms
   psychiatric survivor, psychiatrized, and *consumer/survivor* tend to reflect
   critical perspectives on the experience of psychiatric hospitalization. The
   terms *consumer* or *mental health client* is favoured by those who uncritically
   endorse psychiatric care, while the term *mental health care recipient* tends to
   be more neutral. I use a variety of these terms throughout the chapter,
   usually in ways that reflect the beliefs of the particular constituent discussed.

4 Burstow (2005) helpfully points to the distinctions and overlap between
   the psychiatric survivor movement, anti-psychiatry, and feminism with
   respect to mental health. Historically, the psychiatric survivor movement
   was driven by people who had had experiences of psychiatric institutionalization, whereas the anti-psychiatry movement was driven by professionals and academics who critiqued psychiatry and concepts like 'mental
   illness.' Contemporarily, both movements are led by psychiatric survivors
   but the anti-psychiatry movement is distinct in its altogether rejection of
   the institution of psychiatry. While members of the psychiatric survivor
   movement may be highly critical of the practices of psychiatry, their
   positions on psychiatry vary. What the two movements share 'is a commitment to the centrality of psychiatric survivors, a commitment to appreciate
   difference, an ethic of common support, and, what is fundamental, an
   appreciation that psychiatry is or can be oppressive'(p. 247). While some
   feminists have been actively engaged in these movements, the feminist
   movement as a whole has not taken the abuses of psychiatry as a central
   concern.

5 Interviews with key individuals working in the mental health system
   were conducted in each province and an extensive review of policy documents and reports related to mental health was also undertaken. The
   author would like to acknowledge the Canadian Institutes of Health
   Research for their support in carrying out this research.

6 The DSM is the manual used by mental health professionals to diagnose people.

7 For example, studies have shown that women, disproportionately to men, are prescribed benzodiazepines (Currie, 2003) and receive electroshock two to three times more often (Burstow, 1994).

8 Historically, in Quebec, tensions related to language and sovereignty have had an impact on the relationships between white Quebecois women and those from other racial and ethnic backgrounds in the women's movement.

9 At the time of research L'AGIDD did not have representation in northern Quebec, however, efforts were being made to establish better links with these (predominantly Aboriginal) communities.

10 A focus of policy and resources on people with the most serious and persistent forms of mental illness (usually Axis I diagnoses, according to the DSM; for example, schizophrenia, depression, and other mood disorders) began to be introduced in provincial mental health plans in the 90s to ensure that these individuals did not go without care. A number of factors have contributed to this policy shift in Canada, including concerns that the psychiatric deinstitutionalization movement had left people with the most debilitating illnesses without adequate services.

11 Researchers in BC (including the author) documenting similar issues were invited to address the conference and present their research, which resulted in an important cross-provincial exchange.

12 Under the Liberals 2000–2004 term, a Minister of State for Mental Health was appointed and a Minister's Advisory Council was established. In 2005, when the Liberals began their second term, the position of Minister of State was lost in the new Cabinet shuffle and the council was disbanded.

13 MPA began in the 1970s as a progressive psychiatric survivor-driven organization.

14 The Ministry's Advisory Council on Women's Health has subsequently been eliminated.

REFERENCES

Ad Hoc Working Group on Women, Mental Health, Mental Illness and Addiction. (2006). *Women, Mental Health, Mental Illness and Addiction: An Overview*. Winnipeg, MB: Canadian Women's Health Network.

Anderson, C., & Chiocchio, K. (1997). The interface of homelessness, addictions and mental illness in the lives of trauma survivors. In M. Harris & C. Landis (Eds.), *Sexual Abuse in the Lives of Women Diagnosed with Serious Mental Illness* (pp. 21–38). New York: Harwood Academic Publishers.

Astbury, J. (1996). *Crazy for You: The Making of Women's Madness*. New York: Oxford University Press.

Barnes, M., & Bowl, R. (2001). *Taking Over the Asylum: Empowerment and Mental Health*. Basingstoke, Hampshire: Palgrave.

Barnett, R., White, S., & Horne, T. (2002). *Voices from the Front Lines: Models of Women-Centred Care in Manitoba and Saskatchewan*. Winnipeg, MB: Prairie Women's Health Centre of Excellence.

Blackbridge, P., & Gilhooly, S. (1985). *Still Sane*. Vancouver: Press Gang.

Boyer, M., Ku, J., & Shakir, U. (1997). *The Healing Journey: Phase II Report – Women and Mental Health: Documenting the Voices of Ethnoracial Women Within an Anti-Racist Framework*. Toronto: Across Boundaries Mental Health Centre.

Broverman, I.K., Broverman, D.M., Clarkson, F.E., Rosencrantz, P.S., & Vogel, S.R. (1970). Sex-role stereotypes and clinical judgements of mental health. *Journal of Counselling and Clinical Psychology, 34*(1), 1–7.

Burston, B. (1994). *When Women End Up in Those Horrible Places* (Video). Toronto, Author.

Burstow, B. (2005). Feminist antipsychiatry praxis – women and the movement(s): A Canadian perspective. In W. Chan, D. Chunn, & R. Menzies (Eds.), *Women, Madness and the Law: A Feminist Reader* (pp. 245–258). London: Glasshouse.

Canadian Task Force on Mental Health Issues Affecting Immigrants and Refugees. (1988). *After the Door Has Been Opened*. Ottawa: Minister of Supply and Services.

Caplan, P. (1987a). *The Myth of Women's Masochism*. Scarborough, ON: New American Library of Canada.

Caplan, P. (1987b). The psychiatric association's failure to meet its own standards: The dangers of self-defeating personality disorder as a category. *Journal of Personality Disorders, 2*(178).

Caplan, P. (1995). *They Say You're Crazy: How the World's Most Powerful Psychiatrists Decide Who's Normal*. Reading, MA: Addison-Wesley Longman.

Caplan, P. (2005). Sex Bias in Psychiatric Diagnosis and the Courts. In W. Chan, D. Chunn, & R. Menzies (Eds.), *Women, Madness and the Law: A Feminist Reader*. London: Glasshouse Press.

Chamberlin, J. (1978). *On Our Own: Patient Controlled Alternatives to the Mental Health System*. New York: Hawthorne Books.

Chan, W., Chunn, D., & Menzies, R. (Eds.). (2005). *Women, Madness and the Law: A Feminist Reader*. London: Glasshouse Press.

Chesler, P. (1972). *Women and Madness*. New York: Avon Books.

Chui, L., Morrow, M., Clark, N., & Ganeson, S. (2005). Spirituality and treatment choices by South and East Asian women with serious mental illness. *Transcultural Psychiatry, 42*(4), 630–656.

Church, K. (1997). Business (not quite) as usual: Psychiatric survivors and community economic development in Ontario. In E. Shragg (Ed.), *Community Economic Development: In Search of Empowerment* (2nd ed.). Montreal: Black Rose.

Church, K. (2001). Imagining a better world: 'Working like crazy' on economic security for users of mental health services. Unpublished article.

CPHI National Roundtable. (2003). *Poverty and Health: Links to Action*. Proceedings of the CPHI National Roundtable on Poverty and Health. Ottawa: Canadian Population Health Initiative.

Currie, J. (2003). *Manufacturing Addiction: The Overprescription of Benzodiazepines and Sleeping Pills to Women in Canada*. Vancouver: BC Centre of Excellence for Women's Health.

den Heyer, I.W., Wien, F., Knockwood, J., & Virick, F. (2001). *Mi'kmaq Students with Special Education Needs in Nova Scotia*. Sydney, NS: Mi'kmaq Kina'matnewey.

Doyal, L. (1998). *Women's Health Services*. Buckingham, UK: Open University Press.

Everett, B., Adams, B., Johnson, J., Kurzawa, G., Quigley, M., Wright, M., et al. (2003). *Recovery Rediscovered: Implications for Mental Health Policy in Canada*. Ottawa: Canadian Mental Health Association.

Farley, M., Lynne, J., & Cotton, A.J. (2005). Prostitution in Vancouver: Violence and the colonization of First Nations women. *Transcultural Psychiatry, 42*(2), 242–271.

Federal/Provincial/Territorial Advisory Committee on Population Health. (1996). *Report on the Health of Canadians: Technical Appendix*. Prepared for a meeting of the ministers of health, Toronto.

Federal/Provincial/Territorial Working Group on Women's Health. (1993). *Working Together for Women's Mental Health: A Framework for the Development of Policies and Programs*. Ottawa: Health Canada.

Federal/Provincia/Territorial Advisory Network on Mental Health. (1997). *Review of Best Practices in Mental Health Reform*. Ottawa: Health Canada.

Foucault, M. (1965). *Madness and Civilization: A History of Insanity in the Age of Reason*. New York: Random House.

Gauthier, N., Leclerc, M., Roberge, M.T. (1997). *Écoute-moi quand je parle!*

Rapport du Comité de travail sur les services de santé mentale offerts aux femmes. Quebec: Ministère de la santé et des services sociaux.

Gold, J.H. (1998). Gender differences in psychiatric illness and treatments: A critical review. *Journal of Nervous and Mental Disease, 186*(12), 769–774.

Greaves, L., Varcoe, C., Poole, N., Morrow, M., Johnson, J., Pederson, A., et al. (2004). Mothering under duress: Women caught in a web of discourses. *Journal of the Association for Research on Mothering, 6*(1), 9–20.

Guberman, N. (1990). Les femmes et la politique de sante mentale. *Sante mental au Quebec, XV*(1), 62–84.

Harris, M. (1998). *Trauma, Recovery and Empowerment: A Clinician's Guide for Working with Women in Groups.* New York: Free Press.

Harris, M. (Ed.). (1997). *Sexual Abuse in the Lives of Women Diagnosed with Serious Mental Illness*: New York: Harwood Academic Publishers.

Health Canada. (2003). *The health of Aboriginal women.* Ottawa: Health Canada.

Health Statistics Division. (1998). *National Population Health Survey Overview 1996/97.* Cat. no. 82-567. Ottawa: Statistics Canada.

Howell, H.B., Brawman-Mintzer, O., Monnier, J., & Yonkers, K.A. (2001). Generalized anxiety disorders in women. *Psychiatric Clinics of North America, 24*(1), 165–178.

Kimball, M. (1975). Sex role stereotypes and mental health: Catch 22. In D. Smith and S. David (Eds.), *Women Look at Psychiatry* (pp. 121–142). Vancouver: Press Gang.

Kirby, M. (2006). *Out of the Shadows at Last: Transforming Mental Health, Mental Illness and Addiction Services in Canada*: Final report of the Standing Senate Committee on Social Affairs, Science and Technology. Ottawa: Standing Senate Committee on Social Affairs, Science and Technology.

Kirmayer, L., Brass, G.M., & Tait, C.L. (2001). The mental health of Aboriginal peoples: Transformations of identity and culture. *Canadian Journal of Psychiatry, 45*(7), 607–617.

Lefebvre, J., Lesage, A., Cyr, M., Toupin, J., & Fournier, L. (1998). Factors related to utilization of services for mental health reasons in Montreal, Canada. *Social Psychiatry and Psychiatric Epidemiology, 33*, 291–298.

Lister, R. (2003). *Feminist Theory and Practice of Citizenship.* Paper presented at the German Political Science Association, Mainz, Germany.

McNaughton, E. (1992). Canadian mental health policy: The emergent picture. *Canada's Mental Health, 40*(1), 3–10.

Memoire de L'R des centres de femmes du Quebec. (1997). *Les Femmes Existent! Orientations pour la transformation des services de sante mentale consultation.* Montreal: L'R des centres de femmes du Quebec.

Morrow, M. (2002a). *Violence and Trauma in the Lives of Women with Serious*

Mental Illness: Current Practices in Service Provision in British Columbia. Vancouver: British Columbia Centre of Excellence for Women's Health.

Morrow, M. (2002b). *Women and Mental Health Across the Life Span: Creating a National Cross-Disciplinary Research Agenda and Strategy: A Report to the Canadian Institutes of Health Research.* Vancouver: British Columbia Centre of Excellence for Women's Health.

Morrow, M. (2002c). *Women and Mental Health Across the Lifespan: Creating a National Cross Disciplinary Research Agenda and Strategy.* Vancouver: Report for CIHR Institutes of Gender and Health and Institute of Neurosciences, Mental Health and Addictions.

Morrow, M. (2003a). *Demonstrating Progress: Innovations in Women's Mental Health.* Vancouver: British Columbia Centre of Excellence for Women's Health.

Morrow, M. (2003b). *Mainstreaming Women's Mental Health: Building a Canadian Strategy.* Vancouver: British Columbia Centre of Excellence for Women's Health.

Morrow, M. (2006). *Community Based Mental Health Services in BC: Changes to Income, Employment and Housing Security.* Vancouver: Canadian Centre for Policy Alternatives.

Morrow, M., & Chappell, M. (1999). *Hearing Women's Voices: Mental Health Care for Women.* Vancouver: British Columbia Centre of Excellence for Women's Health.

Morrow, M., Smith, J., Lai, Y., Jaswal, S. (forthcoming). Shifting landscapes: immigrant women and post-partum depression. *Health Care for Women International.*

National Health and Welfare Canada. (1989). *Mental Health for Canadians: Striking a Balance.* Ottawa: National Health and Welfare Canada.

Pavkov, T., Lewis, D., & Lyons, J. (1989). Psychiatric diagnoses and racial bias: An empirical investigation. *Professional Psychology: Research and Practice, 20*(364).

Prior, P.M. (1999). *Gender and Mental Health.* New York: New York University Press.

Rhodes, A., Goering, P., To, T., & Williams, J. (2002). Gender and outpatient mental health service use. *Social Science & Medicine, 54,* 1–10.

Ripa, Y. (1990). *Women and Madness: The Incarceration of Women in Nineteenth-Century France.* Cambridge: Polity Press.

Roberts, R., Roberts, C., & Chen, R. (1997). Ethnocultural differences in the prevalence of adolescent depression. *American Journal of Community Psychology, 25*(1), 95–110.

Romanow, R. (2002). *Building on Values: The Future of Health Care in Canada*. Ottawa: Commission on the Future of Health Care in Canada.

Ross, D.P. (2003). *Policy Approaches to Address the Impact of Poverty on Health: A Scan of Policy Literature*. Ottawa: Canadian Institute for Health Information.

Rush, F. (1980). *The Best Kept Secret: Sexual Abuse of Children*. Upper Saddle River, NJ: Prentice-Hall.

Saraceno, B., & Barbui, C. (1997). Poverty and mental illness. *Canadian Journal of Psychiatry, 42*, 285–290.

Statistics Canada. (2003). Canadian Community Health Survey. Cycle 1.2. Ottawa: Statistics Canada.

Trainor, J., Pomeroy, E., & Pape, B. (1993). *A New Framework for Support for People with Serious Mental Illness*. Toronto: Canadian Mental Health Association.

Trainor, J., Pomeroy, E., & Pape, B. (2004). *A Framework for Support*. 3rd ed. Toronto: Canadian Mental Health Association.

Trainor, J., Shepherd, M., Boydell, K., Leff, A., & Crawford, E. (1997). Beyond the service paradigm: The impact of consumer/survivor initiatives. *Psychiatric Rehabilitation Journal, 21*(2).

Vogel, U. (1994). Marriage and the boundaries of citizenship. In B. van Steenbergen (Ed.), *The Condition of Citizenship* (pp. 76–89). London: Sage.

White, D. (1996). A balancing act: Mental health policy making in Quebec. *International Journal of Law and Psychiatry, 19*(3/4), 289–307.

Wilton, R. (2003). Putting policy into practice? Poverty and people with serious mental illness. *Social Science & Medicine, 58*, 25–39.

Woolsey, L. (1977). Psychology and the reconciliation of women's double bind: To be feminine or to be fully human. *Canadian Psychological Review, 18*(1), 66–78.

World Health Organization. (1986). Ottawa Charter for Health Promotion. *Canadian Journal of Public Health, 77*, 425–430.

14 Between Visibility and Vulnerability: Women and HIV/AIDS

MEREDITH RAIMONDO

In the early years of the epidemic, the activist slogan 'Women don't get AIDS, they just die from it' provided a clear assessment of the gendered impact of HIV infection. Nonetheless, 'women,' as a distinct class, have been visible in varying and often inconsistent ways in AIDS research, policy, and services. The complexity of gendered visibilities is not simply a matter of gender inequality. Rather, it reflects the intersection of multiple forms of structural inequality with a complex set of activist demands with regard to gender. In an important work on the status of women in AIDS discourse, activist and cultural critic Cindy Patton (1994) offered this explanation of the complexity for activist engagements with gender: 'This conflict between different (biologically) and same (socially) is not just a category problem, but the underlying paradox organizing research and policy: we are asking simultaneously for women to be treated as 'the same as' and 'different from' men' (p. 5) That is to say, when activists challenged researchers, social service providers, and policy makers to respond to women, they were not always asking for the same thing in each instance. When women were excluded from participation in clinical trials, for example, activists demanded the same kind of access to treatment and research for all people affected by AIDS. At the same time, however, they offered strong critique of the apparently gender neutral case definition for its failure to account for gynecological symptoms.

This tension, emerging from a complex understanding about the relationship of socially constructed categories, biologically distinct bodies, and structural inequalities, suggests that the AIDS epidemic presents not only a particular challenge to, but also an important opportunity for the women's health movement, with its historical emphasis on grassroots organizing, empowerment, and institutional transformation. While feminist health activism provided an important model for AIDS activism – especially because many women active in AIDS organizing had prior experience in women's health movements – the central category upon which the conceptual framework of 'women's health' rests was not stable in its function or meaning in relationship to AIDS.

Nonetheless, *gender* and *women* remain important concepts for understanding the impact of AIDS. As the pandemic enters its third decade, making useful sense of how to address women's experiences of HIV/AIDS remains a challenging task. As the demographics of those affected continues to change, women make up an increasingly large number of people living with HIV/AIDS. Globally, women comprise around half of the people living with HIV, with the vast majority in developing countries. In Canada, while women remain a smaller fraction of cumulative AIDS diagnoses (16.5 per cent), they represent about a quarter of those who have tested positive for HIV (Centre for Infectious Disease and Prevention Control [CIDPC], 2003g, pp. 2–3). Given gendered constructions of nurturing, many more women are directly impacted by the pandemic as they function as primary caregivers for friends, family members, and lovers living with AIDS.

This last example suggests that statistical scope is not the only reason to retain 'women and AIDS' as an important strategy for drawing attention to the impact of gender on HIV/AIDS. Contemporary feminist thinkers working in intersectional frameworks stress the importance of situating gender in relationship to other axes of difference in order to understand the complex nuances of positionality within institutionalized relations of power (Schneider & Stoller, 1995). At a time when universal platitudes such as 'AIDS is everywhere' or 'Anyone can get AIDS' seem increasingly inadequate for characterizing the uneven impact of HIV locally, nationally, and globally, feminist thinking about difference holds important insights for utilizing categories like 'women and AIDS' to address some of the challenges presented by HIV/AIDS. The history of political engagement with the issue of visibility, the more recent shift to the concept of vulnerability to illuminate the social factors in HIV transmission, and the challenge of understanding the global pandemic transnationally all demonstrate that AIDS remains unthinkable without gender – indeed, without women.

This overview begins with a brief history of the epidemic, highlighting the gendered social construction of AIDS with a particular focus on

---

Text Box 14.1 Women and HIV/AIDS in Canada

- Feminist analysis of 'women and AIDS' foregrounds the dual demand of achievement of equality and attention to difference in research, policy, and practice.
- Feminist concern about *visibility*, which noted the invisibility of some women and the hypervisibility of others, demonstrated the importance of drawing attention to intersections of race, class, gender, and other axes of difference.
- Contemporary models for analysing women's *vulnerability* to HIV infection foreground the role of multiple inequalities in structuring risk and highlight the role of political economy in the production of epidemics.

---

discourses of media and epidemiology (see text box 1). Concern with women's *visibility* in the first decade of the epidemic illustrates the complex and multiple meanings of activist calls to address women with AIDS, suggesting that the uses of the category 'women' varied depending on the issues at hand. By the mid-1990s, understanding the relationship of gender and HIV infection led researchers to explore the concept of *vulnerability* to highlight the social and economic significance of gender differences. As the global pandemic enters its third decade, significant global disparities have suggested that questions of *access* to research, medical care, and basic survival resources are central to understanding the experiences of women with AIDS in both wealthy and poor nations. The examples discussed here highlight the continuing importance of ensuring women's inclusion, while simultaneously remaining attentive to gendered differences in research, policy, and practice.

Epidemiological Quandaries: Vectors, Visibilities, and the Politics of Gender

In an essay first published in 1988, feminist media critic Paula Treichler (1999) noted: 'the AIDS epidemic is simultaneously an epidemic of a transmissible lethal disease and an epidemic of meanings or significa- tion' (p. 11). The vibrant body of AIDS cultural criticism produced in the late 1980s and early 1990s argued that activist responses to AIDS required a simultaneous engagement with the material needs of affected bodies and the complex system of meanings shaping understandings of and responses to the epidemic (Treichler, 1999; Watney, 1994; Patton, 1990; Crimp, 1988). The early and virulent association of AIDS with gay men created a highly politicized context around questions of identity (Yingling, 1997, p. 47). This association of AIDS with identity persisted even as public health researchers attempted to shift to less socially freighted rhetoric, demonstrating Sue Craddock's (2000) point that 'identity categories formed within medical and public discourses bear scrutiny for their capacity to mask power relations' (p. 162).

Even after 20 years of scientific research, epidemiological revision, and activist challenges, the original focus in media, research, and policy on AIDS as a 'gay disease' in North America remains a powerful and consequential cultural logic that continues to link HIV with pathologizing concepts of deviance (Patton, 1985, 1990, pp. 116–117). Treichler (1999) outlined this problem as follows: 'Despite documented cases of AIDS in women from almost the beginning of the epidemic, AIDS was assumed by most of the medical and scientific community to be a "gay disease" and a "male disease" – assumed, that is, to be different from other sexually transmitted diseases' (p. 42). Though the importance of this link cannot be overstated, it is also crucial to note that the hypervisibility of gay men in AIDS discourse was always accompanied by other gendered subjects whose presence was critical in stabilizing a central set of assumptions about HIV/AIDS. In the 1980s, for example, the mass media also offered accounts of vengeful prostitutes wilfully infecting hapless johns, heroic hemophiliacs whose tragic wives remained stoic through their shared tragedy, and desperate Haitian migrants threatening to smuggle HIV across national borders along with their hopes for a better future. Although cultural narratives about AIDS 'carriers' have changed over the course of the epidemic, universal blood screening contributed to the receding importance of consumers of blood products in North America.[1] Thus the broad thematic assumptions developed in these early years remain firmly in place. AIDS was and remains firmly associated with:

- *perversity*, especially sexual perversity as a master trope for those dangerously unnatural appetites that lead to dangerously unnatural uses of the body;

- *criminality*, both legally (as in the case of sex work, intravenous drug use, and undocumented migration) and morally (as in the case of homosexuality, which seemed to violate if not human laws – as in contexts such as Canada where sodomy has been decriminalized – then in terms of laws of nature);
- *mobility*, evident not only in images of anonymous Haitian refugees, but also in the international hype about the so-called 'Patient Zero,' a Canadian flight attendant that the U.S. Centers for Disease Control linked to a number of early cases. In Canada, the sensationalist media frenzy about Charles Ssenyonga, the Ugandan immigrant who died during the course of his trial on charges of criminal negligence for failing to inform his partners of his HIV status, coupled with the trope of the dangerous racialized immigrant with the sexual voracity emphasized in the Patient Zero story;[2]
- *modernity*, in narratives that used AIDS as a trope to symbolize the limits of progress and the imminence of a dystopian future. Such images appeared in a diverse range of domains. For example, the seeming forward progress of biomedicine faltered as a 'cure' remained elusive. Large metropolitan centres, material symbols of futurity, became dangerous epidemic 'epicentres.' Nations in Africa and the Caribbean only recently emerged from the historical domination of colonialism, struggled with the devastating, and the disproportionate impact of AIDS.

Not only did these associations depend on and reinforce each other, they also shaped and were shaped by gender in complex and varying ways. Although the early identity-based categorizations of AIDS cases drew on gendered logics, gender was not, per se, a central category itself. While 'gay' and 'hemophiliac' carried assumptions of masculinity, and 'intravenous drug user' and 'Haitian' appeared to encompass both men and women, none of the categories seemed to highlight female gender identity as an important conceptual issue in relationship to HIV/AIDS, even though it was precisely on these grounds that scientists justified the exclusion of women from drug trials (Treichler, 1999, p. 250).

Despite the importance of gender to many of the categories so visible in epidemiology and mass media in the first years of the epidemic, 'women' did not materialize as a key category for understanding AIDS. And yet women were present in AIDS caseloads from very early in the epidemic, even if their absolute numbers at the aggregate national level did not seem immediately epidemiologically significant in the North American context.[3] Cindy Patton (1994) suggests that broad cultural narratives associating women with innocence were coupled in insidious ways with the representation of specific women with AIDS as deviant, whether as sex workers (one of the few presumptively feminized categories), drug users, or simply as individuals who failed to detect deviance in their male sexual partners. Thus, she notes, the mass media in the 1990s constructed 'women' as a category defined in part by its distance from the epidemic: 'Women do not get AIDS, ran the revamped formula, or, if they do, they are not "women" – at least not normal women' (p. 62). Literary critic Katie Hogan (2001) argues that for this reason, 'invisibility' is not an accurate or useful way to think about the difficulty of articulating 'women' as a category in AIDS discourse. 'Women have always been visible in the AIDS epidemic,' she states, 'but in terms of a particular notion of what counts as "woman"' (p.7). Popular representations of women of colour, working-class women, and sexualized women primarily characterized such women as a threat to others, rather than illuminating their experiences as people at risk of HIV infection (Stockdill, 2003, p. 8; Hammonds, 1997).

Thus, while demanding attention to 'women' was a necessary intervention, it was not because women represented a natural grouping but because this category provided a useful strategy for intervening in AIDS politics. One consequence of the focus on identity in early AIDS epidemiology was the assumption that AIDS would remain primarily within those groups. Such a conclusion was only possible to sustain by examining the aggregate statistics at the level of nation for evidence of a single and uniform epidemic; but as has become evident, there were multiple epidemics taking place in varying states of temporal progression.

This critical context provides a useful framework for considering the changing epidemiology of HIV/AIDS in Canada. Initially, women comprised a relatively low number of the total reported AIDS cases in Canada – less than 10 per cent in the period 1982 to 1986 (Women's Outreach Network, 2000). However, the Centre for Infectious Disease Prevention and Control (CIDPC) analysis of the data through 1999 describes 'the changing face of the Canadian HIV epidemic,' noting worrisome increases among new infections among men who have sex with men, 'an increasing urgency of the situation among Aboriginal populations,' and a continuing serious problem among injection drug users, despite some decline in incidence. The number of women in

Canada living with HIV at the end of 1999 – around 6,800 – represented a 48 per cent increase from the 1996 analysis of the data (CIDPC, 2003e). At the end of 2002, the number had grown to approximately 7,700, a 13 per cent increase from 1999 (Health Canada, 2003). The availability of antiretroviral treatment placed renewed significance on HIV diagnoses rather than on AIDS diagnoses as a more accurate measure of the broad scope of the problem. The percentage of women among newly reported HIV diagnoses grew steadily from 2001 to the first half of 2003 to comprise nearly 25 per cent (CIDPC 2003c).

The initial epidemiological emphasis on identity did little to illuminate women's risk of HIV infection, but the turn to a more behavioural approach to risk had its limitations as well. The obvious problems of an identity-based framework led epidemiologists to focus on behaviors related to HIV transmission, but this change did not eliminate prejudicial associations with identity. Because the two most visible forms of risk behaviour – anal intercourse and injection drug use – seemed determinative of the identity categories they were meant to supplant, they only served to reinforce the association between risk and identity. Moreover, behaviour carried its own implicit gender politics. The plethora of mass media coverage that characterized women as victims – either of devious bisexual men within the North American context, or of development in stories about Africa – implicitly masculinized the concept of behaviour. On the whole, such narratives characterized women's HIV infection as a secondary product of other people's actions, constructing them as the objects. Stories about sex workers remained a clear exception, especially when sex workers were viewed as a vector of transmission from marked risk identities into the 'general population' (Gorna, 1996, pp. 264-272). The other broad exception to this pattern emerged in stories about pediatric AIDS, where violations of normative motherhood served to racialize, masculinize, and queer women with AIDS. Such stories borrowed tropes from accounts of irresponsible reproduction, constructing risk behaviour as a selfish individualism recklessly endangering innocent children (Hammonds, 1990).

Though the focus on behaviour instead of identity was an attempt to find a socially neutral rubric for epidemiology and prevention education, the contentious debates about how to characterize lesbian risk provides one the clearest examples of the difficulty and necessity of gendered analysis. Under a risk behaviour schema, lesbians remained difficult to visualize, since the sexual practices most commonly associated with this identity category seemed relatively safe in terms of HIV transmission. However, this notion reveals several underlying – and, in the case of HIV transmission, enormously problematic – assumptions about human sexuality. Dominant cultural frames treated sexuality as dichotomous (along a clearly articulated homosexual/heterosexual binary), transparent (so that behaviour and identity both reflected and determined each other), and stable (self-identical over time).

However, women who identify as lesbians might engage in any number of behaviours that put them at an increased risk for HIV infection, including injection drug use or sexual encounters with men (either in the context of their intimate lives or in the context of sex work). Epidemiologically, these forms of exposure could be apprehended through established schemas, so long as researchers remained cognizant of the importance of self-identification. What remained challenging was how to translate such analysis into useful and accessible prevention information. For women for whom 'lesbian' represented a primary social identity, HIV prevention materials that addressed them through this category seemed vital. But to be effective, they also needed to address a wide range of behaviours, even if they seemed to fall outside of the conventional boundaries of this gendered sexual category (Hollibaugh, 1998; Stoller, 1998; Alexander, 1996; Patton, 1994). Effective strategies for understanding and preventing HIV transmission must address the complex and often plural character of human sexualities.

Moreover, modes of exposure identified as epidemiologically distinct are often complexly interrelated in the context of women's lives, as the relationship between sexuality and drug use illustrates. Generally, heterosexual transmission accounts for 62 per cent of cases among women in Canada, up from 46 per cent in the period between 1985 and 1996 – a relatively steady 36 per cent of cases were attributed to intravenous drug use (IDU). However, IDU has become a more prominent exposure category in recent years, nearly doubling from the period before 1996 to 2000. A CIDPC epidemiological update suggested: 'The latest national HIV estimates published by CIDPC for 1999 indicate that an estimated 54% of all new HIV infections among women were attributed to IDU' (CIDPC, 2003a). Although HIV/AIDS in Canada is still predominantly associated with urban areas, the report noted a worrisome increase in HIV infection 'outside major urban areas' and proposed that 'given geographic mobility of IDU and their social and sexual interaction with nonusers, the dual problem of injecting drug use and HIV infection is one that ultimately affects all of Canadian society' (CIDPC, 2003a). Despite some declines in the number of new infections attributable to injection drug use, it remains a serious problem, especially when the incidence and prevalence are viewed with attention to differences among populations. While IDU generally accounts for about 30 per cent of infections, it accounts for about 63 per cent of new infections among Aboriginal people (CIDPC, 2003e).

Sexual behavior and drug use often intersect in complex and critical ways. Despite the early associations between sex workers and HIV transmission, studies on sex work indicate a complex interrelationship of variables. For instance, some intravenous drug users enter sex work to access drugs and/or resources, but one study found that 'HIV prevalence among women injectors who reported sex trade involvement ... was not higher than those not involved in the sex trade' (Spittal et al., 2003, p. 192). Causality and correlation are not always easy to distinguish. One study of death among homeless populations reported: 'Among women 18-44 years of age, the most common causes of death were HIV/AIDS and drug overdose' (Cheung & Hwang, 2004, p. 1245). How homelessness or other experiences of poverty might shape various and often multiple forms of risk requires careful analysis. Even the category of 'sex work' is not transparent, since the focus on commercial sex work often fails to account for women's reliance on their sexual partners for food, housing, and other forms of support.

One of the most obvious and consequential outcomes of sustained activist campaigns concerned with women's visibility was the revision of the AIDS case definition to include a wider range of opportunistic infections.[4] The failure to include these infections in the definition resulted in significant undercounting among several broad demographic groups, including women and intravenous drug users. In particular, little attention had been paid to the relationship between HIV disease and gynecological health. Although the inclusion of invasive cervical cancer in the expanded definition was an important step, considerable questions about the basic etiology of HIV remain pressing. The Canadian Women's Health Study, a longitudinal study launched in 1993, is pursuing potential links between HIV and human papilloma virus (HPV) co-infection, an infectious agent suspected of playing a role in cervical cancer. One study determined that 'two-thirds of the women participating in the Canadian Women's HIV Study have HPV infection,' suggesting the importance of analysing the gender implications of co-infection with other sexually transmitted infections. Careful attention to differences within the category 'women' was necessary, given the finding that age is an important variable, with HPV disproportionately affecting women under 30 (Hankins et al., 1999 p. 189).

This example suggests that continued basic research on HIV infection and disease progression remains critical. Assessments of women's 'biological vulnerability' to HIV infection note the higher concentration of HIV in semen than in vaginal fluids, the development of mucous membranes in the vagina and cervix in adolescence, and the possibility of tears and/or sores in the vagina from any number of causes, including sexual violence, inadequate lubrication, or sexually transmitted infections (Nova Scotia Advisory Council on the Status of Women [NSACSW], 2003, p. 5; Buzy & Gayle, 1996, p. 191). Additionally, important questions remain about key issues, including disease course, sex differences in drug toxicities, the impact of biological sex on vaccine development, hormones and HIV, and pregnancy and maternal health (Gilad, Walfish, Borer, & Schlaeffer, 2003, Forum for Collaborative HIV Research, 2002). As only one example, studies have shown that even though progression to disease is similar in men and women, women exhibit lower HIV RNA levels as compared to men, an important indicator for treatment initiation (Napravnik, Poole, Thomas, & Eron, 2002).

Assessing the impact of treatment on biologically distinct bodies is one especially lively area of investigation. Considerable research is currently underway exploring sex differences in relationship to antiretroviral therapy (Ofotokun & Pomeroy 2003; Pernerstorfer-Schoen et al., 2001); as the U.S. National Institutes of Health reports, 'Women also exhibit different characteristics from men for many of the same complications of antiretroviral therapy, such as metabolic abnormalities' (National Institutes of Health, 2004). For example, one study found that women were seven times more likely to experience severe rash when treated with nevirapine (Bersoff-Matcha et al., 2001). Important issues related to hormones, body mass, metabolism, and dosage of antiretroviral drugs remain to be investigated (Pai, Schriever, Diaz-Linares, Novak, & Rodvold, 2004, Galli et al., 2003). One study that examined adherence to the demanding antiretroviral regimens noted that adherence 'during pregnancy may be difficult,' an important problem to address given the number of young women affected by HIV (Burdge et al., 2003, p. 1683). One future direction is the inclusion of transgender people in studies of sex differences, a change which may require the adoption of feminist models about the complexity and plurality of biological sex.

As ongoing debates about HIV testing and informed consent for pregnant women illustrate, policy still remains an important domain for addressing the inclusion of gender analysis. While testing is elective, policies currently vary by province between use of 'opt-in' strategies – where women are tested only if they affirmatively accept, and 'opt-out' strategies – where women are tested unless they ask not to be (CIDPC, 2003f). Screening may be particularly valuable in reaching women who are not yet aware of their HIV status, as it fulfils an important public health mandate by identifying opportunities to prevent perinatal transmission, the major source of pediatric HIV infection. However, such strategies are troubled by the historical tendency to focus on women only in terms of their reproductive capacity and the challenge of addressing the role of gender and other inequalities in shaping the context of informed consent (Scott, 2003, pp. 160–195). Certainly, there are important arguments for seizing opportunities for early detection of HIV infection. However, critics of such testing point out that without strong services in place for women, they may find themselves learning of an HIV diagnosis in a particularly stressful context. Such debates illustrate the critical importance of attending to the context of women's lives as well as to abstract categorical data.

Vulnerability: A Useful Category?

Increased attention to women's issues in AIDS research and policy raised important questions about not just the degree of HIV infection among women, but also the reasons why different women faced increased risk of HIV infection. The concept of vulnerability provides an explanation that emphasizes the social factors shaping the AIDS pandemic. Although widely disseminated rhetoric like 'the spread of AIDS' implies a steady, even expansion of HIV infection across proximate identities and territories, the complex geographic distribution of HIV infection demonstrates how badly such notions have mischaracterized the epidemic (Raimondo, 2003). The Health Canada website description of AIDS reflects a more nuanced understanding, noting that 'the HIV/AIDS epidemic is actually several epidemics, occurring in specific populations' (Health Canada Online, 2004a). What this statement gestures towards, but does not fully reveal, is the ways that 'population' is both a necessary and limited concept that runs the risk of carrying forward the problem of seeing categories as discretely bounded groups. While risk of HIV transmission is not contained by identity categories, it is not universally dispersed. One of the central contemporary challenges of the AIDS epidemic is understanding how and why some people remain at increased risk of infection. How are women at risk? And what important differences exist within this category?

To answer these questions, researchers examining the dynamics of gender in a variety of local contexts offered the theoretical concept of vulnerability, which emphasizes the role of social and economic context in shaping health and sickness. A social perspective allowed researchers to address two related findings: first, that gender inequalities limiting access to resources and power meant that many women found themselves unable to insist that their sexual partners wear condoms, the world's predominant prevention strategy (Farmer, Connors, Fox, & Furin, 1996, pp. 178-179; Ulin, Cayemittes, & Gringle, 1996); and, second, that not all women were equally at risk for HIV infection. Vulnerability offered a way to foreground what doctor and anthropologist Paul Farmer (1999) called those 'historically given (and often economically given) processes and forces that conspire to constrain individual agency' (p. 79). This model situated personal decision-making in social structure, highlighting the importance of structural inequality. The Nova Scotia Advisory Council on the Status of Women (2003), for example, used vulnerability to highlight gender roles, violence, and inequality.

Bringing social context into view draws attention to diversity within the category of women, a strategy that reflects the larger feminist understanding of identity as positionality within fields of power. A closer examination of the epidemiology of HIV/AIDS and women in Canada reveals how necessary it is to attend to differences within broad categories, and not just between them. Ethnicity, race, class, and age are among the significant distinctions shaping rates of HIV infection in women. Aboriginal people in Canada are disproportionately affected by HIV, representing around a quarter of all new diagnoses between 1999 and the first half of 2002 where ethnicity data was available (gaps in reporting, especially for HIV diagnoses, mean the current statistical picture is incomplete) (CIDPC, 2003a; Canadian Aboriginal AIDS Network, 2003). Not only do Aboriginal people report higher rates of HIV infection than white Canadians, gender and age play distinctive roles as well. Women made up nearly 45 per cent of those between 15 and 29 years of age who tested positive for HIV in 2001 (CIDPC, 2003d). Between 1998 and 2002, women comprised 17 per cent of the AIDS cases among whites, but close to half of those among Black Canadians and Aboriginal people (NSACSW, 2003, p. 6).

More local foci may reveal even more worrisome trends, as one fact sheet on the issue noted: 'At a BC clinic which cares for the majority of HIV infected pregnant women in the province, 41 per cent (21/41) of the women under care in 1996 were Aboriginal people' (Canadian Aboriginal AIDS Network, 2000). The CIDPC reported a similar troubling finding, noting that 'a higher proportion of HIV-infected pregnant women who deliver are Aboriginal.' Such data suggests that risk of perinatal transmission is not equally distributed (CIDPC, 2003a). To note such patterns is not sufficient, however. The category of vulnerability holds important utility as a strategy for demonstrating that social context affects risk of infection in ways often masked by broad categories: 'When women are included in HIV/AIDS analyses, it is largely as disembodied categories such as 'prostitutes,' having little bearing on personal identities, practices, or lived experiences' (Craddock, 2000, p. 164). The disproportionate impact of HIV on Aboriginal women directs attention to racism, class inequalities, gender discrimination, and colonialism as forces that distribute disease unequally.

Institutional and structural context provide an explanation for disparities among women. For example, data on HIV rates among incarcerated people in Canada suggests a disproportionate impact on women (NSACSW, 2003; see also DiCenso, Dias, & Gahagan, 2003). This finding suggests at least two related questions: How does gender shape issues of HIV prevention and treatment in the context of incarceration? And how might gender, along with other important social markers such as class, shape the increased risk faced by women who are becoming incarcerated? Indications that HIV infection for women in prison is 'strongly associated with a past history of injection drug use' underscore the importance of multifactoral analysis (Marble, 1997). This example illustrates that while gender is clearly a factor in social vulnerability, it is not the only, or in some cases, the most important factor. A 2001 article in a special issue of the journal *Canadian Woman Studies* on HIV/AIDS on supportive housing for women with AIDS noted that 'at Gladstone [a facility in Toronto], we are faced with supporting women who may not only be HIV positive but are battling an addiction to crack/cocaine or alcohol, may still be actively working the street, and in conflict with the law' (Reynolds, 2001).

An attention to vulnerability requires attention to the complex contexts of women's lives. Contributors to the *Canadian Woman Studies* special issue identified, in a range of contexts, the importance of integrated services and treatments to address the needs of women living with HIV/AIDS, an approach that challenges the dominant tendency to approach AIDS as a discrete health issue. Erin Connell (2001) emphasized the importance of integrating HIV prevention into sexual and reproductive health services, arguing that 'although HIV is a sexually transmitted infection (STI), it has through its politicization and professionalization, become a stand alone issue largely divorced from the rest of sexual and reproductive health' (p. 5). Discussing the Northern Women's Health Outreach Project, Karen O'Gorman (2001) suggested that 'placing the issue of HIV and substance use into a broader context helps to "normalize" the issues, providing safety, decreasing the negative inferences and labeling of those who do access services' (p. 114). Considering HIV services for women with mental illness, Amy Andrews (2001) noted that there are 'few programs that seek to address the multi-faceted material, social, and emotional needs of women living with mental illnesses' (p. 83). Integrating HIV education and prevention with sexual violence prevention is another emerging area of interest (Health Canada, 2004b). Such multifactor analyses and multisector solutions are consistent with the feminist health activists' call to treat women's lives with a holistic perspective (Whittle & Inhorn 2001; see Commonwealth Secretariat 2002, for an example of a gender mainstreaming approach).

But the emphasis on vulnerability also offers important challenges to some of the precepts of women's health organizing. In a comparative study of women's health in Canada and the United States, Feldberg, Ladd-Taylor, Li, & McPherson (2003) argue that 'feminist health activists engaged in three main strategies: education, self-help, and political reform' (p. 27). The first two strategies in particular reflect the importance of agency for feminist thinking and organizing. Vulnerability suggests that education and self-help cannot be employed effectively if structural constraints on agency are not directly addressed. To the extent that prevention and treatment take autonomy and individual empowerment for granted, they run the risk of further marginalizing particular groups of women. Amy Andrews (2001) argues that 'women are often assumed to be individuals who not only have the ability to determine their own health practices, but to also influence the health practices of their families,' which may create barriers for women living with mental illnesses and those living in violence.

While vulnerability has provided a useful tool for shifting discussion of women from an abstract, stable, and uniform category to the power relations that give difference meaning, the cultural association of vulnerability with femininity means that this concept runs the risk of reinforcing broad and problematic gender stereotypes – especially when it is divorced from the analysis of political economy. This problem is most evident in the use of vulnerability to discuss the material particularity of bodies. HIV/AIDS education materials routinely make use of the concept of 'women's biological vulnerability' to describe the increased risk that women face in vaginal intercourse (NSACSW, 2003; United Nations Development Fund for Women [UNIFEM], 2001). While this concept helps draw attention to specific physiological differences, it also runs the risk of repeating the representation of women as the fragile and helpless victims of AIDS. Such modes of talking about the body are too easily stripped of social context and can obscure rather than illuminate the political economies of embodied materialities. It is somewhat ironic that nearly 20 years ago, the scientific theory of the 'rugged vagina' was offered to explain women's imperiousness to HIV infection. Reversing its terms is no more likely to enable useful prevention than the argument that the 'vulnerable anus' demonstrated the inherent dangerousness and deviance of anal intercourse (Treichler, 1999, p. 17; Farmer, 1999, p. 61).

This example suggests that vulnerability functions most usefully when it enables a complex analysis of gender politics rather than simply providing a rhetorical substitute for the category 'women.' The necessity of mapping multiple forms of gendered vulnerabilities is critical not only to meet the needs of diverse groups of men – a category with similar diversity in relation to race, class, sexuality, and age (Lindblad, 2003) – but also to address the long-standing invisibility of transgender people and HIV/AIDS prevention and treatment. Feminist responses to HIV/AIDS have not generally included the particular issues facing transgendered people, even though a Quebec study addressing 'female to male transsexuals and transvestites' recommended the same kind of integrated approach to services feminists have embraced (Namaste, 1999). Gender binaries have failed to illuminate trans issues as gender issues. How might trans men, for example, be included in emerging research on gynecological health and HIV? How might hormonal regimens affect HIV treatment? How might needle exchanges address people obtaining and injecting hormones outside the context of the medical system? The Vancouver High Risk Project, founded in 1993, represents one of the groups playing a leading role in identifying needs of transpeople in relation to HIV/AIDS.[5] Developing a theoretical rubric that tracks the complexity of gender while preserving the politically important task of keeping women's concerns vital remains an important and critical project.

Placing Canada in the Global Pandemic: Transnational Approaches to Access

From a global perspective, the impact of HIV on women has been evident from the first (UNIFEM, 2001) (see text box 14.2). For activists, health practitioners, and researchers confronting AIDS in communities outside of North America, the importance of gender and the centrality of women was never an unexpected discovery. Nonetheless, while women have been *visible* in the global pandemic from its inception, the significance of *gender* as an analytic category has been more contested. As human rights frames gain increasing prominence in the global response to AIDS, however, gender analysis circulates more visibly through the work of organizations like UNAIDS, whose executive director Pierre Piot stated, 'Gender inequality is a fundamental driving force of the AIDS epidemic' (Joint United Nations Programme on HIV/AIDS [UNAIDSb], 2000). The global pandemic has raised important challenges for international AIDS policy and challenged wealthy nations like Canada to address global economic inequalities.

The shift from a focus on women to a focus on gender inequality has represented an important change, but it has also raised complex ques-

---

Text Box 14.2 Women and the Global HIV/AIDS Pandemic

- Transnational analysis of HIV/AIDS draws connections between the most affected people in Canada and those most at risk globally for HIV infection by focusing on issues of access to research, prevention, and treatment.
- Canadian participation in international efforts such as the Global Fund to Fight AIDS, Malaria, and Tuberculosis represents a larger political debate about the role of wealthier nations in addressing the impact of HIV globally.
- Issues of access exist not just in poor nations, but also in wealthy countries where barriers such as education, geography, racism, and other constraints may prevent some people from accessing resources.

tions about the application of universal human rights principles in diverse social and cultural contexts. Ironically, the contemporary global focus on women and AIDS primarily treats gender in its most private and local settings, concentrating on individual agency in sexual decision-making but not on other ways in which gender shapes HIV infection as a transnational health crisis. Gender, for example, seldom enters the heated debate about global drug patents. Contemporary analysis about the possibilities and limits of global feminism seldom find expression in debates about AIDS and human rights (Cook & Dickens, 2002; Bunch, 2001; Grewal, 1999).

One place where gender politics and the global economy clearly meet is in the demand for new women-centred prevention technologies. The traditional reliance on condoms in AIDS prevention raises the problem of limits on women's agency, since gaining a partner's cooperation is not always possible. The so-called 'female condom' (which can be used either vaginally or rectally) thus far has not provided a suitable alternative, given the prohibitive cost, the difficulty of proper insertion, and the visibility and noisiness of the material, which means it cannot be used without a partner's awareness. A more promising line of technological research is in microbicides, gels or foams inserted vaginally or rectally that would target the HIV virus. Such technologies are seen as particularly crucial in cultural contexts where women's status is linked to motherhood. Developing technologies that would prevent HIV infection but allow pregnancy would be a major breakthrough for women in some of the most affected areas. The biggest problem in microbicide research thus far has been funding – unlike high-end HIV treatment drugs, microbicides would be inexpensive and thus have not represented an attractive line of investment for drug companies (UNAIDS, 1998). The case of microbicides suggests that Patton's argument – about the simultaneous importance of demanding attention to the biological distinctiveness of gendered bodies and the need for social equality (here measured by similar levels of investment in research) – continues to have relevance.

Canada, like other wealthy nations, faces pressure to contribute to a solution to the international pandemic, especially in access to treatments. Current international efforts focus on the Global Fund to Fight AIDS, Malaria, and Tuberculosis. The notion of a fund was first seriously proposed at the July 2000 G8 meeting in Okinawa, and met with enthusiastic response. Still even though only the tiniest fraction of people affected by HIV/AIDS could afford and/or access antiretroviral treatments, the fund has struggled to achieve full funding levels. Although initial estimates suggested that US$10 billion a year would be needed to control these three interrelated epidemics, not quite half of that amount has been pledged from the fund's inception in 2001 through 2008. In May 2004, Canada, which currently has a seat on the Global Fund board, doubled its annual pledge for 2005 to CDN $70 million and devoted CDN $100 million to the World Health Organization/UNAIDS '3 by 5' initiative – designed to reach three million people with antiretroviral treatments by 2005 (Global Fund, 2004). Addressing the global problem of 'women and AIDS' had required grappling with the uneven effects of global capitalism and the responsibilities of wealthier nations to the poorest people in the world. The Canadian Strategy on HIV/AIDS includes participation in international organizations and programs as well as focused efforts through the Canadian International Development Agency.

The political economy of globalization, with its acute crisis around access to resources, does not take place only at a distance. 'Many North Americans remained under-served, rather than overpowered, by modern medicine,' noted Feldberg, Ladd-Taylor, Li, & McPherson (2003, p. 23) in their comparative analysis of women's health in Canada and the United States. HIV/AIDS presents a clear example of this problem. Writing about the Northern Women's Health Outreach Project, O'Gorman (2001) argued that 'while some services were available either in a nearby urban setting or within their rural area, a significant number of women were not aware of what those services were or how to access them.' Even as people in developing countries struggle for economic justice, questions of access continue to challenge many people with AIDS in wealthier countries. To the extent that global capitalism exacerbates the divide between the richest and poorest people and distributes such economic positions unequally, the analytic frameworks that illuminate the needs of the large numbers of people infected in poor countries also help explain the increasingly disproportionate effects of HIV on poor people of colour in North America. If, as Daily, Farmer, Rhatigan, Katz, & Furin (1996) argue, 'poverty and its attendant social circumstances are clear risk factors for HIV acquisition' (p. 133), then class remains a significant issue in understanding the continued and growing impact of HIV on particular communities.

Even in Canada, where national health addresses some of the problems with expensive treatments urgent in privatized health systems such as the United States, important questions of access to the benefits of advanced biomedicine remain. For example, a study of women's participation in clinical trials found that while overall women's rate of participation in clinical trials is comparable to that of all people with AIDS, there were barriers to participation for some women related to degree of access to antiretroviral treatments, levels of education, racial and ethnic identity, injection drug use, and regional residence (Hankins, Lapointe, Walmsley, 1998). A study of intravenous drug users concluded that 'access to HIV/AIDS care is most pressing in the developing world, but [it] also presents major challenges in the developed world, even in the context of universal healthcare systems such as Canada's' (Wood et al., 2004, pp. 136–137; see also Walmsley, 1998). This study suggests that questions of access must include not only the material stuff of treatments, but also the creation of a context in which those treatments can be used effectively.

Gender continues to be one of the critical axes for understanding barriers to access even when resources are theoretically available. The NSACSW (2003) reported: 'Focus groups conducted with HIV+ women in Atlantic Canada as recently as 2000 indicated that physicians tend to dismiss women's HIV concerns, even when risk assessments indicate vulnerability' (p. 4). A study on sex workers who inject drugs also noted that 'access issues in this population may need to be carefully examined' (Spittal et al., 2003, p. 193). Such questions apply to prevention as well as treatment, as a study on the limited availability of prevention materials to women in prison demonstrated (Jürgens, 2002).

Models for analysing gender transnationally offer new possibilities for understanding the cultural politics of AIDS, as well as questioning assumptions based on national perspectives (Petchesky, 2003) (see text box 14.3). Inderpal Grewal and Caren Kaplan's (1994) notion of 'scattered hegemonies,' for example, provides a useful model for understanding broad systems of power as well as attending to the complexities and discontinuities in local contexts. Developing frameworks that render visible the connections between the most affected people within Canada and the unfolding global crisis is one strategy for illuminating a lesson that has been clear since the earliest AIDS activism: AIDS is not merely a product of the natural effects of disease, but rather a failure of social justice. Claiming the category 'women' and demonstrating the significance of gender have been and remain important strategies for ensuring that HIV/AIDS research, prevention, education, and treatment address the needs of and become available to the diversity of people facing the effects of HIV infection.

Text Box 14.3 Women and HIV/AIDS: Future Directions in Theory, Policy, and Practice

- Basic science research exploring the differential effects of HIV and HIV treatments on biologically distinct bodies.
- Development of more effective responses to the global pandemic that address the relationship between health outcomes, social structure, and inequality.
- The need for new prevention strategies such as microbicides illuminates the ongoing intersection of attention to gender issues in scientific research as well as analysis of the social and cultural context of prevention and treatment.
- Ongoing concern with the disproportionate risk of women, the needs of transgenderd people, and the role of men in prevention suggest the continued need for feminist models addressing a range of gendered subjects.

In this way, feminist engagement with HIV/AIDS has the potential to contribute to the transformation of models for understanding and responding to epidemic disease. Transnational feminist analysis of the relationship of agency and constraint suggest important strategies for situating individualist prevention strategies in a broader social, political, and economic context. Concern with the power dynamics of transnational institutions and actors may provide models for addressing acute inequalities while simultaneously acknowledging the ways in which global philanthropy and human rights discourse can function to reinforce rather than deconstruct those very inequalities.

In the wake of recent concern about severe acute respiratory syndrome (SARS), it seems more than obvious that global epidemics represent an ongoing public health challenge. Not only is there an urgent need to think through the ways in which the categories at work in various professional discourses operate, but it is also critical to analyse the circulation of such forms of knowledge across the realms of research, policy, and practice. Too often, the identification of a particular population group with epidemic disease serves to heighten stigma and obscure the centrality of social structure to health outcomes. Feminist analysis of the complex and important relationship between bodies, difference, and power represents a rich resource for crafting more effective public health responses.

NOTES

1 An earlier version of this argument is developed in Patton and Raimondo (2002).
2 See, for example, June Callwood's (1995) sensationalist account of the case in her book *Trial without End: A Shocking Story of Women and AIDS*. New York: Knopf. As part of the highly publicized trial, Ssenyonga's lawyer introduced expert witnesses who diagnosed post-traumatic stress based on his experiences of repression in Uganda, one example of the ways in which his identity as an immigrant was highlighted throughout this case (Adamick, 1993).
3 The World Health Organization Global Program on AIDS initially mapped global regionalization patterns that distinguished between Pattern 1 (North America and Europe), composed primarily of gay men and to a lesser extent injection drug users; Pattern 2, mainly characterized by 'heterosexual transmission' and applied most frequently to describe HIV/AIDS in Africa; and Pattern 3, a kind of 'everywhere else' category related to subsequent 'contact with Pattern I/II sites through forces such as tourism and migration, applied significantly to Asia. Although this model was abandoned by the 1990s, it had a significant impact on and established both explicitly and implicitly gendered tropes for global epidemiology (Patton, 2002).
4 Sustained activist campaigns targeting the U.S. Centers for Disease Control in particular led to a revision of the case definition in 1993 in the United States as well as in Canada, Australia, and the European community. In addition to recurrent bacterial pneumonia, pulmonary tuberculosis, and invasive cervical cancer, the U.S. also added a CD4 lymphocyte count less than 200 cells per cubic millimeter, a criteria that Canada did not adopt.
5 Additional information on the High Risk Project, including resources on transgendered people and HIV/AIDS, can be found at http://mypage.direct.ca/h/hrp/index.html#high.

REFERENCES

Adamick, P. (1993 May 11). Man 'buried' truth about HIV London trial told. *Toronto Star*, A20.

Alexander, P. (1996). Women who sleep with women. In L. Long & M. Ankrah (Eds.), *Women's Experiences with HIV/AIDS: An International Perspective* (pp. 43–55). New York: Columbia University Press.

Andrews, A. (2001, December). Missing links: Women, mental illness, and the need for a new model of HIV prevention and sexual health promotion. *Canadian Woman Studies, 21*(2), 82–88. Retrieved 12 May 2004, from http://etextb.ohiolink.edu/bin/gate.exe?f=fulltest&state=h239hs.4.1. Contemporary Women's Issues database http://rave.ohiolink.edu/databases/login/cwis.

Bersoff-Matcha, S.J., Miller, W.C., Aberg, J.A., van der Horst, C., Hamrick Jr., H.J., Powderly, W.G., & Mundy, L.M. (2001, January). Sex differences in nevirapine rash. *Clinical Infectious Diseases, 32*(1), 124–129.

Bunch, C. (2001). Women's human rights: The challenge of global feminism and diversity. In M. DeKoven (Ed.), *Feminist Locations: Global and Local, Theory and Practice* (pp. 129–146). New Brunswick, NJ: Rutgers University Press.

Burdge, D., Money, D., Forbes, J., Walmsley, S.L., Smaill, F., Boucher, M., Samson, L., Steban, M., and the Canadian HIV Trials Network Working Group on Vertical HIV Transmission (2003, 23 June). Canadian consensus guidelines for the care of HIV-positive pregnant women: Putting recommendations into practice. *Canadian Medical Association Journal, 168*(13), 1683–1687.

Buzy, J., & Gayle, H. (1996). The epidemiology of HIV and AIDS in women. In L. Long & M. Ankrah (Eds.), *Women's Experiences with HIV/AIDS: An International Perspective* (pp. 181–204). New York: Columbia University Press.

Callwood, J. (1995) *Trial without End: A Shocking Story of Women and AIDS.* New York: Alfred A. Knopf.

Canadian Aboriginal AIDS Network. (2000). AIDS and Aboriginal Women. Retrieved 11 May 2004, from http://www.linkup-connexion.ca/catalog/prodImages/022302014405_52.pdf.

Canadian Aboriginal AIDS Network. (2003, July). *Strengthening Ties, Strengthening Communities.* Retrieved 20 May 2004, from http://www.caan.ca/english/grfx/resources/publications/strengthening_ties.pdf.

Cheung, A., & Hwang, S. (2004, 13 April). Risk of death among homeless women: A cohort study and review of the literature. *Canadian Medical Association Journal, 170*(8), 1243–1247.

Centre for Infectious Disease Prevention and Control (CIDPC). (2003a, April). HIV/AIDS among Aboriginals persons in Canada: A continuing concern. *HIVAIDS EpiUpdate.* Ottawa: Health Canada. Retrieved 13 May 2004, from http://www.hc-sc.gc.ca/pphb-dgspsp/publicat/epiu-aepi/hiv-vih/aborig_e.html.

Centre for Infectious Disease Prevention and Control (CIDPC). (2003b, April). HIV/AIDS among injecting drug users in Canada. *HIVAIDS EpiUpdate.* Ottawa: Health Canada. Retrieved 13 May 2004, from http://www.hc-sc.gc.ca/pphb-dgspsp/publicat/epiu-aepi/hiv-vih/idus_e.html.

Centre for Infectious Disease Prevention and Control (CIDPC). (2003c, April). HIV and AIDS among women in Canada. *HIV/AIDS Epi Update,* (pp. 18–20). Ottawa: Health Canada Retrieved 10 May 2004, from http://www.hc-sc.gc.ca/pphb-dgspsp/publicat/epiu-aepi/index.html#HIV.

Centre for Infectious Disease Prevention and Control (CIDPC). (2003d, April). HIV and AIDS among youth in Canada. *HIV/AIDS Epi Update.* Ottawa: Health Canada Retrieved 20 May 2004, from http://www.hc-sc.gc.ca/pphb-dgspsp/publicat/epiu-aepi/hiv-vih/youth_e.html.

Centre for Infectious Disease Prevention and Control (CIDPC). (2003e, April). National HIV prevalence and incidence estimates for 1999. *HIV/AIDS Epi Update,* (pp. 1–5). Ottawa: Health Canada. Retrieved 10 May 2004, from http://www.hc-sc.gc.ca/pphb-dgspsp/publicat/epiu-aepi/index.html#HIV.

Centre for Infectious Disease Prevention and Control (CIDPC). (2003f, April). Perinatal transmission of HIV. *HIV/AIDS Epi Update,* (pp. 25–30). Ottawa: Health Canada. Retrieved 10 May 2004, from http://www.hc-sc.gc.ca/pphb-dgspsp/publicat/epiu-aepi/index.html#HIV.

Centre for Infectious Disease Prevention and Control (CIDPC). (2003g, November). HIV/AIDS in Canada. Surveillance report to 30 June 2003, (pp. 1–64). Ottawa: Health Canada Retrieved 21 May 2004, from http://www.hc-sc.gc.ca/pphb-dgspsp/publicat/aids-sida/haic-vsac0603/pdf/haic-vsac0603.pdf.

Commonwealth Secretariat and Maritime Centre of Excellence for Women's Health. (2002). *Gender Mainstreaming in HIV/AIDS: Taking a Multisectoral Approach.* London: Commonwealth Secretariat.

Cook, R., & Dickens, B. (2002). Human rights and HIV-positive women. *International Journal of Gynecology & Obstetrics, 77,* 55–63.

Connell, E. (2001). *Bridging the Gap: Integrating HIV Prevention into Sexual and Reproductive Health Promotion* (pp. 1–5). Retrieved 19 May 2004, from http://www.ppfc.ca/HIV/e/cws_article_English.pdf. First published in *Canadian Woman Studies, 21*(2), 68–71.

Craddock, S. (2000). Disease, social identity, and risk: Rethinking the geography of AIDS. *Transactions of the Institute of British Geographers, 25,* 153–168.

Crimp, D. (Ed.). (1988). *AIDS: Cultural Analysis, Cultural Activism.* Cambridge, MA: MIT Press.

Daily, J., Farmer, P., Rhatigan, J., Katz, J., & Furin, J. (1996). Women and HIV infection: A different disease? In P. Farmer, M. Connors, & J. Simmons (Eds.), *Women, Poverty, and AIDS: Sex, Drugs, and Structural Violence* (pp. 125–144). Monroe, ME: Common Courage Press.

DiCenso, A.M., Dias, G., & Gahagan, J. (2003, 28 March). *Unlocking Our Futures: A National Study on Women, Prisons, HIV, and Hepatitis C.* (Prisoners HIV/AIDS Support Action Network). Retrieved 18 May 2004, from http://www.pasan.org/Publications/Unlocking_Our_Futures.pdf.

Farmer, P. (1999). *Infections and Inequalities: The Modern Plagues.* Berkeley: University of California Press.

Farmer, P., Connors, M., Fox, K., & Furin, J. (1996). Rereading social science. In P. Farmer, M. Connors, & L. Simmons (Eds.), *Women, Poverty, and AIDS: Sex, Drugs, and Structural Violence* (pp. 147–205). Monroe, ME: Common Courage Press.

Feldberg, G., Ladd-Taylor, M., Li, A., & McPherson, K. (2003). Comparative perspectives on Canadian and American women's health care since 1945. In G. Feldberg, M. Ladd-Taylor, A. Li, & K. McPherson (Eds.), *Women, Health and Nation: Canada and the United States Since 1945* (pp. 15–42). Montreal and Kingston: McGill-Queen's University Press.

Forum for Collaborative HIV Research. (2002). *Report of the Workshop: Sex and Gender Issues in HIV Disease.* George Washington University Medical Center. Retrieved 10 March 2004, from http://www.hivforum.org/publications/S&G per cent20Final.pdf.

Fumento, M. (1990). *The Myth of Heterosexual AIDS.* New York: Basic Books.

Galli, M., Gervasoni, C., Ridolfo, A., Trabattoni, D., Santambrogio, S., Vaccarezza, M., et al. (2003, April). Cytokin production in women with antiretroviral treatement-associated breast fat accumulation and limb wasting. *AIDS, 17* (Suppl. 1), S155–S161.

Gilad, J., Walfish, A., Borer, A, & Schlaeffer, F. (2003, 15 August). Gender differences and sex-specific manifestations associated with Human Immunodeficiency Virus infection in women. *European Journal of Obstetrics and Gynecology and Reproductive Biology, 109*(2), 199–205.

Global Fund to Fight AIDS, Tuberculosis, and Malaria (2004, 14 May). *Canada doubles Global Fund pledge for 2005.* (Press release). Retrieved 20 May 2004, from http://www.theglobalfund.org/en/media_center/press/pr_040514.asp.

Gorna, R. (1996). *Vamps, Virgins and Victims: How Can Women Fight AIDS?* London: Cassell.

Grewal, I. (1999, November). 'Women's rights as human rights': Feminist practices, global feminism, and human rights regimes in transnationality. *Citizenship Studies, 3*(3), 337–354.

Grewal, I., & Kaplan, C. (Eds.). (1994). *Scattered Hegemonies: Postmodernity and Transnational Feminist Practices*. Minneapolis: University of Minnesota.

Hammonds, E. (1990, April). Missing persons: African American women, AIDS, and the history of disease. *Radical America, 24*(2), 7–24.

Hammonds, E. (1997). In N. Goldstein, & J. Manlowe (Eds.), *The Gender Politics of HIV/AIDS in Women* (pp. 113–126). New York: New York University Press.

Hankins, C., Coutlée, F., Lapointe, N., Simard, P., Tran, T., Samson, J. & Hum, L. (1999, 26 January). Prevalence of risk factors associated with human papillomavirus infection in women living with HIV. *Canadian Medical Association Journal, 160*(2), 185–192.

Hankins, C., Lapointe, N, & Walmsley, S. (with Canadian Women's HIV Study Group). (1998). Participation in clinical trials among women living with HIV in Canada. *Canadian Medical Association Journal, 159*(11), 1359–1365.

Health Canada. (2003, 1 December). Estimates of HIV prevalence and incidence in Canada. *Canadian Communicable Disease Report 29–27*. Retrieved 20 May 2004, from http://www.hc-sc.gc.ca/pphb-dgspsp/publicat/ccdr-rmtc/03vol29/dr2923ea.html.

Health Canada Online. (2004a). *AIDS*. Retrieved 18 May 2004, from http://www.hc-sc.gc.ca/english/diseases/aids.html.

Health Canada Online. (2004b). *HIV and Sexual Violence Against Women*. Canadian strategy on AIDS. Retrieved 20 May 2004, from http://www.hc-sc.gc.ca/hppb/hiv_aids/you/sex_violence/.

Hogan, K. (2001). *Women Take Care: Gender, Race, and the Culture of AIDS*. Ithaca, NY: Cornell University Press.

Hollibaugh, A. (1998). Transmission, transmission, Where's the transmission? In N. Roth & K. Hogan (Eds.), *Gendered Epidemic: Representations of Women in the Age of AIDS* (pp. 63–71). New York: Routledge.

Joint United Nations Programme on HIV/AIDS (UNAIDSa, 1998, April). *Microbicides for HIV Prevention: UNAIDS Technical Update*. Retrieved 21 May 2004, from http://www.unaids.org/en/in+focus/topic+areas/microbicides.asp.

Joint United Nations Programme on HIV/AIDS (UNAIDSb, 2000, 5 June). *Gender Is Crucial Issue in Fight Against AIDS*. Press release. Retrieved 20 May 2004, from http://www.thebody.com/unaids/gender.html.

Jürgens, R. (2002). HIV/AIDS in prisons: Recent developments. *Canadian HIV/AIDS Policy and Law Review, 7*(2 –3), 13 – 20. Retrieved 25 April 2004, from http://www.aidslaw.ca/Maincontent/otherdocs/Newsletter/vol7no2-32003/vol7no2_3.pdf.

Lindblad, B. (2003). *Men and Boys Can Make a Difference in the Response to the HIV/AIDS Epidemic*. New York: UNAIDS. Retrieved 17 May 2004, from http://www.un.org/womenwatch/daw/egm/men-boys2003/WP4-UNAIDS.pdf.

Marble, M. (1997, 3 March). Rates among women in Canada increasing. *Women's Health Weekly*. Retrieved 5 March 2007, from http://www.newsrx.com/newsletters/Womens-Health-Weekly/1997-03-03/199703033331ww.html.

Masters, W., Johnson, V., & Kolodny, R. (1988). *Crisis: Heterosexual Behavior in the Age of AIDS*. New York: Grove Press.

Namaste, V. (1999). HIV/AIDS and female to male transsexuals and transvestites: Results from a needs assessment in Quebec. *International Journal of Transgenderism*, 3(1, 2). Retrieved 15 May 2004, from http://www.symposion.com/ijt/hiv_risk/namaste.htm.

Napravnik, S., Poole, C., Thomas, J., & Eron, J. (2002). Gender difference in HIV RNA levels: A Meta-analysis of published studies. *Journal of Acquired Immune Deficiency Syndromes*, 31(1), 11–19.

National Institutes of Health. (2004, May). *HIV Infection in Women*. NIAID fact sheet. Retrieved 18 March 2005, from http://www.niaid.nih.gov/factsheets/womenhiv.htm.

Nova Scotia Advisory Council on the Status of Women (NSACSW). (2003, September). *Gender and HIV/AIDS: A Backgrounder* (pp. 1–14). Retrieved 10 May 2004, from http://www.gov.ns.ca/staw/pubs2003_04/genderHIV_Sept2003.pdf.

Ofotokun, I., & Pomeroy, C. (2003). Sex differences in adverse reactions to antiretroviral drugs. *Topics in HIV Medicine*, 11(2), 55 –59.

O'Gorman, K. (2001, December). Northern women's health outreach project. *Canadian Women's Studies*, 21(2), 113–116. Retrieved 23 April 2004, from http://etestb.ohiolink.edu/bin/gate.exe?f=fulltext&state=h239hs.6.1. Contemporary Women's Issues database http://rave.ohiolink.edu/databases/login/cwis.

Pai, M., Schriever, C., Diaz-Linares, M., Novak, R., & Rodvold, K. (2004, May). Sex-related differences in the pharmacokinetics of once-daily saquinavir soft-gelatin capsules boosted with low-dose ritonavir in patients infected with Human Immunodeficiency Virus Type 1. *Pharmacotherapy*, 24(5), 592–599.

Patton, C. (1985, 8 February). Heterosexual AIDS panic: A queer paradigm. *Gay Community News*, 116–117.

Patton, C. (1990). *Inventing AIDS*. New York: Routledge.

Patton, C. (1994). *Last Served? Gendering the HIV Pandemic*. London: Taylor & Francis.

Patton, C. (2002). *Globalizing* AIDS. Minneapolis: University of Minnesota Press.

Patton, C., and Raimondo, M. (2002, March) Guest editors' introduction. *Femmist Media Studies*, 2(1), 5–18.

Pernerstorfer-Schoen, H., Jilma, B., Perschler, A., Wichlas, S., Schindler, K., Schindl, A., et al. (2001, 13 April). Sex differences in HAART-associated dyslipidaemia. *AIDS*, *15*(6), 725–734.

Petchesky, R. (2003). *Global Prescriptions: Gendering Health and Human Rights*. New York: Zed Books.

Raimondo, M. (2003). 'Corralling the virus:' Migratory sexualities and the 'spread of AIDS' in the US media. *Environment and Planning D: Society and Space*, *21*, 389–407.

Reynolds, K. (2001, December). Supportive housing for women living with HIV/AIDS. *Canadian Woman Studies*, *21*(2), 129. Retrieved 23 April 2004, from Contemporary Women's Issues Database.

Schneider, B., & Stoller, N. (Eds.). (1995). *Women Resisting AIDS: Feminist Strategies of Empowerment*. Philadelphia: Temple University Press.

Scott, J. (2003). *Risky Rhetoric: AIDS and the Cultural Practices of HIV Testing*. Edwardsville, IL: Southern Illinois University Press.

Spittal, P., Bruneau, J., Craib, K.J.P., Miller, C., Lamothe, F., Weber, A.E., Li, K., Tyndall, M.V., O'Shaughnessy, M.V., & Schecter, M.T. (2003). Surviving the sex trade: A comparison of HIV risk behaviours among street-involved women in two Canadian cities who inject drugs. *AIDS Care*, *15*(2), 187–195.

Stockdill, B. (2003). *Activism against AIDS: At the Intersections of Sexuality, Race, Gender, and Class*. Boulder, CO: Lynne Rienner.

Stoller, N. (1998). *Lessons from the Damned: Queers, Whores, and Junkies Respond to AIDS*. New York: Routledge.

Treichler, P. (1999). *How to Have Theory in an Epidemic: Cultural Chronicles of HIV/AIDS*. Durham, NC: Duke University Press.

Ulin, P., Cayemittes, M., & Gringle, R. (1996). Bargaining for life: Women and the AIDS epidemic in Haiti. In L. Long, & M. Ankrah (Eds.), *Women's Experiences with HIV/AIDS: An International Perspective* (pp. 91–111). New York: Columbia University Press.

United Nations Development Fund for Women (UNIFEM). (2001). *Turning the Tide: CEDAW and the Gender Dimension of the HIV/AIDS Pandemic*. New York: Author.

Walmsley, S. (1998). The new antiretroviral 'cocktails': Is the stage set for HIV-positive women to benefit? *Canadian Medical Association Journal*, *158*, 339–341. Retrieved 16 May 2004, from http://collection.nlc-bnc.ca/100/201/300/cdn_medical_association/cmaj/vol-158/issue-3/0339.htm.

Watney, S. (1994). *Practices of Freedom: Selected Writing on HIV/AIDS*. Durham, NC: Duke University Press.

Whittle, K., & Inhorn, M. (2001). Rethinking difference: A feminist reframing of gender/race/class for the improvement of women's health research. *International Journal of Health Services*, 31(1), 147–165.

Women's Outreach Network. (2000, April). *HIV and AIDS among Women in Canada*. Retrieved 15 May 2004, from http://www.womenfightaids.com/epistats.html#fig1.

Wood, E., Montaner, J., Braitstein, P., Yip, B., Schecter, M., O'Shaughnessy, M., & Hogg, R. (2004). Elevated rates of antiretroviral treatment discontinuation among HIV-infected injection drug users: implications for drug policy and public health. *International Journal of Drug Policy*, 15, 133–138.

Yingling, T. (1997). *AIDS and the National Body*. R. Wiegman (Ed.). Durham, NC: Duke University Press.

15 Breast Cancer: Lived Experience and Feminist Action

SUE WILKINSON

This chapter addresses one of women's central health concerns – breast cancer – from a critical, feminist perspective (see Wilkinson 2000a, 2004). The first section of the chapter provides a demographic overview of breast cancer in Canada. It presents some incidence and mortality statistics, and considers the ways in which breast cancer incidence, mortality, and risk are influenced by the key social variables of gender, age, social class, race/ethnicity, and sexual identity.

The second – central section – of the chapter offers an empirical analysis of women's lived experience of breast cancer. It draws both on my own (UK-based) focus group research, and on published accounts by Canadian women, to identify some key features of women's experience of receiving and coming to terms with a breast cancer diagnosis. It also explores some of the consequences of such a diagnosis for a woman's life and for the lives of those close to her. This central section illustrates one important feminist strategy for pursuing social change: documenting the commonality and diversity of women's experience, and making sense of this in relation to a broader social and political context.

The final section of the chapter examines both this strategy and a range of other forms of feminist action – particularly as they relate to the Canadian context. These forms of action include: establishing support services; campaigning for improved resources; challenging the invisibility of women with breast cancer through artistic expression; and exposing the link between the profits of the breast cancer 'industry' and environmental risk factors.

Breast Cancer: Incidence, Mortality and Risk

Breast cancer is the most common invasive cancer among Canadian women.[1] Across the country, around 5,400 women died from breast cancer in 2003; and the lifetime risk of being diagnosed with breast cancer in Canada is about one in nine[2] (Bryant, 2003a) – a similar incidence rate to other Western, industrialized countries. These incidence and mortality figures – along with those relating to risk factors for breast cancer – are heavily influenced by gender, age, class, and race/ethnicity.

The biggest risk factor for breast cancer is being a woman (only 1 to 2 per cent of cases diagnosed occur in men); and for 85 per cent of women, the major risk factor is increasing age (Altman, 1996). The older a woman gets, the greater the risk she faces. Other risk factors relate to reproductive history (not having children, a 'late' first pregnancy, a greater number than average number of menstrual cycles); 'lifestyle' factors (e.g., high-fat diet, being overweight, excessive drinking); and the presence of environmental, including workplace,[3] carcinogens. There is only one proven environmental cause of human breast cancer: ionizing radiation (see Brady, 1991). However, research also shows a strong correlation between breast cancer and exposure to other chemicals. The strongest evidence involves natural and synthetic oestrogens (including the pesticide simizane); vinyl chloride (released during the manufacture of polyvinyl choloride (PVC)); and organic solvents, such as methylene chloride (found in paints and paint removers)[4] (Evans, 2002). Although relatively little is known about workplace exposures, studies of occupational risk factors suggest an increased risk of breast cancer for two broad categories of workers: those who regularly handle toxic chemicals (e.g., lab technicians, dental hygienists, paper mill workers, meat cutters, and microelectronics workers), who are disproportionately poor and/or ethnic minority women[5]; and professionals (e.g., teachers, social workers, physicians), who are generally women in higher socio-economic groups (Goldberg & Labreche, 1996; Morton, 1995).[6] Elevated breast cancer incidence among professional women is generally explained in terms of delayed childbearing or not having children. Genetic factors are also implicated in breast cancer risk,[7] although – despite the publicity surrounding the 'breast cancer genes' – BRCA1 and BRCA2 – only 5 to 10 per cent of breast cancers have an identifiable genetic component. Nor is it known, despite recent media 'scares,' whether lesbians' risk of developing breast cancer is greater than that of heterosexual women (see Yadlon, 1997). (For a more extensive discussion of breast cancer risk, see Love, 2000, chapters 14 and 15.)

Breast cancer is still on the rise: the (age-standardized) incidence rate for Canadian women increased by 25 per cent in the 25-year period to 1998, although it is now apparently leveling off. The reason for the increase is unclear, but it may be due to changing reproductive patterns (fewer children, later childbearing) and/or to greater use of screening mammography, leading to more cancer detections (Bryant, 2003b).

Better news is that fewer women are now dying from breast cancer in Canada: The (age-standardized) mortality rate fell by 15 per cent in the 25-year period to 1998, with most improvement in recent years. Again, the reason is unclear, but it is likely due to a combination of increased screening (allowing for detection at an earlier, more treatable, stage), and improvements in cancer treatment (Bryant, 2003a).

This, then, is the national picture, and it is one broadly in line with that in the United States and northern Europe – where breast cancer incidence rates are higher, and mortality rates lower, than in less industrialized nations. However, these overall figures mask both some important variations and some startling omissions.

For example, there are some significant regional differences across Canadian provinces/territories. Breast cancer mortality rates range from a low of 22 deaths per 100,000 women in Saskatchewan to a high of 29 per 100,000 in Nova Scotia, Newfoundland, and Labrador (National Cancer Institute of Canada, 2002). Similarly, five-year relative survival rates range from a low of 76 per cent in Newfoundland and Labrador to a high of 85 per cent in British Columbia, possibly due to differences in mammography utilization (Ellison et al., 2001). To date, there has been no systematic study of the reasons for these differences.

Little is known about differences in breast cancer incidence or mortality across different ethnic or racial groups, because Canadian cancer registries do not systematically collect this information. One exception is the suggestion that rates tend to be lower in Inuit populations (Miller & Gaudette, 1996). Further, little is known about rates in migrant groups as compared to non-migrant groups, despite the general observation that migrants to higher-risk countries (like Canada and Australia) from lower-risk (generally Asian) countries tend to develop higher rates of risk (Kliewer & Smith, 1995). Recent migrant status is (increasingly) associated with low employment rates and with poverty – particularly for members of racialized groups and for women – with largely unknown health consequences (Galabuzi, 2004).

From research conducted outside Canada (particularly in the United States), we know that there are differences in breast cancer incidence and mortality rates due to both race/ethnicity and to socio-economic status. In general, women of colour are at lower risk of receiving a breast cancer diagnosis than are white (non-Hispanic Caucasian) women, but their mortality rate is higher, particularly among African Americans (Love, 2000, pp. 217–218). And in general, poorer women are at lower risk for breast cancer than women of higher socio-economic status, but their mortality rate is higher (Love, 2000, p. 222). The most likely explanation for these differences is differential health care, with lack of health insurance precluding access to health services or ensuring substantial delays – and this, in turn, meaning later diagnosis, poorer treatment, and reduced chance of survival (Kasper, 2000). While the Canadian context is somewhat different, we need the data to enable such systematic comparisons to be made; in addition to urban-rural comparisons, which are also crucial to documenting the consequences of differential access to health care.

Women's Experience of Breast Cancer

What is it like for a woman to receive a breast cancer diagnosis, to deal with its daily realities, and to incorporate its broader implications into her life? Despite some moving autobiographies (e.g., Butler & Rosenblum, 1991; MacPhee, 1994; Lorde, 1980), there has been very little social scientific research addressing this question. Still less research has taken either an experiential/phenomenological perspective or a feminist approach that starts from women's own experience, rather than from a preconceived theoretical framework.

Feminist experiential approaches place women's experiences within a broader social and political context and provide an opportunity to make women's experience central to an understanding of the world. Mainstream research (and culture) has systematically ignored, trivialized, or distorted women's experience by assimilating it into patriarchal models of 'reality' (Kitzinger and Wilkinson, 1997). By contrast, feminist experiential approaches 'reclaim' women's experience in its own right (Brems & Griffiths, 1993), and seek to make visible the diversity of experience in relation to differences of race/ethnicity, class and sexual identity, for example. This approach is in contrast to positivist empiricist research – which limits and constrains responses by means of standardized questions, scales and measures, and loses the individual in statistical summaries. Experiential approaches generate vivid, personal accounts of individual lives and experiences (e.g., Swann, 1997; Stevens, 1998). They may also provide new – and unexpected – insights, second wave feminist analyses of gendered power relations were based, in part, on sharing accounts of experiences, and on making new sense of these through new concepts, such as 'sexual harassment,' 'domestic violence,' or 'marital rape.'[8] Documenting and making sense of experience, and of the diversity of experience, is an essential first step towards social and political transformation.

In this chapter, I will report some key findings from my own research on women's experience of breast cancer. While this work was conducted in England, the findings appear to be broadly applicable, as I will show throughout by comparison with published materials on women's experience of breast cancer in Canada.

Eighty-one women with breast cancer talked with me, and with each other, in a series of focus group discussions. The women were recruited to the study through the clinic of a consultant surgeon specializing in breast surgery, and they were at different stages of their breast cancer 'careers.' They were generally typical of the breast cancer population in being mostly middle-aged or older, and of the particular geographical region in being mostly working-class and white, and from a mix of urban and rural locations. No woman self-identified as other than heterosexual in these groups. The focus groups consisted of wide-ranging and relatively unstructured conversations – often lasting three or four hours – about the experience of living with breast cancer. These conversations were tape-recorded, transcribed, and analysed in a variety of ways. (For more details of the project see Wilkinson, 1998, 2000a; Wilkinson & Kitzinger, 2000.)

Here, I will draw on a preliminary thematic analysis of the data (Wilkinson, 2000b) to highlight four key aspects of what these women told me: their initial reactions to a breast cancer diagnosis; the impact of breast cancer on their relationships; their concerns about treatment, especially surgery; and the broader changes breast cancer had wrought in their lives. I will also draw on data from additional focus groups I conducted with the male partners of some of these women, and with self-identified lesbians talking about their experiences of breast cancer.

Initial Diagnosis

The diagnosis of breast cancer was described by one participant as 'every woman's nightmare.' In general, women reported extreme emotional reactions: they said they were 'devastated,' 'gutted,' or 'poleaxed' (i.e., 'bowled over') by the news. Many described feelings of fear ('terrified,' 'fear-stricken,' 'frightened,' 'paralyzed in me head with fear'), sometimes accompanied by physical reactions such as crying, shaking uncontrollably, or collapsing. Some women recalled their feelings of shock and disbelief ('You don't believe it,' 'I couldn't believe that it could happen to me,' or 'You don't think it's ever going to happen to you, and when it does you just can't believe it'). Others described an inability to take in the information or to react to it ('It didn't register properly,' 'I was in a stupor and I never spoke,' 'I just went numb'). Feelings of detachment were common: one woman said, 'When I was told, it was someone else – it was a long while before I realised it was me.' Others said the experience was like being 'on another planet' or 'in a different world.'

The voices of women in one widely cited Canadian breast cancer anthology (Galambos, 1998) tell a remarkably similar story of fear, disbelief, and frozen disorientation: 'What I remember most is the fear' (p. 13); 'I was stunned' (p. 29); 'I took a breath, and it stuck in my throat. For an instance, I didn't know how to exhale'(p.155); 'I stared into space with disbelief ... I felt as if I were in a foreign world' (pp. 70–71). In another, more recent Canadian anthology (Tocher, 2002), one woman said, 'Life seemed to stop right there' (p. 68); another reported 'I couldn't speak, literally ... All I could do was sort of whine and snort' (p. 60); and a third describes her reaction as 'stunned wonder,' because 'it was all so surreal' (p. 55). And Rosalind MacPhee (1994), diagnosed with breast cancer in Vancouver in 1994, writes of the moment her surgeon first uttered the words 'It is cancer': 'I was in a bubble. I saw his mouth moving and I was aware of the flow of words, but I was unable to process most of the information. He may as well have been speaking in a different language' (p. 41).

Relationships

Women in my study often worried about other people's reactions to their breast cancer diagnosis and sometimes withheld the news for a considerable period of time from those close to them, even altogether from those seen as unable to cope with it (e.g., aged parents,[9] young children). Similarly, one participant in a Canadian study of women with breast and other cancers (Clarke, 1985) delayed telling anyone, including her husband: 'I couldn't tell anyone else. For three months I knew it was serious, but I couldn't tell my husband' (p. 21).

Telling others was carefully managed: women in my study waited until children had finished examinations, or sick colleagues had returned to work. In Clarke's study, one woman waited until her husband had been on a fishing trip in order not to 'ruin' it for him (p. 63), and others 'talked of how they had often felt it was their responsibility to ensure that the conversation flowed smoothly, with the friend, doctor, child, parent, or husband (p. 53).

Women in my focus groups often underemphasized the seriousness of their condition: 'I really did deliberately play it down,' said one woman (talking about her son), 'I thought, he's far away – it would worry him sick.' In order to protect others – especially family members – perceived as vulnerable, women also minimized or hid their own pain, distress, and anxiety: 'I daren't say much to me husband or family for fear of distressing them'; 'You don't want to put your worries on them do you, all the time?'; 'You end up being strong for your friends, your family, because they don't know how to handle it.' One participant commented, 'We become very good at behaving ourselves, especially as women – we're very good at hiding what we feel and just putting on a brave face for everybody else.'

One of Galombos' (1998) contributors also reflected on women's traditional roles: 'As women, we have been brought up to be strong. Our primary place is in the home, not merely for doing the chores, but for being nurturers and caregivers. Our families revolve around us, and it is our basic instinct to protect them. They are dealing with their own fears and concerns about our disease, and we don't want to make things worse. Inevitably, we protect them from our pain, our emotional vulnerability, and the worst of our imaginations' (contributor Beryl MacRae, quoted in Galombos, 1998, p. 36). And one of Clarke's (1985) participants even hid her feelings in order to protect her doctor (who had assured her that her breast lump was not malignant, on four separate visits over a year): 'Whenever any anger came to me, I swallowed it. I just could not hurt him further' (p. 55).

My research participants were often aware of silences around cancer[10]: people around them 'are embarrassed,' 'don't know what to say,' or 'just don't want to know'; work colleagues 'don't mention it at all.' As with cancer generally (Sontag, 1979), women with breast cancer may find that others seem to fear and avoid them (almost three-quarters of Peters-Golden's (1982) respondents reported this experience). 'My neighbours seem to think I'm a leper,' one of my research participants said. 'There's one lady in particular and she always crosses the road ... as though if she touches me she's going to get something.' Another told how her sister (also diagnosed with breast cancer) returning unexpectedly to a friend's house, found the friend 'cleaning the cushion of the settee she'd been sitting on ... as if she thought she could catch the cancer.' Clarke's (1985) participants also reported this fear and avoidance: one reported that an old friend found it very hard to visit her in hospital, 'so she avoided that like the plague ... she wouldn't show. She couldn't face it' (pp. 53-54); another confronted her best friend, who said she was 'too terrified, too frightened' to visit, that she 'just couldn't' (p. 54).

Close friends, family members, and – particularly – partners were often reported as having particular difficulties in coming to terms with a cancer diagnosis. 'My husband took it pretty hard,' said one of Clarke's (1985) participants, 'I think it was harder on him than it really was on me' (p. 60). Others characterized their husbands as 'so distressed' (p. 62), and as 'feeling tremendous grief' (p. 64). Other Canadian women indicated their husbands avoided talking about their diagnosis: 'He would not talk about cancer. He tuned me out if I tried to express my feelings' (contributor in Tocher, 2002, p. 57); sometimes, indeed, (for a time) they absolutely could not cope: 'He was not able to sleep and suffered hallucinations as well as giddiness and depression' (contributor in Tocher, 2002, p. 87); 'My husband's world collapsed' (contributor in Galambos, 1998, p. 59).

In my data, women also described their male partners' reactions in this way: 'My husband was very, very upset'; 'He didn't want to eat, he wasn't sleeping, he was absolutely morose ... he didn't know how to handle it really'; 'It was my husband we were more worried about than anybody.' Another participant's assessment – 'It's a traumatic time, isn't it, for husbands?' – provoked strong agreement from the other women present. Male partners, too, in their own (separate) focus group discussions, echoed this assessment. They described the situation as 'hard to take,' 'frightening,' 'difficult to deal with,' 'very difficult to live with,' and 'a lot of pressure.' My experience of facilitating the partner focus groups was that these were particularly emotionally charged.

Lesbian partners may face an additional difficulty: the assumption that they will be supportive and empathetic, because they share the experience of being a woman, and that is how women are supposed to be. However, many of my research participants explicitly countered this assumption, some expressing the opinion that it may actually be harder for a woman to deal with her female partner's breast cancer because it evokes the possibility of the same thing happening to her. Two participants spoke at length of partners who simply could not cope, describing their relationships as 'very fraught' and subject to 'huge sturm und drang': the latter relationship, in fact, broke up soon after the breast cancer diagnosis.

A recent Ontario study of lesbians' cancer experiences (Lesbians and Breast Cancer Project Team, 2004a) reports similar difficulties: '[My partner and I] didn't hardly communicate, or we didn't talk about the cancer hardly at all' (p. 26); '[The woman I was with] couldn't cope with my emotional reactions. She didn't know what to do'(p. 26). And for lesbians who are neither 'out' to their families of origin (an important alternative source of support for many women with breast cancer), nor integrated into a lesbian community, the resulting emotional isolation may be particularly acute.

Treatment and Appearance Concerns

Most of my research participants had undergone surgery for their breast cancer (35 per cent lumpectomy; 63 per cent mastectomy), usually accompanied by adjuvant therapy – most commonly radiotherapy, together with a course of the synthetic oestrogen-blocker, Tamoxifen[11] (64 per cent). A further 21 per cent had taken Tamoxifen alone. Relatively few had been prescribed chemotherapy, or had chosen 'alternative' treatments.

Women exchanged experiences of treatments and symptoms: the awfulness of not being able to wash for several weeks once 'marked up' for radiotherapy ('the smell was horrid'; 'I felt I ponged from here to here'); the radiotherapy burns and skin irritation ('Bright red, I was, like a tomato'; 'As if I was on fire ... I was sort of burning'); and the weight gain, night sweats, and vaginal itching produced by Tamoxifen ('It was really driving me crazy'; 'All inside was really raw'). Canadian women, too, often emphasize the horrors of radiotherapy: 'The radiation affects you internally, and then it comes to the surface. They tell you it's going to be like a bad sunburn. You think, *Oh, I can handle that*, but inside, where I was radiated, it is still so tender. Under my arm at the site of my surgical incision, my skin was split wide open, really badly burned. And under my breast it was raw – *raw* ... When you put something in a microwave, it cooks from the inside out. That's exactly what it's like' ('Franci,' contributor in Tocher, 2002, pp. 85–86). Francis Martindale (1994) even suggests that the depersonalization, vulnerability, and brutality she experienced during radiotherapy 'called up associations of the gas chambers' (pp. 159–140).[12]

When talking about treatment, my research participants focused most extensively on their feelings about surgery, and its consequences for their physical appearance. The psychosocial oncology and autobio-graphical literatures alike (e.g., Maguire, 1982; Kahane, 1995; Kasper, 1995) suggest that a woman who has lost a breast is 'less a woman,' and my (heterosexual) research participants often spoke as if this were so: 'You're not sort of normal any more ... only half a woman'; 'I just felt like all my womanhood was being taken away and I wasn't going to be a she any more, I was going to be an it.' Similarly, one woman in Clarke's (1985) study described her first reaction to mastectomy as, 'I'd be a neuter' (p. 66); and a contributor to Galambos' (1998) anthology felt 'utterly deformed' (p. 61) – this woman goes on to say that she only 'felt like a whole human being' after breast reconstruction (p. 66).

My research participants commonly expressed fears that without breasts, or with less than perfect breasts, they would be unattractive to, or rejected by, men: 'I'm very aware that there are marriages that break down under the stress ... and what your body looks like'; 'part of it was to do with my husband; I didn't know whether he was going to reject me'; 'I was single and I thought, "Oh well, nobody's ever going to be interested in me ... nobody would want anybody who'd had their breast removed."' Some women sought reassurances from the men around them that they were still attractive and desirable; one woman embarked upon a new love affair within days of surgery.

Heterosexual Canadian women, too, very commonly express such concerns, and seek such reassurances;[13] they ask themselves, 'Will any-one ... want me now that I don't have breasts?' (Tocher, 2002, p. 66); 'who would look at me anyway?' (p. 67). One woman only felt 'like a woman again' after her brother's friends flirted with her (Tocher, 2002, p. 113); another 'went from relationship to relationship' in a desperate search for acceptance (p. 64). Such concerns may well be justified: it is not uncommon for relationships to break down under the strain of breast cancer. One woman said, 'I know too many women who have been abandoned physically, emotionally, and sexually after a mastectomy'(Tocher, 2002, p. 69); another, who organized a radio phone-in program about breast cancer survivors whose husbands had left them reports: 'There were so many women that we couldn't handle all the calls. It was terrible' (Galambos, 1994, p.149).

Lesbians (and older heterosexual women) are often assumed *not* to care about their physical appearance, and, it seems, are even told by some surgeons that they do not 'need' their breasts – presumably be-cause breasts are primarily for attracting men and satisfying them sexually, and maybe occasionally for breastfeeding babies (see Wilkinson

& Kitzinger, 1993, for a discussion of heterosexist assumptions in breast cancer advice and treatment).[14] As one of my lesbian focus group participants said, 'It's very easy for them to whip it off and think it doesn't matter.' Indeed, a lesbian in Toronto recently reports that 'through the course of the conversation [her surgeon] just kind of very glibly said, "well we could just lop the whole thing off"' (Lesbians and Breast Cancer Project Team, 2004b).

But, of course, lesbians' breasts also have a sexual role (and sometimes a maternal one, too), and the appearance, touch, and feel of breasts are often central to lesbians' sex lives. Many of my research participants emphasized this: 'I really like my breasts a lot and I have a really erotic relationship to them'; 'I just love [my partner's] breasts and they do turn me on'; 'I think sexually my nipples are very sensitive; when that's the most exciting part of sex, I get so bloody turned on it can drive me up the wall'; 'I must say I think breasts are, you know, one of the most attractive parts of a woman's body'; 'I love my breasts'; 'They're erotic.'

This message was echoed emphatically by lesbians in the recent Ontario study (Lesbians and Breast Cancer Project Team, 2004a): 'I think lesbians really identify with their breasts, you know, as a sexual thing' (p. 28); 'my Breasts are an intrinsic part of making love to another woman' (p. 37); 'There are women like me who can't have an orgasm without involvement of their nipples'(p. 40); 'My breasts are my core sensuality piece of my body' (p. 64).

Not surprisingly, then, the loss of a breast was also described by many of my lesbian participants as 'devastating.' One woman said of her mastectomy, 'I thought, "Well, you know, this is the end of life as I know it," and I actually, I sort of mourned for the loss of my breast ... I was really very disturbed and distressed about it.' Another, whose lover had developed breast cancer, found it extremely difficult to come to terms with her lover's appearance after her mastectomy: 'I thought it was horrific what the body looks like without a breast ... She looked like she'd been butchered ... The fact that she was flat-chested wasn't the issue, it's the scars.' Lesbians contemplating the possibility of mastectomy said, 'I would just feel so mutilated'; 'It's something that is sexual'; 'in my sex life I would miss it'; 'It's not just your breasts, it's your whole body image – it's the way you feel about your body as a whole afterwards.' There was no suggestion at all that breasts are unimportant or irrelevant to lesbians or that the loss of a breast (or breasts) was – or would be – anything other than traumatic.

And lesbians facing breast surgery worry about their attractiveness to future sexual partners, too (Lesbians and Breast Cancer Project Team, 2004a): 'What if I lost mine ... How horrible would that be? ... Who'd want to touch me?' (p. 28); 'It's hard for me to imagine that another person could love me completely without having all of my body there' (p. 37); 'Who's going to want me, now that I have cancer?'(p. 43); 'You do think you're the ugliest thing on the planet and that no one's ever going to date you' (p. 44); 'Who's going to want someone who has this kind of scar, and is someone going to consider me sexy?' (p. 43). In this respect, at least, lesbians' concerns are apparently not dissimilar to those of heterosexual women.

Life Changes

It was common for women in my focus groups to claim that the experience of breast cancer had completely changed their outlook on life: heightened awareness of mortality and uncertainty about the future made them 'appreciate life,' 'enjoy life,' and 'live for the moment.' One woman said, 'I used to be a person who used to always look into the future. We'd got to save up for when we get older and we ought not to have a big holiday because really, you know, we might need the roof mending. I was that sort of person, but I'm not so much that now. I think to myself, "Oh to heck with it, I might not be here next year."' Many emphasized 'an urgency about life,' a need to 'live life to the full,' to 'do more with your life,' and to 'do it today.' One declared, 'If you wanna do it, I think you've got to go for it.' And go for it they did: new experiences (since cancer) ranged from long-distance travel to scuba diving to flying a plane. Some women got involved in breast cancer support work, education, or activism.

Canadian women, too, talked of 'doing things I've never done before' (Clarke, 1985, p. 108) and developing 'a sense of adventure' (p. 107). They pursued new activities, including flying (Tocher, 2002, pp. 159-160), hiking (p. 172), creative writing (p. 158), attending law school (p. 581), and pursuing the adoption of a child (p. 140). Many emphasized the importance of raising awareness about breast cancer, informally, among their social networks (Galambos, 1998, p. 126), by talking to women's groups (Clarke, 1985, p. 105), by becoming breast cancer spokespersons and outreach workers in immigrant communities (Galambos, 1998, p. 112), or by training as volunteers for breast cancer advocacy and support organizations, including Reach for Recovery (p. 65) and the Breast Cancer Foundation (Tocher, 2002, p. 140).

Others among my research participants told me: 'My priorities in life have changed,' or 'I'm having to reassess what I want to do now' – thus deciding to spend money, rather than to save it; to take a job and become independent for the first time; or to exploit a new-found ability to leave housework undone.[15] Several women described themselves as 'more selfish,' saying, 'You've got to think about yourself'; 'I'm number one now'; 'I feel I have a stronger responsibility to myself'; 'I'm entitled to be able to do something for myself'; and 'I want to do even more now of the things that I want to do.'

One Canadian woman described, as a consequence of breast cancer, 'burying the person who was ready to please everybody before pleasing myself' (Tocher, 2002, p. 145). Now, she says, 'the new me comes first' (p.145). Another felt able to challenge her Orthodox Jewish upbringing, telling her family 'from now on I have to love myself. I come first.' She continued: 'I tried to explain that coming first meant that I would live in the "now." That tomorrow would be today. Whatever it was I had to do, or wanted to do, I was going to do it today ... Putting myself first also meant that I would go back to school' (Gert Batist, in Galambos, 1998, p. 64). (She graduated four years later, at the age of 50, with a BA in Sociology). Others said: 'Now I find what I think comes first' (Clarke, 1985, p. 106); 'I'm going to live the way I want to live' (p. 107); and 'I value me more' (p. 108).

Politics of Breast Cancer: Anger, Art, and Activism

Critical, feminist work on breast cancer has not only made women's own experiences (rather than medical or psychiatric perspectives) central, but it has sought to understand these experiences within their broader social and political context (Kasper & Ferguson, 2000; Wilkinson & Kitzinger, 1993). Feminist analyses have suggested, for example, that a preoccupation with physical appearance, rather than survival,[16] is understandable in the context of a breast-obsessed culture in which women's worth is measured by the size and shape of their breasts: 'Women are awash in cultural images of perfect bodies and beautiful breasts and know full well whether they measure up' (Stewart, 1998, p. 86). (Also see Saywell, 2000, for an analysis of the role of the media in promoting a (hetero)sexualized view of breast cancer.)

Feminists have also shown how this cultural bias is partly constructed by – and is in the interests of – the medical profession itself. One doctor writes (in a text on early detection of breast cancer): 'To the average woman, her breast is the badge of femininity, an important part of allurement to charm her male' (Strax, 1974, cited in Altman, 1996, p. 242). Another is reported to have said brightly (in breaking the news to a woman that she needs a mastectomy): 'It's not the end of the world ... I can make you another one. If you were my wife, I'd want you to have it' (Prior, 1987, p. 20). Around the time of the Second World War, surgeons invented the disease of 'hypomastia' (small breasts); psychiatrists deemed this seriously damaging to a woman's self-esteem; and plastic surgeons came forward with the 'cure,' in the shape of augmentation mammoplasty (Zimmerman, 1998). The ensuing massive demand for silicone breast implants – a product improperly tested, and subsequently proving so harmful to women (see Wilson, 1995, for a Canadian example) – has been identified as a direct consequence of this 'medical construction of need' (Jacobson, 2000). Given this context, it is perhaps unsurprising to find a woman who has undergone a mastectomy suggesting that this constitutes a threat to her body image, femininity, and gender identity; and also to find that it is 'taken for granted that she will want implants to "normalize" her body' (Stewart, 1998, p. 86).

Similarly, in a powerful analysis deriving from her own experience of breast cancer treatment, feminist sociologist Barbara Ehrenreich (2001) identifies the 'relentless brightsiding' of the 'implacably optimistic' mainstream breast cancer culture – serving primarily, she says, to 'tame and normalize' the disease (p. 43) (see also Wilkinson & Kitzinger, 2000, on 'thinking positive' as a moral injunction for breast cancer patients). Ehrenreich suggests that there is not nearly enough anger around at the commercialization of breast cancer – particularly the infantilizing effects of a multitude of ultra-feminine, pink-ribbon-themed breast cancer products – and not nearly enough attention paid to environmental risk factors, including the implication of the major pharmaceutical companies in these risks. This is a point I shall return to later on in the chapter.

The political analysis of personal experience is, however, just one feminist strategy in working for social change. The remainder of this final section examines a range of other forms of feminist action around issues central to a critical, feminist analysis of breast cancer, particularly as these apply in the Canadian context.

The feminist breast cancer movement in Canada shares many features of the larger (and better-known) movement that began in the United States in the 1970s (see Altman, 1996, for historical context). In particular, feminist activists have set up resource centres and support services; have campaigned for increased research funding and improved health care facilities; have used the visual and verbal arts to challenge the widespread invisibility of women with breast cancer; and have exposed commercially driven links between the values and practices of the breast cancer 'industry' and a range of (largely unacknowledged) risks, particularly environmental risks (Batt, 1994).

Providing Support

Providing appropriate support for women with breast cancer has always been central. In the 1970s U.S. movement, many community cancer projects and programs were founded by feminist and lesbian activists. There is a smaller network of these in Canada, although, as in the United States, they tend to be concentrated in large urban centres (e.g., the Willow Breast Cancer Support and Resource Service and the Ontario Breast Cancer Community Research Initiative in Toronto). One issue is the extent to which generic organizations and support groups (i.e., for all types of cancer, or for all women) are sufficient to meet the diversity of women's needs – and there is a need for more organizations/groups specifically designed to support particular groups of women (e.g., First Nations women, Jewish women, lesbian and bisexual women, as are found in Vancouver). The related issue of support for partners – particularly female partners – and others living with, or close to, women with breast cancer has barely been addressed.

One particular kind of support, which reflects both the contemporary emphasis on the role of exercise in recovery from breast cancer, and feminist ideals of sisterhood, is the dragon boating movement (see the contributors to Tocher, 2002, for what this movement means to them). Although the ancient origins of dragon boating lie in Asia, its role in relation to breast cancer rests on pioneering research at the University of British Columbia, in which the strenuous upper-body exercise involved in paddling dragon boats was shown to aid recovery from surgery and radiotherapy (McKenzie, 1988). The original Vancouver dragon boat team of breast cancer survivors – Abreast in a Boat – has now been joined by more than two dozen others across Canada: for example, Survivorship, Island Breaststrokers, NorthBreast Passage (all based in BC), Two Abreast (Montreal), Dragons Abreast (Toronto), Sistership (Calgary), and Chemo Savvy (Winnipeg). Indeed, dragon boating by breast cancer survivors has become an international movement, with, for example, a South Pacific Breast Cancer Regatta held in New Zealand in 2003.

Campaigning for Resources

Another key feminist concern has been the lack of financial resources for breast cancer research and health care facilities. In campaigning for improved resources, Canadian feminists have (like their sisters in the United States) found it expedient to draw explicit parallels between the HIV/AIDS epidemic and the spread of breast cancer. Sharon Batt (1991), for example, invites the reader to compare the 1987 Canadian breast cancer mortality figure (of over 4,000 women) to 'the 417 deaths from AIDS in Canada in the same year' (p. 60). Canadian feminists have also drawn on AIDS activism in finding creative ways to celebrate the struggle against breast cancer and to honour the memory of women who have died. The Life Quilt for Breast Cancer, conceptualized and inaugurated by Judy Reimer (who, sadly, died in October 2002), and designed by British Columbia artist Gay Mitchell, is a tryptich composed of painted and quilted cotton panels. The three centre panels represent stages in the life of a forest: destruction, re-colonization/hope, and re-growth/ healing. Each panel is surrounded by 136 individual squares, created by individual contributors to reflect their personal stories or those of their loved ones. Over 20,000 people have contributed to the making of the Life Quilt, and it has been exhibited at libraries and galleries across Canada.[17]

Challenging Invisibility

Representing personal experience – both verbally and visually – has long been central to feminist political action around breast cancer (Wilkinson, 2001). The central motivation for this is to challenge the widespread invisibility of women with breast cancer (see, for example, Datan, 1989; Lorde, 1980) and to provide both realistic information and messages of hope to others facing such a diagnosis. Consider, for example, Jo Spence's (1986) gritty realism in a series of photographs representing her 'ordinary' woman's body with undisguised scarring, sagging, and stretch marks, and Deena Metzger's (1981) more 'spiritual' pose, arms uplifted to the sky, and with a 'tree of life' tattooed on her mastectomy scar. Both, in their different ways, break the taboo that has long surrounded the representation of the post-mastectomy body.

Similarly, the anthology *Art.Rage.Us.* (Art.Rage.Us, 1998) – a collection of paintings, drawings, poetry and essays by San Francisco women with breast cancer – is an important counter to the expectation of silence and concealment.

I have drawn on a number of autobiographies and anthologies of personal stories by Canadian breast cancer survivors in the central section of this chapter. Here, I want particularly to highlight a unique combination of the verbal and the visual. The recent anthology, *My Breasts, My Choice: Journeys Through Surgery* (Brown, Aslin, & Carey, 2003) began life as a photographic installation in Toronto. By including, alongside personal accounts and images of surgery for breast cancer, accounts and images of breast surgery undertaken for a variety of other reasons, such as chronic pain, gynaecomastia, and gender reassignment; and by including resource materials covering a wide range of approaches to breast health, it is a particularly comprehensive, inclusive, and informative volume.

Exposing the Link between Profit and Risk

One final, and particularly compelling, strand of feminist breast cancer activism has been to expose the – insidious, and often unacknowledged – links between the commercialization of breast cancer and the downplaying of risk, particularly environmental risk. The breast cancer 'industry' is incredibly lucrative: its constitutive parts – 'breast health centres,' mammographic screening services, facilities for radiotherapy and chemotherapy, and extensive drug treatments – represent an estimated income of US$16 billion a year in the United States alone (Ehrenreich, 2001). However, the values and practices of this multinational corporate enterprise have repeatedly come under fire from feminists (Batt, 1994; Clorfene-Casten, 1996; Leopold, 1999), environmentalists, and others.

The primary sponsor of the annual Breast Cancer Awareness Month is the multinational chemical giant AstraZeneca (formerly Zeneca[18]), which manufactures the estrogen-blocking drug Tamoxifen, widely used in the treatment of breast cancer. AstraZeneca also manufactures a range of fungicides and herbicides, including the carcinogen acetochlor; and one of its plants is reportedly the third-largest source of airborne carcinogenic pollution in the United States (Batt & Gross, 1999). Not surprisingly, the literature for Breast Cancer Awareness Month does not mention the possible role of such chemicals in raising breast cancer rates. Activists in San Francisco – including representatives of Breast Cancer Action, Greenpeace, and the Women's Cancer Resource Center – have instituted an annual 'toxic tour' of the cancer industry in the Bay Area to raise awareness of these concealed risks (Klawiter, 2000). They have also been attempting to broaden the focus of the local 'Race for the Cure' and 'Women and Cancer Walk' to encompass 'an environmental justice discourse of cancer prevention' (p. 81), as well as the traditional focus on services and advocacy for women with cancer. Canadian feminists, too, have consistently called for a stronger emphasis on prevention, relative to the prevailing (medical) discourses of 'treatment' and 'cure' (Batt & Gross, 1999).

For the cancer industry, 'prevention' typically signals 'chemo-prevention' – and, here again, attendant risks are typically downplayed. In the mid-1990s, the U.S. National Cancer Institute (NCI) formed an unusual alliance with (what was then) Zeneca to launch a major clinical trial to determine whether Tamoxifen could prevent breast cancer in healthy women deemed at 'high risk' of contracting it (primarily for genetic reasons). Zeneca provided the Tamoxifen and placebos 'free of charge.' Controversially, the trial was halted early, with NCI declaring unequivocally that Tamoxifen can prevent breast cancer in 'high risk' women; this conclusion was disputed by British scientists, and deemed 'more hype than hope' by breast cancer and women's health activists (Evans & Martin, 2000, p. 46).[19] Amid the hype it was barely acknowledged that Tamoxifen has a wide range of side effects (most commonly mimicking menopausal symptoms), and some of these are serious, if relatively rare (e.g., uterine cancer, blood clots in the lungs and large blood vessels, stroke). Annual sales of Tamoxifen in the United States alone generate more than US$265 million for AstraZeneca – and if the drug were prescribed for the 29 million purportedly 'high-risk' women, this would rise to a staggering US$7.6 billion a year (Evans & Martin, 2000). Once again, it appears that women's health is being subordinated to the profit motive of the multinational pharmaceutical companies. NCI has now launched another trial, this time to compare the effects of Tamoxifen and Raloxifen(e) – an osteoporosis-prevention drug manufactured by Eli Lilly (which claims it has fewer negative side effects than Tamoxifen). However, this trial has no placebo group, thus assuming that one of these two drugs can prevent breast cancer in 'high-risk' women, and failing to compare the effects of drug therapy with no chemo-prevention at all (Evans & Martin, 2000). Canadian feminist activists (among others) have also criticized the logic of such trials as 'casting too wide a net' (Batt, 1994, p. 198), for the simple reason that we don't have the knowledge to identify women who are truly 'high risk' – except for those few who have first degree relatives with breast cancer.

Taking a critical, feminist perspective mandates both a focus on women's experience, and a political analysis of that experience, as key components of working for social transformation. However, this brief review cannot do more than illustrate the richness and variety of women's lived experience of breast cancer; and the range of feminist action directed towards better understanding that experience and improving the conditions of women's lives. At the same time, particularly when juxtaposed against the breast cancer statistics with which I began this chapter, it reveals how little is known about – and often by – women with breast cancer, and how much more is needed in terms of research, resources, support, education, and advocacy.

Breast cancer is still on the rise, and will become a personal reality during her lifetime for one in nine Canadian women. It is feared – and for good reason – by every woman. Yet, although its causes are poorly understood, many women are exposed to unnecessary risks. Others do not get appropriate treatment, or their treatment is unacceptably delayed. Many lack support. Resources are severely limited; research is desperately underfunded; and prevention has barely been addressed. As such, breast cancer is surely a priority area for developing critical theory, policy, and practice.

NOTES

1 Although lung cancer is the leading cause of death.
2 The 1 in 9 figure represents *cumulative lifetime risk* up to age 90. Olivotto, Gelmon, & Kuusk (2001, pp. 18–20) provide a clear description of the difference between *lifetime* risk of developing breast cancer, and *annual* risk, which increases with each decade of life.
3 According to Jackson (2004), in Canada 'Experts estimate that anywhere from 10% to 40% of cancers may be caused primarily by workplace exposures' (p. 86).
4 Other chemicals which may also be related to breast cancer include dioxin (created when plastics and chlorine-containing materials are burned); polychlorinated biphenyls (traditionally used in the manufacture of

electrical equipment); and phthalates (used to make plastic soft and flexible). See Evans (2002).

5 And, of course, these women not only suffer exploitation in the labour market, but continue to carry a disproportionate burden of housework and child care, imposing additional stressors. For a recent analysis of the racialization of poverty in Canada, including its effects on health status, see Galabuzi (2004).

6 Although the role of higher social class has been challenged. See Petralia et al. (1998).

7 Women who have a first-degree relative with breast cancer have a 1 in 7 or 1 in 6 (lifetime) risk of developing breast cancer themselves.

8 The subsequent 'postmodern turn' within feminism (as within the academy more generally) has generated considerable epistemological debate about the concept of 'experience' (e.g., Grant, 1993; Scott, 1993; Stanley, 1994). There is a clear split between those who favour a 'realist' epistemology and those who criticize such an epistemology on the grounds that the 'real world' is always socially constructed (see Ramazanoglu, 2002, chaps. 4, 7, for a useful summary of these debates). What sometimes seems to be missing from these debates is the recognition that to claim something as a social construction is not necessarily to deny its reality – in the sense that social constructions can (indeed, do) have real, material effects in the world.

9 In Margaret Atwood's (1981) novel *Bodily Harm*, the character Rennie doesn't tell her mother about her mastectomy.

10 Such silences may be particularly acute in 'traditional' ethnic minority communities, as contributors to the Galambos (1998) anthology write in relation to the immigrant Sinhalese (p.111) and Caribbean (p.125) communities in Toronto. See also Bottorff et al. (2001), Hilton et al. (2001) and Johnson et al. (2004) for the South Asian communities in Vancouver.

11 In Canada, the 'new generation' alternative, Raloxifen(e), which was originally developed as an osteoporosis-prevention drug, is more likely to be prescribed. Clinical trials comparing Tamoxifen and Raloxifen(e) continue in the United States (Love, 2000, pp. 303–305); see last section of this chapter for problems with these.

12 She is not alone in making this association: Jewish lesbian Sandra Butler does so as she looks at her lover Barbara Rosenblum's body marked up for radiation (Butler & Rosenblum, 2000, p. 154).

13 Some women from cultures where long hair is strongly associated with womanhood have described losing their hair through chemotherapy as

more traumatic than losing a breast. See, for example, the account of
immigrant women to Canada from Sri Lanka, in Galambos (1998,
pp. 109–110).

14 For some graphic examples of heterosexism in oncology care, see Lesbians
and Breast Cancer Project Team (2004a); for analyses of heterosexism in
health care more generally, see, for example, Stevens (1992, 1996).

15 This may be a hitherto unrecognized 'side effect' of having breast cancer.
See also contributors to Galambos (1998, p. 54) and Tocher (2002, p. 145).

16 Others have challenged the assumption that appearance is indeed
women's primary concern, reporting data in which women – when asked
about their concerns following a breast cancer diagnosis – more frequently
cite 'future health' than appearance or physical attractiveness
(Meyerowitz, 1981).

17 More information about the Life Quilt can be found at http://www.
starrynight.ca/lifequilt/index.html. Judy Reimer's contribution to
Galambos (1998) describes its genesis (p.189).

18 Zeneca was formerly owned by Imperial Chemical Industries (ICI), one
of the world's largest manufacturers of organochlorines. ICI was sued in
1990 for dumping DDT and PCBs (both banned toxic chemicals) off the
coast of California (Batt & Gross, 1999).

19 Indeed, the feminist National Women's Health Network opposed it
entirely. Physician and board member Adriane Fugh-Berman said the trial
was 'premature in its assumptions, weak in its hypotheses, questionable
in its ethics and misguided in its public health ramifications' (cited in Batt,
1994, p. 194).

REFERENCES

Altman, R. (1996). *Waking Up, Fighting Back: The Politics of Breast Cancer.*
Boston: Little, Brown.

Art.Rage.Us. (1998). *Art.Rage.Us.: Art and Writing by Women with Breast Cancer.*
San Francisco: Chronicle Books.

Atwood, M. (1981). *Bodily Harm.* Toronto: McClelland & Stewart.

Batt, S. (1991). Smile, you've got breast cancer. In J. Brady (Ed.), *1 in 3: Women
with Cancer Confront an Epidemic* (pp. 58–63). Pittsburgh, PA: Cleis Press.

Batt, S. (1994). *Patient No More: The Politics of Breast Cancer.* Charlottetown,
PEI: gynergy books.

Batt, S., & Gross, L. (1999). *Cancer, Inc.* (Sierra, 36(63), pp. 38–41). Retrieved
26 July 2004, from http://www.sierraclub.org/sierra/199909/cancer.asp.

Bottorff, J.L., Johnson, J.L., Venables, L.J., Grewal, S., Popatia, N., Hilton, B.A., et al. (2001). Voices of immigrant South Asian women: Expressions of health concerns. *Journal of Health Care for the Poor and Underserved, 12*, 392–403.

Brady, J. (Ed.). (1991). *1 in 3: Women with Cancer Confront an Epidemic*. Pittsburgh, PA: Cleis Press.

Brems, S., & Griffiths, M. (1993). Health women's way: Learning to listen. In M. Koblinsky, J. Timyan, and J. Gay (Eds.), *The Health of Women: A Global Perspective* (pp. 255–273). Boulder, CO: Westview Press.

Brown, B., Aslin, M., & Carey, B. (2003). *My Breasts, My Choice: Journeys Through Surgery*. Toronto: Sumach Press.

Bryant, H. (2003a). Breast cancer in Canadian women. *Women's Health Surveillance Report: A Multi-Dimensional Look at the Health of Canadian Women* (pp. 1–13). Retrieved 23 February 2004, from the Canadian Institute for Health Information. http://secure.cihi.ca/cihiweb/products/CPHI_Women'sHealth_e.pdf.

Bryant, H. (2003b). Breast cancer in Canadian women. *Women's Health Surveillance Report: A Multi-Dimensional Look at the Health of Canadian Women* (pp. 25–26). Retrieved 23 February 2004, from the Canadian Institute for Health Information. http://secure.cihi.ca/cihiweb/products/CPHI_Women'sHealth_e.pdf. (Summary report available from Health Canada, Population and Public Health Branch, Ottawa K1A 1B4.)

Butler, S., & Rosenblum, B. (1991). *Cancer in Two Voices*. San Francisco: Spinsters Book Company.

Butler, S., & Rosenblum, B. (2000). Blood money: August-November 1885. In V.A. Brownworth (Ed.), *Coming Out of Cancer: Writings from the Lesbian Cancer Epidemic* (pp. 150–165). Seattle, WA: Seal Press.

Clarke, J.N. (1985). *It's Cancer: The Personal Experiences of Women Who Have Received a Cancer Diagnosis*. Toronto: IPI Publishing.

Clorfene-Casten, L. (1996). *Breast Cancer: Poisons, Profits and Prevention*. Monroe, ME: Common Courage Press.

Datan, N. (1989). Illness and imagery: Feminist cognition, socialization and gender identity. In M. Crawford & M. Gentry (Eds.), *Gender and Thought: Psychological Perspectives*. New York: Springer-Verlag.

Ehrenreich, B. (2001). Welcome to cancerland. *Harper's, 303*, 45–53. Retrieved 26 July 2004, from http://www.findarticles.com/p/articles/mi_mllll/is_1818_303/ai_79665310/print.

Ellison, L.F., Gibbons, L. (with the Canadian Cancer Survival Analysis Group). (2001). Five year relative survival from prostate, breast, colorectal and lung cancer. *Health Reports, 13*, 23–34.

Evans, N. (2002). *State of the Evidence? What Is the Connection Between Chemicals and Breast Cancer?* San Francisco: Breast Cancer Fund and Breast Cancer Action. Available from: info@breastcancerfund.org.

Evans, N., and Martin, A.R. (2000). *Pathways to Prevention. Eight Practical Steps – from the Personal to the Political – Toward Reducing the Risk of Breast Cancer.* 2nd. ed. San Francisco: Breast Cancer Fund. Available from info@breastcancerfund.org

Galabuzi, G-E. (2004). Social exclusion. In D. Raphael (Ed.), *Social Determinants of Health: Canadian Perspectives* (pp. 235–251). Toronto: Canadian Scholars' Press.

Galambos, A. (1998). *An Unexpected Journey: Women's Voices of Hope after Breast Cancer.* Charlottetown, PEI: gynergy Books.

Goldberg, M.S., & Labreche, F. (1996). Occupational risk factors for female breast cancer: A review. *Occupational and Environmental Medicine, 53,* 145–156.

Grant, J. (1993). *Fundamental Feminism: Contesting the Core Concepts of Feminist Theory.* London: Routledge.

Hilton, B.A., Grewal, S., Popatia, N., Bottorff, J.L., Johnson, J.L., Clarke, H., et al. The desi ways: Traditional health practices of South Asian women in Canada. *Health Care for Women International, 22,* 553–567.

Jackson, A. (2004). The unhealthy Canadian workplace. In D. Raphael (Ed.), *Social Determinants of Health: Canadian Perspectives* (pp. 79–94). Toronto: Canadian Scholars' Press.

Jacobson, N. (2000). *Cleavage: Technology, Controversy, and the Ironies of the Man-made Breast.* New Brunswick, NJ: Rutgers University Press.

Johnson, J.L., Bottorff, J.L., Browne, A.J., Grewal, S., Hilton, B.A., & Clarke, H. (2004). Othering and being othered in the context of health care services. *Health Communication, 16,* 253–271.

Kahane, D.H. (1995). *No Less a Woman: Femininity, Sexuality and Breast Cancer.* 2nd ed. Alameda, CA: Hunter House.

Kasper, A.S. (1995). The social construction of breast loss and reconstruction. *Women's Health: Research on Gender, Behavior and Policy, 1,* 197–219.

Kasper, A.S. (2000). Barriers and burdens: Poor women face breast cancer. In A.S. Kasper & S.J. Ferguson (Eds.), *Breast Cancer: Society Shapes an Epidemic* (pp. 183–212). New York: St Martin's Press.

Kasper, A.S., & Ferguson, S.J. (2000). *Breast Cancer: Society Shapes an Epidemic.* New York: St Martin's Press.

Kaufert, P.A. (1998). Women, resistance and the breast cancer movement. In M. Lock and P. Kaufert (Eds.), *Pragmatic Women and Body Politics.* Cambridge: Cambridge University Press.

Kitzinger, C., & Wilkinson, S. (1997). Validating women's experience? Dilemmas in feminist research. *Feminism & Psychology, 7,* 566–574.

Klawiter, M. (2000). Racing for the cure, walking women and toxic touring: Mapping cultures of action within the Bay Area terrain of breast cancer. In L.K. Potts (Ed.), *Ideologies of Breast Cancer: Feminist Perspectives* (pp. 63–97). London: Macmillan.

Kliewer, E.V., and Smith, K.R. (1995). Breast cancer mortality among immigrants in Australia and Canada. *Journal of the National Cancer Institute, 87,* 1154–1161.

Leopold, E. (1999). *A Darker Ribbon: Breast Cancer, Women and Their Doctors in the Twentieth Century.* Boston: Beacon Press.

Lesbians and Breast Cancer Project Team. (2004a). *Coming Out About Lesbians and Cancer.* Retrieved 30 June 2004, from Ontario Breast Cancer Community Research Initiative Web site: http://dawn.thot.net/lbcp.

Lesbians and Breast Cancer Project Team. (2004b). *Coming Out About Lesbians and Cancer.* Retrieved 30 June 2004, from Ontario Breast Cancer Community Research Initiative. http://dawn.thot.net/lbcp. Summary report available from Willow Breast Cancer Support and Resource Services in Toronto. info@willow.org.

Lorde, A. (1980). *The Cancer Journals.* London: Sheba Feminist Publishers.

Love, Susan M., with Lindsey, K. (2000). *Dr Susan Love's Breast Book.* 3rd ed. Cambridge, MA: Perseus Publishing.

MacPhee, R. (1994). *Picasso's Woman: A Breast Cancer Story.* Vancouver: Douglas & McIntyre.

McKenzie, D. (1998, 25 August). Abreast in a boat: A race against breast cancer. *Canadian Medical Association Journal, 159*(4).

Maguire, P. (1982). Psychiatric morbidity associated with mastectomy. *Experientia, 41,* 373–380.

Martindale, F. (1994). My (lesbian) breast cancer story: Can I get a witness? In M. Oikawa, D. Falconer, & B.R. Wainrib (Eds.), *Resist: Essays Against a Homophobic Culture* (pp. 137–150). Toronto: Women's Press.

Metzger, D. (1981). *Tree.* Culver City, CA: Peace Press.

Meyerowitz, B.E. (1981, August). Postmastectomy concerns of breast cancer patients. Paper presented at the American Psychological Association Annual Convention, Los Angeles.

Miller, A.B., and Gaudette, L.A. (1996). Breast cancer in circumpolar Inuit 1969–1988. *Acta Oncologica, 35,* 577–580.

Morton, W.E. (1995). Major differences in breast cancer risk among occupations. *Journal of Occupational and Environmental Medicine, 37,* 328–335.

National Cancer Institute of Canada. (2002). *Canadian Cancer Statistics 2002.* Toronto: National Cancer Institute of Canada. Available from Statistics Canada. http://www.ncic.cancer.ca.

Olivotto, I., Gelmon, K., & Kuusk, U. (2001). *Breast Cancer*. Vancouver: Intelligent Patient Guide.

Peters-Golden, H. (1982). Breast cancer: Varied perceptions of social support in the illness experience. *Social Science & Medicine, 15E*, 257–265.

Petralia, S.A, Fena, J.E., Freudenheim, J.L., Marshall, J.R., Michalek, A., Brasure, et al. (1998). Breast cancer risk and lifetime occupational history: Employment in professional and managerial occupations. *Occupational and Environmental Medicine, 55*, 43–48.

Prior, A. (1987). Personal view. *British Medical Journal, 295*, 920.

Ramazanoglu, C., with Holland, J. (2002). *Feminist Methodology: Challenges and Choices*. London: Sage.

Rosenthal, M.S. (1997). *The Breast Sourcebook*. Los Angeles: Lowell House.

Saywell, C. (with Beattie, L., & Henderson, L.) (2000). Sexualized illness: The newsworthy body in media representations of breast cancer. In L.K. Potts (Ed.), *Ideologies of Breast Cancer: Feminist Perspectives* (pp. 37–62). London: Macmillan.

Scott, J.W. (1993). Experience. In J. Butler and J.W. Scott (Eds.), *Feminists Theorize the Political*. London: Routledge.

Sontag, S. (1979). *Illness as Metaphor*. London: Allen Lane.

Spence, J. (1986). *Putting Myself in the Picture: A Political, Personal and Photographic Autobiography*. London: Sheba Feminist Publishers.

Stanley, L. (1994). The knowing because experiencing subject: Narratives, lives and autobiography. In M. Lennon & M. Whitford (Eds.), *Knowing the Difference: Feminist Perspectives in Epistemology*. London: Routledge.

Stevens, P.E. (1992). Lesbian health care research: A review of literature from 1970 to 1990. *Health Care for Women International, 13*, 91–120.

Stevens, P.E. (1996). Lesbians and doctors: Experiences of solidarity and domination in health care settings. *Gender & Society, 10*, 24–41.

Stevens, P.E. (1998). The experience of lesbians of color in health care encounters: Narrative insights for improving access and quality. *Journal of Lesbian Studies, 2*, 77–94.

Stewart, M.W. (1998). *Silicone Spills: Breast Implants on Trial*. Westport, CT: Praeger.

Swann, C. (1997). Reading the bleeding body: Discourses of premenstrual syndrome. In J.M. Ussher (Ed.), *Body Talk: The Material and Discursive Regulation of Sexuality, Madness and Reproduction* (pp. 176–198). London: Routledge.

Tocher, M. (2002). *How to Ride a Dragon: Women with Breast Cancer Tell Their Stories*. Toronto: Key Porter Books.

Wilkinson, S. (1998) Focus groups in health research: Exploring the meanings of health and illness. *Journal of Health Psychology, 3,* 329–348.

Wilkinson, S. (2000a). Feminist research traditions in health psychology: Breast cancer research. *Journal of Health Psychology, 5*: 359–372.

Wilkinson, S. (2000b). Women with breast cancer talking causes: Comparing content, biographical and discursive analyses. *Feminism & Psychology, 10,* 431–460.

Wilkinson, S. (2001). Breast cancer: Feminism, representations and resistance. *Health, 5,* 269–277.

Wilkinson, S. (2004). Feminist contributions to critical health psychology. In M. Murray (Ed.), *Critical Health Psychology* (pp. 83–100). New York: Palgrave Macmillan.

Wilkinson, S., & Kitzinger, C. (1993). Whose breast is it anyway? A feminist consideration of advice and 'treatment' for breast cancer. *Women's Studies International Forum, 16,* 229–238.

Wilkinson, S., & Kitzinger, C. (2000). Thinking differently about 'thinking positive': A discursive approach to cancer patients' talk. *Social Science & Medicine, 50,* 787–811.

Wilson, L. (with Brown, D.). (1995). *A Woman in My Position: The Politics of Breast Implant Safety.* Toronto: New Canada Press.

Yadlon, S. (1997). Skinny women and good mothers: The rhetoric of risk, control and culpability in the production of knowledge about breast cancer. *Feminist Studies, 23,* 645–667.

Zimmerman, S.M. (1998). *Silicone Survivors: Women's Experiences with Breast Implants.* Philadelphia: Temple University Press.

16 Selling 'The Change': A Comparison of the Dangers of Hormone Replacement Therapies in Profit versus National Health Care Delivery Systems

BRIAN RICHTER AND CINDY PATTON

Women approaching menopause or on hormone replacement therapy to deal with symptoms of menopause and aging faced disturbing questions Tuesday after a major U.S. study said the risks of the treatment were too high to justify long-term use.

In fact, scientists conducting what was meant to be an 8½-year study on whether HRT protects postmenopausal women against heart disease pulled the plug more than three years early. It had become clear the combination of estrogen and progestin didn't protect, but raised the risk of heart attack, stroke and blood clots among users. The increased risk of breast cancer was already known.

The take-away message? If you are using HRT to stave off heart disease during or after menopause, don't. (Branswell, 2002)

The announcement yesterday that a hormone replacement regimen taken by six million American women did more harm than good was met with puzzlement and disbelief by women and their doctors across the country.

A rigorous study found that the drugs, a combination of estrogen and progestin, caused small increases in breast cancer, heart attacks, strokes and blood clots. Those risks outweighed the drugs' benefits – a small decrease in hip fractures and a decrease in colorectal cancer. Many of the 16,000 women in the study, supported by the National Institutes of Health, opened letters yesterday telling them to stop the drugs. In light of the findings, the study had come to a halt. (Kolata & Peterson, 2002)

Slamming on the Breaks

On 9 July 2002, North America's millions of female baby boomers, now solidly within the 'menopause spectrum' awoke to news of a scientific discovery that was said to affect their ability to age gracefully and healthfully. Media reported that the first prospective study (Women's Health Initiative Trials [WHI]) of the side effects of a drug that had been widely prescribed for 70 years had been abruptly halted when the drug's risks seemed to outweigh its benefits. 'Shocked' a decade or two earlier when the Pill that had partly enabled the sexual liberation of their generation came under attack, boomer women were now described in the media as 'panicking' and 'confused';[1] they wanted to know what they were supposed to do *now*. But as we will detail in a moment, while North American media agreed that women needed to consult their doctors, the subtle difference in how the Canadian and U.S. media represented what that encounter might entail speak to larger and more fundamental differences between a medical system that promotes the right to health care for all versus one that rests on the right to choose by a smaller number of citizens.

In the wake of the storm of advice lay several larger and in some ways more vexing questions than the individualistic 'What-should-a-woman-do?' The answer to these larger questions formed the context of individual advice-giving, and enabled the long-standing and general disregard for women's health to be transformed into an apparent debate about women's right to drugs. Perhaps, unsurprisingly, there was an uncomfortable juxtaposition of objective and subjective threats. On one hand, it might make sense to weigh osteoporosis-reduction *benefit* against cancer *risk*, since both could result in shortened lifespan. But not everyone agreed that relief of 'menopause symptoms' (poor sleep, depression, hot flashes, vaginal dryness) were important enough to continue using the drugs in the face of apparently increased risk of cancer, stroke, and heart attack. But the asymmetry in the risk calculus goes unquestioned: asking 'who gets to decide which aging effects count?' would have forced reporters to enter the fray about whether menopause symptoms are 'real' or only the fabrication of pouting middle-class women.[2] The refusal to open up this debate meant that advice itself was curiously asymmetric, pitting subjective body-states against objective measures of ill health. In this framing of the HRT debate, HRT advocates had to argue for the utility of symptom relief by minimizing the degree of risk, while those who thought the risks too great had to minimize the degree and significance of symptoms.

The reportage also reduces differences among women to a matter of idiosyncrasy: who knows why some women have problems and others don't? In the absence of any other description of the possible variations among women – race and class in the largest sense; diet, smoking, alcohol consumption, and exercise in the realm of practices; habits widely known to vary by race and class – we are left to imagine either that, beyond individual quirks, all menopausal women are the same, or that the media are primarily concerned with white, middle-class women.[3] Indeed, the emphasis on the damage of menopause symptoms on careers and the suggestion that this is the central crisis in women's lives reinforces our supposition that the media see the debate about HRT as principally a white, middle-class women's 'problem.' Indeed, although it is nearly impossible to determine rates of prescription of HRT by race and class, much less rates of adherence to HRT by race and class, several factors make it likely that the media are imagining middle-class white women when they quiz doctors, advocates, and policymakers about the meaning of the drugs and their newly recognized side effects, if only because white, middle-class women are more likely to access medical care – and thus are more likely to be offered pharmaceuticals – than their poorer and darker sisters. When we discuss the varying media representations of women's relationships to their doctors, it becomes even clearer that the bodies of concern are those of middle-class women, since we can hear in the debates about rights and choice the concerns about these issues that are more germane to privileged women.[4]

But even more troubling was the question of how one of the most widely prescribed drugs in North America, in use in some form for more than 70 years, had never undergone the kind of testing that consumers assume is a basic requirement of drug licensure, indeed, many have argued, a form of scientific research that is a moral responsibility of scientists and government regulators.

In discussing what is self-evidently a women's health issue, it is impossible to assess the media coverage of the end of the HRT trials without acknowledging feminist critiques of the medicalization of menopause (Seaman & Seaman, 1977; Lock, 1991, 1998; Worcester & Whatley, 1992; Coney, 1994; Hunt, 1994; Wilkinson & Kitzinger, 1994; Wiley, Taguchi, & Formby, 2003); the gendered construction of medical knowledge (Zola, 1972; Wilkinson & Kitzinger, 1994; Bell, 1995; Van Wijk, Vliet, & Kolk, 1996; Malterud, 1999); and the analysis of the social construction of the idea that women's bodies are inherently labile and women's mental states determined by their biologic fluctuations (Coney, 1994; Findlay & Miller, 1994). But which side in the debate about whether – or how – individuals should continue HRT is the 'feminist' side? The debates pit a feminist-influenced critique of medicine misused against a (neo)liberal feminist position that argues that women can make their own decisions about their health care. The variations in these positions hinge on the ontological status of 'menopause symptoms': are they real? And if real, pervasive? And if pervasive, threatening to quality of life? And if threatening, of the order of threat that only medical intervention can eradicate?

While the women and doctors represented in the media findings are cautious about making strong statements about the reality and significance of 'menopause symptoms,' the tone of the media coverage does the work of re-establishing women's bodies as indeed the locus of unpleasant, even nation-threatening flux. For example, a *Maclean's* article cites one physician as saying: 'If women stop hormones abruptly we'll have a nation full of women having horrible hot flashes, night sweats, insomnia, irritability and mood swings.' *Maclean's* (More harm, 2002) reports a second doctor suggesting that 'the brain gets used to high estrogen levels and it reacts just like an addict's brain reacts when their drug of choice is withdrawn. You need to sort of de-condition the brain.' Similarly, *Newsweek* writer Claudia Kalb (2002) quotes a physician describing her patients' reaction to stopping their HRT: 'I'm getting women calling up and saying, "I can't function, I can't sleep, I can't think straight and I can't have sex"' (p. 53). Finally, an *Edmonton Journal* reporter (Branswell, 2002) quotes a physician who dramatizes the severity of going 'cold turkey' off HRT: 'In my experience, the hot flashes that are provoked by a woman who stops estrogen suddenly are the most difficult of any in the world to treat.' Taken together, these indirect descriptions of the female body and mind under siege from hormone 'imbalance' serve less to dramatize the reality of menopause symptoms than they serve to subtly question whether menopausal women possess the rationality to consent to taking potentially harmful drugs. But reporters never directly raise the issue of the disqualifying effect of menopause on women's ability to exercise their rights as a citizen (in Canada, one with a right to care; in the United States, one with a right to choose). Instead, both countries focus on directing women to seek advice from doctors. But while the media coverage in the United States and Canada is quite similar, the status of doctors as knowledge translators differs. At first glance, we might regard the Canadian coverage as placing an over-reliance on doctors' authority. But closer examination suggests that this is likely due to a more fundamental difference in the two systems' understanding of how to distribute health care. Thus, we draw particular attention to the subtle juxtaposition of Canadian women, who have a right to have their health interests protected by science and the state (as embodied by the doctor, funded through a largely public system), and U.S. women, who are accorded a 'right to choose' health option even if that means disregarding the advice of their doctor, whose interests align not with the state, but with the health care market that pays her or him. We want to position the media representation of the HRT debate not only in the context of feminist health concerns, but specifically in the context of debates about which consumers are able to direct the course of scientific research and evaluate its results on their own. This places our analysis in the trajectory of feminist debates about whether we can have good science in a market model (investigating questions arising from consumer interests), and whether we need knowledge intermediaries to assess the significance and public health implications of scientific study results.

We want to turn now to an overview of how HRT emerged as a treatment, and how it gained such widespread use in North America without ever undergoing major trials. We then return to the question of the media representation of doctors' authority with respect to protecting women's right to care versus enacting women's right to choose.

History of HRT

The switch from HRT as treatment to HRT as preventative therapy has occurred without debate or justification. It is a shift of the profoundest significance, yet has gone unremarked and undiscussed. (Coney, 1994, p. 207)

The history of hormone replacement therapy in North America is not a simple one; indeed, even the term *hormone replacement therapy* is not entirely accurate, since the drugs that are prescribed to 'replace' hormones lost at menopause, do not actually function identically to those the body creates on its own. In part because pharmaceutical companies can only create huge profits if their products can be protected by patent (for example, you cannot patent soybeans – another agent commonly used for symptomatic relief – unless you have genetically engineered them), the various products are composed of synthesized estrogen. For example, the highly popular Premarin, manufactured by Wyeth-Ayerst, is derived from pregnant mare urine. These estrogens do not actually replicate the body's 'natural' rhythmic, cyclical production of hormones (Wiley, Taguchi, & Formby, 2003), and thus they might more accurately be viewed as *introducing* a substance that has similar but not identical functions, rather than replacing or supplementing a substance in decline.

The idea of delaying the end of menstruation runs across cultures and time, but what were initially women's subcultural practices became a Western medical obsession at more or less the dawn of modern medicine in the early twentieth century. In its traditional form, coping with women's 'old-age' conditions entailed remedies derived from the urine of pregnant women or from plant sources. But in the 1930s, menopause, now constructed as a 'stage' in women's lives, became definitively medicalized, with attendant symptoms – hot flashes, fatigue, headaches, vaginal dryness, and sexual 'problems' – that the emergent pharmaceutical industry promised it could alleviate. Applying the then-new scientific discovery of hormones and their role in human biology (the critical breakthrough of the mid-twentieth century, much like mapping the genome has been at the millennium), most of the early 'menopause' drugs were designed to replace estrogen, a theoretical and practical solution that continued to be the primary focus of this line of research and manufacturing until the 1960s.

In the 1960s, researchers began to experiment with combinations of hormones beyond estrogen supplementation. Progesterones and progestins became common agents to combine or alternate with estrogen. Even testosterone, which is often viewed as a 'male' hormone, was included in HRT drug combinations. One liquid HRT drug produced in the 1970s by Ayerst, Mediatric, included estrogen along with testosterone, vitamins, methamphetamine hydrochloride, and 15 per cent alcohol (Seaman & Seaman, 1977). The industry also invested significant research and development dollars in different modes of delivering hormones: by the 1990s, HRT could be prescribed in the form of oral pills, liquids, patches, and transdermal creams.

The first medical model HRT drugs were developed in the early twentieth century, well before contemporary systems for animal and human trials of pharmaceutical agents. There were a range of laws governing potions and patent medicines; however, agencies like the American Food and Drug Administration (FDA) still debate what is a 'food' (hence, supplement) and what is a drug. The line between the two is easiest to see when an aetiologic agent – say the flu or HIV – attacks the body; here, the body cannot cope, and drugs are designed to eliminate or mitigate the effects of a germ. In an important sense, while the thalidomide case spurred on the development of more rigorous drug-testing standards, it is really the antibiotic or antiviral, or more recently anticancer, agent that most clearly appears as a 'drug.' As the huge industry of 'holistic' products reveals, with immune system enhancers and hormone system balancers, the line between drug and food is very difficult to draw. It is easy to see, then, how a pharmaceutical agent that developed alongside the scientific and ethical regulation of drugs might have escaped rigorous trials. After all, were not doctors and their pharmaceutical helpmates just giving back to women what nature had taken away?

But the potential problems associated with recalibrating the aging process did not go unremarked. As early as the 1940s, clinicians noticed that endometrial cancer might be a potential side effect for women who were taking estrogen HRT drugs, an observation that did not prompt actual research until the 1970s. Indeed, it turned out to be the case that estrogen supplementation was causing many women to overstimulate the endometrium (Coney, 1994). The solution? Add progestogen to estrogen, causing a menstrual bleed that helped prevent the development of endometrial hyperplasia (Coney, 1994).

This was the first of a series of major, widely reported problems with HRT, the first time that the growing industry had to actively allay women's fears that the cure might be worse than the condition. This might have been a small problem if HRT had remained as it began: primarily prescribed for short-term use to treat common effects of menopause, such as hot flashes, anxiety, and other conditions associated with this phase of aging. But HRT manufacturers and physicians who liked the drugs extended the claims of HRTs role in women's health. From the mid-1960s until the mid-1970s, HRT began to be prescribed for much longer periods of time in an attempt to guarantee women eternal beauty and the ability to maintain their femininity, which has been intertwined with perceived worth and value as a woman. From the mid-1970s until the beginning of the 1980s, HRT was marketed as a way to experience symptom-free menopause, enabling women to stay in the workplace and enjoy their older years. Finally, in the early 1980s, HRT began to be marketed as a means for escaping chronic disease (MacPherson, 1993). Significantly, through this progression of rationales for taking HRT, the status of the agents as drugs becomes increasingly firmly entrenched. No longer a beauty aid, HRT was a major missile in the armament against cardiovascular disease, some cancers, and osteoporosis – newly represented as a major threat to active middle-aged women's mobile lifestyle.

It is under the guise of disease prevention that the number of women to whom HRT was prescribed skyrocketed. Pharmaceutical companies took a nearly cradle-to-grave approach to the management of female hormones. Not only should girls go on birth control early (even after

Depoprovera shots – which were supposed to 'protect' against pregnancy for up to three months – proved controversial and potentially dangerous, the patch continued to appeal to worried moms who feared their daughters might be unable or unwilling to follow through on a daily regimen of birth control pills), but at the very hint of menopause, all women should start HRT to prevent osteoporosis, breast cancer, and heart disease.

After the Women's Health Initiative (WHI) trials, it is now widely accepted that only the claims about osteoporosis hold any truth, but even here, the fit between medical definition and cultural construction raise questions about whether the use of HRT for this purpose is necessary for more than a tiny minority of women. It is important to note that prior to the 1960s, osteoporosis was medically catalogued and viewed as a type of general bone disease (Van Keep, 1990). Most women were advised to drink plenty of milk and engage in weight-bearing exercise. It is clear that men and women lose some bone density with age, and that after menopause many women lose at a faster rate. However, that is a far cry from the suggestion that all women run the risk of major bone breakage simply because they are past menopause. Nevertheless, in the wake of criticism about HRT's association with some forms of cancer, the pharmaceutical companies began to market HRT as not *a* way to stave off bone loss, but the *best* way. In 1986, manufacturers fought for and obtained U.S. FDA permission to include bone loss prevention on HRT usage labels (Wiley et al., 2003). While there are no clear data to tell us why HRT is prescribed in particular cases, most women who regularly access care report that at the least mention of menopause, but certainly by the time they reached age 45, their physician had taken it upon her or himself to mention the potential of HRT to prevent future bone loss, without regard to family history or lifestyle. It is no surprise, then, that within a few years of labelling HRT for bone loss prevention, U.S. sales of the major 20 estrogen drugs equalled nearly a half-billion dollars (Risks vs. benefits, 1992).

Studying HRT and the Problem of Labelling

We do not want to suggest that the various forms of HRT never underwent any scientific evaluation; rather, we want to contextualize the kind of research that had been conducted on the evolving types of HRT. It is important to understand that there are two major routes to assessing drug efficacy and side effects. First, a new agent can be put through its paces, first in animal models, next in very limited human toxicity trials, and, finally, in clinic trials designed to see if the agent actually works (these may be either placebo-controlled, or, if a treatment standard already exists, the drug goes head-to-head with its competitor to see if it works better). In this ideal model, most side effects are defined in the toxicity phase, although others may appear in the controlled trials.

If an agent is already in use, researchers can gather data on the experience with the drug in real-life clinical settings. While this looks like the classic clinical trial phase, there is little ability to control these studies, since the reason an individual doctor prescribes a drug and the reason an individual takes it may not be clear for any number of reasons, including physician off-label uses. One of the chief opportunities and problems in this type of research is the 'labelled' versus 'unlabelled' use of approved drugs. The 'label' tells doctors and consumers the ailments that a drug has been tested for; however, doctors commonly make the decision to use a drug labelled for one thing to treat something else. As consumers, we are ambivalent about this practice: on one hand, we like drugs to have been tested for the disease for which we are undergoing treatment, on the other, if a drug is available and it makes theoretical sense to use it for an ailment we have, we would probably rather go ahead and take the drug than wait the years it might take to be retested and approved for the second ailment. Thus, any drug – even one rigorously tested for an initial labelled use – could find itself in the situation of being widely used – and only later evaluated – for a second, unlabelled use. As a simple example, the use of aspirin, labelled as an analgesic, for 'blood thinning' – and, in fact, for many an unwanted side effect – and eventually for prevention of cardiovascular problems, is a story of unlabelled use, followed – like HRT – by testing for the efficacy of these unlabelled uses, followed by label changes.

HRT got to its present state both because it predates by decades the 'new agent' testing and labelling protocols, and because it was easy to prescribe for non-labelled uses. Thus, huge numbers of North American women have used HRT at one point or another, enabling large-scale studies to be constructed from groups who were already using HRT. While many of these epidemiologic studies suggested there might be 'problems' with the drugs, their main contribution was to determine whether the claims for the drugs' benefits actually held up (Wiley et al., 2003). And, of course, unlike clinical trials, which control for confounding factors in order to determine if a drug works, epidemiologic studies are designed to find broad patterns in 'natural' settings.

Even given the vast numbers of women who have been prescribed HRT, it is difficult to construct a good epidemiologically based study since no one really knows why or how faithfully – or even whether – most women actually take their HRT. Although the number of written and filled prescriptions can be tracked, these numbers tell nothing of the actual reasons a particular doctor prescribes the drug to a particular woman, nor whether a given woman took the drug as prescribed. For example, although HRT drug labels did not mention the reduction of risk of heart disease, this was a major rationale for long-term use among women in the 1990s (Off-Label drug use, 1997).

Although adherence is a complex phenomenon to study, it appears that many women do not stick to the prescribed dosage of HRT. There are myriad and changing reasons for non-adherence. Unless a woman has had her uterus removed, she is usually prescribed some amount of progestogen to reduce the chance of endometrial cancer, but this often leads to unwanted bleeding. Much like taking aspirin for a headache, women who recognize a close connection between symptoms and their resolution with drugs may take HRT according to their own schedule. Indeed, a Massachusetts Women's Health Survey in the mid-1980s found that 20 per cent of women prescribed HRT stopped taking the drug after nine months, and that 20 to 30 per cent of the women surveyed never had their prescriptions filled because they were not convinced of the benefits or certain of the risks (Ravnikar, 1987). A friend of ours related her own HRT story, articulating a mode of resistance that is likely familiar to most women. 'The doctor just kept insisting that I take hormones, even though I didn't want to, so I finally just smiled and said I would. I never filled it. My next visit after the refills would have run out, the doctor wrote me another prescription, which I did not fill.' As many feminist critics of health care have noted, women appear simultaneously passive in relation to their doctors, and, at the same time, quite willing to define their own treatment. Research on adherence generally now suggests that patients are far less likely to do what their doctors tell them than clinical trials and epidemiologically based outcome studies assume. Given the significance of the doctor in both prescribing HRT and in facilitating the conduct of epidemiologic trials, we want now to turn to the post-WHI media coverage of 'what women should do.'

'See Your Doctor'

Both the American and Canadian press urged women to talk to their doctor before making any sudden change in their HRT regimen. But the tone of this common admonition varied considerably between the two nations' presses. The Canadian press presented the doctors as compassionate, decisive, and willing to take the time to explain a woman's options. The *Calgary Sun* (Linton, 2002) was typical of this representation of the calm and helpful doctor: '"Do not panic," says cardiologist Dr Beth Abramson. She advises women to make an appointment with their doctor ("an elective, not an emergency appointment") and to use the meeting as an opportunity to discuss their whole heart health risk profile and ways they can be proactive about their health. "Don't immediately stop taking this stuff. Don't go cold turkey," says Dr Elaine Chin, a family physician and co-founder of the Beresford Group, a multidisciplinary health, wellness, and beauty facility. Doing so, she warns, may result in rebound hot flashes, night sweats, and mood swings. "You will feel horrible, as stopping hormones too quickly shocks the system"' (p. 35).

Similarly, the Montreal *Gazette* (Carroll, 2002) suggests that doctors, if not eager to help their HRT patients, would have to step in and play the crucial role of medical counsellor:

> A scientific bombshell has blown some conventional medical wisdom out of the water this week. The case illustrates once again that there's no substitute for informed individuals making their own decisions.
>
> But the research does lead us inexorably to the conclusion that every woman for whom HRT might be appropriate needs to inform herself fully, in consultation with her doctor, about the potential benefits and risks in her own case.
>
> Doctors, rushed and over-burdened though they might be, are going to have to answer a lot more questions about this therapy, and that is as it should be. (p. A6)

Another Montreal *Gazette* article (Assessing HRT risks, 2002), represents women as capable of calmly assessing the study results, and, if anything, being stoked into panic by the press:

> 'The panicky response comes as much from what the women don't know as what they have learned about the cancelled study,' says Dr Morrie Gelfand, co-director of the McGill University Health Centre menopause clinic at the Jewish General Hospital.
>
> 'We've had a hundred calls – it's very bad,' Gelfand said yesterday. 'There is an important issue at stake, and the patients are grabbing onto the sensational headlines.'

... But women should take a closer look at the study results and talk to their doctors before jumping to conclusions about HRT use, said Gelfand, president of the North American Menopause Society.

Many women don't even know if they are taking the specific hormone combination raising concerns in the U.S., Gelfand noted. (p. B2)

In subtle contrast to these representations of doctors as knowledge-able information brokers, willing to calm their patients in the face of a media-generated panic, the American news outlets suggest that doctors will only give women confusing advice about the relative risks and benefits of HRT. Reporter Susan Brink, in a 29 July 2002 *US News and World Report* story, puts it this way: The study, '... leaves women in a quandary. Should they take a drug that could stave off the fracture-prone bones of osteoporosis, yet lead to heart trouble, breast tumors, and possibly – according to another new study – ovarian cancer? (p. 62).

Business Week answers his question with a hard-line consumerist position that suggests less that women *can* sort through material, than that 'the person swallowing the pill' has to just make up her mind. Alluding to long-standing debates about HRT, this *Business Week* writer (Arnst, 2002) importunes:

The hue and cry over hormones shows no signs of abating. Anti-estrogen crusaders are crowing that a huge study on hormone replacement therapy (HRT) proves the drugs raise the risks of breast cancer and heart disease. Beleaguered women who found relief from the torments of menopause through HRT say the dangers are overblown. In the end, the study spot-lights an underappreciated medical axiom: There is no such thing as treatment without risk. And patients must figure out for themselves if the risk is worth taking.

Don't assume your doctor has the answer. Physicians may try to 'First, do no harm,' but those are difficult words to practice by, given that any two doctors may strongly disagree on exactly what causes harm. Where does that leave the patient? With another set of words to live by: 'Know thyself.'

Often, the benefits outweigh the risks. But only the person swallowing the pill can make that determination – not a doctor, not society, and not some stranger quoted on TV. (p. 74)

Unlike the Canadian fantasy of a woman and her doctor calmly discussing options in the context of some shared sense of common good, the above author questions doctors' utility, and even willingness to give patients clear directions. Instead, the consumer is asked to dig deep and make a decision about whether a product is more helpful than harmful. Importantly, the Canadian media tend to focus on the study's research questions – Does HRT protect against cardiovascular events? – while the American media blur the question of the use of HRT against the 'torrents of menopause' with the question of the safety of HRT's expanded uses. Indeed, in the quotes above, we see Canadian Dr Abramson coaching women to place the question of HRT use in 'their whole heart health risk profile and ways they can be proactive about their health,' while the *Business Week* writer, having intimated that doctors aren't going to be much help, can only offer the advice to 'know thyself.'

This small difference in how the media position the doctors' advice rests on two underlying assumptions about how medical choices should be made. First, the right-to-care position suggests that everyone, regardless of personal ability to understand medical information or level of medical need, should receive an appropriate level of care. In this framework, it doesn't really matter if women are plagued by the hot flashes, sleeplessness, and depression that are said to curse them in menopause. These states, which might be seen to diminish their ability to make rational decisions, do not disqualify the woman from making a reasonable decision about whether or how to take HRT: there to safeguard her decision-making is her physician. (We would likely have other things to say about how well physicians deal with women's bodies, but that is a different debate than the question of the national ethos regarding the right to – rather than the ability to actually get – care.)

By contrast, in the right-to-choose model, the individual's capacity to make a rational decision has everything to do with how the for-profit system works. The right-to-choose model is especially problematic when debates about the criterion of effective citizenship – a conceptualization in American democracy that hinges on rationality, defined by literacy, sanity, whiteness, participation in the economy, and so on – collide with choice rhetoric and profit motives, as they do in neoliberalism, the guiding principle in most U.S. social policy, and, increasingly, in Canadian policy debates. Neoliberalism argues that social issues, like financial ones, can best be handled by market forces. In the case of medicine, the market is understood less explicitly in financial terms than in quality of life terms, although it is obvious that the financial incentives for one treatment versus another depend on the overall cost of maintaining different standards of quality for people occupying different social positions. Here, individual patients are understood to make choices about their care that include how much they like their providers, how they understand the efficacy of particular treatments, and whether they – or understand themselves to be responsible to – minimize costs and maximize health. 'Choosing' among the different forms of health insurance (for those who have any choice) becomes a kind of calculated bet about one's ability to stay healthy without intervention from the medical system versus the odds one will experience catastrophic illness beyond prediction or control. Unfortunately, while right-to-choose rhetoric seems to suggest that patients – in this case, menopausal women – have the ability to sort through medical materials; if they do not (because they are hormone crazed), that is not the fault of the medical system or their doctors, but due to a flaw in their personality (they are not tough enough to be one of those women who, as one writer put it, 'sails through menopause'). What the feminist-sounding, right-to-choose position obscures is the extent to which doctors' inclination towards magic bullets and drug companies inclination towards profits, have misframed the larger question of healthy aging. Once a medico-epistememological framework is in place (Let's fix aging with a pill!), consumers can only 'choose' between the different products that promise to fulfil the now-self-evident solution. By contrast, the right-to-care model leaves open the question of alternative ways of thinking about the larger question of how to improve a woman's ability to age, considering the possibility that there may be different answers to specific concerns with cardiovascular and cancer risk, and her overarching concern with maintaining a sex life, general levels of physical activity, and paid work post-menopause.

Truth or Confusion

In fairness to the many reporters who covered the HRT story in U.S. and Canadian journals, there was some discussion of both the political economy of health care and the possibility that age-related osteoporosis, hot flashes, increased cardiovascular risk, and cancer might each have its own cure. The *Toronto Star* (A stake, 2002), convinced by the study, suggested that criticism of the results arose equally from two sources: 'This week, the question was answered definitively when a major, government-funded U.S. study showed that HRT significantly increases risk of breast cancer, heart disease and stroke. The problem is that there are two enormously powerful motivations to downplay or obfuscate the results and both are at work now: vanity and greed' (p. F02).

A more exceptional analysis suggests that the meaning and significance of the study depend on various medical professionals' understanding of how to deal with the complex of aging issues that HRT was supposed solve in one pill. Dr Utian of the Menopause Society (Kolata & Peterson, 2002) said he was not surprised that an active debate seemed to be emerging. 'There are an awful lot of interests at stake here beyond women's health,' he said. 'There are investigators with research grants, NIH grants and grants from the pharmaceutical industry. There are academics with careers to build.' Added to that, he said, are medical specialists – gynaecologists are comfortable with hormones, internists with statins to lower cholesterol and protect against heart disease, bone experts with drugs like bisphosphonates to protect against osteoporosis. 'It's not just a matter of what the data says,' Dr Utian added. 'Truth is opinion' (p. A1).

Additionally, there was some coverage of the impacts of HRT prescription and labelling as well as alternative options for treatment of menopausal symptoms. By mid-2003, the FDA required drug companies to update the labels and instructions for all HRT drugs to include findings and warnings from the WHI study. Health Canada also guaranteed to update their labels with new warnings after reviewing the WHI findings.

These changes, along with the reported findings of the WHI study, resulted in a dramatic drop in the level of prescriptions for two of the most popular HRT drugs, Prempro (combined estrogen and progestins) and Premarin (estrogen) in Canada and the United States, having dropped 66 per cent and 33 per cent respectively (Vanderhaeghe, 2004). There are several other major studies underway to analyse combinations not tested in the WHI study (although one of these trials was also halted in 2003, and another in 2004),[6] and doctors continue to debate narrow conditions under which they will prescribe HRT.

And, not insignificantly, the many alternatives to HRT are more widely discussed, with attention to the different means available to deal with both menopause symptoms and with combating chronic disease. Diet and plant or herb supplements are often suggested as alternatives for those women who do not want to take HRT. One approach is a low-fat diet with plenty of fruits and vegetables, regular exercise, taking recommended amounts of vitamin D and calcium, and using herbs that naturally ease transitions to lower estrogen levels, including black cohosh, flaxseed, red clover, or dong quai (Do-it-yourself, 2001). Other approaches focus more on maintaining a strong exercise routine and generally healthy lifestyle, which may help with some of the symptoms, but certainly contribute to combating osteoporosis and cardiovascular disease. In addition, healthy-lifestyle advocates who want to de-medicalize women's aging point out that only women who have long had appropriate nutrition and adequate exercise will be able to evaluate whether, in their perimenopause years, their bodies have become unbalanced (Lonsdorf, 2004). The *New Harvard Guide to Women's Health* has started to promote massage and meditation as legitimate and effective ways to deal with many of the mood, anxiety, and physiological symptoms of menopause (Patz, 2004).

Whether it is a combination of the alternative methods of dealing with menopause or a combination of these with some form of medicalized HRT, the WHI trial media event has increased debate and prompted existing government and non-profit groups' efforts to make more information available to women. Routine suggestion to women of a certain age that they begin to think about HRT is now likely to be met with more open questioning. However, as our analysis here suggests, while the media was quick to raise an apparently feminist flag in the face of the WHI trial results, the representation of women as repositories of either a right to protection or a right to choice suggests that women's health activists have a great deal more work ahead.

Conclusion

Although U.S. and Canadian media responses to the WHI trials and findings share many similarities, it is the subtle differences which are the most interesting and telling of underlying systemic differences. The Canadian responses took a slightly more serious tone in response to the WHI findings, they presented the findings in a very straightforward manner. Although the articles in general do not preach for women to end their use of HRT, on balance they suggest that if women are taking HRT for preventative disease purposes, they should not.

The Canadian press also was more supportive of discussing options, evidence, risks, and benefits with doctors, and reinforced the idea that doctors are largely responsible for ensuring their patients' well-being and that they should be a major resource for informing and helping women. Of the few benefits that the articles acknowledged that HRT provides, there was a moderate degree of discussion concerning alternative sources to help provide these benefits without using HRT. Most of the articles did not dismiss HRT, but seemed to emphasize that women should approach its use with some caution and skepticism. Interestingly, the responses suggest that the Canadian health agencies/medical groups did not place as many restrictions/guidelines on HRT, but rather placed faith in the doctor/patient relationship as the level at which decisions about use and safeguarding of the patients should occur.

Alternatively, we feel the U.S. media responses conveyed a more confusing and uncertain tone. Although some of the responses blamed the media for sending confusing messages to women about the stopped WHI study, the articles did little to help resolve that confusion. Women were provided with very few productive avenues for dealing with their confusion or finding information, reinforcing the message that there are too many contradictions flying about.

By placing far more agency/responsibility on the women solely, de-emphasizing (and at times arguing against) reliance upon doctors for information about whether or not to start/continue using HRT, the U.S. articles articulate a health care system which privileges choice, even if no alternatives are offered. So where the federal government and medical agencies may place more restrictions/suggestions on labels and guidelines for use, this is not an effort to protect women, but to displace decision-making onto women rather than their doctors, in essence, holding women responsible if they deviate for their own reasons from the decisions dictated by the formal guidelines.

De-medicalizing women's bodies – and, especially, combating the 'one pill' approach to a range of ailments, some of which we would agree are well handled in the medical model – while at the same time demanding that pharmaceutical companies continue to find non-toxic ways to support women's health – requires treading a thin line: we want *both* to be protected from scientific and manufacturing practices that we have little means to evaluate on our own, and we want to exercise our knowledge and power to choose among health care options. But at present, and in striking contrast when we look across the forty-ninth parallel, the very ideology of health care systems seems incapable of accommodating both.

NOTES

1 The comparison to this cohorts' early brush with lung clots in the short run and increased cardiovascular risk in the long run does not go entirely unnoticed in the media reports. However, instead of suggesting these

women have a lot of history with poorly designed drugs to regulate their hormone cycles, a CBC broadcast on 10 July 2002 has Dr Terry O'Grady, an obstetrician and gynecologist at the Health Sciences Centre in St John's saying: 'Women shouldn't make any rash decisions. I just have this fear that, like when you get a birth control pill scare, everybody stops their birth control pills and the next thing, you have this big increase in the abortion rate because everybody got pregnant.'

2 There is both a feminist and a biologist version of this position – and of course, feminist/biologist. The feminist argument suggests that menopause is an Anglo-American cultural construction designed to oppress women; the biologists argue that women in other cultures, especially Asia, don't seem to have these symptoms, leading to speculation about the role of phytoestogens in non-Anglo-American diets.

3 The significance of race/ethnic difference and differences in habits have not been widely investigated, although some differences are alluded to in some studies. The most systematic analysis has been done by researchers associated with the Postmenopausal Health Disparities Study, which collected clinical data on hundreds of women. In one paper arising from the study published in the wake of the WHI trial termination, researcher Judith S. Gavaler (2003) reviews biomedical and social data to suggest that the 'one dose fits all' model relies on the assumption that there are few patterned differences in the extent to which women achieve the target estrogen levels when they are under treatment. Rather than contesting the WHI findings, she suggests that in current clinical practice, some women are overtreated – increasing the potential side effects for no reason – or undertreated, decreasing the anti-osteoporosis benefits.

The overall findings of the research project are that 'race/ethnic group plays a role in the response to HRT'; that is, in how successfully women who do take it achieve the target level of estrogen. The study highlights the level and problem of non-compliance, but equally importantly, points to additional factors that affect the metabolic process of creating estrogen. Very important is the role of alcohol, which raises testosterone levels, and hence raises estrogen levels slightly, since women's bodies convert testosterone when estrogen levels drop. In addition, the study points to the potential role of phytoestrogens in modulating estrogen; for example, soy and components of red wine play the role of improving – through several related biochemical processes – the level of estrogen. Finally, the study shows that body mass index (BMI) plays a role, since fat cells are implicated in the process of generating the circulating level of hormones. She also notes that some of these same agents are independently helpful in blocking processes that enable or accelerate the development of cancer cells. In the study, compliance, alcohol consumption, and BMI were all positive predictors of achieving estrogen levels on conventional dosing schemes, even irrespective of race/ethnicity.

Although the implications of this study are not fully spelled out, we can easily recognize that the positive predictors are all likely to vary by socio-economic class and likely by ethnicity/race (if the later is itself tied to class). Pierre Bourdieu's (1984) monumental work on class and taste, though conducted in the 1960s, demonstrates unequivocally that diet, exercise, and body-size preferences are directly related to class, not because the poor eat badly – which may be truer today where McDonald's is the most economical place to eat – but because subcultural norms inculcate tastes.

Future research on HRT 'in use' must consider the relationship between culture and biology, and consider how patterned differences may occur. Feminism has had some difficulty contesting the idea that 'biology is destiny,' and this has likely been nowhere more contentious than in areas like motherhood and menopause. But we should be in a theoretical and scientific position today to recognize that cultural practices – for example, high consumption of red wine – intersect with biological processes, in this case the production of hormones, and that this intersection must be made explicit if, as Gavaler argues, women are to benefit, when they can, from pharmaceutical interventions. Still hopeful about the role of HRT, Gavaler in the end advocates for using tests to measure hormone levels, rather than relying on identifying a level of 'symptom relief' as a means of reducing vasomotor symptoms and providing any protective benefits, while seeking to keep dosage below the threshold of causing negative side effects.

4 The women's movement concept of 'choice' was developed in relation to attaining safe and legal abortion for all women regardless of race or social and economic status. In the early years of the abortion movement, inability to get an abortion was viewed as something of a leveller of privilege. Tied to the nineteenth-century feminist abolitionists analysis of white men's abuse of Black women, second wave white feminists worked hard to understand, in particular, Black women's experience of and desire for the option of abortion. However, as neoliberalist market/consumerist under-standing of choice had, by the 1990s, overtaken the earlier human rights version of choice, differences in individual women's ability to exercise the supposed 'choices,' determined by class, race, cultural, and social barriers, is less likely to be considered. In fact, human rights and choice are often in conflict in economies of scarcity; 'goods' like health services, distributed (at

least in social democracies) at the level of the state rather than in the market, must trade off the greater ability of the rich to access ('choose') from a range of services to which the poor only barely have a right (and at minimum level). The concept of access to care has lost some of its power in rights' rhetoric as access has been rewritten as a specification of choice.

5 As reported by many new sources, the WHI shut down the memory arm branch of the HRT study in May of 2003 because it found an increased risk of dementia in women 65 and older who took combination therapy. Additionally, in early February 2004, the WHI shut down an estrogen-only portion of the trial, involving 11,000 women with hysterectomies, because while there was found to be no apparent positive or negative affect on the heart, the data shows that estrogen alone increases the risk of stroke, enough so that the agency deemed these otherwise healthy women were at too great a risk to continue their HRT therapy (Another HRT, 2004).

REFERENCES

Another HRT trial halted. (2004, 3 March). *Health 24 News*. Retrieved 4 August 2004, from http://www.health24.com/news/Menopause/1-928,26786.asp.

Arnst, C. (2002, 29 July 29). But don't run screaming from hormone therapy. *Business Week, 3793*, 73.

Assessing HRT risks. (2002, 11 July). *The Gazette* (Montreal), p. B2.

Bell, S.E. (1995). Gendered medical science: Producing a drug for women. *Feminist Studies, 21*(3), 469–500.

Bourdieu, P. (1984). *Distinction: A Social Critique of the Judgment of Taste.* R. Nice (Trans.). London: Routledge. (Original work published as *La distinction: critique sociale du jugement,* 1979).

Branswell, H. (2002, 10 July). New study shakes trust in hormone therapy. *Edmonton Journal*, p. A2.

Branswell, H. (2002, 10 July). Study details risks of hormone therapy. *Times Colonist* (Victoria, BC), p. A1.

Brink, S. (2002, 29 July). Stronger bones without hormones. *US News and World Report, 133*(4), 62.

Carroll, A. (2002, 11 July). Relax, women told: No reason to panic over hormone therapy, expert says. *The Gazette* (Montreal), p. A6.

Coney, S. (1994). *The Menopause Industry: How the Medical Establishment Exploits Women.* Alameda, CA: Hunter House.

Do-it-yourself menopause remedies. (2001). *Prevention, 53*(7), 7.

Findlay, D., & Miller, L. (1994). Through medical eyes: The medicalization of women's bodies and women's lives. In B. Singh Bolaria & H. Dickinson (Eds.), *Health, Illness and Health Care in* Canada (pp. 276–306). Toronto: Harcourt Brace.

Gavaler, J.S. (2003). Thoughts on individualizing Hormone Replacement Therapy based on the postmenopausal health disparities study data. *Journal of Women's Health, 12*(8), 757–768.

Hunt, K. (1994). A 'cure for all ills'? constructions of the menopause and the chequered fortunes of hormone replacement therapy. In S. Wilkinson & C. Kitzinger (Eds.), *Women and Health: Feminist Perspectives* (pp. 141–165). London: Taylor & Francis.

Kalb, C. (2002, 4 November). Coping after HRT. *Newsweek, 150*(19), 53.

Kolata, G., & Peterson, M. (2002, 10 July). Hormone replacement study a shock to the medical system. *New York Times*, p. A1.

Linton, M. (2002, 15 July). HRT in the balance: New study sheds light on hormone replacement. *Calgary Sun*, p. 35.

Lock, M. (1991). Contested meanings of the menopause. *The Lancet, 337*, 1270–1272.

Lock, M. (1998). Anomalous ageing: Managing the postmenopausal body. *Body and Society, 4*(1), 35–61.

Lonsdorf, N. (2004). Natural HRT: Herbal and ayurvedic approaches. *Positive Health, 31*, 34.

MacPherson, K.I. (1993). The false promises of hormone replacement therapy and current dilemmas. In J. Callahan (Ed.), *Menopause: A Midlife Passage* (pp. 145–159). Indianapolis: Indiana University Press.

Malterud, K. (1999). The (gendered) construction of diagnosis interpretation of medical signs in women patients. *Theoretical Medicine and Bioethics, 20*(3), 275–286.

More harm than good. (2002, 22 July). *Maclean's, 115*(29), 36–37.

Off-label drug use. (1997). *Harvard Women's Health Watch, 5*(2), 2–3.

Patz, A. (2004). A women's health bible gets a makeover. *Health, 18*(5), 65–67.

Ravnikar, V.A. (1987). Compliance with hormone therapy. *American Journal of Obstetrics and Gynecology, 156*, 1332–1334.

Risks vs. benefits: How does hormone replacement therapy measure up? (1992). *National Women's Health Report, 14*(4), 1–4.

Seaman, B., & Seaman, G. (1977). *Women and the Crisis in Sex Hormones*. New York: Bantam Books.

A stake in the heart of HRT or too much at stake? (2002, 12 July). *Toronto Star* (Ontario Edition), p. F02.

Van Keep, P.A. (1990). The history and rationale of hormone replacement therapy. *Maturitas, 12*, 163–70.

Van Wijk, C., Vliet, K., & Kolk, A. (1996). Gender perspectives and quality of care: Towards appropriate and adequate health care for women. *Social Science & Medicine, 43*(5), 707–720.

Vanderhaeghe, L. (2004). Menopause misery sends women back to HRT. *Canadian Journal of Health and Nutrition, 259,* 8.

Wiley, T.S., Taguchi, J., & Formby, B. (2003). *Sex, Lies, and Menopause.* New York: HarperCollins.

Wilkinson, S., & Kitzinger C. (Eds.). (1994). *Women and Health: Feminist Perspectives.* London: Taylor & Francis.

Worcester, W., & Whatley, M. (1992). The selling of HRT: Playing on the fear factor. *Feminist Review, 41,* 1–26.

Zola, I. (1972). Medicine as an institution of social control. *Sociological Review, 20,* 487–504.

17 Women's Health and Cardiovascular Care: A Persistent Divide

LYNNE E. YOUNG

Since 1995, there have been 136 heart transplants in B.C., 106 men and 30 women. That means that 78 per cent of recipients are male; the North American average is 73 per cent.

Men received far more referrals for [heart] transplant than women – 730 compared to 252 for women since 1996 ... The issue of inequality has never even been raised at the society [notes Greenwood of the BC Transplant Society] ... There is 'no evidence at all' of gender bias in the allocation of organs. (Dedyna, 2004)

Cardiovascular science and practice are deeply rooted in 'modern' philosophical traditions that focus on the individual as the unit of concern; hold to positivist scientific and professional practices that are decontextualized and 'value-free'; and position the researcher or professional as expert in women's health-related matters. Women's health, on the other hand, is philosophically located in postmodern/poststructural paradigms that focus on women's gendered experience; contextualize that experience; make explicit the values underpinning research and practice; and locate women as the experts on their own health. If cardiovascular care and women's health were philosophically aligned, would there be no evidence of gender-bias in the heart transplant arena as noted in the opening citation?

Cardiovascular disease (CVD) was long held to be a disease that primarily afflicted males, hence cardiovascular research and practice are deeply infused with male bias. In cardiovascular care arenas, females as spouses of men with CVD are recognized as caregivers, sometimes not in positive light. Thus, the cardiovascular arena is a site of particular interest in the women's health arena both from the perspective of research and practice involving women with cardiovascular disease, and from the perspective of appreciating the toll that it takes on women's health to be partners in care for others with cardiovascular disease. This chapter begins by locating the concept of health in the cardiovascular field, then provides an overview of the epidemiology of women and cardiovascular disease. Following this, the evolution of thought about women and cardiovascular disease is discussed in order to place in historical context the 'moment of awareness,' about 1989, in which it became evident that females were absent from cardiovascular science. Two case examples that explore the issue of women in the cardiovascular arena are then presented. The first case example is a review and critique of the heart transplant literature, which reveals that females are less likely to be heart transplant recipients than males at a ratio of 4:1. The second case example, taken from a research program designed to explore low-income lone mothers' risk for CVD, emphasizes the social processes and factors that underlie risk for CVD. The chapter concludes with reflections on issues arising throughout this chapter related to what is necessary to move the women's health agenda forward in the cardiovascular field.

Background to the Issue

Cardiovascular disease is the major cause of death of men and women, with a global epidemic underway that in future years will affect the lives of men and women throughout the world (American Heart Association [AHA], 2003; Heart and Stroke Foundation of Canada [HSFC], 2003; Levenson, Skerrett, & Gaziano, 2002; Mathers, Sadana, Salomon, Murray, & Lopez, 2001). CVD encompasses a constellation of conditions, including coronary artery disease; stroke; congestive heart failure; high blood pressure; diseases of the arteries such as aneurysms, rheumatic fever/rheumatic heart disease; and congenital cardiovascular defects (AHA, 2003). While CVD is often considered to be a disease of the elderly, it is the second leading cause of death of many North Americans aged 45 to 65, and the third leading cause of death for those aged 22 to 45; thus, the indirect costs of CVD to society are staggering (HSFC, 2003; Levenson et al., 2002).

CVD has traditionally been considered a male disease, yet recent research suggests that women are not only as vulnerable as men to this condition, but women also spend approximately twice as many more years disabled than their male counterparts with diseases such as CVD (Mathers et al., 2001). For Canadian women, the estimated direct costs of CVD in 1993 were $3.43 billion. Estimated indirect costs for women from CVD in 1993 were set at $4.72 billion for lost productivity due to illness or disability, or loss of future earnings due to premature death (HSFC, 2003). However, the calculation of indirect costs of CVD does not include the indirect costs of CVD in terms of the loss of women's unpaid work as informal caregivers and community volunteers.

In North America, rates of CVD have steadily declined since the 1960s, with about 25 per cent of the reduction attributed to lifestyle risk (smoking, physical inactivity, high fat diet), 29 per cent related to early diagnosis and treatment, and 43 per cent attributed to improved tertiary care (AHA, 2003). However, the reduction in rates of CVD have a gendered nature. In the United States, in 1984, the rates of CVD were about the same for men and women. In 2001, the rates of CVD had declined dramatically for men and remained about the same for women, yielding overall an ever-increasing gap between men and women with regard to rates of CVD (AHA, 2004). Currently, the prevalence of CVD in men and women in the U.S. is almost the same after age 55 (AHA, 2003b).

In Canada, a similar widening gap in rates of CVD is evident between men and women, with the point estimate of rates of mortality from CVD the same for men and women in 1993, with an ever-widening actual and projected gap projected to 2016 (HSFC, 2003). Interestingly, when one reviews the statistics for the Economic Burden of Illness in Canada (EBIC, 1998), there are glaring differences between expenditures on cardiovascular disease for males compared with females. In 1998, whereas the percentage of costs for diagnostics for cardiovascular diseases was 17.6 per cent for males, it was 12.7 per cent for women, a difference of 5 per cent in diagnostic expenditures. Out of 20 categories, the only other category in which there were notable expenditures of one gender over another (with the exception of pregnancy) was in the category of injury, where the expenditures on males were about 5 per cent greater for males than for females. Given that the rates of CVD are almost equal in men and women in Canada, these differences suggest a systematic gender-related process that underpins decisions about CVD diagnostic services.

Over the past 15 years, socio-economic status (SES) has been identified as a CVD risk factor for women and men in developed countries (AHA, 2004; HSFC, 2003). That SES is a risk factor for CVD brings to light the influence of social processes on the pathways to CVD (Seemans & Crimmins, 2001). A new term has emerged to describe prevention that addresses social and economic factors, *primordial prevention*. In cross-country comparisons of mortality rates in women aged 35 to 74 in 36 countries relative to the Gross Domestic Product (GDP), 8 of the 10 countries with the highest death rates for total CVD ranked below 24 other countries in terms of GDP (AHA, 2004; HSFC, 2003; World Bank, 2004). Of 10 countries with the lowest rates of total CVD in women, all 10 countries ranked in the top 22 for world GDP. At the national level, Canadian, U.S., and British cross-sectional studies suggest that CVD risk factors cluster in low-income women (Young, James, & Cunningham, 2004; Young Cunningham, & Buist, 2005; Ebrahim, Montaner, & Lawlor, 2004). At the neighbourhood level, in a U.S. study of atherosclerotic[1] risk in communities, Borrell, Diez Roux, Rose, Catellier, & Clark (2004) found that CVD mortality decreased with economic advantage for whites and African Americans. Associations between neighbourhood socio-economic characteristics were stronger for white women than for men in this study. African American women and men demonstrated higher age-adjusted mortality rates for CVD than white men and women.

Race and ethnic differences regarding CVD are apparent for U.S. and Canadian women. While CVD is the leading cause of death for U.S. women of white, Black, Hispanic, Asian/Pacific, American Indian/ Alaska Native groups, there are differences in patterns of disease. For example, in 2000, the death rates from CVD when comparing U.S. Black women with white women were 397.1 to 285.8 per 100,000 (AHA, 2004). Patterns such as this suggest that for marginalized women, future success in preventing and addressing cardiovascular disease may well lie in a society's capacity to address the socio-economic determinants of heart health, yet, research and practice in the CVD field is squarely focused on reducing lifestyle/behavioural risk and related interventions. To better understand why this is the focus of the field, it is illuminating to reflect on definitions of health as they are employed in the CVD field.

Health Defined in the Cardiovascular Field

What is most compelling about the concept of health is not how it is defined, but rather, how health as a discourse in a particular field of concern shapes research and practice (Young & Wharf-Higgins, 2004). In North America, health is currently conceptualized within two major discourses: the medical model and the systems view. In the medical model, health is conceptualized as the absence of disease, whereas in the systems view, health is understood to be constructed through the interrelatedness and interdependence of all phenomena (Capra, 1982). Health in the cardiovascular field falls squarely within the medical view of health as evidenced by the dominance of interventions designed to address clinical risk or behavioural risk for, or to 'cure' CVD. In contrast, women's health falls within a systems view of health. Acccording to the Ontario Women's Health Council (2004), health 'involves women's emotional, social, cultural, spiritual, and physical well-being that is determined by biology as well as the social, political, and economic contexts of women's lives. This definition of women's health acknowledges the centrality and validity of women's perceptions and life experiences of health and illness; the values and knowledge of women; and the role of women both as users and providers of health care.' If applied to cardiovascular women's health, such a definition would expand the conceptual lens well beyond the behavioural and biological to the social and economic determinants; the lived experience of women's cardiovascular health; and even to the roles of women as caregivers of those dealing with the sequels to cardiovascular diseases. Redefining health in such a way in the cardiovascular field might go some way to shifting the discourse to better serve the interests of women, in particular marginalized women.

Evolution of Thought about Women and Cardiovascular Disease

Discourses shape how health is defined, and in turn how health care is practiced, as well as the evolution of thought about women and cardiovascular disease. It has long been recognized that women are susceptible to atherosclerosis, a primary underlying pathological process of cardiovascular disease. As early as 1912–1913, Sherman noted that the elderly become more or less sclerotic, a condition often found in elderly women. However, despite this knowledge, the medical gaze remained squarely on males, possibly because of the economic implications of the effects of atherosclerosis on working men. When women were discussed in the literature they were often talked about in terms of the impact of CVD on their childbearing role. For example, in the early part of the twentieth century, Frederick Holden, advocating for birth control or sterilization of certain women with heart disease, wrote, 'A woman has a distressingly decompensated heart. It is known that each succeeding pregnancy leaves her heart muscle weaker and weaker, and finally she passes out, leaving a brood of children for somebody else to bring up' (Lerner, 1994, p. 374). This theme of valuing women for their family-related work was evident in not only the professional but also the lay literature from the late 1950s to the mid-1960s, when women's role as homemakers and caregivers was emphasized (King & Paul, 1996; Miller & Kollauff, 2002). For example, from 1959 to 1967, the American Heart Association sponsored programs with titles such as 'Hearts and Husbands' and 'Cardiac Wives' (Miller & Kollauff, 2002, p. 256).

The kinds of heart disease experienced by women are also often underemphasized. For example, women suffer from cardiac valvular disease in unequal proportions to men (Devereaux, 2001). In the United States, the National Hospital Discharge data in 1987 estimated that 123,000 patients were discharged with aortic or mitral valve disease, 79 per cent of whom were women. Devereaux (2001) notes that in 1987 about 46,000 heart valve replacements were performed, of which 60 per cent were in women, and that in comparison with the 518,000 surgical procedures that were performed for coronary artery disease, women comprised only 29 per cent of recipients. Yet, during the 1980s atherosclerotic heart disease (AHD) remained the focus of care in the cardiovascular area, a condition more common in males. This phenomenon is not surprising, since before 1986 minimal attention was paid to women's health beyond that related to the reproductive system (Miller & Kollauf, 2002).

Several defining moments can be identified that represented shifts in discourse towards serving the interests of women's health more broadly. In 1971, a seminal publication appeared that brought to media attention the issues of women and cardiovascular disease that further emphasized socio-economic and racial influences. The *Green Bay Press-Gazette* of 16 December 1971 reported the results of an American Heart Association panel discussion of physicians who noted that 'some women have socioeconomic protection against high risks, but that aggressive, Type A personalities may be at higher risk. [The release] ... also noted that black women are more susceptible to heart disease than white women' (Miller & Kollauf, 2002, p. 256). While this defining moment was commendable in shifting the focus in the cardiovascular arena to the interface between women, socio-economic status, and race by drawing attention to the risk of 'aggressiveness,' it framed the presentation in a way that contributed to the discourse that served those who had an interest in keeping women working in the home.

Throughout the 1970s and early 1980s, and even now in many publications, the professional cardiovascular literature does not reveal gender differences, thus obscuring gender-related issues. The gendered nature of CVD was first addressed in North America in 1986 when the US National Heart, Lung, and Blood Institute sponsored a professional seminar on women and heart disease. While gender is reported now in the CVD field more consistently than even five years ago, race and SES are seldom reported, leaving issues related to marginal societal status impossible to deconstruct. For example, when I requested information about race, gender, and heart transplantation from the Canadian Organ Replacement Register (CORR) for this chapter, in March 2005, the response was that while the CORR collects this data, the data are poorly reported and not easily categorized.

Opening spaces for discussions about women and cardiovascular disease catalyzed professional and grassroots activities. One notable grassroots activity in the United States was undertaken by a nurse, Bonnie Hartman Arkus, in response to the death of her mother in 1986. Once Ms Arkus learned that women have a death rate three to four times that of men undergoing open-heart bypass surgery, she took action to raise awareness and advocate for change. In 1992, Ms Arkus and her group incorporated the Women's Heart Foundation (WHF) as a charitable organization to advance research and education for women's health. On the professional side, in 1989 a policy-level conference was held entitled, 'First National Conference on Women and Heart Disease,' which included topics such as epidemiology, treatment and evaluation of heart disease, educational needs of women, American Heart Association recommendations, and signs and symptoms specific to women (Miller & Kollauff, 2002).

These early actions engendered a flurry of documents and conferences addressing the topic of women, heart disease, and stroke. In Canada, the Heart and Stroke Foundation of Canada (HSFC) played a leading role in moving the women's cardiovascular health agenda forward. In 1997, the HSFC produced a blueprint for action that called for the development of reliable data to guide clinical decision-making and pubic health recommendations. Then in 1999 the HSFC, in partnership with the Medical Research Council of Canada (now the Canadian Institutes of Health Research), funded over 20 postdoctoral fellows from a wide range of disciplines to build research capacity to develop knowledge in the area of women, heart disease, and stroke. In 2000, the HSFC in partnership with a number of other agencies hosted the First International Conference on Women, Heart Disease, and Stroke in Victoria, BC. A mandate of the conference was to craft a Declaration on Women, Heart Disease, and Stroke (ABFICWHDS, 2000). In February 2005, the Second International Conference on Women Heart Disease and Stroke

Text Box 17.1 The 2000 Victoria Declaration: Women, Heart Diseases, and Stroke

Recognizing that heart diseases and stroke are the leading cause of death among women in the developed world and are fast approaching the same status in the developing world; that gender inequity, poverty, illiteracy, unemployment, and lack of access to health services influence women's health; that taking appropriate action to address these and other underlying determinants of health is required; and that promoting a healthy lifestyle would help prevent heart diseases and stroke, the *Advisory Board of the First International Conference on Women, Heart Disease and Stroke calls upon*:

- Women and men
- Health, media, education, and social science professionals, and their associations
- The scientific research community
- Government agencies concerned with health, education, trade, finance, culture and recreation, commerce, agriculture, and the private sector
- International organizations, agencies concerned with health and economic development, and community health coalitions
- Voluntary health organizations
- Employers and their organizations

to marshall their efforts and invest resources in the prevention and management of heart diseases and stroke among women in both developed and developing countries, and *to adopt the following five values* as the foundation for the development, implementation, and evaluation of all policies, programs, and services:

- Health as a fundamental human right
- Equity
- Solidarity in action
- Participation
- Accountability

Source: Advisory Board of the First International Conference on Women, Heart Disease and Stroke, Victoria, BC, 10 May 2000. Retrieved 9 March 2005, from http://www.cwhn.ca/resources/victoria_ declaration/.

was convened. (Abstracts from this conference are available online at http://circ.ahajournals.org/cgi/reprint/111/4e40.pdf.)

In support of 'getting the word out,' the lay literature has reflected a growing interest in the topic of women and heart disease. Miller & Kollauf (2002) report that from 1987 to 1995, the *Readers' Guide to Periodical Literature* had 35 citations on the topic of women and heart disease in magazines commonly read by female consumers, for example, *Good Housekeeping* and *McCall's*. A study conducted by Clark, Feldberg, & Rochon (2002) designed to analyse content about women's health in academic journals found that in traditional medical journals such as the *Lancet*, less than 20 per cent of the articles reported on women's health, and only 6 per cent of these focused on heart disease. In contrast, in women's health journals such as *Women and Health*, 41.5 per cent addressed non-traditional women's health topics, with 8 per cent of the articles addressing heart disease. Moyer, Vishnu, & Sonnad (2001) compared the coverage of women's health topics in women's magazines (*Women's Day* and *Good Housekeeping*) to articles in major medical journals (JAMA and NEJM) for six months in 1997. Less than 18 per cent of medical journal articles addressed women's health topics. Heart disease was addressed in 2.5 per cent of articles in both categories of publications. The authors of this study also point out that in the women's magazines the source of evidence is seldom reported. Clearly, there is a need for increased research and scholarship in the area of women and cardiovascular disease, as well as stronger links between the two to ensure that what is disseminated in the lay literature contributes to women's health. Now, the word is beginning to reach the public: heart disease is not only a disease of men; women are at risk, too. However, the adequacy and reach of reporting are suboptimal.

Behind these shifts, feminist scholarship and action was a catalyst (King & Paul, 1996). Currently in Canada and the United States, the women's health agenda calls for inclusion of women in clinical trials to explore gender differences in disease states, and to use methodologies that bring to light women's experiences of health and illness (King & Paul, 1996; Health Canada, 1999). Some policy-level action has been taken to increase women in clinical drug trials. In 1982, women were under-represented in cardiovascular drug trials at a ratio of about 2:1 (Merkatz, 1994). Following policy implementation by the U.S. Federal Drug Agency (FDA), the FDA conducted surveys and determined that the extent to which populations such as women were included in new drug applications in 1988 was increased for some drugs. In Canada, in

1996, the Women in Clinical Trails policy was announced, with Health Canada charged with monitoring the implementation of this policy (Health Canada, 1999).

In the next section, two examples are offered to illustrate how the social construction of women in the CVD field, and the concomitant socialization of health care professionals and researchers, has and continues to, influence women's health in cardiovascular arenas. First is a discussion about the inequities evident in the heart transplant field that illustrates ongoing androcentricity; and second is an illustration that brings forward the centrality of shifting the focus from behavioral risk factors to social risk factors if the interests of marginalized women are to be served in the CVD field.

Women and Heart Transplantation: Inequities in Women's Health

Gender bias in the treatment arena in CVD care is well-documented (Aaronson, Sanford Schwartz, Goin, & Mancini, 1995; Beery, 1995; Canning, Dew, & Davidson, 1996; Dong, Ben-Shlomo, Colhoun, & Chaturvedi, 1998; Moser, 1997; Randall, 1993). There is no question that men are more likely than women to be the recipients of transplanted hearts as evidenced by international and local statistics that are consistent in reporting a ratio of about 4:1, males to females, as heart transplant recipients (BCTS, 2002; ISHLT, 2001). Furthermore, it is females (spouses, daughters, or sisters) who, in 85 to 90 per cent of cases, contribute personal resources as caregivers to HT recipients (Canning, Dew, & Davidson, 1996; Dew et al., 1998). These data, when considered side by side, give one pause to consider whether women are treated equitably in the heart transplant field.

Women's access to heart transplant is related to the physiology of gender differences; how parameters are set for determining success of heart transplant programs; and women's willingness to accept the heart transplant procedure (Young & Little, 2004). Perceived and presenting physiological gender differences related to age of disease onset, disease progression and coexisting illnesses, potential for pregnancy following HT, and anatomical size of the heart and blood vessels impact cardiovascular treatment decisions on the pathway to heart transplantation (Cupples, 1997; Rankin, 1992; Sheifer, Escarce, & Schulman, 2000; Carlson, 2002). That women are 10 to 15 years older than men when presenting with heart disease is a truth that guides practice. However, this truth is contested by authors who suggest that since women present symptomatically differently than men, they may have disease but it is not recognized (Arslanian-Engoren, 2000; Beery, 1995; Cerrato, 1998; Culic, Eterovic, Miric, Rumboldt, & Hozo, 2000; Phillips, 1997). Consequently, some women may go untreated for long periods of time, and when they finally do present they are older and have more concurrent conditions than their male counterparts, rendering them ineligible for cardiac transplantation (Costanzo et al., 1995; King & Paul, 1996; Moser, 1997). Another physiological difference that interferes with women's access to HT is the smaller size of women's blood vessels. The equipment and instruments developed for open-heart surgery are based on the larger anatomical structures of men and may not be adaptable to the smaller structures of women (Beery, 1995; Cochran & Panos, 2002; Cupples, 1997) .

Since heart transplant programs are funded according to their demonstrated success, surgeons may be unwilling to risk including women as HT candidates because they are perceived to be at greater risk for a failed procedure than men. Cochran & Panos (2002) report that surgeons hold a generalized bias against women, evident in comments such as, ' If it weren't for operating on women, my complications would be half what they are now' (p. 372). These authors comment: 'Generally speaking, surgeons view women as higher risks and as having more complications than men in all of cardiac surgery' (p. 372). It is interesting to review age/gender data.

> For calendar year 2003 for all heart transplant recipients (includes combination transplants and all grafts):
> Females (N=35), mean age 37.6 (sd 20.2); median age 42
> Males (N=122), mean age 46.9 (sd 18.0); median age 53
> (Consultants Kim Badovinac, Canadian Organ Replacement Register (CORR) Personal communication). 9 March 2005.

Do these data reflect the opinion that older women are at increased risk for morbidity and mortality than men?

Barriers to women's access to HT extend beyond hospital walls. A study by Aaronson (1995) found that women were more likely to refuse the offer of heart transplant than men at a ratio of 3:1; however, the study did not report reasons for refusal. Given that the median annual earnings of women in the United States is about 78 per cent that of their male counterparts (Rathje, 2002), the cost of heart transplantation may be well out of reach for most women, but may be affordable for men. Of note is the fact that the women who have the highest mortality rates for heart disease, African American women (Casper et al., 2000), are the very women who are more likely to have lower earnings and live in poverty, and are less likely to be in professional and managerial jobs. In Canada, where access to health care is more equitable than in the U.S., there remain significant costs to families related to lengthy dislocation and drug expenses (Young, Janosek, & MacKenzie, 2000)

Understanding gender inequities in the HT field is challenging, since statistics may be reported in a gender neutral manner. When statistics are categorized, the two categories that appear are 'Adult' and 'Child.' Access to statistics on race, ethnicity, and socio-economic status (SES) are not readily available in the heart transplant field, yet these factors may impact significantly on women's access. No data or research reports age, at assessment for HT, categorized according to gender, making it difficult to discern the extent of gender inequality.

Paradoxically, while women are less likely to be recipients of heart transplants, they bear the burden of informal caring work (King & Koop, 1999; Young et al., 2000; Young & Little, 2004). Research suggests that caring for a spouse following a heart transplant negatively impacts women's health (Bohachick, Reeder, Taylor, & Auton, 2001; Stukas, et al., 1997). Yet, there is no recognition of the contributions of women as informal caregivers of men, and the contribution of this work to the successful recovery of the heart transplant recipient, and in turn to the success of the heart transplant program and its surgeons. Thus, while social accolades and significant financial rewards are laden on the mostly male members of the medical teams, the contributions of the mostly female informal caregivers are invisible.

Lone Mothers' Risk for Cardiovascular Disease: Illustrating Social Risk

Heart transplantation occurs at the extreme high-tech end of the prevention-to-intervention continuum in the cardiovascular field. Exploring women's health issues as they relate to CVD at the opposite end (that is, primordial prevention) is also informative. To this end, in this section, a research program that explored low-income, lone mothers' risk for cardiovascular disease is discussed (Young, James, & Cunningham, 2004; Young et al., 2005).

As mentioned previously, the dominant discourse in the prevention area of cardiovascular care is located within an individual, behaviorist, perspective. Thus, since 1986, Canadians have been inundated with media messages about how to reduce risk for heart disease by eating right, exercising regularly, avoiding obesity, and by not smoking or stopping smoking (Young, 1997). In addition, in the 80s and 90s, throughout the developed world, workplace, school, and community-based interventions that educated people about these risks and risk reduction strategies were launched and evaluated. Such interventions have been effective in reducing heart disease and some risk factors in some segments of the population but not for others (Winkleby, 1994). A review of research on CVD risk factors shows that most studies are designed to explore a single lifestyle risk factor, for example, smoking. Yet, most such studies conclude that people at the lowest end of the SES scale are at highest risk for CVD related to their lifestyles, relative to the risk factor under investigation.

To develop knowledge about marginalized women's risk for CVD, a participatory research project was launched that convened lone mothers, academic researchers, and health promoters from Canada and the United States, as well as Canadian national and provincial government personnel. Through working with a population whose lives are largely shaped by social policy – family, education, and welfare policies – the plan was to generate knowledge that had the potential to link social policies and women's heart health. To ensure that women's voices were reflected in the research, we designed the study to be participatory, using both quantitative and qualitative methods with a view to opening spaces for mothers' voices in policy-making arenas. We included qualitative methods to ensure that women's voices were present in the data, and quantitative methods to ensure that we could have a dialogue with policy makers and program planners who generally hold quantitative research in higher regard.

Gustavsen's (2001) view of participatory research in which network development is paramount was used as a guide. Therefore we developed partnerships among various sectors catalysing a partnership-driven research program that blended qualitative with quantitative studies while connecting low-income lone mothers from diverse geographic areas with numerous health professionals, including nurses, physicians, health promoters, and epidemiologists, who convened to generate knowledge about low-income lone mothers' risk for cardiovascular disease.

The purpose of the quantitative research (Young et al., 2004; Young et al., 2005) was to compare select lifestyle risks (smoking, obesity, physical activity) and clinical risks (diabetes, hypertension, hypercholester-olemia, C-reactive protein) for cardiovascular disease, with socio-demographic, health, and psychosocial variables in partnered versus lone mothers. We also examined the relationship between partner sta-tus and clinical CVD or cardiovascular heart disease (CHD) event (heart attack, heart failure, or stroke), using the third National Health and Nutrition Examination Survey (NHANES III) and the National Popula-tion and Health Survey (NPHS) of 1998–99. In these secondary analy-ses, we began by identifying lone and partnered mothers. Then, using weighted logistic regression, we compared the prevalence of CVD risk factors, self-reported health, and sociodemographic variables (NHANES III, n = 1446 women <60, lone = 43 per cent, partnered 57 per cent: NPHS n = 2184, lone = 22 per cent, partnered = 78 per cent). Multivari-ate modelling examined the relationship between partner status and CVD or CHD events.

Lone mothers live in poverty, report low education status and poor health, and are socially isolated or lack social support, more often than partnered mothers. Further, in the Canadian analysis, the results indi-cated that lone mothers are more distressed and suffer from depression more frequently than partnered mothers. In U.S. mothers, obesity was the most prevalent lifestyle risk, whereas in Canadian mothers it was smoking. While lone mothers in both countries have a slight advantage over partnered mothers for physical activity levels, all mothers were at increased risk for CVD in both countries because of low levels of physi-cal activity. Whereas, the Canadian analysis did not allow us to analyse the data for ethnicity (the numbers in groups were too small), the U.S. data did allow for such an analysis in a limited way. U.S. lone mothers were more likely to report that they were non-Hispanic Black or Mexi-can American than partnered mothers suggesting a relationship be-tween ethnicity and lone motherhood. Surprisingly, given the age of the sample, in the NHANES III analysis, mothers who had experienced a CVD event were 3.28 (95 per cent CI 3.24, 3.31) times more likely to be lone mothers. When adjusting for age, poverty-related variables, self-reported health, body mass index, and family history of myocardial infarction, mothers who reported having experienced a CVD event remained 1.81 (95 per cent CI 1.80-1.84) times more likely to be a lone mother. U.S. mothers with clinical factors (diabetes, high C-reactive protein [CRP], hypercholesterolemia, and hypertension) were 1.31 times (95 per cent CI 1.31, 1.31) more likely to be a lone mother. Since this research used cross-sectional analyses, cause and effect cannot be inferred. However, the results point to a possible causal pathway of women's health that implicate macro-level factors.

Turning now to the qualitative study (Wharf-Higgins, Young, Naylor & Cunningham, 2006) our participatory approach proved to be enriching. Low-income lone mothers contributed to focus group and personal interviews (N=38). Mothers represented considerable diversity in terms of geographic location, race, ethnicity, levels of poverty, rural/urban, and age (17–54). Settings for the interviews varied and included participants' homes (for the individual interviews), community-based support groups, a teen mothers group, and a transition home for homeless families. The mothers represented not only women on welfare or social assistance, but also the working poor (annual income of about $15,000 CDN per year), and those employed at slightly below the poverty line ($30,000 CDN). Women were offered a small stipend to cover the expenses incurred for their participation. Interviews were taped and transcribed according to usual protocols. Following each interview (focus or individual), women were invited to participate in the analysis of the interview in which they participated. Four women volunteered to participate in the analysis of data from their interviews. These women were paid for their efforts at the rate commensurate with hourly wages of a research assistant.

The academic research team of four worked individually and collectively with the data, guided by the women's analyses. (It is notable that there were aspects of the analysis that only became evident to the academic researchers through the women's analyses.) Themes and patterns were identified by the collective. The lead researcher then put it all together using the McKinlay and Marceau (2000) upstream-midstream-downstream conceptual framework to interpret the findings that were then vetted by the lone-mother analysts for accuracy and effectiveness. The overriding pattern that reflected the low-income, lone mothers' discussions, and the higher-order interpretive category, was that the women felt *out of the mainstream* of everyday life, socially and as citizens. They felt excluded by the policies and professional practices that shaped their everyday lives. The women's accounts fleshed out the particularities of the causal pathways between cardiovascular lifestyle risk behaviors and macro-level policies and practices.

Taken together, these studies identify a population of concern for primordial prevention in the cardiovascular arena. Lone mothers' lives are shaped by exclusionary social policies and practices that influence their capacity for heart health, suggesting the need for research on

casual pathways to CVD that begins with taken-for-granted social policies and practices. The participatory approach brought together researchers from a wide range of disciplines and settings, and made space
for women's voices that deepened understandings. Not surprisingly,
the theme evident in the analysis of women and heart transplantation –
that women's family work is invisible and not valued – was evident in
these studies.

Surfacing Issues: Gender and HT; Women, SES, and CVD

Whose interests are served in the cardiovascular science and practice?
Heart transplantation is the tip of an iceberg. The iceberg itself is chilling – are women equally as valued as men in cardiovascular science
and practice? The evidence suggests otherwise. Since statistics show
clearly that men receive more cardiovascular diagnostic services than
women, and males and females have equal rates of CVD, what systemic
inequities mitigate against women achieving optimal CVD health? If
there are inequities, are all women treated the same or do other types of
systemic discriminations intersect with gender to affect the cardiovascular health of marginalized women, such as poor, illiterate, immigrant
women? And what about women's caregiving? Heart transplantation
provides an example of women's unpaid work: not only do women
contribute to the health of their male loved ones through caregiving;
but, by extension, these same women also contribute to the careers of
largely male transplant physicians, who benefit financially from the
success of their heart transplant programs.

Regarding the behavioural risk-factor approach to risk reduction in
the CVD field, while the approach has been successful for some groups
such as the well off and well educated, for others, such as those living in
poverty, lifestyle risk reduction has not been as effective. While much
attention is focused on behavioural risk factors, knowledge generated
using rigorous methods over a number of decades suggests that socio-
economic conditions shape these behaviours, yet little attention is paid
to this phenomenon in science or practice. Thus, the CVD risk-reduc-
tion discourse remains located in a largely decontextualized view of
disease risk. Lack of attention to, and interest in, the macro-level influences on cardiovascular health is a highly resistant problem, one that
will undoubtedly reproduce rather than disrupt social processes that
contribute to inequalities for women in cardiovascular arenas. On the
other hand, since cardiovascular disease is such a prevalent health

condition in Canada, if circumstances shift such that funding agencies focus knowledge development pertinent to the influence of macro-level social processes and dominant practices on women's health in the cardiovascular field, much needed theoretical and empirical knowledge will be generated that has potential to bridge between dominant discourses of health – the biomedical and social determinants perspectives.

Women's Health and Cardiovascular Care: Closing the Gap

Women's health is a relatively new idea in the cardiovascular arena. Professional and research practices in the cardiovascular field are deeply rooted in androcentric, patriarchal, and capitalist values, beliefs, and opinions. Shifting these will be akin to moving mountains. Yet, because cardiovascular disease is a major cause of death and disability for women in the developed and developing world, those concerned about women's health must begin to work together to move this agenda forward. Because cardiovascular practice is focused on a 'body part,' a legacy of the Cartesian view and an unpopular philosophical position in the women's health arena, does it attract the same levels of attention and respect as other areas of scholarship in women's health? If not, this collection is a starting point to synergize collaborations and open new spaces for dialogue to begin the daunting task of closing the gap between women's health and cardiovascular science and practice. The common theme evident in the two case examples – that women's family work is invisible and not valued – may be an important bridge between the women's health movement and cardiovascular care to focus action.

NOTE

1 Atherosclerotic refers to a degenerative disease of the arteries that in later stages results in narrowing of the arteries and compromised blood flow.

REFERENCES

Aaronson, K.D., Sanford Schwartz, J., Goin, J.E., & Mancini, D.M. (1995). Sex differences in patient acceptance of cardiac transplant candidacy. *Circulation, 91*, 2753–2761.

Advisory Board First International Conference on Women, Heart Disease and Stroke. (2002). The 2000 Victoria Declaration: Women, heart disease, and stroke. Victoria, BC, 8–10 May 2000. *CVD Prevention* (2000), *3*, 174–327.

American Heart Association (2003). Congestive heart failure. Heart disease and stroke statistics – 2003 update. Retrieved 1 Sept 2003, from http://www.americanheart.org/downloadable/heart10590179711482003HDSStatsBookREV7-03.pdf.

American Heart Association (2004). Heart disease and stroke statistics – 2004 update. Retrieved 2 July 2004, from http://www.americanheart.org/presenter.jhtml?identifier=1200026

Arslanian-Engoren, C. (2000). Gender and age bias in triage decisions. *Journal of Emergency Nursing, 26*, 117–124.

Beery, T.A. (1995). Gender bias in the diagnosis and treatment of coronary artery disease. *Heart and Lung, 24*, 427–435.

Bohachick, P., Reeder, S., Taylor, M.V., & Anton, B.B. (2001). Psychosocial impact of heart transplantation on spouses. *Clinical Nursing Research,10*, 6–25.

Borrell, L.N., Diez Roux, A.V., Rose, K., Catellier, D., & Clark, B.L. (2004). Neighbourhood characteristics and mortality in the Atherosclerosis Risk in Communities Study. *International Journal of Epidemiology, 33*, 398–407.

British Columbia Transplant Society. (2002). Heart transplantation statistics. Vancouver: BC Transplant Society.

Canning, R.D., Dew, M.A., & Davidson, S. (1996). Psychological distress among caregivers to heart transplant recipients. *Social Science & Medicine, 42*, 599–608.

Capra, F. (1982). *The Turning Point: Science, Society, and the Rising Culture.* New York: Simon & Schuster.

Carlson, K.J. (2002). Approach to the patient and her family. In P.S. Douglas (Ed.), *Cardiovascular Health and Disease in Women* (2nd ed., pp. 3–7). Toronto: W.B. Saunders.

Casper, M.L., Barnett, E., Halverson, J.A., Elmes, G.A., Braham, V.E., Majeed, Z.A., et al. (2000). *Women and Heart Disease: An Atlas of Racial and Ethnic Disparities in Mortality.* 2nd ed. CDC Office for Social Environment and Health Research, West Virginia University. Greenburg, PA: Chas Henry Printing.

Cerrato, P. (1998). Women and heart disease. *RN, 61*(11), 40–43.

Clark, J.P., Feldberg, G.D., & Rochon, P.A. (2002). Representation of women's health in general medical versus women's health specialty journals: A content analysis. *BMC Women's Health, 20*, 5.

Cochran, R.P., & Panos, A. (2002). Coronary artery by-pass surgery. In P.S.

Douglas (Ed.), *Cardiovascular Health and Disease in Women* (2nd ed., pp. 372–382). Toronto: W.B. Saunders.

Costanzo, M.R., Augustine, S., Bourge, R., Bristow, M., O'Connell, J.B., Driscoll, D., & Rose, E. (1995). Selection and treatment of candidates for heart transplantation. Retrieved January 2003, from http://www.americanheart.org/presenter.jhtml.

Culic, V., Eterovic, D., Miric, D., Rumboldt. Z., & Hozo, I. (2000). Gender differences in triggering of acute myocardial infarction. *American Journal of Cardiology, 85*, 753–756.

Cupples, S.A. (1997). Cardiac transplantation in women. *Critical Care Nursing Clinics of North America, 9*, 521–533.

Dednya K. (2004). Study gets to heart of gender inequality: UVic researcher finds inequity in transplant numbers. *Times Colonist* (Victoria). (Friday, 2 July 2004), D6.

Devereux, R. (2001). Valvular heart disease. In Pamela S. Douglas (Ed.), *Cardiovascular Health and Disease in Women* (2nd ed., pp. 405–425). Toronto: W.B. Saunders.

Dew, M.A., Goycoolea, J.M., Stukas, A.A., Switzer, G.E., Simmons, R.G., Roth, L.H., & Di Martini, A. (1998). Temporal profiles of physical health in family members of heart transplant recipients: Predictors of health changes. *Health Psychology, 17*, 138–151.

Dong, W., Ben-Shlomo, Y., Colhoun, H., & Chaturvedi, N. (1998). Gender differences in accessing cardiac surgery across England: A cross-sectional analysis of the health survey for England. *Social Science & Medicine, 47*, 1773–1780.

Ebrahim, S., Montaner, D., & Lawlor, D.A. (2004). Clustering of risk factors and social class in childhood and adulthood in British women's heart study: Cross sectional analysis. *British Medical Journal, 5*. Retrieved 19 August 2005, from http://bmj.bmjjournals.com/cgi/content/full/328/7444/861.

Economic Burden of Illness in Canada (EBIC) – On-Line. (1998). Selected costs. All diagnostics – males and females. Retrieved 12 July, from http://ebic-femc.hc-sc.gc.ca/help_e.php?Lange.

Gustavsen, B. (2001). Theory and practice: The mediating dosscourse. In P. Reason & H. Bradbury (Eds.), *Handbook of Action Research* (pp. 17–26). Thousand Oaks, CA: Sage.

Health Canada. (1999). Women's Health Strategy. Ottawa: Health Canada.

Heart and Stroke Foundation of Canada. (1997). *Women, Heart Disease, and Stroke in Canada: Issues and Options*. Ottawa: HSFC.

Heart and Stroke Foundation of Canada. (2003). *Growing Burden of Heart Disease and Stroke in Canada*. Ottawa: HSFC.

International Society for Heart and Lung Transplantation. (2001). Retrieved January 2003, from http://www.ishlt.org/.

King, K.M., & Koop, P.M. (1999). The influence of the cardiac surgery patient's sex and age on the caregiving received. *Social Science & Medicine, 48,* 1735–1742.

King K.M., & Paul, P. (1996). A historical review of the depiction of women in cardiovascular literature. *Western Journal of Nursing Research, 18,* 89–101.

Lerner, B.H. (1994). Constructing medical implications: The sterilization of women with heart disease or tuberculosis, 1905–1935. *Journal of the History of Medicine and Allied Sciences, 49,* 362–379.

Levenson, J.W., Skerrett, P.J., & Gaziano, J.M. (2002). Reducing the global burden of cardiovascular disease: The role of risk factors. *Preventive Cardiology, 5,*188–199.

Mathers, C.D., Sadana, R., Salomon, J.A., Murray, C.J., & Lopez, A.D. (2001). Healthy life expectancy in 191 countries, 1999. *Lancet, 357*(9269), 1685–1691.

McKinlay, J., & Marceau, L. (2000). US public health and the 21st century: Diabetes Mellitus. *Lancet, 356,* 757–761.

Miller, C.L., & Kollauf, C.R. (2002). Evolution of information on women and heart disease 1957–2000: A review of archival records and secular literature. *Heart and Lung, 31,* 253–261

Moser, D.K. (1997). Heart failure in women. *Critical Care Nursing Clinics of North America, 9,* 511–519.

Moyer, C.A., Vishnu, L.O., & Sonnad, S.S. (2001). Providing health information to women. *Int J Technology Assessment in Health care, 17,* 137–145.

Ontario Women's Health Council. (2004). Public Education. Retrieved 22 July 2004, from http://www.womenshealthcouncil.on.ca/.

Phillips, L. (1997). Women, men, and treatment for heart disease. *Hospital Technology Scanner, 16*(2), 4–5.

Randall, T. (1993), The gender gap in selection of cardiac transplantation candidates: Bogus or bias? *Journal of the American Medical Association, 269,* 2718–2720.

Rankin, S.H. (1992). Psychosocial adjustments of coronary artery disease patients and their spouses: Nursing implications. *Nursing Clinics of North America, 27,* 271–284.

Rathje, K. (2002). Male versus female earnings: Is the gender wage gap converging? *Expert Witness Newsletter, 7.* Retrieved 9 March 2005, from http://www.economica.ca/ew71p2.htm.

Seemans, T.E., & Crimmins, E. (2001). Social environment effects on health and aging: Integrating epidemiological and demographic approaches and perspectives. *Annals of the Academy of Sciences, 954,* 88–117

Sheifer, S.E., Escarce, J.J., & Schulman, K.A. (2000). Race and sex differences in the management of coronary artery disease. *American Heart Journal, 5,* 848–857.

Stukas, Jr., A.A. Dew, M.A., Switzer, G.E., DiMartini, A., Kormos, R.L., Griffith, B.P., & Thurau, R. (1997). Perceived gender bias in the treatment of cardiovascular disease. *Journal of Cardiovascular Nursing, 15,* 124–127.

Wharf-Higgins, J., Young, L.E., Naylor, P.J., & Cunningham, S. (2006). Out of the mainstream: Low-income lone mothers' life experiences and perspectives on heart health. *Health Promotion Practice, 7,* 221–233.

Winkleby, M.A. (1994). The future of community-based cardiovascular disease prevention. *American Journal of Public Health, 84,* 1369–1372.

Women's Heart Foundation. (2004). Retrieved 15 July 2004, from http://www. womens heartfoundation.org/content/About_WHF/history_of_whf.asp.

World Bank. (2004). World Development Indicators data base: Total GDP July 2003. Retrieved 10 July, from http://www.worldbank.org/data/ databytopic/GDP.pdf.

Young, L.E. (1997). Family influence on individual health-related decisions in response to a heart-health initiative. Unpublished doctoral dissertation. University of British Columbia, Vancouver.

Young, L.E., Cunningham, S., & Buist, D. (2005). Lone mothers are at higher risk for cardiovascular disease compared to partnered mothers. Data from the National Health and Nutrition Examination Survey III (NHANES III). *Health Care for Women International, 26,* 604–621.

Young, L.E., James, A., & Cunningham, S. (2004). Lone motherhood and risk for cardiovascular disease: The National Population Health Survey, 1998– 99. *Canadian Journal of Public Health, 95*(5),329–335.

Young, L.E., & Little, M. (2004). Women and heart transplantation: An issue of gender equity? *Health Care for Women International, 25,* 436–453.

Young, L.E., & Wharf–Higgins, J. (2004). Concepts of health: Discourses, determinants, lay perspectives, and the role of the community health nurse. In L. Stamler, & C. Yiu (Eds.), *Community Health Nursing: A Canadian Perspective* (pp 73–85). Don Mills, ON: Pearson Education Canada.

Young, L.E., Janosek, S.V., & McKenzie, L. (2000) Family health promotion in cardiovascular care. *Canadian Journal of Cardiovascular Nursing, 11*(4), 10–18.

18 From Global to Local and Over the Rainbow: Violence Against Women

OLENA HANKIVSKY AND COLLEEN VARCOE

The Natashas have been shipped all over the world ... They line the streets of the red-light districts in Austria, Italy, Belgium and Holland. They stock the brothels in South Korea, Bosnia and Japan. They work nude in massage parlours in Canada and England. They are locked up as sex slaves in apartments in the United Arab Emirates, Germany, Israel and Greece. They star in peep shows and seedy strip clubs in the United States ... Day in and day out, the Natashas are forced to service anywhere from ten to thirty men a night. The money they make goes to their 'owners.' They live in appalling conditions, suffering frequent beatings and threats. Those who resist are severely punished. Those who refuse are sometimes maimed or killed. (Malarek, 2003, p. 3)

I take my baby with me because I cannot tolerate this situation. So we went to the transition house ... So we lost the house. I lost my car. So I cannot go back to work because of my daughter. I have nobody. And then they tried to put me [on] welfare, and then they say, 'No, you cannot take the welfare, you gonna go to the EI.' And then I go to the EI and then they say, 'No, because you quit the job, you go to the welfare.' So I don't know where to go. So I stay in one transition house to another. And I go to the food bank to get something else for me and my daughter. (Survivor [pseudonym], interview, 2001)

Lots of girls in my school go to rainbow parties. The girls all wear different colours of lipstick. The idea is that at the end of the night, the guy with the most colours on his [penis] wins. You pretty much have to go if you want to have any [boy] friends. (Canadian high school student, interview, 2004)

Over the last two decades, violence against women has been recognized as a violation of human rights, an important health policy issue, and a problem with enormous socio-economic costs to society. As the varied quotes above suggest, violence against women has multiple dimensions and is a problem at local to global levels. Progress has been made in terms of understanding violence, developing legal and policy responses, and establishing appropriate programs and services. However, the problem endures and remains a global epidemic. Violence against women is so pervasive that, as the above quotes suggest, social practices seem increasingly tolerant of such violence.

Violence against women is present in every country, cutting across boundaries of culture, class, education, income, ethnicity, and age (United Nation Children's Fund [UNICEF], 2000). Specific groups of women are more vulnerable, including minority groups, women who live in poverty, indigenous and immigrant women, refugee women, women in institutions and detentions, women with disabilities, female children, and elderly women. This vulnerability arises due to the relative social, political, and economic power and freedom such groups have in comparison to more dominant groups within any given population.

Globally, one in three women will be raped, beaten, coerced into sex or otherwise abused in her lifetime (United Nations Development Fund for Women [UNIFEM], 2003a). In Canada, over 50 per cent of Canadian women surveyed had survived at least one incident of sexual or physical violence in their lives (Statistics Canada, 1993). Violence is a daily occurrence. For example, each day 6,000 women are genitally mutilated in North Africa. This year, over 15,000 women will be sold into sexual slavery in China. Suitors and husbands will horribly disfigure 200 women in Bangladesh. Family members and in-laws will murder more than 7,000 women in dowry disputes in India (Amnesty International, 2001).

The incidence and prevalence of violence against women remain constant. At the same time, gender-based violence has become a much more complicated phenomenon to assess and address. Partly this is because research completed to date has led to a more nuanced comprehension of the different patterns and experiences of violence among various groups of women, both nationally and internationally. In addition, violence against women is being intensified and transformed by growing inequalities and commodification of sexual relations associated with globalization, as well as a general decrease in human security internationally. UNIFEM (2003b) maintains that violence against women is as much a global pandemic as HIV/AIDS and malaria.

While it has been understood in most Canadian jurisdictions that any effective response to violence against women requires multisectoral

---

Text Box 18.1 Violence Against Women Is a Global Issue

Violence against women is now internationally recognized as a social problem with serious social and health implications for women.

- The World Bank estimates that in industrialized countries, sexual assault and domestic violence take away almost one in five healthy years of life of women ages 15-44 (World Health Organization, 1997, 2002).
- One-fifth to three-quarters of women have experienced physical or sexual violence since age 15, most of it inflicted by male partners (WHO, 2005).
- 40–70% of homicides of women are committed by intimate partners (Heise, Ellsberg, & Gottemoeller, 1999).
- Globally, about 20% of women, and 5 to 10% of men suffered sexual abuse when they were children (World Health Organization, 2004).

---

coordination, committed resources, and support from the highest levels in government, recent changes in policy, both nationally and internationally, suggest that new strategies are required – strategies that transcend national borders and are accompanied by sufficient political will to result in meaningful action. Feminist scholars and theorists in particular have recognized the need to better understand the meaning and consequences of interacting social hierarchies for women's experience of violence (Price, 2005).

This chapter outlines the problem of violence against women in Canada, situating the problem within wider socio-political and economic contexts, and within the wider global context. We describe the current social response to violence against women, identifying some of the theoretical, political, and practical challenges and strategies for eliminating violence against women.

Violence Against Women

In its Declaration on the Elimination of Violence Against Women, the United Nations General Assembly (1993) defined violence against women as:

Any act of gender-based violence that results in, or is likely to result in, physical, sexual, or psychological suffering to women, including threats of such acts, coercion or arbitrary deprivation of liberty, whether occurring in public or private.

It encompasses but is not limited to physical, sexual, and psychological violence occurring in the family, including battering, sexual abuse of female children in the household, dowry related violence, marital rape, female genital mutilation and other traditional practice harmful to women, non-spousal violence, and violence related to exploitation, physical, sexual, and psychological violence occurring within the general community, including rape, sexual abuse, sexual harassment and intimidation at work, in education institutions, and elsewhere; trafficking in women and forced prostitution; and physical, sexual, and psychological violence perpetrated or condoned by the state, wherever it occurs.

As can be seen from the above definition, violence against women encompasses a wide range of abuses and harms. The language used in relation to violence against women is an important and ongoing issue. Terms such as *domestic violence, family violence, spousal abuse,* and *interpersonal* or *intimate partner violence* obscure the gendered nature of violence. WHO (World Health Organization, 2004) points out that while women can be violent, international research consistently shows that women bear the brunt of interpersonal violence. Other terms such as *woman abuse* or *wife abuse,* while pointing to the gendered nature of violence, obscure the fact that there are actual people committing violence. Other terminology, such as 'male violence against women,' emphasizes the gendered nature of violence and identifies the gender of most perpetrators of violence, but seems to have an individualizing tone, drawing attention away from the pervasive and widespread nature of violence against women in the media, in institutions, in widespread social practices, and in language, as well as in the behaviour of individuals. The network of influences that result in social tolerance of coercive sex, whether it is the kidnapping of women for use in sexual slavery, or participation in 'rainbow parties' by adolescents, are complex, multifaceted, and pervasive.

As these varied terms illustrate, the language that is used to discuss violence against women is important because such language conveys understandings about the causes and nature of violence. Across disciplines, theorists have endeavoured to understand violence by focusing attention on and seeking causal explanation for violence within three spheres: individuals, couples or dyads, and society (Bograd, 1988; Gelles & Loseke, 1993). Stark and Flitcraft (1991) labelled these three perspectives the interpersonal model, the family violence model, and the gender-politics model.

Early understandings of violence against women focused on individuals and interpersonal relationships, emphasizing the psychology of the victim and perpetrator, and their interrelationships. These theories tended to focus on the characteristics of victims and thus diverted attention from the situation to the victim, and treated women's reasonable responses to unreasonable situations as pathological (Wardell, Gillespie, & Leffler, 1983). More recent psychological theories shifted examination of causes of violence to the psychopathology of the perpetrator, but do not routinely attend to power, gender relations, and other forms of oppression. Importantly, Dobash and Dobash (1992) argued that the media has popularized the focus on the individual in ways that perpetuate common understandings of violence as strictly a problem of abnormal individuals who need psychiatric help. This focus on the psychology of individuals suggests that violence is an aberrance of a few men, rather than a predominant pattern of behaviour, and it excuses men, implicates women, and concludes that the differences between abused and non-abused women are the causes rather than the consequences of abuse (Bograd, 1988). Causal explanations of violence related to the psychology of the individual leave power and gender relations unexamined and consider violence in isolation from the social and historical contexts in which it occurs. The normalization of violence and coercive sex are not addressed through such lenses.

The second set of perspectives on violence explains the causes of violence as located within couples and families. These perspectives dominated most early research on violence (Silva, 1994), tended to be gender neutral, to treat power inequities as only one factor among many, and to explain violence as resulting from external stresses and breakdown of the family, rather than as a part of most normally functioning families (Bograd, 1988; Stanko, 1988). As with the focus on individuals, the focus on dyads or families does not draw attention to the influence of the social context or the role of women in society and families.

Gender-political or 'feminist' perspectives explain violence as arising from the social context, and contribute an analysis of the influence of gender and power relations to theorizing violence (Yllö, 1993). Feminist perspectives take into account the gendered nature of violence. However, feminist perspectives have been criticized by some (e.g., Dutton, 1994; Gelles, 1993; Letellier, 1994) as inadequate for understanding violence because such explanations are seen as limited to a single caus- ative factor (patriarchy). Others (e.g., Crenshaw, 1994; Mahoney, 1994; Miller, 1994; Mosher, 1998; Phillips, 1998; Renzetti, 1994; Tolman & Bennett, 1990) argue that while violence is deeply gendered, other interacting forms of oppression (such as oppression based on race, class, disability) are critical to understanding violence against women. In particular, Black feminists have emphasized how 'race' cannot be separated from gender in analyses of violence against women (e.g., hooks, 1984; Razack, 1998), leading to calls for the use of an 'intersect- ing oppression perspective' which considers how other forms of op- pression are magnified by one another and magnify the violence in women's lives (Crenshaw, 1994; Mosher, 1998; Varcoe, 1996; 2002). Rather than focusing on individuals and on discrete acts of violence, inter- sectionality (see the Introduction, this collection, for a more general discussion of the concept) focuses on the social context to explain violence against women. Rather than focusing solely upon gender, attention is turned to a culture of violence that encompasses the vio- lence of racism, poverty, heterosexism, and other forms of inequity. From this perspective, the experience of violence is seen as being influenced profoundly by the intersections of multiple social locations of privilege and oppression. This perspective, which we use in this chapter:

• Shifts from individual to social explanations of violence against women
• Shifts away from assigning blame and responsibility to women who are victims of violence
• Turns attention to structural inequalities as causing and perpetuat- ing violence against women
• Focuses on the importance of social policy in reducing and ending violence against women

Violence Against Women in Canada

Similar to most countries around the world, in Canada, violence against women is a pervasive problem of epidemic proportions (see Text Box 18.2). The most comprehensive national study of the problem remains the 1993 Violence Against Women study, conducted by Statistics Canada

---

Text Box 18.2   Violence Against Women in Canada Is Widespread

- 50% of Canadian women have experienced at least one incident of sexual or physical violence (Statistics Canada, 1993).
- 19% of women experience violence after leaving a relationship,
  and for 43% of those the violence began or escalated after
  leaving (Canadian Centre for Justice Statistics, 1993).
- 29% of never-married/common law partnered women report
  being physically assaulted by a current or former partner since
  the age of 16 (Statistics Canada, 1993).
- 25% of all violent crimes reported to a sample of police services in 2001 involved cases of family violence, 2/3 were
  violence committed by a spouse or ex-spouse and 85% of the
  victims were female (Statistics Canada, 2003, 23 June).
- 1999 data showed that at least half a million children had
  heard or witnessed a parent being assaulted during the previous 5 years (Statistics Canada, 2000).

---

and analysed by numerous researchers (e.g., Johnson, 1996; Kerr &
McLean, 1996; Rodgers, 1994). A review by Clark and DuMont (2003)
illustrates that in Canada, data on the prevalence of violence against
women is very limited and of poor quality. However, Statistics Canada
produces an annual report drawing on a range of surveys and detailing
some aspects of the problem (Statistics Canada, 1996-2004). In 2003, this
report showed that one quarter of all violent crimes reported to police
in 2001 involved 'family violence,' and that from 1995 to 2001, the rate
of incidents of spousal violence reported by police increased steadily.
Although the term *family violence* obscures the fact that the vast majority
of these crimes (85 per cent) were committed against women, the report
contains overwhelming evidence of the gendered nature of the problem. The abuse and violence that girls and women have experienced
within institutional settings has also been recognized (Feldthusen,
Hankivsky, & Greaves, 2000; Law Commission of Canada, 2000). Further, there is increasing recognition of the levels of violence within
same-sex relationships (e.g., Renzetti, 1996; Ristock, 2002).

Violence against women in Canada has tremendous impacts on the
health of women, the health of their children, and on the economy (see
Text Box 18.3). Nearly 2,600 spousal homicides (which includes legally

---

Text Box 18.3 Some of the Health, Social, and Economic Impacts of Violence Against Women

Physical and mental health implications include:

- Acute physical injuries, unwanted pregnancies and miscarriages (Gielen et al., 2000; Campbell, 2002).
- STDs including HIV/AIDS (Gielen et al., 2000; Martinet al., 1999; Zierler, 1997).
- Psychological trauma and poorer mental health (e.g., Cascardi, O'Leary, & Schlee, 1999; Herman, 1992; Mouton, Rovi, Furniss, & Lasser, 1999).

Social impacts include:

- Poverty (Raphael, 2000; Weinreb, Goldberg, Bassuk, & Perloff, 1998).
- Homelessness (Bassuk et al. 1997; Browne & Bassuk, 1997).
- Lost educational/employment opportunities, loss of safety (Jones et al., 1999; Robertson, 1998).
- Decreased self-esteem (Murphy & Cascardi, 1999; Browne, 1993, 1997).

Economic costs include:

- Over $4.2 billion annually in Canada, spanning social services/education, criminal justice, labour/employment, and health (Greaves, Hankivsky, & Kingston-Riechers, 1995).

---

married, common-law, divorced, and separated spouses) were recorded in Canada between 1974 and 2000, the majority of which (77 per cent) have been against women (Canadian Centre for Justice Statistics, 2000). The stress and emotional burden placed on women who are not able to leave an abusive relationship often manifest themselves in an increase of physical/mental illness and disease (Campbell, Kub, & Rose, 1996; Day, 1995; Gerlock, 1999).

The costs of violence to women themselves, to their children, to the health care system, and to the economy more generally, are enormous in

Canada (Day, 1995; Greaves, Hankivsky, & Kingston-Riechers 1995). Women experience a wide range of health impacts as a consequence of violence, including injuries, chronic pain, depression, and post-traumatic stress disorder, gastrointestinal problems such as irritable bowel syndrome, and gynaecological problems, including pelvic inflammatory disease (Ali et al., 2000; Campbell, 2002; Champion, Piper, Holden, Korte, & Shain, 2004; Coker, Smith, King, & McKeown, 2000; Green, Flowe-Valencia, Rosenblum, & Tait, 1999; Reilly & Warshaw, 1998). Over their lives, abuse survivors experience more surgical interventions, physician and pharmacy visits, hospital stays, and mental health consultations than other women even when controlling for other factors affecting health care utilization (Heise, Ellsberg, & Gottemoeller, 1999). Children of abused women are often abused (Bowker, Arbitell, & McFerron, 1988; Edleson, 1999; Margolin, 1998; Stark & Flitcraft, 1991), and many who witness violence experience similar problems to those of children who have been directly abused, including emotional and behavioural problems (Fantuzzo et al., 1991; Fantuzzo & Mohr, 1999; Jaffe, Wolfe, & Wilson, 1990; Knapp, 1998; Statistics Canada, 2003). The effects of these impacts on women and children are manifest in higher costs for the health care and social services systems (Yodanis, Godenzi, & Stanko, 2000). Moreover, friends and neighbours who offer victims assistance and shelter often become targets of violence themselves (Amnesty International, 2004).

Violence against women and its impacts are not borne equally by all groups of women in Canada. As Yuval-Davis (1997) argues, 'Not all women are oppressed and/or subjugated in the same way or to the same extent, even within the same society at any specific moment,' and this of course extends to the issue of violence against women where issues of intersectional subordination need to be recognized (Crenshaw, 1994). Accordingly, an intersectional lens provides an effective tool for analysing the way that different categories of identity within specific contexts produce different vulnerabilities and experiences of abuse. Aboriginal women, women of colour, lesbians, women with disabilities, young girls, and older women face multiple forms of discrimination and are at higher risk for violence (Day & McMullen 2005). For example, 8 in 10 Aboriginal women in Ontario reported having personally experienced violence (Gurr, Mailloux, Kinnon, & Doerge, 1996), a stark consequence of historical and ongoing colonization of aboriginal people (for a fuller discussion see Chapter 4, this collection). The meaning and consequences of the abuse that Aboriginal women experienced within residential schools is only just starting to be understood (see Dion-Stout & Kipling, 2003; Smith, Varcoe, & Edwards, 2005).

Women with disabilities are at least 1.5 to 2 times as likely to be abused as non-disabled women (Stimpson & Best, 1991; Sobsey, 1988). At the same time, these women have limited access to appropriate health and social services, and when they attempt to seek help they often experience physical and attitudinal barriers (Womendez & Shneiderman, 1991). For example, 'less than two-thirds of shelters for abused women report being accessible to women with disabilities' (Status of Women Canada, 2003).

Moreover, there is a growing awareness that trans-women, like non-trans-women, are vulnerable to sexual and physical assault, harassment, and other forms of misogynist brutality. In 1999, Carrie Davis, director of GenderPac (Gender Public Advocacy Coalition) in the United States, reported that almost 60 per cent of transgendered and trans-sexual people are victims of violence (cited in Darke & Cope, 2002, p. 33). In a 1998 survey in Portland, Oregon, 50 per cent of the transgendered respondents reported having been assaulted or raped by a partner; 31 per cent identified as survivors of domestic violence (Courvant & Cook-Daniels, 1998). In 1995, post-operative MTF transsexual Tawni Sheridan was harassed, verbally abused, and denied access to the women's washroom at a popular gay lounge, B.J.'s, in Victoria, British Columbia. Ironically, pre-operative MTF transsexuals who are expected to use women's washrooms as a condition of 'life in the female role' prior to surgery, often face derision and physical attacks in public places.[1]

Immigrant women face the compounding effects of migration, and many also face discriminatory language barriers and racialization (for a fuller discussion see Chapter 8, this collection). Many fear being ostracized from their communities or deportation by immigration authorities if they disclose their abuse (Smith, 2004). Immigrant women additionally have less access to supports, and available supports are less appropriate (Agnew, 1998; Hyman et al, 2004; Jiwani, 2000; D.L. Martin, & Mosher, 1995; McDonald, 1999; Miedema & Wachholz, 1998; Mosher, 1998). When women who have few supports and financial resources leave abusive partners they often experience increased poverty (Gurr et al., 1996; Raphael, 2000, 2002; Weinreb, Goldberg, Bassuk, & Perloff, 1998), hunger, and homelessness (Bassuk et al., 1997; Browne & Bassuk, 1997; Ontario Association of Interval and Transition Houses, 1998; Robertson, 1998). Access to appropriate social, economic, and political support is critical to fostering the personal change and growth that can occur after leaving an abusive partner (Campbell, Rose, Kub, & Nedd, 1998; Langford, 1996; Wuest & Merritt-Gray, 1999, 2001), and to recovery following sexual assault (e.g., Davis & Brickman, 1996; Druacker, 1999; Suleman & McLarty, 1997).

Historical Overview of the Social Response to Violence Against Women

In 1982, Margaret Mitchell, MP for Vancouver East, brought the issue of violence against women to the Canadian House of Commons, citing estimates that 1 in every 10 women experiences violence in their intimate relationships every year. Other Members of Parliament responded with laughter and derision. This reaction may not be surprising given that in Canada it was legally permissible for a man to rape his wife until 1983, when Bill C-127 introduced a three-tiered offence of 'sexual assault,' to ensure that all forms of assault would be dealt with under the law (Levan, 1996).

The social response to violence against women has been driven largely by women themselves, with the 'battered women's movement' emerging in the late 1960s (Dobash & Dobash, 1992). As Morrow outlines in relation to the women's health movement more generally (see chapter 2, this collection), the response to violence against women has been marked by shifting tensions between the role of the women's movement and the role of the government. Despite the ongoing debate among feminists regarding engagement with the state (Brown 1995; chapter 1, this collection), the reality is that 'women who are survivors of physical and sexual violence are often dependent on state-funded organizations and social welfare as they attempt to leave violent partnerships and re-establish their lives' (Morrow, Hankivsky, & Varcoe, 2004, p. 3). The state, its institutions, and funded programs and services are therefore invaluable to the well-being, security, and survival of women. At the same time, community members and activists have an important role to play in continuously keeping the issue of violence against women in the public eye, lobbying, and providing critique and service alternatives. In particular, such activists and community members can promote intersectional analyses that widen understanding of violence as a complex social issue affected by all forms of discrimination and oppression.

Starting as early as the 1970s, in Canada and internationally, initiatives have been undertaken by women and governments to prevent and respond to violence against women. In 1973, the first rape crisis centres opened in Vancouver and Toronto. That same year, Interval House, one of the first shelters for abused women, opened in Toronto (Armour & Stanton, 1990). In 1979, the UN produced the first international document that identified violence against women as a priority issue. In 1982, the National Clearinghouse on Family Violence was established in Canada, followed by the Family Violence Prevention Division in the Department of Health and Welfare in 1986.

More significant changes in Canada started taking place in the late 1980s. In 1988, the federal government launched a Family Violence Initiative. Three years later, in 1991, a Royal Commission – the Canadian Panel on Violence Against Women – was established, largely in response to the 1989 Montreal Massacre of 14 young women at the L' École Polytechnique by Marc Lépine. In many ways this event was a catalyst. Feminists drew on the event as an example of the daily assaults and killings that women experience each year (Levan, 1996). In 1992, five Family Violence and Violence Against Women Research Centres were funded. In 1996, the federal government set up five Centres of Excellence for Women's Health by Health Canada. These centres link up with the violence centres, community-based groups, service providers, and academic researchers on the social determinants of women's health, including violence against women.

Importantly, these initiatives have developed a more comprehensive understanding of violence against women, including understanding how racism, classism, poverty, ageism, ableism, geography, and heterosexism interact to compound violence against women in Canada (e.g., see British Columbia Task Force on Family Violence, 1992; Biesenthal, Sproule, & Plocica, 1997; Jiwani, 2000; Minister's Advisory Council on Women's Health, 1999). Violence against women has been recognized as a social issue, an economic issue (Greaves et al., 1995), a health issue, an education issue, a justice issue, and a human rights issue. In addition, international coalition-building around the issue of violence against women is particularly well-developed and has contributed to growing awareness of the issue, as well as to the development of conventions and policies that have improved the lives of women globally (Morrow et al., 2004). And, advances in information and communication technologies have facilitated the organized fight against gender-based violence and made possible the sharing of research internationally.

The United Nations, in particular UNIFEM, Amnesty International, and the World Health Organization, have been leaders in these endeavors. For example, in 1993, the UN Declaration on the Elimination of Violence Against Women was adopted. The declaration states that violence against women 'is one of the crucial social mechanisms by which women are forced into a subordinate position compared with men.' Two years later the Beijing Declaration and Platform for Action was adopted by 189 nations at the Fourth Conference on Women. As of 2000, 118 countries along with Canada had developed national action plans to implement commitments made to the Beijing Platform, in particular to combat violence (United Nations Division for the Advancement of Women, 2001). The 25th of November is now celebrated as the International Day for the elimination of violence against women. International human rights courts and tribunals now recognize that the pain and suffering resulting from rape are consistent with torture. They also recognize rape and other forms of sexual abuse as war crimes and crimes against humanity under the Geneva Conventions (Amnesty International, 2004).

At an Impasse? Current Social Responses to Violence Against Women

Despite growing awareness of the problem, and progress in the social response, violence against women continues, seemingly unabated, and adequate solutions have not yet been devised (Amnesty International, 2001; Lee, Sanders Thompson, & Mechanic, 2002; Levan, 1996). Despite numerous reports with concrete recommendations in Canada, few of those recommendations have been enacted, especially within the health care system (Morrow & Varcoe, 2000). While the flurry of activity in the late 1980s and 1990s resulted in important initiatives, some of which have been sustained, there has been little recent innovation in developing policy and practice in the area of violence. Progress has been limited by myths, stereotypes, and ideologies, and by global trends including reductions in social welfare spending, the spread of religious fundamentalism, and the commodification of women.

Myths, Stereotypes, and Ideologies

To develop future strategies, it is essential to understand the extent to which harmful myths, stereotypes, and other misunderstandings continue to undermine prevention and intervention efforts. For example, some in the general public still believe that women 'ask for' or 'deserve' to be abused (Cross, 2000; DuMont & Parnis, 1999; Ehrlich, 2001). Consent is an issue that is still not well understood despite campaigns such as 'No means no.' Others do not understand why women do not 'just leave,' and therefore blame them for staying within an abusive situation. Still others believe that only certain groups of poor and racialized women experience abuse. For instance Varcoe (2001) has noted how this stereotype carries over into the medical system, affecting how patients are assessed and treated by nurses. Alcohol and drugs are often seen as reasonable excuses for violent behaviour. Some think that, with time, abusive situations will improve and that families need to stay together. The relationship between tolerance of violence generally and violence against women specifically, is often overlooked. For example, although research has shown that children who are exposed to violent television are proportionately more prone to violence when older (e.g., Zimmerman, Glew, Christakis, & Katon, 2005) few steps are taken to limit such exposure.

Perhaps most disturbing is the growing perception, evidenced by reduced government support, that violence against women is no longer a pressing social issue. Not only do such cultural 'stories' support the elimination or reduction of services, they further perpetuate structural inequalities that permit violence against women, children, and other vulnerable populations. Indeed, it is such social and cultural norms that help to create a climate in which violence is encouraged or inhibited (Krug, Mercy, Dahlberg, & Zwi, 2002).

Various myths, stereotypes, and ideologies support new and emerging modes of violence as both national and international developments and policy changes intersect with violence against women to create new areas of concern. For example, the liberal ideology of 'choice' is compatible with the entrenchment of neo-liberalism (meaning emphasis on individual choice and freedom within a free market economy) and massive cuts to the social welfare system. Women may be seen as 'choosing' to live in poverty, to stay with abusive partners, or to engage in sex work. This combination has had particularly grave consequences for women who experience violence, especially those who are most vulnerable due to their socio-economic status (Morrow, Hankivsky, & Varcoe, 2004; Ontario Association of Interval and Transition Houses, 1996, 1998). In addition, international pressures associated with economic globalization have also created conditions for the commodification of women, (particularly those who live in poverty), sex, and violence against women to flourish. Intersectional analyses draw attention to these ideologies and the ways in which these global trends affect women and limit their 'choices' differently depending on their social locations.

Transforming the Social Welfare State and Violence Against Women

Since the early 1990s, governments have reduced significantly their spending on supports and social policy initiatives in the area of violence against women, along with other programs dedicated to women's issues (Morrow et al., 2004). Existing resources are simply not being dedicated to policies and actions to end violence. In Canada, this process began with the introduction of the Canada Health and Social Transfer in 1995, which, along with unprecedented social spending cuts in the areas of health, education, and social welfare, also removed national standards for the delivery of social services. While spending levels have increased since 1995, the ideology of the previous decade, which emphasizes private solutions to social problems, remains entrenched (Bashevkin, 2002; Jayasuriya, 2002).

Within this neo-liberal policy environment, it is becoming more difficult to make arguments for attending to the needs of women who experience violence. This challenge is evidenced in the fundamental restructuring and cuts to violence-related programs and services for women in the provinces of Ontario, Alberta, and British Columbia (Morrow et al., 2004; Ontario Association of Interval and Transition Houses, 1996, 1998). While in some places violence-specific services such as transition houses have remained intact, the social welfare, housing, and legal services that are required to escape, prevent, or decrease violence are reduced or eliminated. The rationale for spending cuts is premised on an argument of cost-savings and increasing international competitiveness, even though it has been demonstrated that cuts to programs and services for women who are abused do not lead to savings. As Yodanis, Godenzi, and Stanko (2000) correctly point out, 'It is *not* the ... services to victims which cause the costs. Violence causes the costs. Therefore the costs will only be reduced when violence is reduced' (p. 274).

Driven by the intention to reduce spending on social services and programming, and supported by liberal individualism, government approaches to the problem of violence become superficial, inadequate to the magnitude of the problem, and trivialize and individualize violence without considering that it is a social problem of epidemic proportions (Salmi, 1993). While existing programs and services need to be continually evaluated for their efficacy, any substantial reduction to violence intervention and prevention funding will not provide meaningful savings to provinces. To assume that cutting services will reduce costs is using logic that not only is faulty, but also is extremely short-sighted. Reductions to services and programs have enormous effects and concomitant costs in all areas of policy. And, if existing funding can no longer provide adequate crisis intervention, one must consider what kinds of priorities and values are being placed on basic needs and safety and the quality of human life. The preoccupation with cost cutting needs to shift to a consideration of the costs of cutting (Education Wife Assault [EWA], 1997).

Globalization and the Commodification of Women

These federal and provincial policy changes in Canada have not occurred in isolation. They mirror the dismantling of welfare states internationally and the parallel developments associated with globalization. Globalization, and especially economic globalization, has significantly altered gender relations and provided the context for many new forms of violence against women.

First, although it has led to some improvements, economic globalization has compounded social inequities overall. For women, their access to basic needs like food, shelter, education, and health care has eroded. Feminization of poverty has also increased, putting women at higher risk of violence. According to the WHO (2002), poverty acts as a marker for various social conditions that combine to increase women's risk of experiencing violence. For instance, in Canada, the restructuring of the economy has caused unemployment and created more precarious, poorly paid employment for women (Bakker, 1996; Vosko, 2000). Elsewhere, a new generation of jobs for women in export-processing, free trade zones, and world market factories have been created. Often, however, this work is insecure, demeaning, and extremely poorly remunerated. Moreover, it can be extremely dangerous. For example, in Mexico, women working in maquiladors – assembly plants owned by multinational companies on the U.S.-Mexican border – risk sexual exploitation and death. To escape poverty and income insecurity, many women bypass the formal sector and engage in 'transactional' or 'survival' sex in exchange for money, goods, food, shelter, or other gifts' (Amnesty International, 2004, p. 40).

Many women search for employment and better lives abroad. When they do, they are often at risk of violence and abuse. For example, migrant domestic workers experience both exploitation and violence. Amnesty International (2004) reports that in 'case after case, women migrant domestic workers describe how they are forced to work 18–20 hours a day, expected to sleep in corners or corridors, raped with regularity and beaten' (p. 46). The mail-order bride trade has also increased, creating marital relations 'marked by bonds of subordination, which keep the brides under the yoke of their consumer-husbands and sometimes engender situations of spousal violence' (Langevin & Belleau, 2000, p. 2). Other women find themselves being trafficked. Trafficking involves the recruitment and/or transportation of another person for the purposes of exploitation and abuse, such as forced prostitution (UNIFEM, 2003a). It is a distinct manifestation of globalization that has created a world in which everything becomes marketable and everything becomes a commodity – including women's bodies and their sexual services.

According to UNICEF, globalization has made trafficking easier as it has become less difficult for traffickers to transport women across borders (2001). Each year, roughly two million girls between the ages of 5 and 15 are trafficked, sold, or coerced into prostitution (Lederer, 1996). Trafficking in women and girls for the purpose of sexual exploitation is a growing phenomenon around the world. It is considered to be one of the fastest growing international criminal enterprises, with a worth over $7 billion (U.S.) annually (Hughes, 2000). Trafficking, and the sex trade more generally, makes women and girls vulnerable to violence (Paci, 2002). The burgeoning sex trade has made two million sex workers potential carriers of HIV, STDs, and AIDS (World Council of Churches, 2002).

Despite some misconceptions, trafficking is also a Canadian problem. In Canada, trafficking in people represents a market of $120 million to $400 million, affecting 8,000 to 16,000 illegal immigrants annually (Guéricolas, 2000, p. 27). Canada is both a destination and transit country for women trafficked from China, South Korea, Thailand, Cambodia, the Philippines, Latin America, Russia, and Eastern Europe (U.S. Department of State, 2003). In response, Canada has signed a UN Protocol to Prevent, Suppress, and Punish Trafficking in Persons, Especially Women and Children, supplementing the UN Convention against Transnational Organized Crime. It has also created an Interdepartmental Working Group to oversee the country's anti-trafficking policies.

Second, the global rise and spread of fundamentalism has also influenced the rise of violence against women. Among other ideological developments, the increase in fundamentalist movements has created a backlash against the quest for women's equality. Cultural, religious, and ethnic movements have attempted to reassert traditional roles, and in the process 'justify or excuse violence against women in the name of religion, cultural, custom, and tradition' (Amnesty International, 2004, p. 35). Despite critiques by cultural relativists, who argue that social mores should outweigh universal rights, a human rights framework remains important for addressing the subordination of women, and especially for combating abusive and violent practices and behaviours.

Third, increased tensions and conflicts internationally have led to the militarization of many societies. This trend has significant implications for gender-based violence against women. During times of conflict, civil unrest, and post-conflict situations, women and girls are at increased risk of being raped and forced to sell their bodies to access means of survival (WHO, 2002). Rape is a weapon of war, a tool used to achieve military objectives such as ethnic cleansing, spreading political terror, breaking the resistance of a community, rewarding soldiers, intimidation, or extracting information. Many forms of violence that women suffer during armed conflict are gender specific in both nature and result. Recent investigations have clearly demonstrated that in multiple conflict situations, the targeting of victims and forms of the abuse during armed conflict were based on gender as well as other identity markers, such as ethnicity or race (Amnesty International USA, 2004). Women and children are also the majority of refugees fleeing these situations. Again, although Canada is not currently 'at war,' these impacts are directly relevant to Canadians. Women who come to Canada as refugees or immigrants often have been victims of violence. Further, Canada annually sends personnel around the globe as 'peacekeepers.' And, as Malarek (2003) has documented, peacekeeping personnel routinely have been implicated in fostering and sustaining trafficking and sexual exploitation of women and girls.

In all the above-mentioned trends resulting from globalization, women from racial or ethnic minorities are disproportionately affected. They face multiple forms of discrimination – not just gender discrimination. As a result, they are at increased risk for poverty and marginalization. As globalization deepens, approaches to violence must take on an intersectional methodology whereby the intersection of gender oppression with race, ethnicity, age, caste, class, religion, culture, language, sexual orientation, and immigrant or refugee status are recognized and examined in the research process and in terms of policy and program development. For example, trafficking flourishes in developing countries 'because of the compound effects of poverty, gender discrimination and lack of access to resources that are maintained through the collusion of the market, the state, the community and the family unit' (UNIFEM, 2003b, p. 77). Indeed, traffickers target certain groups of women, namely ethnic minorities, refugees, illegal immigrants, uneducated individuals, and women looking for financial support. Adequate responses to trafficking must therefore respond to all the converging factors that *create* the necessary conditions for this form of violence to continue to thrive.

Feminists and other social justice groups have concluded that women's human and equality rights are being significantly eroded by these developments. As a result of trade liberalization, women's underpaid and unpaid – caring or domestic – labour is exploited, and their access to basic needs like food, shelter, education, and health care is eroded. These changes are profound and compounded for women who are marginalized by poverty, racism, disability, and violence.

Conclusion: Where Do We Go from Here?

What has been learned to date is that any adequate solution to the problem of violence against women needs to be supported by the eradication of power imbalances more generally. According to UNIFEM's executive director, Noeleen Heyzer, 'Gender inequality fuels violence against women, and the power imbalances it creates are not easily rectified' (UNIFEM, 2003a). This of course necessitates understanding differences among women and critiquing generalized notions of gender relations (Yuval-Davis, 1997). There are growing calls for multi-causal, multidisciplinary approaches that strive to understand violence as the convergence of factors at individual, cultural, political, and socio-economic levels (Harway & O'Neill, 1999; Heise et al., 1999). While initiatives to date have focused upon individual victims and perpetrators of violence, future efforts must concentrate on cultural, political, and social change.

Increasingly, feminists and other social justice advocates are challenging the lack of resources committed to the problem of violence against women; the damaging effects of restructuring the traditional welfare state; the 'logic' of globalization and its concomitant impact on the commodification of women's bodies, work, and sexual services internationally; and the relationships among this commodification, corporatization, and the media. Work to combat these trends, and efforts to support human rights, food security, and economic security will contribute to ending violence against women.

Women's health and freedom from violence will be improved as their economic, political, and social circumstances improve. A fuller understanding of the health effects of violence requires attention to the relationships among personal, social, economic, and political factors; ongoing abuse; and health and well-being (Barnett, 2000, 2001; Robertson, 1998). And as Sexwale and Matlanyane (1994) put it, 'We ought to acknowledge that although many forms of violence against women are common across the board, some forms and/or their incidence are strictly related to one's positioning in terms of the diversity of our realities' (p. 200). Such understanding, embedded within an intersectional feminist framework of analysis, will support calls for changes to the circumstances of women's lives.

NOTE

1 In another drastic 'cost-saving' move, the BC Liberals forced the closure of the Gender Clinic at Vancouver Hospital in May 2002. The closure means the loss of BC's only accredited referral service for SRS (sex reassignment surgery), as well as its centralized hormone, electrolysis, and counselling services for transgenders and transsexuals in the province.

REFERENCES

Agnew, V. (1998). *In Search of a Safe Place: Abused Women and Culturally Sensitive Services*. Toronto: University of Toronto Press.

Ali, A., Toner, B., Stuckless, N., Gallop, R., Diamant, N., Gould, M., et al. (2000). Emotional abuse, self-blame, and self-silencing in women with irritable bowel syndrome. *Psychosomatic Medicine 62*(1), 76–82.

Amnesty International. (2001). *Broken Bodies, Shattered Minds: Torture and Ill Treatment of Women*. London Amnesty: International Publications.

Amnesty International. (2004). *It's in Our Hands: Stop Violence Against Women*. London: Amnesty International Publications.

Amnesty International USA. (2004). *Violence Against Women in Armed Conflict:*

A Fact Sheet. Retrieved 21 August 2004, from http://www.amnestyusa.org/ stopviolence/factsheets/armedconflict.html#top.

Armour, M., & Stanton, P. (1990). *Canadian Women in History: A Chronology*. Toronto: Green Dragon Press.

Bakker, I. (1996). *Rethinking Restructuring: Gender and Change in Canada*. Toronto: University of Toronto Press.

Barnett, O.W. (2000). Why battered women do not leave. Part 1: External inhibiting factors within society. *Trauma, Violence and Abuse, 1(4)*, 343–372.

Barnett, O.W. (2001). Why battered women do not leave. Part 2: External inhibiting factors-social support and internal inhibiting factors. *Trauma, Violence and Abuse, 2(1)*, 3–35.

Bashevkin, S. (2002). *Welfare Hot Buttons: Women, Work and Social Policy Reform*. Toronto: University of Toronto Press.

Bassuk, E.L., Buckner, J.C., Weinreb, L.F., Browne, A., Bassuk, S.S., Dawson, R., et al. (1997). Homelessness in female-headed families: Childhood and adult risk and protective factors. *American Journal of Public Health, 87*(2), 241–249.

Biesenthal, L., Sproule, L.D., & Plocica, Z. (1997). *Violence Against Women in Rural Communities in Canada: Research Project Backgrounder*. Ottawa: Research and Statistics Division, Department of Justice Canada.

Bograd, M. (1988). Feminist perspectives on wife abuse: An introduction. In K. Yllö & M. Bograd (Eds.), *Feminist Perspectives on Wife Abuse* (pp. 11–26). Newbury Park, CA: Sage.

Bowker, L.H., Arbitell, M., & McFerron, J.R. (1988). On the relationship between wife beating and child abuse. In K. Yllö & M. Bograd (Eds.), *Feminist Perspectives on Wife Abuse* (pp. 158–174). Newbury Park, CA: Sage.

British Columbia Task Force on Family Violence. (1992). *Is Anyone Listening? Report of the British Columbia Task Force on Family Violence*. Victoria: Ministry of Women's Equality.

Brown, W. (1995). *States of Injury: Power and Freedom in Late Modernity*. Princeton: Princeton University Press.

Browne, A. (1993). Violence against women by male partners: Prevalence, outcomes, and policy implications. *American Psychologist, 48*(10), 1077–1087.

Browne, A. (1997). Violence in marriage: Until death do us part? In A.P. Cardarelli (Ed.), *Violence Between Intimate Partners: Patterns, Causes and Effects* (pp. 48–69). New York: Allyn & Bacon.

Browne, A., & Bassuk, S.S. (1997). Intimate violence in the lives of homeless and poor housed women: Prevalence and patterns in an ethnically diverse sample. *American Journal of Orthopsychiatry, 67*(2), 261–278.

Campbell, J. (2002). Health consequences of intimate partner violence. *Lancet, 359*, 1331–1336.

Campbell, J., Kub, J.E., & Rose, L. (1996). Depression in battered women. *JAMWA, 51*(3), 106-110.

Campbell, J., Rose, L., Kub, J., & Nedd, D. (1998). Voices of strength and resistance: A contextual and longitudinal analysis of women's responses to battering. *Journal of Interpersonal Violence, 13*, 743–762.

Canadian Centre for Justice Statistics. (1993). *Violence Against Women Survey highlights and Questionnaire Package*. Ottawa: Statistics Canada.

Canadian Centre for Justice Statistics. (2000). *Family Violence in Canada: A Statistical Profile*. Ottawa: Statistics Canada.

Cascardi, M., O'Leary, K.D., & Schlee, K.A. (1999). Co-occurrence and correlates of posttraumatic stress disorder and major depression in physically abused women. *Journal of Family Violence, 14*(3), 227–249.

Champion, J.D., Piper, J., Holden, A., Korte, J., & Shain, R.N. (2004). Abused women and pelvic inflammatory disease. *Western Journal of Nursing Research, 26*(2), 176–191.

Clark, J.P., & Du Mont, J. (2003). Intimate partner violence and health: A critique of Canadian prevalence studies. *Revue Canadienne de Sante Publique/ Canadian Journal of Public Health, 94*(1), 52–58.

Coker, A.L., Smith, P.H., King, M.R., & McKeown, R.E. (2000). Physical consequences of physical and psychological intimate partner violence. *Archives of Family Medicine, 9*(5), 451–457.

Courvant, D., & Cook-Daniels, L. (1998). *Tran and Intersex Survivors of Domestic Violence: Defining Terms, Barriers, and Responsibilities*. Survivors' Project, NE Fargo #10 2, Portland, OR.

Crenshaw, K.W. (1994). Mapping the margins: Intersectionality, identity politics, and violence against women of color. In M.A. Fineman & R. Mykitiuk (Eds.), *The Public Nature of Private Violence* (pp. 93–118). New York: Routledge.

Cross, P. (2000). *Defining Consent: What Does R. V. Ewanchuk Mean for Us?* Toronto: Ontario Women's Justice Program.

Darke, A. & Cope, A. (2002). *Trans Inclusion Manual for Women's Organizing: A Report for the Trans/Women Dialogue Planning Committee and the Trans Alliance Project*. Vancouver.

Davis, R.C., & Brickman, E. (1996). Supportive and unsupportive aspects of the behavior of others toward victims of sexual and nonsexual assault. *Journal of Interpersonal Violence, 11*(2), 250–262.

Day, S., & McMullen, N. (2005). *A Decade of Going Backwards: Canada in the Post-Beijing Era*. Canadian Feminist Alliance for International Action.

Retrieved 10 February 2005, from, http://www.fafia-afai.org/images/pdf/ B10_0105.pdf

Day, T. (1995). *The Health-Related Costs of Violence Against Women in Canada*. London, ON: Centre for Research on Violence Against Women and Children.

Dion-Stout, M., & Kipling, G. (2003). *Aboriginal People, Resilience and the Residential School Legacy*. Ottawa: Aboriginal Healing Foundation. Retrieved January 2005, from, http://www.ahf.ca/newsite/english/pdf/ resilience.pdf.

Dobash, R.E., & Dobash, R. (1992). *Women, Violence and Social Change*. London: Routledge.

Druacker, C.B. (1999). Knowing what to do: Coping with sexual violence by male intimates. *Qualitative Health Research, 9*(5), 588–601.

DuMont, J., & Parnis, D. (1999). Judging women: The pernicious effect of rape mythology. *Canadian Women Studies, 19*(102),102–109

Dutton, D. (1994). Patriarchy and wife assault: The ecological fallacy. *Violence and Victims, 9*(2), 167–182.

Edleson, J.L. (1999). The overlap between child maltreatment and woman battering. *Violence Against Women, 5*(2), 134–154.

Education Wife Assault (EWA). (1997). *Education Wife Assault Newsletter* 7(Winter).

Ehrlich, S. (2001). *Representing Rape: Language and Sexual Consent*. London: Routledge.

Fantuzzo, J.W., & Mohr, W.K. (1999). Prevalence and effects of child exposure to domestic violence. *The Future of the Children, 9*(3), 21–32.

Fantuzzo, J.W., DePaola, L.M., Lambert, L., Martino, T., Anderson, G., & Sutton, S. (1991). Effects of interparental violence on psychological adjustment and competencies of young children. *Journal of Consulting and Clinical Psychology, 59*, 258–265.

Feldthusen, B., Hankivsky, O., & Greaves, L. (2000). Therapeutic consequences of civil actions for damages and compensation claims by victims of sexual abuse. *Canadian Journal of Women and the Law, 12*(1), 66–116.

Gelles, R.J. (1993). Introduction. In R.J. Gelles & D.R. Loseke (Eds.), *Current Controversies on Family Violence* (pp. 1–9). Newbury Park, CA: Sage.

Gelles, R.J., & Loseke, D.R. (1993). *Current Controversies in Family Violence*. Newbury Park, CA: Sage.

Gerlock, A. A. (1999). Health impact of domestic violence. *Issues in Mental Health Nursing, 20*(4), 373–385.

Gielen, A.C., Fogarty, L., O'Campo, P., Anderson, J., Keller, J., & Faden, R. (2000). Women living with HIV: Disclosure, violence, and social support. *Journal of Urban Health, 77*(3), 480–491.

Gordon, M. (2000). Definitional issues in violence against women: Surveillance and research from a violence research perspective. *Violence Against Women*, 6(7), 747–783.

Greaves, L., Hankivsky, O., & Kingston-Riechers, J. (1995). *Selected Estimates of Costs of Violence Against Women*. London, ON: Centre for Research on Violence Against Women and Children.

Green, C.R., Flowe-Valencia, H., Rosenblum, L., & Tait, A.R. (1999). Do physical and sexual abuse differentially affect chronic pain states in women? *Journal of Pain and Symptom Management*, 18(6), 420–426.

Guéricolas, P. (2000). Géographie de l'inacceptable. *Gazette des femmes, 22* (1) 27–31.

Gurr, J., Mailloux, L., Kinnon, D., & Doerge, S. (1996). *Breaking the Links between Poverty and Violence Against Women*. Ottawa: Health Canada.

Harway, M., & O'Neill, J.M. (Eds.). (1999). *What Causes Men's Violence Against Women?* Thousand Oaks, CA: Sage.

Heise, L., Ellsberg, M., & Gottemoeller, M. (1999). *Ending Violence Against Women. Population Reports*. Series L, No. 11. Baltimore: John Hopkins University School of Public Health. Population Information Program (December).

Herman, J.L. (1992). *Trauma and Recovery*. New York: Routledge.

hooks, b. (1984). *Feminist Theory: From Margin to Center*. Boston: South End Press.

Hughes, D.M. (2000, Spring). The internet and sex industries: Partners in global sexual exploitation. *Technology and Society Magazine*, 35–42.

Human Rights Watch. (2002, November). *Hopes Betrayed: Trafficking of Women and Girls to Post-Conflict Bosnia and Herzegovian for Forced Prostitution, 14* (9).

Hyman, I., Guruge, S., Mason, R., Gould, J., Stuckless, N., Tang, T., et al. (2004). Post-migration changes in gender relations among Ethiopian immigrant couples in Toronto. *Canadian Journal of Nursing Research, 36*(4), 74–89.

Jaffe, P., Wolfe, D., & Wilson, S. (1990). *Children of Battered Women*. Newbury Park, CA: Sage.

Jayasuriya, K. (2002). The new contractualism: Neo-liberal or democratic? *Political Quarterly, 73*(3):309–20.

Jiwani, Y. (2000). *Race, Gender, Violence and Health Care: Immigrant Women of Colour Who Have Experienced Violence and Their Encounters with the Health Care System*. Vancouver: Feminist Research, Education, Development and Action.

Johnson, H. (1996). *Dangerous Domains: Violence Against Women in Canada*. Scarborough, ON: International Thomson Publishing.

Jones, A.S., Gielen, A.C., Campbell, J.C., Schollenberger, J., Dienemann, J.A., Kub, J., et al. (1999). Annual and lifetime prevalence of partner abuse in a sample of female HMO enrollees. *Women's Health Issues, 9*(6), 295–305.

Kerr, R., & McLean, J. (1996). *Paying for Violence: Some of the Costs of Violence Against Women in BC.* Victoria: Ministry of Women's Equality.

Knapp, J.F. (1998). The impact of children witnessing violence. *Violence Among Children and Adolescents, 45*(2), 355–364.

Krug, E.G., Mercy, J.A., Dahlberg, L.L., & Zwi, A.B. (2002). World Report on Violence and Health. *Lancet 360,* 5 October, 1083–1088.

Langevin, L., & Belleau, M. (2000). *Trafficking in Women in Canada: A Critical Analysis of the Legal Framework Governing Immigrant Live-in Caregivers and Mail-Order Brides.* Ottawa: Status of Women Canada. Retrieved 12 August 2004, from http://www.swc-cfc.gc.ca/pubs/066231252X/index_e.html.

Langford, D. (1996). Predicting unpredictability: A model of women's processes of predicting battering men's violence. *Scholarly Inquiry for Nursing Practice, 10*(4), 371–385.

Law Commission of Canada. (2000). *Institutional Child Abuse: Restoring Dignity: Responding to Child Abuse in Canadian Institutions.* Ottawa: Minister of Public Works and Government Services.

Lederer, L.J. (1996, August). National legislation on child pornography and international trafficking. Unpublished document. Center on Speech, Equality and Harm, University of Minnesota Law School, Minneapolis.

Lee, R.K., Sanders Thompson, V.L., & Mechanic, M.B. (2002). Intimate partner violence and women of color: A call for innovations. *American Journal of Public Health, 92*(4), 530–535.

Letellier, P. (1994). Gay and bisexual male domestic violence victimization: Challenges to feminist theory and responses to violence. *Violence and Victims, 9*(2), 95–106.

Levan, A. (1996). Violence against women. In Janine Brodie (Ed.), *Women and Canadian Public Policy* (pp. 319–354). Toronto: Harcourt Brace.

Mahoney, M.R. (1994). Victimization or oppression? Women's lives, violence, and agency. In M. Fineman & R. Mykitiuk (Eds.), *The Public Nature of Private Violence* (pp. 59–92). London: Routledge.

Malarek, V. (2003). *The Natashas: The New Global Sex Trade.* Toronto: Viking.

Margolin, G. (1998). Effects of domestic violence on children. In P.K. Trickett & C.J. Stellenbach (Eds.), *Violence Against Children in the Family and the Community* (pp. 57–101). Washington, DC: American Psychological Association.

Martin, D.L., & Mosher, J.E. (1995). Unkept promises: Experiences of immigrant women with the neo-criminalization of wife abuse. *Canadian Journal of Women and the Law, 8,* 3–44.

Martin, S.L., Matza, L.S., Kupper, L.L., Thomas, J.C., Daly, M., & Cloutier, S. (1999). Domestic violence and sexually transmitted diseases: The experience of prenatal care patients. *Public Health Reports, 114*(3), 262–268.

McDonald, S. (1999). Not in the numbers: Domestic violence and immigrant women. *Canadian Woman Studies / Les cahiers de la femme, 19*(3), 163–167.

Miedema, B., & Wachholz, S. (1998). *A Complex Web: Access to Justice for Abused Immigrant Women in New Brunswick*. Ottawa: Status of Women Canada.

Miller, S.L. (1994). Expanding the boundaries: Toward a more inclusive and integrated study of intimate violence. *Violence and Victims, 9*(2), 183–194.

Minister's Advisory Council on Women's Health. (1999). *Moving Toward Change: Strengthening the Response of British Columbia's Health Care System to Violence Against Women*. Victoria: Ministry of Health and Ministry Responsible for Seniors, Government of British Columbia.

Morris, M. (2002). *Violence Against Women and Girls: A Fact Sheet*. Ottawa: Canadian Research Institute for the Advancement of Women (CRIAW).

Morrow, M., & Varcoe, C. (2000). *Violence Against Women: Improving the Health Care Response: A Guide for Health Authorities, Health Care Managers, Providers and Planners*. Victoria: Ministry of Health.

Morrow, M., Hankivsky, O., & Varcoe, C. (2004). Women and violence: The effects of dismantling the welfare state. *Critical Social Policy, 24*(2), 358–384.

Mosher, J.E. (1998). Caught in tangled webs of care: Women abused in intimate relationships. In C.T. Baines, P.M. Evans, & S.M. Neysmith (Eds.), *Women's Caring: Feminist Perspectives on Social Welfare* (2nd ed., pp. 139–159). Toronto: Oxford University Press.

Mouton, C., Rovi, S., Furniss, K., and Lasser, N. (1999). The associations between health and domestic violence in older women: Results of a pilot study. *Journal of Women's Health and Gender-Based Medicine, 1*(9), 1173–1179.

Murphy, C.M., & Cascardi, M. (1999). Psychological abuse in marriage and dating relationships. In R.L. Hampton (Ed.), *Family Violence Prevention and Treatment* (2nd ed., pp. 198–226). Beverly Hills, CA: Sage.

Ontario Association of Interval and Transition Houses. (1996). *Locked In, Left Out: Impacts of the Progressive Conservative Budget Cuts and Policy Initiatives on Abused Women and Their Children in Ontario*. Toronto: OAITH.

Ontario Association of Interval and Transition Houses. (1998). *Falling Through the Gender Gap: How Ontario Government Policy Continues to Fail Abused Women and Their Children*. Toronto: Ontario Women's Justice Network.

Paci, P. (2002). *Gender in Transition*. Washington, DC: World Bank, Human Development Unit, Eastern Europe and Central Asia Region.

Phillips, D.S.H. (1998). Culture and systems of oppression in abused women's lives. *Journal of Obstetrical and Gynaecological Nursing, 27*, 678–683.

Price, L.S. (2005). *Feminist Frameworks: Building Theory on Violence Against Women.* Halifax: Fernwood.

Raphael, J. (2000). *Saving Bernice: Battered Women, Welfare, and Poverty.* Boston: Northeastern University Press.

Raphael, J. (2002). Keeping battered women safe during welfare reform: New challenges. *Journal of the American Medical Women's Association, 57*(1), 32–35.

Razack, S. (1998). What is to be gained by looking white people in the eye? Race in sexual violence cases. In S. Razack (Ed.), *Looking White People in the Eye: Gender, Race and Culture in Courtrooms and Classrooms* (pp. 56–87). Toronto: University of Toronto Press.

Reilly, M.A., & Warshaw, C. (with Center for Research on Women and Gender/ The University of Illinois at Chicago). (1998). *Health Aspects of Violence Against Women.* Prepared for the US Public Health Services Office on Women's Health and the US Department of Health and Human Services.

Renzetti, C.M. (1994). On dancing with a bear: Reflections on some of the current debates among domestic violence theorists, *Violence and Victims, 9*(2), 195–200.

Renzetti, C.M. (1996). *Violence in Gay and Lesbian Domestic Partnerships.* New York: Haworth Press.

Ristock, J.L. (2002). *No More Secrets: Violence in Lesbian Relationships.* New York: Routledge.

Robertson, A. (1998). Shifting discourses on health in Canada: From health promotion to population health. *Health Promotion International, 13*(2), 155–166.

Rodgers, K. (1994). Wife assault: The findings of a national survey. *Juristat: Service Bulletin, 14*(9), 1–22.

Salmi, J. (1993). *Violence and Democratic Society.* London : Zed Books.

Sexwale, B., & Matlanyane, M. (1994). Violence against women: Experiences of South African domestic workers. In H. Afshar & M. Maynard (Eds.), *The Dynamics of 'Race' and Gender: Some Feminist Interventions* (pp. 196–221). London: Taylor & Frances.

Silva, N. (1994). Towards a feminist methodology in research on battered women. In A. J. Dan (Ed.), *Reframing Women's Health: Multidisciplinary Research and Practice* (pp. 290–298). Thousand Oaks, CA: Sage.

Smith, D., Varcoe, C., & Edwards, N. (2005). Turning around the intergenerational impact of residential school on Aboriginal people: Implications for health policy and practice. *Canadian Journal of Nursing Research, 37*(4), 39–60.

Smith, E. (2004) *Nowhere to Turn? Responding to Partner Violence Against Immi-*

grant and Visible Minority Women. Ottawa: Canadian Council on Social Development.

Sobsey, D. (1988). Sexual offenses and disabled Victims: Research and practical implications. *Vis-à-Vis: A National Newsletter on Family Violence, 6*(4). Winter.

Stanko, E.A. (1988). Fear of crime and the myth of the safe home: A feminist critique of criminology. In K. Yllö & M. Bograd (Eds.), *Feminist Perspectives on Wife Abuse* (pp. 75–88). Newbury Park, CA: Sage.

Stark, E., & Flitcraft, A. (1991). Spouse abuse. In M. Rosenburg & M. Fenely (Eds.), *Violence in America: A Public Health Approach* (pp. 123–155). New York: Oxford University Press.

Statistics Canada. (18 November 1993). The Violence against women survey. *The Daily*. Ottawa: Ministry of Industry.

Statistics Canada. (1996–2004). *Family Violence in Canada*. Retrieved August 2004, from http://www.statcan.ca

Statistics Canada. (2000). *Family Violence in Canada: A Statistical Profile 2000*. Ottawa: Centre for Justice Statistics.

Statistics Canada. (2003, 23 June). Family violence. *The Daily*, Retrieved Ausgust 2004, from http://www.statscan.ca/.

Statistics Canada. (2003, 1 December). Witnessing violence: Aggression and anxiety in young children. *Statistics Canada – The Daily*. Retrieved August 2004, from http://www.statcan.ca/.

Status of Women Canada. (2003). *Fact Sheet: Statistics on Violence Against Women in Canada*. Ottawa: Status of Women.

Stimpson, L., & Best, E. (1991). *Courage Above All: Sexual Assault and Women with Disabilities*. Prepared for DisAbled Women's Network (DAWN). Toronto: Dawn.

Suleman, Z., & McLarty, H. (1997). *Falling Through the Gaps: Gaps in Services for Young Women Survivors of Sexual Assault*. Vancouver: Feminist Research, Education, Development and Action Centre (FREDA).

Tolman, R.M., & Bennett, L.W. (1990). A review of quantitative research on men who batter. *Journal of Interpersonal Violence, 5*, 87–118.

UNDAW. (2001). *From Beijing to Beijing +5: Review and Appraisal of the Implementation of the Beijing Platform for Action* (pp. 13–14). New York: United Nations Division for the Advancement of Women.

UNICEF. (2000). *Domestic Violence Against Women and Children*. Florence, Italy: Innocenti Research Centre. www.unicef-icdc.org/publications/pdf/digest6e.pdf.

UNICEF. (2001). *Profiting from Abuse*. New York: United Nations Children's Fund.

UNIFEM. (2003a). *Not a Minute More*. New York: United Nations Development Fund for Women.

UNIFEM (November 2003b). *International Day to Eliminate Violence Against Women: Message by Noeleen Heyzer*. Retrieved 21 August 2004, from, http://www.ykliitto.fi/aineisto/unifem251103.htm.

United Nations General Assembly. (1993). *Declaration on the Elimination of Violence Against Women*. A/RES/48/104, adopted by the UN General Assembly, 20 December 1993.

U.S. Department of State. (2003, June). Trafficking in persons report. In *Canadian Council for Refugees*. (2004). *The Situation of Trafficking in Canada According to the US Report on Trafficking in Persons*. Retrieved 21 August 2004, from http://www.web.net/~ccr/situation_canada.htm.

Varcoe, C. (1996). Theorizing oppression: Implications for nursing research on violence against women. *Canadian Journal of Nursing Research, 28*(1), 61–78.

Varcoe, C. (2001). Abuse obscured: An ethnographic account of emergency nursing in relation to violence against women. *Canadian Journal of Nursing Research, 32*(4), 95–115.

Varcoe, C. (2002). Inequality, violence and women's health. In B.S. Bolaria & H. Dickinson (Eds.), *Health, Illness and Health Care in Canada* (3rd ed., pp. 211–230). Toronto: Nelson.

Vosko, L. (2000). *Temporary Work: The Rise of a Precarious Employment Relationship*. Toronto: University of Toronto Press.

Wardell, L., Gillespie, D.L., & Leffler, A. (1983). Science and violence against wives. In D. Finkelhor, R. Gelles, G. Hotaling, & M. Straus (Eds.), *The Dark Side of Families* (pp. 69–84). Beverly Hills, CA: Sage.

Weinreb, L., Goldberg, R., Bassuk, E., & Perloff, J. (1998). Determinants of health and service use patterns in homeless and low-income housed children. *Pediatrics, 102*(3, Pt. 1), 554–562.

Women's EDGE. (2002). *Framework for Gender Assessments of Trade and Investment Agreements*. Washington, DC: Women's EDGE.

Womendez, C., & Shneiderman, K. (1991). Escaping from the abuse: Unique issues for women with disabilities. *Sexuality and Disability, 9*(3), 273–279.

World Council of Churches. (2002, February). *Economic Globalization Equals Violence Against Women*. Retrieved 21 August 2004, from, http://www2.wcc-coe.org/pressreleasesen.nsf/index/pu-04-05.html.

World Health Organization. (1997). *Violence Against Women: A Priority Health Issue*. Geneva: World Health Organization, Family and Reproductive Health.

World Health Organization. (2002). *World Report on Violence and Health*. Geneva: World Health Organization.

World Health Organization. (2002). *World Report on Violence.* E.G. Krug, L.L. Dahlberg, J.A. Mercy, A. Zwi, & R. Lozano (Eds.). Geneva: World Health Organization.

World Health Organization. (2004). *The Economic Dimensions of Interpersonal Violence.* Switzerland, Geneva: World Health Organization, Department of Injuries and Violence Prevention.

World Health Organization. (2005). *Multi-country Study on Women's Health and Domestic Violence against Women: Initial results on prevalence, health outcomes and women's responses* http://www.who.int/gender/violence/who_multicountry_study/summary_report/en/index.

Wuest, J., & Merritt-Gray, M. (1999). Not going back: Sustaining the separation in the process of leaving abusive relationships. *Violence Against Women,* 5(2), 110–133.

Wuest, J., & Merritt-Gray, M. (2001). Beyond survival: Reclaiming self after leaving an abusive male partner. *Canadian Journal of Nursing Research, 32*(4), 79–94.

Yllö. K. (1993). Through a feminist lens: Gender, power and violence. In R.J. Gelles & D.R. Loseke (Eds.), *Current Controversies on Family Violence* (pp. 47–62). Newbury Park, CA: Sage.

Yodanis, C., Godenzi, A., & Stanko, E. (2000). The benefits of studying costs: A review and agenda for studies on the economic costs of violence against women. *Policy Studies, 21*(3), 263–276.

Yuval-Davis, N. (1997). *Gender and Nation.* London: Sage.

Zierler, S. (1997). Hitting hard: HIV and violence against women. In N. Goldstein & J.L. Manlowe (Eds.), *The Gender politics of HIV/AIDS in Women : Perspectives on the Pandemic in the United States* (pp. 207–221). New York: New York University Press.

Zierler, S., & Krieger, N. (1997). Reframing women's risk: Social inequalities and HIV infection. *Annual Reviews of Public Health, 18,* 401–436.

Zimmerman, F.J., Glew, G.M., Christakis, D.A., & Katon, W. (2005). Early cognitive stimulation, emotional support, and television watching as predictors of subsequent bullying among grade-school children. *Archives of Pediatric and Adolescent Medicine, 159*(4), 384–388.

19 Women's Access to Maternity Services in Canada: Historical Developments and Contemporary Challenges[1]

CECILIA BENOIT, DENA CARROLL,
AND RACHEL WESTFALL

Pregnancy and childbirth are core female events fundamental to the survival of the human species, yet the social organization of these events shows amazing variation across time and place. One obvious dimension of this variation concerns the care women have available to them to help make a successful transition to motherhood. While specialized care provided by medical doctors falls within this domain, an additional form of maternity care that is often overlooked in our technologically focused society is women's desire for social support or 'social care' in their local communities. Few would dispute that access to medical specialists and advanced technology have been of positive benefit for women experiencing difficult pregnancies, achievements associated with the urbanization and scientization of modern life. Yet social support from family members, extended kin, neighbours, and primary care providers such as lay midwives and *doulas*[2] has been in the past and remains today fundamental to the health of all childbearing women, regardless of biological condition. This is the case not only in high-income countries such as Canada, but around the world, and is promoted by the World Health Organization (WHO) as well as other key international organizations working to improve the health and well-being of women and girls in their home countries.

Below we give evidence that social support is a key *social determinant of health* (Raphael, 2004) for childbearing women in Aboriginal and non-Aboriginal societies alike, and continues today to be central to what women say they want with regard to maternity care services (Bourgeault, Benoit, & Davis-Floyd, 2004; De Vries, DeVries, Benoit, Van Teijlingen, & Wrede, 2001). Not all Canadian women have access to social support at the community level, however; rather, the evidence shows that social support, much like other social determinants, is stratified along lines of social class, ethnicity and race, and geographical location, among other factors. While much of the feminist literature on pregnancy and child-birth has highlighted the 'patriarchal' underpinning of medicine and depicted the female midwife as women's 'natural' ally during preg-nancy and childbirth (e.g., Oakley, 1984; Witz, 1992), in this chapter we use an intersectional approach to analyse important differences among women. In particular, we show that social support remains a privilege predominantly of white middle-class women residing in Canada's bet-ter-off urban areas where an array of maternity care options are avail-able, often free of charge.

Because of the rich and distinct historical records relating to mater-nity care systems in Aboriginal and non-Aboriginal communities across Canada, as well as the fact that there are clear differences among Cana-dian women of non-Aboriginal and Aboriginal statuses with regard to access to high-quality maternity care, including access to midwives, we discuss each separately while highlighting overarching themes com-mon to all women.

Maternity Care in Aboriginal Communities

Prior to contact with European settlers, there existed an informal sys-tem of maternity care across Canada's diverse Aboriginal communities. Pregnant women had access to an extensive local network of family members, neighbours, and healers who embraced a world view where birthing was considered a cultural and spiritual process rather than an individual act or medical event. One such healer was the traditional birth attendant or midwife, who was typically trained through a lengthy apprenticeship that included technical as well as extensive socio-cultural training. The midwife's role was typically reserved for female elders who had personal childbearing experience, and who held posi-tions of respect and honour in their communities. Fiske (1992) states, when writing about the pre-contact Carrier peoples of British Colum-bia: '[R]eproductive roles were central to women's claims to social prominence. Carrier women who successfully raised their families and provided care and nurturance to the needy became influential as family spokespersons. The wisdom of older women was proclaimed in legend and song and institutionalized in the valued role of the grandmothers of the tribe (p. 201).'

Although seldom occupying the role of midwife until their own children were grown, candidates tended to be chosen much earlier on for apprenticeship. Young girls, for example, often attended the births of their female relatives in order to build a solid basis of both technical skills and local knowledge of rituals, language, customs, herbal medicines, and spiritual norms related to reproduction. According to one elder, the young apprentice was sometimes taught to recognize the 'birth energy,' described as a special communication between the labouring woman and her baby (Benoit & Carroll, 1995).

Boas (1966), in his Kwakiutl ethnography, described the complex social organization of pregnancy and childbirth in Aboriginal societies on the Pacific Northwest coast, including the traditional stories and dances, such as the Atlak'im masks and Legends of the G*exsem of the Kwakiutl people, used to illustrate the spiritual and cultural connection between midwife, mother, and newborn. Boas relates that pregnant women were also required to follow specific regulations, rituals, and obligations; pay careful attention to their activities; and avoid certain social networks and foods, in order to ward off danger to their babies. Other related cultural practices included naming the baby and his/her relationship to the environment, and refraining from intervening in the natural process of growth by not cutting the baby's hair (Boaz, 1966). Among the Cree, the midwife's tasks included gathering wood, making and beading the *tikinagan* (cradle board), preparing the 'birthing hands,' honouring the placenta, using traditional medicines to aid birth, preparing the rabbit skins, gathering moss, and preparing special foods (Kioke, 2000).

The midwife was also closely involved with the newborn's family circle during the four-week post-partum 'healing period,' and midwifery care was often extended throughout the child and mother's life cycles. The small size of the communities and the close proximity of the people were important factors facilitating this type of care. In addition, the midwife oversaw a variety of preparations for labour and delivery and the welcoming of the new baby into the community.

When colonial governments began taking an interest in Aboriginal health care provision, this community-based and culturally appropriate care was undermined, and the organization of maternity care became isolated from other aspects of community life. Beginning in the late nineteenth century, Aboriginal family structures were negatively impacted by the imposition of colonial laws and policies aimed at assimilation of Canada's Aboriginal peoples (Waldram, Herring, & Young, 1995). Aboriginal peoples became defined as federal responsibility under the 1876 Indian Act, and the federal government assumed an increasingly large role in the lives of Aboriginal people on reserves. Indian agents, employed by the federal government, were appointed to oversee the affairs of Aboriginal communities; they often worked hand in hand with medical doctors brought in from the outside. Christian missionaries were an additional powerful force in Aboriginal people's lives. Many Aboriginal midwives and other healers increasingly found themselves threatened, punished, or brushed aside by one or other of these foreigners (Wells, 1994). Of course, there were exceptions. Such was the case of one Tsimshian midwife from Vancouver Island, Mary Wiha, who died in 1917 at the age of 87. Her obituary, in the *Prince Rupert Evening Empire* of 27 December 1917, made note of the fact that she 'practiced for years the profession of midwife, and was most successful, treating upwards of 200 cases without a single mishap. Her services were greatly appreciated by the medical men on the coast at that time' (see Atkinson, 2003). The obituary suggests that midwife Mary Wiha continued to hold a vital place in her Aboriginal community even with the presence of colonial agents.

However, in many other parts of British Columbia, midwives were frequently treated as charlatans and their original birthing practices dismissed as outdated and even harmful to pregnant women in their community. Elders were discouraged from passing traditional knowledge to the young. Eventually, the government established residential schools, where Aboriginal children, often against their own and their parents' will, were sent away to be educated in non-Aboriginal traditions, languages, and customs (Hiebert, 2003).

As part of a general federal strategy to provide primary care to Aboriginal peoples, by the late 1950s Health and Welfare Canada had established nursing stations in rural and northern Aboriginal communities. Pre- and post-natal care was provided by station nurses, many who were immigrant nurse-midwives. The research literature is mixed regarding their effectiveness in meeting the social care as well as the more technical needs of local women. Some report that the nurse-midwives remained 'outsiders,' failing to work with traditional midwives and gain the confidence and trust of the pregnant women they had come to serve (Waldram et al., 1995). Yet other researchers note that some nurse-midwives, especially those who remained for long periods, became accepted into the community and respected by local healers and childbearing women (Hiebert, 2003).

New federal government policies in the early 1970s led to the closing down of most nursing stations. The combination of factors mentioned above meant that Aboriginal women no longer had viable alternatives at the community level to deliver their babies close to their homes. Instead, they were placed under increasing pressure to leave their communities and deliver their babies in large hospitals located in distant urban settings. Some resisted and continued to give birth in their own communities, attended by elder midwives and/or members of their family and community (O'Neil & Kaufert, 1996). For those women who left their communities to give birth, loneliness and disruption of their families' lives were commonplace (Daviss, 1997). They travelled, usually by plane and without their families, to urban centres where they were attended by English-speaking professional nurses and physicians who knew little about the language and traditions of Aboriginal peoples. This remains the situation in most remote communities to this day.

Maternity Care in Settler Communities

Immigrant groups began settling in present-day Canada in the 1700s. Over time, settlers began to develop systems of maternity care that were a combination of customs and traditions learned in their countries of origin and the practices found in their new homeland. In some cases, Aboriginal midwives provided much needed services to colonial settlers (Biggs, 2004).

As in Aboriginal communities, the traditional lay midwives who emerged to care for childbearing women in settler communities were mostly older women who had little or no formal education but who nevertheless demonstrated strong skills, were well integrated into their ethnically diverse local communities, and sometimes were informally 'elected' by the women they served (Biggs, 2004; Mitchinson, 2002). One of the first references to lay midwifery in this part of the world appears in a deed published by a Mr Massicotte 'which reveals that the women of Ville-Marie [Montreal], in solemn concave assembled, on February 12th, 1713, elected a midwife Catherine Guertin for the community' (Abbott, 1931, p. 28).

Physicians' capacity to influence government legislation over health matters, including the organization of care for pregnant women, began as early as 1795 in Upper Canada (present-day Ontario) with the introduction of the first Medical Act to regulate the practices of 'physic' and 'surgery.' This act essentially made it illegal to practise midwifery without an official license to do so. Due to the impracticality of such a ruling, the small degree-holding, urban-based segment of the medical profession was left vulnerable to public criticism and the act was eventually repealed in 1806 (Canniff, 1894, p. 22). From 1806 to 1866, traditional lay midwifery remained immune from the licensing laws of the Ontario Medical Board. However, by 1866, permission awarded by the provincial government to unlicensed female midwives had been withdrawn and midwifery practice was henceforth restricted exclusively to academia-trained physicians. Medical schools were closed to women until the latter part of the nineteenth century, no female physicians were licensed in Ontario until the 1880s, and few women worked in this capacity for many decades to come. Thus, licensed male physicians enjoyed an official monopoly over childbirth and other medically designated health events (Biggs, 1983). Nonetheless, even in the larger urban areas of Ontario, competition between physicians and midwives as to who had authority for home births continued for several decades after Confederation. Although physician-attended births were eventually to become the norm, for some time midwives continued to attend women in rural and remote areas of the province, as well as the urban poor who could not afford physician attendance fees.

Outside Ontario, midwives in other settler communities remained active much longer. In Quebec, for example, traditional lay midwives (*sage-femmes*) continued to remain unregulated in legislative terms, and were controlled by local clergy and by birthing women themselves. In 1879, the Quebec College of Physicians and Surgeons, following events in Ontario, placed midwifery practice in the hands of physicians (Laforce, 1990). Nevertheless, for the next half-century, Quebec midwives in rural areas were permitted to practice, provided that their competence was physician-certified. Such was the case as well in New Brunswick and Saskatchewan, where as late as 1924 at least 50 per cent of births were not attended by medical doctors (Biggs, 1983).

In Central Canada in the 1930s, prominent Canadian health reformers started advocating for 'health teams' composed of midwives, physicians, and public health nurses working out of community clinics. However, medical and nursing associations, worried that competition from midwives might reduce work for their own memberships, lobbied against these recommendations. Ultimately, the hospital-based physician-obstetrical nurse team replaced the community midwife as primary attendant during childbirth, initially among the urban middle classes and eventually reaching other sectors of society. The commonly adopted perspective promoted by the medical and nursing professions was that 'the art of midwifery belongs to prehistoric times' (Biggs, 1983, p. 32). Nonetheless, women continued to aid one another during pregnancy and in childbirth. Though obstetrical nurses were officially subordinate to doctors and were denied the technical training required to be effective autonomous birthing care providers, in practice many continued to serve as women's primary attendant at birth, sometimes with the attending physician's acquiescence. While physicians were able to lay claim to the territory of childbirth, they were, in practice, unable to service the entire population. In reality, physician services were available to those who could afford them, and to those who did not reside in areas which were geographically remote or too sparsely populated to support a successful physician's practice.

Accordingly, in the mid-twentieth century, as was the case in Aboriginal communities, the Federal government made special provision for nurse-midwives to practice in remote non-Aboriginal communities where physician services were unavailable (Bourgeault & Fynes, 1997).

The historical record is even more complex when we look at settler communities in the western and eastern provinces of Canada. Access to formal health care and trained health professionals (including midwives as well as physicians) was limited in relation to how far women lived from towns and villages. Often stories arose about male relatives who were forced to travel large distances to 'fetch' the midwife, if time and weather permitted, while the woman laboured alone or perhaps with a neighbour standing by. Mrs Elizabeth Akitt of Edmonton, Alberta, who was attended by a doctor and a nurse with midwifery training, indicated: 'I know what lots of women have gone through by not having a doctor. Sometimes, there was just a neighbour; no midwife' (cited in Rasmussen, Rasmussen, Savage, & Wheeler, 1976, p.78). In recalling the beginning of labour, a first-generation settler in Alberta indicated to Eliane Leslau Silverman (1984) that 'some good friends were with us; one of them wasn't exactly a midwife, but people used to call her that' (p. 66). Eileen Lillian Cleary of Beaver Harbour, Halifax County, Nova Scotia, helped deliver seven of her nieces and nephews in the late 1940s and early 1950s out of both necessity and generosity, and also helped seven other local women birth their babies (Karen Robb, personal communication, July 2003).

Traditional maternity care practices also survived well into the twentieth century in Newfoundland and Labrador, which have arguably better records of this form of health care for childbearing women than anywhere else in the country (McNaughton 1989). Midwives from

Canada's most easterly province were often given the epithet of 'granny' or 'auntie,' signalling the wisdom and practical skill that comes with age and experience, as well as denoting the respect that these women often held within their outport and rural communities. Like their Aboriginal counterparts, many Newfoundland and Labrador traditional midwives learned their craft from female relatives or senior midwives as well as via personal experience (most had given birth themselves, often many times over); they thus learned by observation and simply by 'doing the work.' According to one granny midwife from the west coast of the island: 'I first learned to doctor the women and others in the village from my dear mother. I learned to give a newborn a steeped brew from weeds – caraway seeds perhaps [and to be] always present during birth, consoling and guiding the mother' (cited in Benoit, 1990, p.185). Newfoundland and Labrador midwives were often called upon to provide an array of nursing services to local families, most of whom had no access to professional forms of health care: 'I had to do the other things besides bringing along babies 'cause there was no nurse there for a long time. So I had to do that work too. When anybody got sick, they'd call' (cited in Benoit, 1991, p. 57). Similarly, accordingly to midwife Aunt Gertie Legge from Heart's Delight in eastern Newfoundland, 'we understood sickness and set bones and everything, and even did animals' (cited in Benoit, 1983, p. 23). Clara Tarrant, a granny midwife from St Laurence, Newfoundland, described her experience this way: 'I got into a situation when I just had to [do midwifery] and there was nobody but myself. I had been at a birth and had seen deliveries and I had children. Seeing is believing but feeling is the naked truth' (cited in Benoit, 1983, p. 24).

As on the Island of Newfoundland, until well into the twentieth century, most Labrador families resided in small fishing villages or rural farming communities separated from each other by considerable distances. Access to the services of local midwives was crucial to survival. Bertha Anderson or 'Aunt Bertha,' as she was affectionately known in her home community of Makkovik, Labrador, was one such local midwife; she travelled by dog team, boat, or overland 'to answer a call of mercy' (Chard, 1978). Susan Andersen (1914-2000), another local Labrador lay midwife, is recorded as having delivered 50 babies in her lifetime, many of them at the 'White Elephant,' a multi-purpose building located in Makkovik where women from nearby fishing villages came to deliver their babies.

While variation existed in skill level and dedication to task, what stands out about these examples of 'social care' from the prairies and eastern coastal communities is the willingness of female elders to provide technical care and social support to birthing women in need. Often there was little or no remuneration for these culturally relevant services that emerged from within local communities themselves. In regions where physicians were unable or unwilling to set up practices, and nursing stations did not exist, women rarely went entirely without care, and traditional systems of midwifery were perpetuated. As shown next, this went on largely unnoticed by health policy makers, whose ultimate aim was to extend physician and hospital services to Canadian women and their families.

Medicare and the Solidification of Medical Dominance

Federal and provincial governments eventually responded to inequities in access to physician and hospital services through the establishment of a system of universal health coverage. First, in 1957, the federal government of Canada introduced the Hospital Insurance and Diagnostic Act. This act provided for a number of medical services associated with hospitalization and medical testing. The payment structure determined by the federal government was a cost-matching scheme whereby provincial governments were reimbursed 50 per cent for some fixed portion of the expenditures. Of crucial importance, however, physicians' fees were not covered under the act of 1957. Universal health insurance finally arrived in Canada with the passage of the federal Medical Care Act of 1968 (implemented in 1972). The act teamed national principles with provincial administration through an innovative program, eventually known as 'Medicare.' Importantly, under this second act, physicians' fees were insured. Thus, pregnant women in Canada, for the first time, had free access to physician and hospital services. The 'conditions' or five fundamental principles of the Medicare plan included universality (everyone would be covered), portability (from province to province), comprehensiveness, accessibility, and public administration.

It is crucial to note that, though initially resistant to the implementation of a 'socialized' health care system for Canada (there was even an infamous doctors' strike to protest the government Medicare plan), physicians across the country eventually gained much by this new welfare state policy. First of all, their services were reimbursed through the public purse, thereby virtually guaranteeing them economic security. Secondly, Medicare solidified physicians' dominance over maternity care services, granting them a virtual monopoly over the provision of the country's care of pregnant women. This monopoly was reinforced by the first point – the reimbursement of physicians but not midwives for services rendered – thus limiting women's choices regarding style of care. Thirdly, physicians retained their right to remain private entrepreneurs, establishing their practices wherever they deemed appropriate, where they would provide a range of medical services to women that physicians themselves, not the women, decided upon as necessary. This point is notable as it did nothing to alleviate the preexisting disparity in the availability of physician services between rural and urban areas. Finally, hospitalization of childbirth had long been a goal of the Canadian medical profession. Medicare solidified the medically dominated hospital as the linchpin to the entire maternity care system. One important reason for physicians to promote hospital birth rather than domiciliary care was the need for physicians to be able to use substitute health providers to assist them in the care of birthing women and their newborns. Canadian physicians thus gave their support to the training of obstetrical nurses (rather than community midwives), a strategy that was supported by the nursing lobby itself (Benoit & Carroll, 2005).

It should be noted here that it is a common misconception that the rise in physician attendance at births led to lower rates of maternal mortality. This belief has been critically examined by a number of authors. In the Canadian context, Suzann Buckley's (1988) examination of Ottawa birth records from the 1930s illustrated how socio-economic factors played a large role in determining the likelihood that a woman (and her baby) would survive childbirth. Similarly, Strong-Boag and McPherson (1986) considered the trend towards hospital deliveries in Vancouver between 1919 and 1939. Their statistics demonstrate that maternal mortality rates dropped at a rate that exceeded the increase in hospital births over this period of time. British Columbia had the highest rates of hospital birth in the country over that time span, at 84.4 per cent of live births by 1940, yet the province had one of the highest maternal mortality rates, with Vancouver's rates of hospitalization and maternal mortality exceeding those of rural areas. These studies indicate that in Canada, like elsewhere, the trend towards hospitalization and physician attendance was not a 'cure' for the problem of childbirth-related mortality; rather, it served the professional interests of the medical profession.

Challenges to Medical Dominance of Maternity Care

Compared to most other developed welfare states, Canada has been a laggard in regard to establishing public funding for midwifery services, as well as state recognition of midwives as a viable health profession vital to women's maternity care (Wrede, Benoit, & Sandall, 2001). Recent developments in the last two decades have resulted in decreasing physicians' dominance over maternity care services. Studies in both Aboriginal and non-Aboriginal communities indicate that childbearing women are keen to take advantage of viable options to physician attendance and hospital birth if they are available in their own communities. However, as shown below, many difficulties remain before the kind of social care available to Canadian women in earlier times again becomes a reality for all.

Revival in Aboriginal Communities

Many Aboriginal women in remote reserve communities have expressed their dissatisfaction with the lack of community-based maternity care available to them. In recent decades, birthing women have been separated from their families and communities due to a government policy of evacuation of all pregnant women to urban centres in their final weeks of pregnancy. In some communities, Aboriginal women have lobbied for local, culturally appropriate maternity care services, and such options now exist in a few places. Quebec was the first Canadian province to allow a remote, northern Aboriginal community to set up a birthing centre; the Puvirnituq Maternity Centre (PMC) was opened in the mid-1980s as a pilot project. This unique program has been successful in allowing Inuit women to give birth among their own people; it makes use of midwives from the local community, ensuring that women have access to Inuit birth attendants who can communicate in Inuktitut. In 2000, Inuit midwives cared for approximately 70 to 80 Inuit women at the PMC. For these women, to give birth on their traditional land without facing legal action, attended by maternity care providers who can speak to them in their own native tongue, is a major step forward. Unfortunately, recent provincial legislation in Quebec recognizes only five existing trained Nunavik Inuit midwives, restricts their membership to the Nunavik territories, and denies membership in the Quebec Order of Midwives to any other Aboriginal midwives. Aboriginal midwives in Quebec are campaigning to change this ruling and have Inuit maternity care workers recognized as fully certified midwives, without restrictions on where they may practice (Benoit & Carroll, 2005).

Other Aboriginal birthing initiatives include the birthing and training centre in Southern Ontario known as the Tsi Non:we Ionnakeratstha ('the place they will be born') Ona:grahsta' (Cayuga word for 'a Birthing Place'). The centre, which receives provincial funding, is located on Six Nations Reserve in Hagersville. This unique arrangement incorporates traditional practices with modern-day midwifery services, and also offers a three-year training program for Aboriginal midwives. Although the Six Nations midwives do not currently have hospital privileges, they hold formal provincial (Ontario) certification as 'Aboriginal midwives.' In 2002, there were two full-fledged community midwives on staff at the centre and two Aboriginal midwife apprentices overseeing nearly 200 births.

An example from British Columbia is the Rankin Inlet Birth Centre (RIBC), which, while not yet sanctioned under provincial legislation, nevertheless provides vital, culturally unique services to local women. Legislation to allow professional designation for Aboriginal midwives in British Columbia is missing, thus limiting future access to community-based services. It is telling that before midwives were certified in the province, Sheway, a health centre in Vancouver's Downtown Eastside (DTES), provided general medical but also midwifery services to inner-city pregnant women, a large proportion of whom were of Aboriginal background (Benoit, Carroll, Chaudhry, 2003). However, since provincial legislation legitimizing certified midwifery in the province has been passed, this practice was discontinued in the DTES. The limited number of trained Aboriginal midwives in the province is also a major barrier to access; mainstream education programs in British Columbia, but also in Ontario and Quebec, are struggling to address the diversity and cultural effectiveness of education and training programs at the community level. Recent developments in Manitoba that provide a variety of gateways to training look promising (Robinson & Kaufert, 2004).

In short, Aboriginal midwifery programs have been established in a handful of locations, yet Aboriginal midwives remain vastly under-represented in midwifery training programs overall. Moreover, traditional Aboriginal knowledge and practices are diminishing due to the limited number of elders who speak the language and can transmit the ways of knowing to the younger generations.

New Maternity Care Options in Other Communities

Much of the pressure for change in non-reserve areas of Canada emerged in the late 1960s and early 1970s, a time that was marked by a general lessening of trust in professional authority, an unprecedented decline in respect for medicine, and a growing recognition of the emotional, social, and spiritual components of life, and healing in particular (Barrington, 1985). Many Canadian women and their partners became aware of how childbirth practices differed internationally, and they began to question whether physician attendance and birth in the hospital setting should be the only options available to childbearing families. This was the origin of the contemporary Home Birth Movement, the proponents of which hold that childbirth in most instances should occur at home without medical intervention, and should be celebrated as a woman's achievement and an occasion for celebration with partners, close family, and friends. This movement first occurred among counterculture groups, but soon spread to mainstream society as well.

Canadian independent lay midwifery originated in the late 1960s to early 1970s on the West Coast. In the Kootenay region of British Columbia, for example, childbirth statistics from the late 1970s show a startling and radical departure from mainstream birthing procedures. Nearly 8 per cent of all births in the Selkirk District (centred on Nelson) during this period took place at home under the care of midwives, compared to 1 to 2 per cent in other health districts in the province (Barrington, 1985, p. 87).

By the mid-1980s, most larger urban areas across Canada had women's groups advocating for midwives, including in Quebec where *sage-femmes* emerged in 1979 (Barrington, 1985, p.37). Of the women who chose to become midwives in the early years of the Home Birth Movement, very few were formally trained or certified to do this work. While they augmented their experience with weekend workshops, observation, and labour coaching in hospitals and occasionally short courses taken outside the country, the style of practice of most of these midwives was very informal (Lyons, 1981). Many of their clients were or became their friends. Payment, if any, was worked out based on the ability to pay and sometimes took the form of barter. Prenatal visits were usually informal and took place at irregular intervals. At the births, there were often other friends attending, with the midwife acting as only one player in the event. Midwives not only supported the mother but also helped care for other children, prepared food, or cleaned up during and after the birth. There were often strong links between personal child-bearing experience and the midwife's occupational calling. Women who had themselves undergone traumatic and alienating birth experiences, or who had given birth at home or assisted a friend or neighbour in a home birth, subsequently trained in midwifery (Burtch, 1994).

Emerging from the Home Birth Movement were several small yet vocal childbirth groups formed by consumers and their midwives in the United States and later in Canada. These groups challenged the necessity of 'routine' obstetrical practice and questioned the effectiveness and possible iatrogenic (harm-causing) effects of intervention. Many instead pushed for 'family-centred' maternity care, which included childbirth education and assistance for home birth parents. A number of organized lobbies were formed, including the Home Oriented Maternity Experience (HOME), the Association of Childbirth at Home International (ACHI), the National Association for Parents and Professionals for Safe Alternatives in Childbirth (NAPSAC), and the International Childbirth Education Association (ICEA). Many of these largely U.S.-based groups had and continue to have Canadian members and Canadian chapters, including NAPSAC in Ontario, Association for Safe Alternatives in Childbirth and Birth Unlimited in Calgary, and Association for Safe Alternatives in Childbirth in Edmonton and in Nova Scotia. Other local groups also formed, such as Naissance Renaissance in Quebec and Choices in Childbirth in Ontario. Political pressure from such organizations brought about legislative changes in many provinces, paving the way for the inclusion of formally trained midwives in the public health care systems of some provinces.

Legislative changes did not occur synchronously across the country, as each province has jurisdiction over its own health care services. To this day, independent lay midwives continue to practice in some areas of Canada that have not yet passed new legislation enabling certified midwifery to establish itself, while in many communities neither lay nor certified midwives are available. Where midwifery has become regulated, a new type of midwife – the certified midwife – has emerged. Currently five provinces – Ontario, British Columbia, Alberta, Quebec, Manitoba – have certification procedures in place for midwives. In Alberta, midwives are regulated, but not publicly funded (James, 1997; Bourgeault et al., 2004). In contrast, midwifery services are covered under provincial health care plans in Ontario, British Columbia, Quebec, and Manitoba. Saskatchewan has passed a Midwifery Act, but the act has yet to be proclaimed.

Styles of midwifery care also vary between the provinces. In Quebec, certified midwives are largely salaried practitioners working in birthing centres, and homebirth attendance is not covered under current legislation (Hatem-Asmar & Blais, 1997; Vadeboncoeur, 2004). By contrast, in Ontario and British Columbia, certified midwives are paid per client's course of care, and are permitted to attend births either in clients' homes or in hospital. Both Ontario and British Columbia have adopted a 'woman-centred care' midwifery model which emphasizes continuity of care (with the same midwife or team of midwives caring for the woman throughout her course of care), informed choice (whereby the woman is given the information she needs to make decisions regarding diagnostic tests, interventions, and procedures), and choice of birthplace (home or hospital, for those who qualify for home birth on the basis of their obstetrical history, health, and other criteria). Certified midwives working in these two jurisdictions are paid by the course of care, per client file, and they tend to work in independent group practices of two, three, and as many as eight midwives as part of a team.

In Ontario and British Columbia, the demand for midwifery care exceeds the availability of midwives in most regions. To complicate matters, certified midwifery care does not meet the needs and expectations of all women. Some women say they find the services offered by certified midwives to be overly 'medicalized,' as care is oriented around the same diagnostic tests, procedures, and timelines used by the medical profession (Westfall & Benoit, 2004). Some women have expressed a desire for more traditional forms of social care, like that provided by lay midwives in earlier historical periods; these women have continued to seek out lay midwives (Westfall, 2002).

In Manitoba, midwives are regulated and funded, and multiple routes of entry into midwifery training are available to ensure midwives have practiced in many different settings. Manitoba midwives also have both hospital and home birth privileges. In 2000, the first group of twelve midwives was registered in Manitoba as certified, paid by salary (unlike the paid-by-client midwives of Ontario and British Columbia) and directly employed by provincial health authorities. Discussions are currently being undertaken with rural health authorities to expand into First Nations communities. The absence of midwifery care services in traditionally under-serviced Aboriginal and rural communities has not gone unnoticed, and perhaps the utilization of salaried care providers will help to alleviate the problem in Manitoba. Currently, though, for women in remote areas, midwifery services remain unattainable. Women from such regions continue to travel long distances to give birth in urban hospitals, or they rely on the assistance of lay midwives in their communities or give birth unattended.

Even for urban women, the restructuring of maternity care services has only affected the lives of a few. On one hand, certified midwives have been awarded public legitimacy, and urban women in a number of provinces have gained greater choice in regard to both primary childbirth attendant and place of birth, making social care once again an option. Nevertheless, the small number of midwife-attended births in Canada hardly signifies a revolutionary change from earlier decades of medical dominance over maternity care. The overall Canadian figure for midwife-attended births is still less than 5 per cent.

It should also be noted that public funding of midwifery services in some provinces has been accompanied by a reduction in federal health care funding for maternity and other health care services. One result has been sharp discontent among Canadian family physicians and obstetricians, who still provide the bulk of maternity care in Canada. Not surprisingly, this has led to a decline in the number of medical practitioners willing to take on new maternity clients. The resulting 'physician shortage' has especially left rural pregnant women, as well as their counterparts in the low-income areas of large cities, in an unenviable situation: there are too few physicians willing to attend to these women's prenatal and childbirth needs; at the same time the women cannot access publicly funded midwives, who remain too few in numbers and who mainly serve an urban clientele. At the same time, immigrant midwives have found it very difficult to gain certification in the provinces where colleges of midwives have been established, leaving pregnant women from the country's diverse ethnic and racial communities without access to midwives who speak their own language and understand their maternity care traditions (Nestel, 2004). Meanwhile, postpartum care is, for the most part, neglected under the current system of health care delivery. While the care of women following childbirth was continuous with birthing care in traditional community-based midwifery systems, it has never been an important part of medical health care. Further, recent moves to early discharge from hospital following birth have not been accompanied by increased community-based resources.

Conclusions

As is clear from the above historical overview, midwives of different types have been active in what is now Canada before the arrival of

European settlers and up to the current time, providing crucial technical care but also social support to enhance the health and well-being of women and babies. Historically, this care has been community-based and culturally appropriate for the client population. Yet, substantial resources have been spent in Canada to fund the professions of obstetrics and gynaecology and to provide hospital care for birthing women, though this style of care has neglected women's social needs. Despite important reductions in maternal and infant mortality and morbidity, significant problems remained even after the country had established its public health care system in the early 1970s. In addition to the neglect of social care, remote regions of the country have been chronically under-serviced, and choice of style of maternity care has predominantly remained the privilege of urban women. Women in some remote Aboriginal communities have lobbied successfully for community-based, culturally appropriate care, whereas others continue to give birth routinely in urban centres, in isolation from their families and communities. Similarly, women in non-reserve communities have lobbied for more socially oriented care, and have championed midwives as the solution to the shortcomings of the hospital-based, physician-managed standard of care. Efforts to alleviate these problems through the integration of midwifery care into the health care system have thus far been insufficient, as midwives are too few in number, they are concentrated in urban centres, and their services are not equally available in all provinces. Future health planning will need to address these shortcomings.

NOTES

1 This chapter is based in part on information found in Benoit and Carroll (1995, 2005) and Carroll and Benoit (2004).
2 A doula is a person trained and experienced in childbirth who provides continuous physical, mental, and informational support to a woman during labour, birth, and the immediate post-partum period. Doulas also sometimes provide care for families in the first week, including household help, advice with newborn care, and feeding and emotional support.

REFERENCES

Abbott, M. (1931). *The History of Medicine in the Province of Quebec*. Montreal: McGill University Press.

Atkinson, M. (2003). 'The Mother of this Place': (Paykw) Mary Wiha, Professional Midwife and Tsimshian Role Model. Prince George, BC: University of Northern British Columbia.

Barrington, E. (1985). Midwifery Is Catching. Toronto: NC Press.

Benoit, C. (1983). Midwives and healers: The Newfoundland experience. Healthsharing, 5 (1), 22–26.

Benoit, C. (1990). Mothering in a Newfoundland community: 1900–1940. In K. Arnup, A. Levesque, & R. Roach Pierson (Eds.), Delivering Motherhood: Maternal Ideologies and Practices in the 19th and 20th Centuries (pp. 173–189). London and New York: Routledge.

Benoit, C. (1991). Midwives in Passage: The Modernisation of Maternity Care. St John's, NFLD: Memorial University, Institute of Social and Economic Research.

Benoit, C., & Carroll, D. (1995). Aboriginal midwifery in British Columbia: A narrative still untold. Western Geographic Series, 30, 221–46.

Benoit, C., & Carroll, D. (2005). Canadian midwifery: Themes from past to present. In C. Bates, D. Dodd, & N. Rousseau (Eds.), On All Frontiers: Four Centuries of Canadian Nursing (pp. 27–41). Ottawa: University of Ottawa Press and Canadian Museum of Civilization.

Benoit, C., Carroll, D., & Chaudhry, M. (2003). In search of a healing place: Aboriginal women in Vancouver's Downtown Eastside. Social Science & Medicine, 56, 821–833.

Biggs, C.L. (1983). The case of the missing midwives: A history of midwifery in Ontario from 1795–1900. Ontario History, 65(2), 21–35.

Biggs, C.L. (2004). Rethinking the history of midwifery in Canada. In I. Bourgeault, C. Benoit, & R. Davis-Floyd (Eds.), Reconceiving Midwifery: Emerging Models of Care (pp. 17–45). Montreal and Kingston: McGill-Queen's University Press.

Boas, F. (1966). Kwakiutl Ethnography. H. Codere (Ed.). Chicago: University of Chicago Press.

Bourgeault, I., & Fynes, M. (1997). The Integration of Nurse- and Lay Midwives in the US and Canada. Social Science & Medicine, 44(70), 1051–1063.

Bourgeault, I., Benoit, C., & Davis-Floyd, R. (Eds.). (2004). Reconceiving Midwifery: The New Canadian Model of Care. Montreal and Kingston: McGill-Queen's University Press.

Buckley, S. (1979). Ladies or midwives? Efforts to reduce infant and maternal mortality. In Kealey, L. (Ed.), A Not Unreasonable Claim: Women and Reform in Canada, 1880s – 1920s (pp. 131–149). Toronto: Women's Press.

Buckley, S. (1988). The search for the decline of maternal mortality: The place of hospital records. In W. Mitchinson, & J.D. McGinnis (Eds.), *Essays in the History of Canadian Medicine* (pp. 148–197). Toronto: McClelland & Stewart.

Burtch, B. (1994). *Trials of Labour: The Re-emergence of Midwifery.* Montreal and Kingston: McGill-Queen's University Press.

Canniff, W. (1894). *History of the Medical Profession in Upper Canada, 1783–1850.* Toronto: W. Biggs.

Carroll, D., & Benoit, C. (2004). Aboriginal midwifery in Canada: Merging traditional practices and modern science. In I. Bourgeault, C. Benoit, & R. Davis-Floyd (Eds.), *Reconceiving Midwifery: The New Canadian Model of Care* (pp. 263–286). Kingston and Montreal: McGill-Queen's University Press.

Chard, S. (1978). Tribute to Aunt Bertha: Bertha Anderson, Makkovik, 1872–1950. *Them Days Magazine* 4(1), 56–58.

Daviss, B. (1997). Heeding warnings from the canary, the whale and the Inuit: A framework for analyzing competing types of knowledge about childbirth. In R.E. Davis-Floyd & C.F. Sargent (Eds), *Childbirth and Authoritative Knowledge: Cross Cultural Perspectives* (pp. 441–473). Berkeley: University of California Press.

De Vries, R., Benoit, C., Van Teijlingen, E., & Wrede, S. (Eds.). (2001). *Birth by Design: Pregnancy, Maternity Care and Midwifery in North America and Europe.* London: Routledge.

Fiske, J. (1992). Carrier women and the politics of mothering. In G. Creese & V. Strong-Boag (Eds.), *British Columbia Reconsidered: Essays on Women* (pp. 198–216). Vancouver: Press Gang.

Hatem-Asmar, M., & Blais, R. (1997). Opinions of certified and lay midwives in Quebec: Perspectives on the future of their profession. In F. Shroff (Ed.), *The New Midwifery: Renaissance and Regulation* (pp. 311–332). Toronto: Women's Press.

Hiebert, S. (2003). Ncn Otinawsuwuk (receivers of children): Taking control of birth in Nisichawayasihk Cree Nation. (Doctoral dissertation, University of Manitoba, 2003). *Dissertation Abstracts International, 65*(03), 1277.

James, S. (1997). Regulation: Changing the face of midwifery? In F. Shroff (Ed.), *The New Midwifery: Reflections on Renaissance and Regulation* (pp. 181–200). Toronto: Women's Press.

Kioke, S.J. (2000). Revisiting the past ... Discovering traditional care and the cultural meaning of pregnancy and birth in a Cree Community. Masters of Science thesis, School of Nursing, Queen's University, Kingston, ON. *Dissertation Abstracts International, 38*(03), 606.

Laforce, H. (1990). The different stages of the elimination of midwives in Québec. In K. Arnup, A., Levesque, & R. Roach Pierson (Eds.), *Delivering*

Motherhood: Maternal Ideologies and Practices in the 19th and 20th Centuries (pp. 36–50). London and New York: Routledge.

Langford, N. (1995). Childbirth on the Canadian Prairies, 1880–1930. *Journal of Historical Sociology, 3*, 278–302.

Lyons, L. (1981). Today – I'm coming out of the closet. In *Midwifery Is a Labour of Love* (pp. 30–34). Vancouver: Maternal Health Society.

McNaughton, J. (1989). The role of the Newfoundland midwife in traditional care, 1900–1970. Doctoral dissertation, Memorial University, St Johns. *Dissertation Abstracts International, 54*(03), 1050.

Mitchinson, W. (2002). *Giving Birth in Canada, 1990–1950.* Toronto: University of Toronto.

Nestel, S. (2004). The boundaries of professional belonging: How race has shaped the re-emergence of midwifery in Ontario. In I. Bourgeault, C. Benoit, & R. Davis-Floyd (Eds.), *Reconceiving Midwifery: The New Canadian Model of Care* (pp. 287–305). Kingston and Montreal: McGill-Queen's University Press.

Oakley, A. (1984). *Captured Womb.* London: Blackwell.

O'Neil, J., & Kaufert. P. (1996). The politics of obstetric care: The Inuit experience. In W. Mitchinson, P., Bourne, A., Prentice, G., Cuthbert Brandt, B., Light, & N. Black (Eds.), *Canadian Women: A Reader* (pp. 416–429). Toronto: Harcourt Brace.

Raphael, D. (Ed.). (2004). *Social Determinants of Health: Canadian Perspectives.* Toronto: Canadian Scholars Press.

Rasmussen, L., Rasmussen, L., Savage, C., & Wheeler, A. (Eds.). (1976). *A Harvest Yet to Reap: A History of Prairie Women.* Toronto: Women's Press.

Robinson, K., & Kaufert, P. (2004). Midwifery on the prairies: Visionaries and realists in Manitoba. In I. Bourgeault, C. Benoit, & R. Davis-Floyd (Eds.), *Reconceiving Midwifery: The New Canadian Model of Care* (pp. 204–220). Kingston and Montreal: McGill-Queen's University Press.

Silverman, E.L. (1984). *The Last Best West: Women on the Alberta Frontier, 1880–1930.* Montreal and London: Eden Press.

Strong-Boag, V., & McPherson, K. (1986). The confinement of women: childbirth and hospitalization in Vancouver, 1919–1939. *BC Studies,* 69/70, 142–174.

Vadeboncoeur, H. (2004). Delaying legislation: The Quebec experiment. In I. Bourgeault, C., Benoit, & R. Davis-Floyd (Eds.), *Reconceiving Midwifery: The New Canadian Model of Care* (pp. 91–110). Kingston and Montreal: McGill-Queen's University Press.

Waldram, J., Herring, D., & Young, T.K. (1995). *Aboriginal Health in Canada:*

Historical, Cultural and Epidemiological Perspectives. Toronto: University of Toronto Press.

Wells, R. (1994.) *Native American Resurgence and Renewal.* Metuchen, NJ: Scarecrow Press.

Westfall, R. (2002). The state of midwifery in British Columbia. *Midwifery Today, 62* (Summer), 51–55.

Westfall, R., & Benoit, C. (2004). The Rhetoric of 'Natural' in Natural Childbirth. *Social Science & Medicine, 59* (7): 1397–1408.

Witz, A. (1992). *Professions and Patriarchy.* London: Routledge.

Wrede, S., Benoit, C., & Sandall, J. (2001). The state and birth/The state of birth: Maternal health policy in three countries. In R. De Vries, R. DeVries, C. Benoit, E. Van Teijlingen & S. Wrede (Eds.), *Birth by Design: Pregnancy, Maternity Care and Midwifery in North America and Europe* (pp. 28–50). London: Routledge.

20 Relocating Care: Home Care in Ontario

PAT ARMSTRONG

A qualitative change is underway in health care. Care is being relocated – not just physically, but socially, ideologically, and psychologically as well. Social and economic forces within and outside health care are contributing to this relocation. Corporations searching for new profit sources, governments intent on eliminating debts and deficits, and media promoting individual responsibility account for just some of these forces. Because such forces are global, the overall patterns in health care reforms have significant similarities. Nevertheless, they tend to play out differently in different places. Indeed, such forces are evident in and realized in particular places, where local histories, conditions, relations, and cultures influence practices.

This chapter uses a feminist political economy perspective to examine how these forces play out in the particular case of Ontario home care. For feminist political economists (Andrew, Armstrong, Armstrong, Clement, & Vosko 2003), analysis begins with the powerful economic, social, and ideological forces, and the resistance to them, that shape the conditions for reforms. These are processes that have a history simultaneously influenced by global pressures and local responses, by past practices, and by current cultures. Often these forces, and the resistance to them, have contradictory results. Victory can turn into loss, and some successes may simultaneously produce harmful and beneficial affects or have a differential impact on different groups. Thus, this chapter begins by setting the historical context for the relocation of care and by exploring some of the contradictions in order to make sense of the kinds of relocation of care underway in Canada. This approach draws our attention to both questions of power and the question of contradictory pressures that shape care in particular places.[1]

The second part of this chapter focuses on the relocation of care to the home. Using the example of Ontario home care, it analyses three kinds of relocation. It explores in turn the shift from institutional to home care, the shift from public and non-profit to for-profit delivery, and the shift among paid providers that relocates responsibility for care.

What makes political economy feminist is the recognition that all social structures, processes, and relations are profoundly gendered, as well as classed and racialized. Gender is understood not simply as difference. Rather, gender is also understood as pervasive inequality in all aspects of life. This means that not only formal economies but also households and communities are taken into account in the analysis. All these developments are thus understood within the context of unequal, gendered relations (Clement & Myles, 1994).

The shift in care that is taking place both nationally and internationally is primarily about women, given that women provide the overwhelming majority of both paid and unpaid care and constitute the majority of patients needing care. Women not only provide more hours of unpaid care compared to men, they also travel farther to provide care, provide more demanding forms of care, and are much more likely than men to look after people with multiple functional limitations and children with disabilities (Morris, 2004). While women account for 80 per cent of the health care labour force, they remain a minority at the most senior levels of the medical hierarchy and in decisions about health care policy (Armstrong & Armstrong, 2003) . Moreover, the jobs at the bottom of the hierarchy are disproportionately done by racialized and immigrant women (Armstrong & Laxer, 2006).

The relocation of care has been promoted both by those who seek more responsive, public care and by those who seek reduced costs and more for-profit care (Baranek, Deber, & Williams, 2004, chap. 1). However, this chapter argues that the relocation of care in the Ontario case too often means increasing inequality among women as providers and patients, lower-quality care, and fewer choices for most women.

Forces of Change

By the beginning of the 1970s, Canadians had universal access to publicly funded hospital and doctor care. Insurance coverage included all medically necessary services, with mainly male doctors defining what was necessary care. Private payment of fees for these services was prohibited, making hospital and doctor care free to the specific user.

Medicare eliminated 'the commercial insurance concepts of deductibles, non-insurable conditions, limitations with respect to age, employment, or membership in groups and experience rating' (Taylor, 1987, p. 235). Care was primarily delivered by either non-profit, charitable, or municipal hospitals while doctors mainly practiced as independent professionals whose fees were paid by the public system (Armstrong and Armstrong, 2003). At the same time, Malcolm Taylor (1987) suggested that the relative success of the publicly funded health care system amounted to a blank cheque for doctors and hospitals as it led to a substantial growth in the use of both. But, as research in 1973 demonstrated (Enterline, McDonald, Davignon, & Salter, 1973), it also allowed people to seek help for important medical symptoms that had previously gone untreated or had been treated too late. In sum, although doctors became very influential within this arrangement, the public system was delivered mainly by private non-profit organizations and independent practitioners, which allowed all individuals – especially women with limited resources – to gain access to care.

However, this expansion in public care also invited some criticism of the system. Academics such as Ivan Illich (1975) began to write about what he called 'the epidemic of modern medicine' and 'the medicalization of daily life' (p. 7). Illich saw this growing dependency on health care as the culprit for an increasing range of 'sickening' problems for three reasons: first, it produces clinical damages, or what we call iatrogenic health consequences; second, it obscures political conditions that make us unhealthy; and third, it takes away power from the individual (p. II). This political economy critique played an important role in what has come to be known as the determinants of health approach. From this perspective, health care is only one among many factors contributing to health, and the way care is organized can undermine health rather than promote it. Food, shelter, jobs, and joy – or what Illich essentially describes as political conditions – are understood as more significant factors in the health of populations (see Evans, Barer, and Marmor, 1994; Marmot and Wilkinson, 1999; Raphael, 2004).

While male academics like Illich were calling attention to medicalization, so too were the women's health movement (see Morrow, Chapter 1, this collection) and some female academics (Doyal, and Pennell, 1979). In the 1960s, a group in Montreal flaunted both health authorities and the law by publishing a birth control guide designed to empower women. This was just the beginning of what became the Women's Health Press, one of many women's groups challenging dominant care practices. In *No Longer Patient*, Susan Sherwin (1992) summed up their perspective in writing that 'the institution of medicine has been designed in ways that reinforce sexism, and the effects of medical practice are often bad for women' (p. 7). Thus, despite the fact that women made up the majority of patients, the overwhelming concentration of power in the hands of the mainly male doctors, in combination with a reliance on drugs, surgery, and institutional care, resulted in fundamental flaws in care. Similar issues were raised by community groups concerned about the quality of care for those with mental health problems (Simmons, 1990) and those with disabilities.

At the same time that these groups were developing critiques of care practices and structures, care providers were getting organized. The male doctors in charge had, for over a century, been represented by a professional organization, The Canadian Medical Association (Naylor, 1986). This representation contributed significantly to their power and to the frequent association of health care with doctor care. But most of those who did the daily care work were women. Indeed, then as now, nearly four out of five health care providers were women (Armstrong & Armstrong, 2003, chap. 4). Moreover, managerial practices were no less sexist than care practices. The work of caring was associated with women's 'innate' nurturing. It was presumed to be done for love rather than money, and the product of nature rather than education.

Although women in nursing had begun demanding increased recognition and wage improvements for over a century, their agenda was somewhat hampered by a number of factors, including the predominance of employment in small workplaces or private homes, a high turnover that resulted from the requirement to leave due to marriage, the enrolment of many nurses in religious orders, and the dominance of male doctors (Coburn, 1987). Finally, given the influence of the Nightingale tradition, coupled with a training program that was limited to highly controlled hospital environments, women were unable to effectively challenge their subordinate position in the health care system (Bates, Dodd, & Rousseau, 2005, Pt. 6). However, women gradually became more successful in their struggle as they began to move out of the hospital training schools and amassed in large numbers to meet the growing demand for public institutional care. They were also helped by the success of the women's movement on issues such as the right to work after marriage and access to birth control. By the end of the 1970s, the majority of women health care professionals were unionized and women's wages, job security, and working conditions all improved significantly (White, 1993).

By the late 1970s, governments had become increasingly concerned about the rising costs of health care, especially as the long post-war economic boom began to fade. In 1977, the federal government announced it would no longer pay for half of all hospital and physician expenditures and created a new formula that would limit federal spending. The provinces would in turn respond to the federal government cutbacks by instituting reforms of their own. The most obvious were in mental health services, where the number of psychiatric beds was significantly reduced. The deinstitionalization strategy was justified in a variety of ways (Simmons, 1990, chap. 9). First, new drugs and changing attitudes allowed people to leave the institutions. Second, deinstitutionalization would allow people to become more independent, lead more dignified lives, and integrate into the community. Third, it was what people with diagnoses of mental illness wanted. Fourth, it was believed that it would save money. In other words, the relocation of people outside institutions seemed to respond to both critiques of the system and new developments in technology while cutting spending as well. But the other half of what the critics saw as essential to the move – namely, more support for community services – did not appear. It was a pattern that would become increasingly familiar. Progressive critiques from those seeking empowerment and equity became the justification for reforms that often undermined those goals.

In the 1990s, additional federal cutbacks followed, culminating in the dramatic reductions of the 1995 Canada Health and Social Transfer. At this point, the justification was primarily fiscal, as the debt load had created a crisis for governments. Social programs, along with the 'big government' they represented, were blamed for much of this debt. Yet, according to a Statistics Canada publication, 'Expenditures on social programs did not contribute significantly to the growth of government spending relative to GDP' (Mimoto & Cross, 1991, p.1). Rather, the debt was largely the result of the way the debt was financed, and the way taxes were reduced for some corporations and individuals. And, although the debt load was clearly an issue, it is important to note that the debt was much larger after the Second World War, when Canada undertook the development and expansion of social programs (Chorney, 1996, p. 358).

Nevertheless, overspending on social programs was the initial justification for drastic cuts. But it was not the only one. More and more, governments at all levels began talking about transforming the state. Instead of notions about market failure that led to the expansion of the state after the Great Depression and the Second World War, there was increasing discussion of government failure. As was the case with mental health reforms, these critiques drew on feminists and other critics of past practices who saw the state as a venue that serves only to reinforce patriarchal and other unequal relations. Essentially, these progressive debates were informed by demands for greater responsiveness and improved quality of services (Seidle, 1995). State discourses co-opted these progressive positions and moved beyond the critics to argue that states should steer not row (Osborne & Gaebler, 1992), and instead of providing services, governments should stick to their core business of establishing conditions for free markets. Under an approach to government called 'new public management,' the accepted assumption was that governments should not do anything that some other organization or individual could do. In other words, families and individuals should take more responsibility for everything, including their own health care. This philosophy was combined with a profound faith in competition, markets, and private sector practices. These concepts were defined as necessarily efficient and effective, as well as applicable to virtually every area of the public sector. Thus, governments were committed to pursuing business-oriented strategies by adopting entrepreneurial practices inside their operations. Canada signed on to trade agreements that reflected and reinforced these assumptions (Hankivsky & Morrow, 2004).

Yet, such assumptions denied evidence indicating that for-profit methods in health care are often not only more expensive and less efficient, but also inappropriate for adequate care (Devereaux et al., 2004; Pollack, 2004). In making these assumptions, policy makers ignored evidence suggesting a connection between for-profit methods and increased inequality, especially for women (Armstrong et al., 2002). They also ignored evidence showing that such methods often undermine workers' health, leading to high absentee rates. Worse still, little attention was paid to the frequent charges, convictions, and out-of-court settlements for fraud among for-profit services in health care (Guyatt, 2003; Pollack, 2004). Nevertheless, provinces and territories responded to federal cutbacks and their growing costs by following new public management strategies of their own, along with managerial and organizational practices taken from the private sector.

This move to restructure government and government expenses in health care was linked to economic developments at both local and global levels. As corporations faced falling profits in traditional industries such as manufacturing and resource extraction, they increasingly looked for new sources of investment in services. Health care delivery proved to be an obvious choice, dominated as it was by non-profit (and often small) or public organizations. Hence, health services represented significant opportunities for investment if governments could be convinced to leave the field or at least open new areas to profit. In order to capitalize on these new investment opportunities, corporations began to pressure governments to privatize public services. Corporations argued, without demonstrating, that the methods of the private sector were more efficient and thus could both address rising health care costs and improve services. Corporations were limited, however, by the strong support for public care. Such support reflected the success of the system in delivering high-quality services on an equitable basis.

Meanwhile, the notion of social determinants of health became increasingly popular. Various government reports on health care reform began with a determinants of health approach. A 1991 Ontario report identified six factors as determinants of health: social environments, physical environments, psychological environments, productivity, wealth, and health care (Ontario Premier's Council on Health Strategy, 1991). This report, like those in other provinces, concluded that spending more on health care was not the answer, given that other factors were at least as important to health. The social determinants became a justification for reducing care funding. As with mental health services, however, governments failed to follow through on addressing social determinants. For example, the number of homeless rose, as did income inequality, just as the importance of shelter and income for health was established. Moreover, governments ignored the ways these determinants operated within health care and for the mainly female care providers. Social, physical, and psychological environments are at least as important for care providers and patients as they are for those who are well and employed in other sectors. Yet, health care was treated as if it was an isolated factor that influences only those seeking care.

Initial arguments for a determinants of health approach saw all factors as not only integrally related but also as only understandable within the context of the political economy. However, most recent reports tend to define social and economic determinants as separate, independent variables. As Blake Poland and others (Poland, Coburn, Robertson, & Eakin, 1998) have argued, such approaches ignore the political economy context as well as the way health is influenced by the same forces that shape the overall society. In the process, this framing of health determinants obscures political conditions such as income and gender inequality, racism, and free markets that make us unhealthy (see

Illich, 1975). It obscures how determinants of health operate in and through gender, and fails to consider how health is also determined by the social, political, and economic arrangements within health care services.

Nevertheless, some of the ideas promoted by women's groups and other organizations were eventually embraced by reformers. For example, the feminist critique of medicalized birth contributed to significant changes in birthing practices. Women were no longer separated from their babies at birth. Instead, babies were placed in cots beside their mother's bed. Hospital stays were dramatically shortened, with women increasingly sent home within 24 hours of giving birth. Midwifery was legalized and was even covered by the public system in some Canadian provinces, including Ontario (see Benoit, Carroll, & Westfall, Chapter 19, this collection). Yet, as was the case with de-insitutionalization and the adoption of a social determinants of health approach, these changes left out crucial elements. Women wanted more choices about birth, not just less medical intervention. What they got instead was some limited choice over the length of hospital stays and minimal improvements in post-natal care. For women without support at home, or no home, a rush out of the hospital was a problem rather than a solution. Moreover, shorter patient hospital stays have not meant less medicalization. Indeed, the Canadian Institute for Health Information (2004) reports that medical interventions have in fact become more common for women giving birth.

Workers also saw contradictory consequences of their efforts. When nurses succeeded in gaining some improvement in working conditions and better pay, employers responded by re-classifying some tasks to be done by women with less formal training for less pay. When these workers organized themselves into unions that won better contracts, they too saw their work carved up and given to lower-cost providers. Certain nursing tasks went first to nursing aides, then to assistants, then to generic workers. Other jobs were divided among cleaners, dietary aides, and porters. Care work was relocated among workers, with immigrant women and those from racialized and Aboriginal groups often assigned the lowest-paid jobs (Armstrong & Laxer, 2006). Finally, among the best organized and the best paid hospital workers, there was increasing pressure to send work to long-term care facilities, where pay and training were less; or to the home, where much of the work was done without pay by women. Care itself was thus relocated, much of it simply sent home.

Workers' success has also become a justification for more service delivery by the for-profit sector. This position has been made quite explicit in a *National Post* Op-Ed piece by Senators Michael Kirby and Wilbert Keon (10 August 2004), both members of the Senate Committee on Health, Science and Technology. While making their argument for subjecting health care delivery to competition, they cited 'the rigid work rules that apply in publicly owned hospitals, as well as the higher salary scales of public institutions,' and warned that a move to the public sector 'will strengthen the monopoly bargaining position of the health care workers involved.' Furthermore, as they argue in their report for the Institute for Research on Public Policy: 'Competition would encourage hospitals to contract out nonmedical services in order to improve productivity and reduce costs' (p. 4).

Relocating care to the for-profit sector divides these mainly female workers both from other workers in the hospitals and from others doing similar work. In the United Kingdom, such strategies led to an 'institutional apartheid' that threatened both morale and patient care (Sachdev, 2001, p. 33). There was a dramatic reduction in the terms of conditions for employment, especially for women (p. 5). Moreover, the impact on women was more extensive in terms of job security, wages, and morale, resulting in a widening of the gender gap. Recent research in British Columbia indicates not only the deterioration in women's work, but also the disproportionate impact on immigrant women and women from racialized groups (Cohen & Griffen-Cohen 2004).

In sum, forces from both within and outside health care have transformed care. A social determinants of health approach challenged the medicalization of daily life, as did the women's movement and other groups supporting deinstitutionalization and different kinds of care. Unions improved the conditions for the mainly female labour force, challenging the notion of medical dominance as well as commonly held ideas about the value of women's work. But these same successes are being used to justify both the relocation of care and practices that undermine women's gains. Government debt and rising health costs have allowed critiques of public sector practices to gain ground. Free markets, personal responsibility, and for-profit service delivery are offered as the solution to both rising costs and non-responsive care. In the process, care is being relocated from non-profit to for-profit organizations, from higher-paid workers to lower-paid workers, from hospitals to long-term facilities or the home, and from a public to a private responsibility. By relocating care from the collective to the individual, these developments encourage a new way of thinking about health. Women paid to do the work lose out to women who are expected to do it without pay or training, suggesting little skill is involved in care. In the, process women as a group suffer, both because gains in the health care working conditions are lost and because women are conscripted into care in their private lives.

Home Care

Home care is fundamentally about the relocation of care. Although the relocation is often presented as a response to public demand, the form it takes often increases inequality by reducing the choices and power of those who give and receive care. Thus, despite the fact that women make up the majority of providers and those needing care, women also comprise the majority of the population that are left with reduced choices. Hence, tensions often accompany this relocation of care; some of these result from the establishment of false dichotomies that can be addressed, while others are inherent in the very nature of home care. The following sections explore various aspects of this relocation using Ontario as an example. Although the funding and delivery of home care differs from province to province, Ontario has features that are common to many provinces, but has also seen more privatization of home care services than in some other jurisdictions. These factors make Ontario useful for exploring the impact of reforms.

From Institutions to Homes

The most obvious relocation is that from institutional to home care. This is often set up as a clear choice between bad institutions and good homes. As Nancy Guberman (2004) explains, the dichotomy character-izes institutional care as 'cold, unfeeling, regimented and without free choice' (p. 77). Care is about technical intervention provided by high-paid professionals. Homes, on the other hand, are presented as warm places of love, with lots of freedom and no schedules. Care is provided by those who give spontaneously out of love.

   The dichotomy was obvious in press coverage in a recent announce-ment that Ontario would close the remaining institutions for those with developmental disabilities. A former resident is quoted as saying that 'no one should live in a place not of their choosing, be forced to go to the bathroom on schedule, have everything done on schedule. Get up at

6 o'clock whether you have to or not. Go to bed at 9 o'clock whether you have to or not' (Mackie & Philip 2004, p. A8). The Minister for Social Services justified the move in terms of the benefits of home care: 'Today, families want greater choice and flexibility in getting the supports and services they need to care for their family members at home' (cited in Mallan 2004, p. A3). But the alternatives are not that simple, nor the options so dichotomous. There are several reasons why this relocation is not simply about a move from bad to good.

First, some people do not have homes to go to or at least do not have homes that can provide support. The women's movement has been convincing in its argument that homes are not always havens in a heartless world for many women but rather are characterized by violence, poverty, and other forms of oppression (Morris, 2004). Homes may be physically unsuited for care with no private space, bathrooms up long stairs, kitchen counters too high, and doorways too narrow for those who are wheelchair bound. Even when homes provide a safe location for care, women have a host of domestic and social responsibilities in the home that can make the provision of good care to people who are ill or disabled difficult in a household environment. And, when women are unable to do the domestic work most women do, the tasks may go undone and may create care places that are no longer healthy, especially for the vulnerable ill or disabled. This is particularly the case for elderly women, many of whom live alone.

Second, when paid care is provided in the home, it may well enforce the same kind of schedule as the one so eloquently described by the former resident of the institution cited above. Publicly paid home care providers work on a schedule too, and usually only appear for fixed periods each day. For those unable to walk, this can determine hours of eating, sleeping, and toileting without much possibility of support in-between. The unpaid female providers who are expected to fill in the gaps also have to fit this schedule and are left little alternative about providing the care. In other words, care in the home does not guarantee choice. Furthermore, the contracting out of home care services in Canada means there is little continuity in care. Each contract period can mean a new crew of women to provide care. Poor working conditions and managerial practices in for-profit firms result in a high turnover in staff. Those with resources can pay for extra care and get more choices, but few can afford this option for long. Women in particular are unlikely to have the resources to buy care.

Ontario has introduced a self-managed care program that allows individuals or families to arrange their own service provision (MacAdam 2003, p. 4). Thus, either those with care needs, or their families, then determine the quality of care, the tasks provided, and the timing of services. While this policy does allow care recipients more choices, the choices are limited by the low financial contributions from government, perhaps reflecting the low value attached to this traditional women's work. The policy may also reduce care choices for the mainly female providers because they are seldom covered by the protection of a union contract. Many of these unprotected female providers are from immigrant and racialized groups. Finally, it is often family members rather than those with care needs who determine the nature of care.

Third, care at home as the only option promotes a very private notion of care. It can reinforce the argument that care is an individual, family, and female responsibility rather than a collective one. In the process, collective provision becomes the alternative for failures in private care, much like welfare. Women in particular are held responsible for care and are the ones who are most likely to rely on subsidized care (Grant et al., 2004). So sending people home – or those they care for home – may not always be the best option. It may be a suitable one for those with the human support and the economic resources, but this is not the case for significant numbers of the population needing care, most of whom are women, and many of whom also happen to be the most vulnerable women.

Fourth, institutions allow people to share the work and resources among skilled providers. Health care analysts and activists have increasingly come to recognize the importance of teamwork in care provision. Institutions bring together such teams, allowing them to contribute their different skills by providing an integrated approach to care. Providers can support each other socially and psychologically as well as physically. They can also combine their strength to ensure decent working conditions. Institutions also have the resources to purchase and use expensive equipment that can assist a number of those with care needs. In contrast, paid home care providers most often work alone, often in unfamiliar and inappropriate places. Perhaps even more importantly, though, home care, especially unpaid home care, places the burden mainly on women untrained for the work. The assumption is too often made that any woman can provide care by virtue of being a woman, even when that care is highly technical as is increasingly the case. Thus, for some, paid home care or care by family and friends may be the best of all options, but this is hardly universal.

Fifth, the dichotomy relieves institutions from the pressure to change in ways that can improve care. Conditions in hospitals have been deteriorating with the advent of recent reforms. Hospitals are cleaned less often, call bells go unanswered, and crowding contributes to the spread of infection, as does the increasing use of staff untrained for health care. The relatively recent outbreak of SARS in Ontario was just one indication of the threat institutions can represent. An Ontario government report (Smith, 2004) on long-term care facilities revealed problems in terms of staffing, the quality and continuity of care, and public accountability. However, if the answer is to send people home more quickly or to avoid institutions as much as possible, there is less pressure to ensure there is enough staff to provide good care. Similarly, the rigid institutional rules for eating, sleeping, and using the bathroom may go unchallenged instead of altered to help make facilities better places for care (Armstrong & Daly, 2004).

Meanwhile, homes face very little supervision or oversight in the provision of care. It is assumed both that they are private and that women know how to provide care. There are few clear standards for safe homes or for appropriate regulations to ensure that the care provided is sufficient. Moreover, because care is hidden in the household, racist, sexist, and violent practices may be hidden as well (Morris, 2004). Although home care is becoming more complicated, the amount of paid support has not increased sufficiently to fill the need. Worse still, adequate assessment and help to overcome poor home conditions is even less likely. Providing high-quality care requires paying attention to all the determinants of health. The determinants of health literature demonstrates that safe environments are those where everyone is clean and well-fed, where working conditions are decent and stable, and where people have some control over their care and conditions. This is not always the case in homes or institutions. And safe environments thus far have not been the focus of reforms.

The point here is not that the dichotomous representation should be reversed; that is to say, that institutions provide better care than homes. Rather, the point is to problematize the dichotomy and create a continuum of good care. The notion that care at home is necessarily better is often about class or gender privilege. It is most frequently the best care for men with resources and partners. Those who have resources may well be better off at home under most circumstances or at particular points in time. But we cannot make that assumption without investigating the particular situation. Home care needs to be a question, not an answer. Does it work for this person and their household under these circumstances? Does it work for the care providers? Does it make sense as a societal choice? Similarly, the notion that institutions are necessarily bad needs to be challenged, as do their practices. Raising these issues could help ensure that these institutions are not simply the poor option for the poor, who work and live within them. Instead, we need a continuum of care choices that stretch from homes through community supports such as respite care or day care to supportive housing, group homes, and institutions that are responsive to the needs of both providers and those with care needs. The relocation of care from institutions to homes guarantees neither good care nor more choices. Nor does it promote equity for providers or those with care needs. We cannot eliminate the tensions inherent in the options, but we can reduce the differences within and among them, as well as create an improved range of options.

From Provider to Provider

The term *provider* is used in two ways in health literature. One form refers to the organizations that hire care workers, while the other refers to the people who provide care. This section looks at relocation in terms of both kinds of providers because they are integrally related.

Until 1996, Ontario public home care was provided mainly by three medium-sized, non-profit organizations, although a large number of small organizations were also involved in home care. The government purchased these services through 74 placement coordination services and regional home care programs (Picard, 1999a). By far, the largest group providing nursing services was the Victoria Order of Nurses (VON). Most of their nurses were unionized, as were some of those in the other two large provider organizations that covered more of the homemaking services, such as cooking, cleaning, and shopping. In 1996, the Ontario government established 43 Community Care Access Centres (CCACs) designed to coordinate services and manage the open bids to contract out services. While the old, non-profit organizations were allowed to bid, the process was open to for-profit companies and the rules favoured their entry through various regulations and conditions for bidding (Armstrong, 2001). Increasingly, large, for-profit organizations have been winning the contracts.

This compulsory bidding process not only made provider organizations compete with each other, but it also pitted individual providers against each other. The for-profit companies are mostly non-unionized and many have a policy of hiring only part-time or casual employees. This means low wages and benefits, as well as no job security. These companies are rapidly driving the unionized providers out of the marketplace. Investigating home care in a series of articles for the *Globe and Mail*, André Picard (1999b) claimed that 'there is a parallel between the plight of homemakers today and that of nurses in the 1960s. The virtually all female profession, after so long being taken for granted, organized and unionized. Nurses became a force within the health-care system. Today, they are fighting the battle all over again, albeit on a much smaller scale, to have community nursing recognized' (p. 5).

Homemakers and personal support workers are having an even more difficult battle. Part of their difficulty can be traced to their gender. The skills involved in cleaning, cooking, shopping, and bathing have been associated with women for so long that there is an assumption that any woman can be hired to do the work, thus making any woman eligible to do the job. Often it is racialized and immigrant women, whose other job skills are under-recognized in the Canadian market, who fill these jobs. Companies have used this assumption of skill, along with government policy that has enthusiastically embraced competition and profit, to dramatically lower wages and working conditions. The Ontario government has acknowledged this emphasis on costs over care. 'According to a formula developed by the previous government, CCAC's are required to evaluate all proposals based on both quality and price. But since this policy was created, there have been significant concerns that the formula places a disproportionate premium on the lowest cost bidder. In an era of restraint, this may not sound like a bad thing. But from the perspective of the patient, the lowest cost does not necessarily equal the best' (Ontario Government, 2004b, p. 23). The scale of the contract changeover is creating instability in the home care labour force and in the homes of the patients they serve.

In just one year, the wages for homemakers dropped by two dollars an hour and were prevented from going lower only by a floor on homemakers' wages set by the government (Picard, 1999a). In their new plan for community care, the government has promised to review the competitive bidding process; however, the emphasis seems to be on adjusting the process rather than on eliminating the profit motive that leads to these practices.

Meanwhile, access centres are paying for fewer and fewer services for the growing numbers who are in need of care. For example, people in need cannot receive more than two hours of care a day after the first 30 days of service (MacAdam, 2003, p. 5). Homemaker services in particular have been reduced, leaving too many people without clean and safe places of care. Women are especially likely to go without these services because it is assumed that they will somehow manage to get them done, and because many cannot afford to pay for such services. Centres refer many of those requesting care, or needing more care than the public sector will provide, to private, for-profit services. Workers in these centres are in competition with those paid by the public sector, and are not covered by the Ontario government minimum wage for public homemaker services.

The compulsory bidding process has contributed significantly to tensions between unionized and non-unionized, publicly funded and privately financed workers. Indeed, a competitive strategy is increasingly justified as a means of countering the gains made by unionized workers (see earlier citation by Kirby & Keon, 2004). The impact is profoundly gendered, undermining years of gains for women. It is hard to see these developments as creating choices for many of those who work in care or for those who receive care. These tensions could be reduced through unionization and through an emphasis on quality standards and skills in the bidding process, or by an abandonment of the bidding process and the profit motive.

Both profit seekers and those who seek cost reductions have primarily promoted market strategies for paid care. However, some providers, academics, and policy makers have been arguing for changes in the regulations regarding the sorts of qualifications that are required of caregivers. Professional governing bodies are central in determining the licensing and scope of practice for doctors, nurses, therapists, and technicians. Unions negotiate duties for others not governed by professional regulations. Professional regulations determine both who can enter a profession and the necessary qualifications for specific types of care, while unions enhance workers' control over workloads and workspaces. However, such regulations also help protect the public by guaranteeing that the necessary skills are in place. Regulations may also prevent reforms that encourage such things as nurses doing more of doctors' work or nursing aides doing more of nurses' work. While shifts such as giving nurses more of doctor's work may seem like a sensible relocation of responsibility, there are contradictory interests involved. On the one hand, alterations in these regulations may enhance and recognize workers' skills while reducing overall costs because lower-paid workers do the job. However, it can also mean deskilling and a reduction in the quality of care, as well as in wages commensurate with skills.

Much of the shift in home care has been to unregulated providers without union contracts. Home support workers, personal care workers, and attendants provide an increasing amount of the care in the home. While many are very skilled at their jobs, there is little guarantee that this is the case. Given that care is hidden within the household, the lack of regulation calls into question the quality of the work.

But these are not the only relocations and tensions among providers. There has also been an enormous shift in care responsibilities from paid to unpaid providers. This is mainly a shift from women with pay to women without pay. A 2002 study found that 77 per cent of family caregivers for those with chronic health problems or disabilities were women (Decima Research, 2002). Nearly half of these unpaid providers gave medications, over a quarter did daily dressing, and one in four gave daily baths, while one in five assisted with feeding, toiletry, and walking (Decima Research, 2002, Table 1). Thus, care work is relocated from women paid and trained for the work to those who are not. The nature of home care is changing as well. Much of the work that is now being sent home, such as intravenous feeding and the attachment of oxygen masks, is not about sending care back home. Such care was never provided in the home. Further, unpaid home care now involves caring for the very frail elderly and those with disabilities, who did not survive with these conditions in the past (Armstrong & Kits, 2004).

Not surprisingly, the impact of care relocation to the home is greater on women than it is on men. Women provide more and different kinds of care compared to men, with women taking the overwhelming majority of responsibility for direct personal care (Morris, 2004). Women's paid work is more affected, and so is their mental and physical health. While both women and men incur financial costs from homecare, there are more long-term costs for women. Equally important, this impact is not evenly distributed across the female population. Those with less formal education and those with lower income provide more care (Morris, 2004). Decima (2002) reports that while 'the profile of family caregivers largely mirrors the Canadian population in terms of language and ethic background,' they 'tend to have household incomes below the national average' (p. 3). In other words, class is critical and the relocation of care to the household means that those women with the least resources have the fewest choices. For example, there is an emerging research indicating that Aboriginal women who provide care are particularly disadvantaged (Morris, 2004, p. 101).

While there may be a commonly held assumption that women have the skills as well as the time and the desire to provide care, significant numbers of women are in the paid labour force and rely on that income to live. This work often leaves them with little time, energy, or desire to take on unpaid caregiving. In any case, they are given less and less choice in the matter. Women told Prime Minister Chretien's National Forum on Health (1997) – a group that consulted widely on the future of health care in Canada – that they did not want to be 'conscripted' into care (p. 19). Women are being freely compelled to provide the necessary labour as caregivers. Yet, while women may feel responsible for care, they are also held responsible for care by ideas about women, by the lack of alternatives, and by policies that in effect make them provide care. This does not mean that all women do not want to provide care. Rather, women simply want both choice and supports. They want some control over what kinds of care they provide, for how long, and under what circumstances.

The relocation of care from higher-paid to lower-paid women, and from women with pay to those without, both increases inequality among women and reduces the choices of many women. It also reinforces the idea that this is work any woman can do, rather than skilled work that requires both formal learning and appropriate payment. The move to for-profit motives and practices contribute substantially to these developments. To a lesser extent they are driven by the search to save money for the state and for better quality care in the home. And there is considerable doubt whether the latter two goals can be achieved through for-profit means.

From States to Corporations, Families, and Individuals

This relocation from public to for profit methods and means sets the context for a discussion of another kind of relocation. Responsibility for care payment is being shifted from the state to families and individuals. Meanwhile, paid providers are being asked not only to do more work, but also to accept less pay. At the same time, responsibility for decision-making is relocated to corporations and to those with financial means to pay for care.

The Canada Health Act provides for universal access to necessary doctor and hospital care, without fees. It is based on notions of rights, equity, and justice. No one who is sick or disabled should be doubly burdened by concerns about paying for care or prevented from receiving care because of its cost. It is also based on insurance principles that recognize that everyone is at risk and that shared risks are cheaper for everyone. As taxpayers in Canada, we all contribute to the cost of care, and our single-payer, tax-based system is widely seen as the most efficient and just method for meeting this human need. Increasingly, however, Canadians are being told that public care is not sustainable and that costs must be reduced if care is to be guaranteed. The aging of the population is largely blamed, but so are demands from paid providers and inefficiencies within the system.

Because labour accounts for the largest single expenditure in health care, Canadians share an interest in keeping wages and benefits under control. However, this goal conflicts with the interests of those who provide paid care. So does the shift to unpaid care in the home. It also conflicts to some extent with the goal of quality care because quality requires skilled, secure, and decently compensated workers who have some control over their labour. A significant body of research has demonstrated that investment in a skilled nursing force improves health care and reduces risks (Sibbald, Shen, and McBride, 2004). At the same time, other research shows that when contracting companies reduce wages and benefits and disregard training, health care services become more hazardous to our health. Health care professionals currently have the highest illness and injury rates among industries in Canada (Canadian Institute for Health Information, 2001), in large measure because we have tried to make providers work harder for fewer rewards. As is the case with selecting where care is to be provided, there is a trade-off between the interests of taxpayers and providers that needs to be balanced rather than resolved by choosing one over the other.

However, it is in this context of appealing to taxpayers over concerns about rising costs and sustainability that for-profit managerial practices, market competition, and for-profit delivery have been promoted. The notion is that this will produce better quality at cheaper prices. Yet, there is no evidence to support this claim. Instead, there is evidence indicating that costs rise while quality, transparency, and access decline. Fraud, primarily linked to services charged for but not provided, or inferior services to those promised, has been common (Pollock, 2004). Meanwhile, wages, benefits, and job security decline, except for those in the most senior management positions who enjoy significant pay increases. More money goes to profit than to care.

Rehearsing this evidence here is relevant because it is important to remember that while the costs of providing health care have not been reduced, less money continues to be allocated towards direct care provision. It is also relevant to the relocation of power. More of the companies involved in delivering home care are large, powerful organizations that are close to becoming monopolies. A growing number are foreign-owned. These companies resist sharing any information with the public, claiming confidentiality is necessary to remain competitive. At the same time, under free trade rules, the introduction of commercial care opens our health care to any foreign providers and severely limits the possibilities for returning care to the public realm or even to public control. Thus, the relocation of care to for-profit providers relocates decision-making from the public to the private realm, and from Canada to international markets, where giant corporations have the most influence.

Home care has also been presented as the cheaper alternative, one that will also save taxpayers money. But rather than saving money for Canadians, the shift in care location is more about a shift in costs to families and individual women than it is about saving money overall. Peter Coyte (2000) estimates that private payment for home care services rose between 1995 and 2000 to account for 20 per cent of total revenue. This is partly because the prohibition against fees does not extend to homecare. Ontario does provide some nursing and housekeeping services without fees, but these are seldom enough to respond to needs. Few could afford the approximately $3,000 a week for 24-hour home care, the cost even at current low-wage rates. In sum, while the government may pick up some of the tab, it rarely covers all of it.

With home care, costs have been relocated along with care from institutions to households and individuals. Families now have complicated care in their midst, with individuals and their households bearing more of the costs of this care. Some of these costs are financial while others are psychological, social, or physical. The discourse is about family care, but the costs are borne disproportionately by women. While the government has put some more money into home care, the expenditures have not kept up with care needs (Grant et al., 2004). Women in particular are likely to go without care, in part because they are the majority of the elderly, in part because they often outlive their older spouses, in part because they have fewer financial resources, and in part because assumptions are made about women's capacity to care for themselves (Morris, 2004). Women are also more likely to pay the financial costs now and in the future for providing or receiving care. In many cases, women who provide care cannot easily combine this work with full-time paid work. This, in turn, means lower wages, fewer opportunities for promotion, and lower pensions (Fast, Eales, and Keating, 2001). It also means greater inequality among women because some women can afford to buy care.

Home care is cheaper than institutional care in large measure because costs are shifted to households and individuals. It is also cheaper because much of the work is unpaid labour performed mainly by women, and because people often get less, and less skilled, care. The decisions about how much care they get through the state is not made by those households, and is often made according to criteria they had no share in developing.

In sum, home care is not only relocating where care happens, it is also about relocating decision-making. Corporations have more say; citizens less. Fewer costs are collectively shared; more are borne by families with members who are ill or disabled. In the process, the discourses and ideas about care are transformed. Care becomes more and more an individual responsibility and a commodity to be bought and sold.

From Some Care Recipients to Others

Finally, there has also been a relocation from care for seniors – who mainly needed some help in order to stay home – to those who require post-operative or palliative care, and those with long-term daily care needs.

In the past, home care was mainly for those who needed assistance with daily living and some help from a public health nurse. Today, those responsibilities are shifted primarily to volunteers or unpaid caregivers or left undone. Instead, allocation of home care often reflects the more pressing needs of those just leaving hospital or those nearing death who are given higher priority, in keeping with the medical model. 'In Toronto, during a one-year period – 1998 to 1999 – there was a 5 per cent increase in acute-care home care clients and a corresponding reduction in chronic-care clients' (MacAdam, 2003, p. 6). Clinical care takes priority over homemaking services. Yet, research in British Columbia (Hollander and Tessaro, 2001) has demonstrated that homemakers are critical to the health of those with non-clinical care needs. In the process, non-clinical care needs are pitted against clinical care needs. As Susan Wagner (cited in Picard, 1999c, p. 3), a nursing professor at the University of Saskatchewan and board member of Saskatoon District

Health, put it: 'Everybody is so focused on the acute side that care for the frail elderly and those with chronic conditions [has] taken a big hit. We're going to pay heavily for that down the road.' Thus, such a shift creates tensions between those who provide care and those who need care, as it becomes even more difficult to satisfy the needs of each within such constrained resources.

Conclusions

Relocating care has consequences. The move to home care in Ontario is about much more than a physical relocation. It marks and promotes a fundamental shift in our thinking about care and our care practices. The relocation of responsibility and service delivery increases inequality among women and reduces their choices, while altering the balance of power in favour of corporations and away from individuals, families, and states. Critiques of health care that came from academics, unions, and social movements have been used to justify these developments. But it is not the shift to home care that primarily causes these outcomes. Rather, it is the context of market strategies and for-profit means. In the process, the critics' goals of equality, choice, and responsiveness of care have been lost.

NOTE

1 For a concise explanation of contradiction in Marx, see Bottomore, 1983, pp. 93–94. For a feminist perspective, see Armstrong and Armstrong, 1983.

REFERENCES

Andrew, C., Armstrong, H., Armstrong, P., Clement, W., & Vosko, L.E. (Eds.). (2003). *Studies in Political Economy: Developments in Feminism*. Toronto: Women's Press.
Armstrong, H. (2001). Social cohesion and privatization in Canadian health care. *Canadian Journal of Law and Society, 16*(2), 65–81.
Armstrong, P., & Armstrong, H. (1983). Beyond sexless class and classless sex: Towards feminist Marxism. *Studies in Political Economy, 10*, 7–44.
Armstrong, P., & Armstrong, H. (2003). *Wasting Away. The Undermining of Canadian Health Care*. Toronto: Oxford University Press.

Armstrong, P., & Daly, T. (2004). *There are Not Eough Hands: Conditions in Ontario's Long Term Care Facilities*. Report prepared for the Canadian Union of Public Employees. Toronto.

Armstrong, P., & Kits, O. (2004). A hundred years of caregiving. In K. Grant & M. Boscoe (Eds.), *Caring For/Caring About: Women, Home Care and Unpaid Caregiving*. Aurora, ON: Garamond Press.

Armstrong, P., & Laxer, K. (2005). *Producing a Portrait of Ancillary Workers in the Health Care Sector*. www.yorku.ca/nnewh/ 3ProducingaPortraitofAncillary WorkersinHCIntro.pdf.pdf.

Armstrong, P., & Laxer, K. (2006). Mapping precariousness in the Canadian health industry: Privatization, ancillary work, and women's health. In L. Vosko (Ed.), *Precarious Employment: Understanding Labour Market Insecurity in Canada*. Montreal and Kingston: McGill-Queen's University Press.

Armstrong, P., Amaratunga, C., Bernier, J., Grant, K., Pederson, A., & Willson, K. (2002). *Exposing Privatization: Women and Health Care Reform*. Aurora, ON: Garamond Press.

Baranek, P.M., Deber, R.B., & Williams, A.P. (Eds.). (2004). *Almost Home: Reforming Home and Community Care in Ontario*. Toronto: University of Toronto Press.

Bates, C., Dodd, D., & Rousseau, N. (Eds.). (2005). *On All Frontiers: Four Centuries of Canadian Nursing*. Ottawa: University of Ottawa Press.

Bottomore, T., Harris, L., Kieran, V.G., & Miliband, R. (Eds.). (1983). *A Dictionary of Marxist Thought*. Cambridge, MA: Harvard University Press.

Canadian Institute for Health Information. (2001). *Canada's Health Care Providers*. Ottawa: Author.

Canadian Institute for Health Information. (2004). *Giving Birth in Canada: A Regional Profile*. Ottawa: Author.

Chorney, H. (1996). Debts, deficits and full employment. In R. Boyer & D. Drache (Eds.), *States Against Markets: The Limits of Globalization*. London: Routledge.

Clement, W., & Myles, J. (1994). *Relations of Ruling*. Montreal and Kingston: McGill-Queen's University Press.

Coburn, J. (1974). 'I see and am silent': A short history of nursing in Ontario, 1850–1930. In D. Coburn, C. D'Arcy, & G. Torrence (Eds.), *Health and Canadian Society* (2nd ed., pp. 441–462). Markham, ON: Fitzhenry & Whiteside.

Cohen, M., & Griffin-Cohen, M. (2004). The politics of pay equity in the BC health care system: The roles of government, multinational corporations and unions. *Canadian Women's Studies, 23*(3,4), 72–77.

Coyte, P. (2000). *Home Care in Canada: Passing the Buck*. Toronto: University of

Toronto Home Care Evaluation and Research Centre, Department of Health Administration.

Decima Research. (2002). *National Profile of Family Caregivers in Canada – 2002.* Ottawa: Author.

Devereaux, P.J., Heuls-Ansdell, D, Lacchetti, C, Maines, T., Burns, K., Cook, D., Ravindran, N., Walter, S.D., McDonald, H., Stone, S., Patel, R., Bhandari, M., Schünemann, H., Choi, P., Bayoumi, A., Lavis, J., Sullivan, T., Stoddart, G., & Guyatt, G. (2004). Payments for care at private for-profit and private not-for-profit hospitals: A systematic review and meta-analysis. *Canadian Medical Association Journal, 170*(12), 1817–1824.

Doyal, L., & Pennell, I. (1970). *The Political Economy of Health.* London: Pluto.

Enterline, P., McDonald, A., Davignon, L., & Salter, R. (1973). The distribution of medical services before and after 'free' medical care. *Medical Care, 11*(4), 269–286.

Evans, R.G., Barer, M.L., & Marmor, T.R. (Eds.). (1994). *Why Are Some People Healthy and Others Not? The Determinants of Population Health.* New York: Aldine De Gruyter.

Fast, J., Eales, J., & Keating, N. (2001). *Economic Impact of Health, Income Security and Labour Politics on Informal Caregivers of Frail Seniors.* Ottawa: Status of Women Canada.

Grant, K., Amaratunga, C., & Armstrong, P. (Eds.). (2004). *Caring For/Caring About: Women, Home Care and Unpaid Caregiving.* Aurora, ON: Garamond Press.

Guberman, N. (2004). Designing home and community care for the future: Who needs to care? In K. Grant, M. Boscoe, A. Pederson, & K. Willson (Eds.), *Caring For/Caring About: Women, Home Care and Unpaid Caregiving.* Aurora, ON: Garamond Press.

Guyatt, G. (2003). Fraud is part of for-profit health care. *Hamilton Spectator* (21 March), A17.

Hankivsky, O. & Morrow, M. (2004). *Trade Agreements: Home Care and Women's Health.* Ottawa: Status of Women Canada.

Hollander, M., & Tessaro, A. (2001). *Evaluation of Maintenance and Prevention Model of Home Care: Final Report.* Victoria, BC: Hollander Analytical Services.

Illich, I. (1975). *Medical Nemesis.* Toronto: McClelland & Stewart.

Kirby, M.J.L., & Keon, W. (2004). Why competition is essential in the delivery of publicly funded health care services. *Policy Matters, 5*(8), 4–32.

MacAdam, M. (2003). Home care: It's time for a Canadian model. *Healthcare Papers.* Retrieved 7 October 2003, from http:www.longwoods.com/hp/fall/lead.html.

Mackie, R., & Philip, M. (2004). Developmental disability homes to be closed. *Globe and Mail* (10 September), p. A8.

Mallan, C. (2004). Centres for the disabled closing. *Toronto Star* (10 September), p. A17.

Marmot, M., & Wilkinson, R.C. (1999). *Social Determinants of Health*. New York: Oxford University Press.

Mimoto, H., & Cross, O. (1991). The growth of the federal debt. *Canadian Economic Observer* (June), 1–17.

Morris, M. (2004). What research reveals about gender, home care and caregiving: Overview and case for gender analysis. In K. Grant, M. Boscoe, A. Pederson, & K. Willson (Eds.), *Caring For/Caring About: Women, Home Care and Unpaid Caregiving*. Aurora, ON: Garamond Press.

National Forum on Health. (1997). *Canada Health Action: Building on the Legacy. Synthesis Report and Issues Paper*. Public Works and Government Services. Ottawa: Author.

Naylor, D. (1986). *Private Practice/Public Payment*. Montreal & Kingston: McGill-Queen's University Press.

Ontario Government. (2004a). *News Backgrounder*. http://www.newswire.ca/ontario/GPOE/2004/07/06/c0758.htm.e.htm.

Ontario Government. (2004b). *Ontario's Health Transformation Plan: Purpose and Progress*. Speaking notes for the Honourable Minister of Health and Long-Term Care. St Lawrence Market, Toronto, 9 September.

Ontario Premier's Council on Health Strategy. (1991). *Nurturing Health. A Framework on the Determinants of Health*. Toronto: Author.

Osborne, D., & Gaebler, T. (1992). *Reinventing Government: How the Entrepreneurial Spirit is Transforming the Public Sector*. Boston, MA: Addison-Wesley.

Picard, A. (1999a). Wide open competition saves money but draws fire. In the series Behind Closed Doors: The Struggle over Homecare. *Globe and Mail*. http://www.globeandmail.com/series/homecare/feature3.html (27 March), pp. 1–3.

Picard, A. (1999b). Hard wages: Why workers don't stay. In the series Behind Closed Doors: The Struggle over Homecare. *Globe and Mail*. http://www.globeandmail.com/series/homecare/feature3.html (27 March), pp. 1–3.

Picard, A. (1999c). Research is skimpy on how much is saved. In the series Behind Closed Doors: The Struggle over Homecare. *Globe and Mail*. http://www.globeandmail.com/series/homecare/feature3.html (27 March), pp. 1–3.

Poland, B., Coburn, C., Robertson, A. & Eakin, J. (1998). Wealth, equity and home care: A critique of the 'Population Health' perspective on the determinants of health. *Social Science & Medicine*, 46(7), 785–798.

Pollack, A.M. (2004). *NHS plc*. London: Verso.

Raphael, D. (Ed.). (2004). *Social Determinants of Health*. Toronto: CPSI.

Sachdev, S. (2001). Contracting culture: From CCT to PPPs. In *The Private Provision of Public Services and Its Impact on Employment Relations*. London: UNISON.Seidle, F.L. (1993). *Rethinking the Delivery of Public Services*. Montreal: Institute for Research on Public Policy.

Sherwin, S. (1992). *No Longer Patient: Feminist Ethics and Health Care*. Philadelphia: Temple University Press.

Sibbald, B., Shen, J., & Mcbride, A. (2004). Changing the skill mix in the health care workforce. *Journal of Health Services Research and Policy, 9* (Suppl. 1), 28–38.

Simmons, H. (1990). *Unbalanced Mental Health Policy in Ontario, 1930–1989*. Toronto: Wall & Thompson.

Smith, M. (2004). *Commitment to Care: A Plan for Long-Term Care in Ontario*. Toronto: Minister of Health and Long Term Care.

Taylor, M. (1987). *Health Insurance and Canadian Public Policy*. Montreal and Kingston: McGill-Queen's University Press.

White, J. (1993). *Sisters and Solidarity*. Toronto: Thompson Educational.

Contributors

Alisha Apale
Health Care Management
Université de Montréal

Pat Armstrong
Department of Sociology and Women's Studies
York University

Cecilia Benoit
Department of Sociology
University of Victoria

Susan Boyd
Studies in Policy and Practice
University of Victoria

Annette Browne
School of Nursing
University of British Columbia

Dena Carroll
Aboriginal Health Consultant
Victoria, BC

Lisa Diedrich
Women's Studies Program
Stony Brook University

Gweneth Hartrick Doane
School of Nursing
University of Victoria

Jane Friesen
Department of Economics
Simon Fraser University

Olena Hankivsky
Public Policy Program and Institute for Critical Studies in
Gender and Health
Simon Fraser University

Cynthia Mathieson
Department of Psychology
University of British Columbia, Okanagan

Marina Morrow
Faculty of Health Sciences and Institute for Critical Studies in
Gender and Health
Simon Fraser University

Kamrun Nahar
School of Nursing, Department of Social and Preventative Medicine
Université de Montréal

Cindy Patton
Department of Women's Studies and Department of Sociology
Simon Fraser University

Meredith Raimondo
Comparative American Studies
Oberlin College

Colleen Reid
British Columbia Centre of Excellence for Women's Health

Brian Alan Richter
Health Research and Methods Training Facility
Simon Fraser University

Victoria L. Smye
School of Nursing
University of British Columbia

Wilfreda E. Thurston
Department of Community Health Sciences
Faculty of Medicine, University of Calgary

Colleen Varcoe
School of Nursing
University of British Columbia

Bilkis Vissandjée
School of Nursing, Department of Social and Preventative Medicine
Université de Montréal

Rachel Westfall
Health and Social Services
Government of Yukon

Sue Wilkinson
Department of Social Sciences
Loughborough University

Lynn Elizabeth Young
School of Nursing
University of Victoria